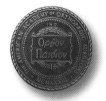

American Academy of Orthopaedic Surgeons

OKU
Orthopaedic Knowledge Update:

Pediatrics

3

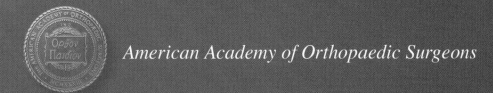

American Academy of Orthopaedic Surgeons

OKU
Orthopaedic Knowledge Update:

Pediatrics

3

Edited by
Mark F. Abel, MD

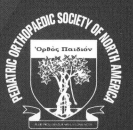

Developed by the
Pediatric Orthopaedic Society
of North America

Published 2006 by the
American Academy of Orthopaedic Surgeons
6300 North River Road
Rosemont, IL 60018
1-800-626-6726

Third Edition
Copyright ©2006
by the American Academy of Orthopaedic Surgeons

ISBN 10: 0-89203-353-3
ISBN 13: 978-0-89203-353-9
Printed in the USA
Library of Congress Cataloging-in-Publication Data

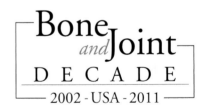

Acknowledgments

Editorial Board
OKU: Pediatrics 3

Mark F. Abel, MD
Alfred R. Shands, Jr. Professor, Orthopaedic Surgery
Division Head, Pediatric Orthopaedics Director,
  Motion Analysis & Motor Performance Laboratory
University of Virginia, Kluge Center
Charlottesville, Virginia

William G. Mackenzie, MD, FRCS(C), FACS
Acting Chairman
Pediatric Orthopaedic Surgery
Alfred duPont Hospital for Children
Wilmington, Delaware

Mark J. Romness, MD
Assistant Professor
Department of Orthopaedics
University of Virginia
Charlottesville, Virginia

Paul D. Sponseller, MD, MBA
Riley Professor and Head, Pediatric Orthopaedics
Johns Hopkins Medical Institutions
Baltimore, Maryland

Kit M. Song, MD
Associate Professor and Assistant Director
Pediatric Orthopaedics
Children's Hospital and Regional Medical Center
University of Washington School of Medicine
Seattle, Washington

Pediatric Orthopaedic Society of North America
Board of Directors, 2005-2006

David Aronsson, MD
  President
Perry Schoenecker, MD
  President Elect
Baxter Willis, MD
  Vice President
John Dormans, MD
  Secretary
James Roach, MD
  Treasurer
Scott J. Mubarak, MD
  Past President

John Birch, MD
  Member at Large
Stephen Albanese, MD
  Member at Large
Mininder Kocher, MD
  Member at Large
R. Dale Blasier, MD
  Historian

American Academy of Orthopaedic Surgeons
Board of Directors, 2006-2007

Richard F. Kyle, MD
  President
James H. Beaty, MD
  First Vice President
E. Anthony Rankin, MD
  Second Vice President
William L. Healy, MD
  Treasurer
Gordon M. Aamoth, MD
Leslie L. Altick
Dwight W. Burney III, MD
John T. Gill, MD
Joseph C. McCarthy, MD
Norman Y. Otsuka, MD
Andrew N. Pollak, MD
Matthew S. Shapiro, MD
James P. Tasto, MD
Kristy Weber, MD
Stuart L. Weinstein, MD
Ken Yamaguchi, MD
Karen L. Hackett, FACHE, CAE *(Ex Officio)*

Staff

Mark Wieting, *Chief Education Officer*
Marilyn L. Fox, PhD, *Director, Department of
  Publications*
Lisa Claxton Moore, *Managing Editor*
Keith Huff, *Senior Editor*
Kathleen Anderson, *Associate Senior Editor*
Mary Steermann, *Manager, Production and Archives*
Sophie Tosta, *Assistant Production Manager*
Susan Morritz Baim, *Production Coordinator*
Michael Bujewski, *Database Coordinator*
Suzanne Schneider, *Graphics Coordinator*
Courtney Astle, *Production Assistant*
Karen Danca, *Production Assistant*
Anne Raci, *Page Production Assistant*

Contributors

Mark F. Abel, MD
Alfred R. Shands, Jr. Professor, Orthopaedic Surgery
Division Head, Pediatric Orthopaedics Director,
  Motion Analysis & Motor Performance Laboratory
University of Virginia, Kluge Center
Charlottesville, Virginia

Peter J. Apel, MD
Department of Orthopaedic Surgery
Wake Forest University
Winston-Salem, North Carolina

Corrie T. M. Anderson, MD, FAAP
Professor of Anesthesiology and
  Adjunct Professor of Pediatrics
University of Washington School of Medicine
Department of Anesthesiology and Pain Medicine
Children's Hospital and Regional Medical Center
Seattle, Washington

Vincent Arlet, MD
Director, Scoliosis and Spine Surgery
Department of Orthopaedic Surgery
University of Virginia
Charlottesville, Virginia

Donald S. Bae, MD
Instructor of Orthopaedic Surgery
Harvard Medical School
Department of Orthopaedic Surgery
Children's Hospital
Boston, Massachusetts

John S. Blanco, MD
Children's Orthopaedics of Atlanta
Children's Healthcare of Atlanta at Scottish Rite
Atlanta, Georgia

Henry G. Chambers, MD
Clinical Associate Professor
Orthopaedic Surgery
University of California at San Diego
San Diego, California

Ernest U. Conrad III, MD
Professor of Orthopaedics
Chair, Department of Pediatric Orthopaedics
Children's Hospital Seattle
Seattle, Washington

Kirk W. Dabney, MD
Attending Pediatric Orthopaedic Surgeon
Department of Orthopaedics
Nemours/Alfred I. duPont Hospital for Children
Wilmington, Delaware

Peter A. DeLuca, MD
Connecticut Orthopaedic Specialists
Branford, Connecticut

Keisha M. DePass, MD
Department of Orthopaedic Surgery
Johns Hopkins Hospital
Baltimore, Maryland

Mohammad Diab, MD
Associate Professor
Chief, Pediatric Orthopaedics
Department of Orthopaedic Surgery
University of California, San Francisco
San Francisco, California

Martin M. Dolan, MD
Department of Orthopaedic Surgery
Children's Hospital/Harvard Medical School
Boston, Massachusetts

John P. Dormans, MD
Chief of Orthopaedic Surgery
Children's Hospital of Philadelphia
Professor of Orthopaedic Surgery
University of Pennsylvania School of Medicine
Philadelphia, Pennsylvania

François Fassier, MD, FRCSC
Director, Pediatric Orthopaedics
McGill University
Chief of Staff
Shriners Hospital, Canada
Montreal, Quebec, Canada

J. Dominic Femino, MD
Assistant Professor of Clinical Orthopaedics
University of Southern California–Keck School of
  Medicine
Childrens Hospital of Los Angeles
Los Angeles, California

John M. Flynn, MD
Childrens Hospital of Philadelphia
Philadelphia, Pennsylvania

Reggie C. Hamdy, MD, MSc, FRCSC
Associate Professor of Orthopaedic Surgery
McGill University
Assistant Chief of Staff
Shriners Hospital, Canada
Montreal, Quebec, Canada

Daniel Hedequist, MD
Assistant Professor of Orthopaedic Surgery
Department of Orthopaedic Surgery
Harvard Medical School
Boston, Massachusetts

John E. Herzenberg, MD
Rubin Institute for Advanced Orthopaedics
Sinai Hospital
Baltimore, Maryland

Daniel G. Hoernschemeyer, MD
Assistant Professor
Department of Orthopaedic Surgery
University of Missouri
Columbia, Missouri

Travis Hunt, MD
Orthopaedic Spine Fellow
Department of Orthopaedic Surgery
University of Virginia
Charlottesville, Virginia

Joseph G. Khoury, MD
Pediatric Orthopedic Surgeon
Shriners Hospitals for Children
Erie, Pennsylvania

Mininder S. Kocher, MD, MPH
Associate Director, Division of Sports Medicine
Department of Orthopaedic Surgery
Children's Hospital, Boston
Harvard Medical School
Boston, Massachusetts

Arabella I. Leet, MD
Assistant Professor
Division of Pediatric Orthopaedics
Department of Orthopaedics
Johns Hopkins University
Baltimore, Maryland

Freeman Miller, MD
Attending Pediatric Orthopaedic Surgeon
Department of Orthopedics
Nemours/Alfred I. duPont Hospital for Children
Wilmington, Delaware

Eric S. Moghadamian, MD
Department of Orthopaedic Surgery
University of Missouri
Columbia, Missouri

Leslie Moroz, BA
Clinical Research Coordinator
Division of Orthopaedic Surgery
Children's Hospital of Philadelphia
Philadelphia, Pennsylvania

Monica Paschoal Nogueira, MD
Assistant Professor
Pediatric Orthopaedics
Hospital Beneficência Portuguesa
Hospital do Servidor Público Estadual
Pediatric Orthopaedics–Limb Lengthening
  and Reconstruction
Sao Paulo, Brazil

Bradford W. Olney, MD
Professor and Chief of Pediatric Orthopedics
Children's Mercy Hospital
University of Missouri-Kansas City School of Medicine
Kansas City, Missouri

Ronald P. Pfeiffer, EdD, LAT, ATC
Professor and Co-Director
Center for Orthopedic and Biomechanics Research
Department of Kinesiology
Boise State University
Boise, Idaho

Kristan A. Pierz, MD
Assistant Professor
Department of Orthopaedic Surgery
Connecticut Children's Medical Center
Hartford, Connecticut

Mark J. Romness, MD
Assistant Professor
Department of Orthopaedics
University of Virginia
Charlottesville, Virginia

Benjamin D. Roye, MD, MPH
Attending Surgeon
Division of Pediatric Orthopedics
Beth Israel Medical Center
New York, New York

James O. Sanders, MD
Chief of Staff
Shriners Hospitals for Children
Erie, Pennsylvania

Dietrich Schlenzka, MD, PhD
ORTON Orthopaedic Hospital
Invalid Foundation
Helsinki, Finland

Christopher I. Shaffrey, MD
Professor of Neurosurgery
Professor of Orthopaedic Surgery
Department of Neurosurgery
University of Virginia
Charlottesville, Virginia

Kevin Shea, MD
Boise, Idaho

Brian G. Smith, MD
Assistant Director
Department of Orthopaedics
Faculty Practice Plan
Connecticut Children's Medical Center
Hartford, Connecticut

Paul D. Sponseller, MD, MBA
Professor and Head, Pediatric Orthopaedics
Johns Hopkins Medical Institutions
Baltimore, Maryland

Lynn T. Staheli, MD
Emeritus Professor
Department of Orthopedics
Children's Hospital and Regional Medical Center
Seattle, Washington

Michael D. Sussman, MD
Staff Surgeon
Former Chief of Staff
Shriners Hospital for Children
Portland, Oregon

Jeffrey D. Thomson, MD
Director, Department of Orthopaedic Surgery
Connecticut Children's Medical Center
Harford, Connecticut

Michael G. Vitale, MD, MPH
Childrens Hospital of New York
New York, New York

Peter M. Waters, MD
Professor of Orthopaedic Surgery
Associate Chief, Pediatric Orthopaedic Surgery
Harvard Medical School
Children's Hospital
Boston, Massachusetts

Jacob Weinberg, MD
Department of Orthopaedic Surgery
Children's Hospital, Boston
Harvard School of Medicine
Boston, Massachusetts

Janet L. Zahradnik, MD
Associate Professor
Department of Orthopaedic Surgery
Connecticut Children's Medical Center
Hartford, Connecticut

Preface

The third edition of *Orthopaedic Knowledge Update: Pediatrics* builds on the success of previous editions. The goal was to provide a review text for general orthopaedic surgeons and residents in training that would update evidence-based treatment guidelines in pediatric orthopaedics. The editors and authors distilled current and past information to provide what is essential for practicing general orthopaedics. Thus, the text can be also used as a reference source. The bibliography includes classic articles that continue to influence treatment as well as an annotated bibliography with updated references published within the past 4 years. Repetition was minimized to be succinct. However, the first section covering General Pediatric Orthopaedics introduces conditions and concepts used in the general assessment of pediatric patients, and some of these conditions and concepts are expanded further in other chapters. The chapter on Assessing and Treating Musculoskeletal Pain was expanded to emphasize the diagnosis of "pain syndromes"; otherwise, the topics covered are similar to prior editions.

The high quality of this book is a result in large part to the efforts of the section editors—Kit M. Song, MD, William G. Mackenzie, MD, Mark J. Romness, MD, and Paul D. Sponseller, MD, MBA—each a leader in the field and an experienced author. They have chosen a panel of expert chapter authors who have volunteered their efforts on behalf of the American Academy of Orthopaedic Surgeons. Great credit and thanks also goes to the publications staff at the Academy, particularly Marilyn Fox, PhD, Lisa Claxton Moore, and Keith Huff. We hope that the readers find this a useful resource in caring for children with musculoskeletal disorders. I welcome suggestions to make future editions as helpful as possible.

Mark F. Abel, MD
Editor

Table of Contents

Section 3: Lower Extremity Conditions

Section Editor: Mark J. Romness, MD

Section 4: Pediatric Trauma

Section Editor: Paul D. Sponseller, MD, MBA

Section 5: Spine

Section Editor: Mark F. Abel, MD

Section 1

General
Pediatric
Orthopaedics

Section Editor:
Kit M. Song, MD

Chapter 1

Motor Development in Orthopaedics

Lynn T. Staheli, MD

Introduction

Motor development is the acquisition of the capability to move and interact with the environment. If the musculoskeletal and neurologic systems are intact, the development of this capacity increases throughout the period of growth. Variations in motor development are common, and these variations concern parents and often result in the orthopaedist being consulted.

Variability is a characteristic of all living things; therefore, variability in motor development in children is to be expected. This variability follows a developmental pattern. Intoeing resolves and infants become bowlegged and then knock-kneed before the limbs achieve adult alignment. The infant is flatfooted and the arch usually develops with time. Why children go through these development sequences is unclear. The overall effect is a progressively increasing efficiency, precision, and speed in performing functional tasks. In contrast, conditions such as cerebral palsy or tibia vara cause pathologic deviations that interrupt normal development, cause disability, and require treatment.

The challenge for the orthopaedist is to understand normal motor development and to identify and effectively treat pathologic conditions. To do so, it is important for the orthopaedist to be able to differentiate physiologic variations from disease. Equally important is acquiring the ability to effectively deal with the family's concerns and to protect the child from the harmful effects of unnecessary and ineffective treatments. To enhance communications, definitions of relevant terms are provided in Table 1.

Evaluation

Establishing an accurate diagnosis is the most important component of management. Every child requires an accurate diagnosis, but few require treatment. An accurate diagnosis differentiates normal from pathologic. Understanding normal development and knowing the range of normal facilitate the differentiation of normal variability from disease. Initial examination is performed in two steps: the whole child is assessed with a screening examination and then focus is given to the area of concern.

Most errors in diagnosis are a direct result of omitting the initial screening examination.

Screening Examination

The child should be examined in a gown that allows inspection of the whole child, while respecting the modesty of the child and the sensitivity of the family. For greater efficiency, the patient's history could be taken while the screening examination is performed.

History

Questions should be asked about the child's developmental history, and problems during pregnancy and delivery should be identified. It should be determined whether the standard motor milestones (sitting, walking, talking, etc) were achieved at the normal ages. Sitting usually occurs between 3 and 6 months, walking between 10 and 16 months, and talking by 2 years of age. Normal range references are provided in Figure 1. It should also be determined whether other members of the family have the condition. For example, femoral antetorsion often presents in both the mother and daughter (Figure 2). Flatfeet are frequently familial.

Height and Weight

While taking the medical history, the orthopaedist should determine whether the child appears normal in height and weight, whether the body is proportionate, and whether the child looks like the biological parents or siblings. For example, familial rickets cause bowlegs or knock-knees and a short stature that will be apparent in the parents and the child. The child's height and weight should be compared with normal growth charts (Figure 3). Concern typically arises when the child's height is below the fifth percentile because this may suggest an underlying metabolic or other systemic disorder (such as osteochondral dysplasias). Weight above the 95th percentile is associated with tibia vara, slipped capital femoral epiphysis, and an increased risk of complications after surgical treatment.

Table 1 | Definitions of Terms

Developmental variations	Occur in otherwise normal children, tend to spontaneously resolve over a period of months or years, cause little or minimal potential for long-term disability, seldom bother children, but commonly concern parents. These variations are commonly overtreated.
Pathologic deviations	Caused by an underlying disease. These deviations are rare, often become more severe with time, delay motor development, often cause pain, and limit function and fixed deformity. Early diagnosis is important and treatment is usually required.
Normal	That which falls within 2 SDs of the mean for the age and gender of the child. Features falling outside this normal range may or may not be a source of disability. Most diseases result in deviations that fall outside the normal range.
Evidence-based management	Based on scientific evidence rather than tradition, convention, or common practice.
Vulnerable child syndrome	An iatrogenic condition usually resulting from inappropriate treatment in infancy or childhood that causes parents to become overprotective and restrictive, and children to feel defective. This results in a lowered self-esteem in childhood and increased potential for functional disorders in adult life.
Appropriate treatment	Treatment that is both necessary and effective. Necessary, as the condition poses the potential for causing disability, and effective, as the treatment results in improvement beyond what occurs naturally with growth and development.
Genetic-based disorders	Conditions common in families such as femoral antetorsion, or have a clear genetic basis such as achondroplasia.

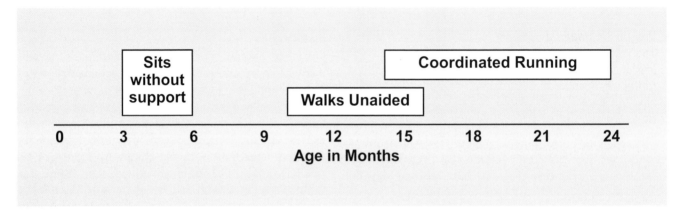

Figure 1 The acquisition of motor skills chart shows the range of normal for acquiring sitting, walking, and running skills. Sitting is typically acquired between 3 and 6 months, walking between 10 and 16 months, and running between 14 and 24 months.

Lower Limb Angulation

Limb alignment should be assessed clinically and care should be taken to clearly separate rotational and angulatory alignment by observing the child in the anatomic position. The child should stand with the knees straight ahead and forearms supinated. Alignment should be assessed in each plane: the frontal or coronal plane for varus and valgus, the sagittal plane for flexion or extension, and the transverse plane for internal and external rotation. Bowing of the tibia is described as apex anterior or posterior bowing. Some tibial deformities occur in intermediate planes, causing posteromedial or anterolateral bowing.

Frontal plane deformity should be assessed by positioning the patella directly forward and observing limb alignment. A visual assessment is typically made with the child standing. The symmetry, severity, and location of the deformity should be noted. The alignment of the two limbs is compared, and the location of the deformity is determined. Deformities may be generalized or focal. Focal deformities include tibia vara, posttraumatic injuries, and pathologic bowing of the tibia. Generalized deformities usually suggest a systemic or generalized musculoskeletal problem such as achondroplasia or rickets.

If the alignment appears abnormal, the child should be assessed in the supine position. The intramalleolar distance for valgus and the intracondylar distance for varus should be measured. To obtain the intramalleolar distance, the child's knees should be positioned with the soft tissues approximated and the distance between the malleoli measured. Measurements up to approximately 8 cm are within the normal range (Figure 4).

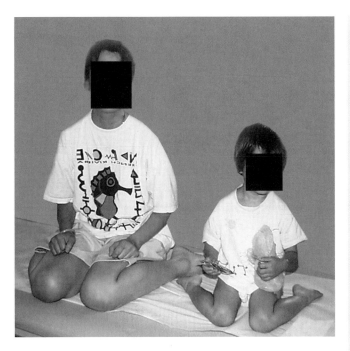

Figure 2 Photograph of a mother and daughter showing the typical sitting posture caused by familial femoral antetorsion.

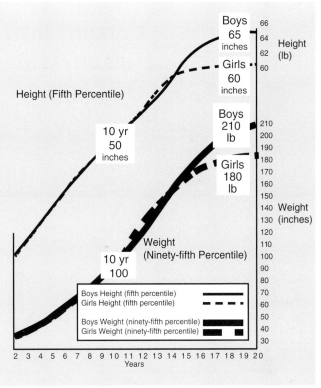

Figure 3 The minimum normal height and maximum normal weight by age chart shows the 5th percentile for height and the 95th percentile for weight in boys and girls. At age 10 years, the lower range of normal height is 50 inches for both boys and girls. At the end of growth, the upper range of normal weight is 210 lb for boys and 180 lb for girls.

Diagnostic Imaging Studies

The separation of pathologic and physiologic deformity can usually be made clinically. When uncertainty exists, radiographs should be obtained. Radiographs are usually diagnostic for rickets, osteochondrodystrophies, tibia vara, and other pathologic instances of tibial bowing. To plan surgical correction, full-length radiographs of the extremity should be obtained to assess the mechanical axes and level(s) of the deformity. It is essential that the radiographs are taken with the lower limbs anatomically positioned. If necessary, the orthopaedist should be present when radiography is performed to be certain the limbs are properly positioned. For children with severe deformities, separate radiographs of each limb should be obtained.

The common causes of pathologic deformity include tibia vara, rickets, osteochondrodystrophies such as achondroplasia, and posttraumatic deformity. If tibia vara is suspected, the metaphyseal-diaphyseal angle should be measured (Figure 5). This is the angle formed by a right angle to the metaphysis and the diaphysis. Angles between 10° and 16° are considered questionable, and angles above this range are diagnostic of pathologic deformity.

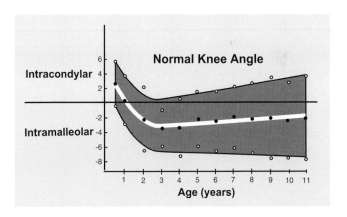

Figure 4 The knee angle development chart shows the normal knee angle in children during the first decade of life. Clinical measures in centimeters between the knees in varus alignment or between the malleoli in valgus alignment are shown. The mean is shown by the white line and the range of normal by the shaded area. Note that the knees are usually in varus in the first year and become valgus in the second year. The range of normal of up to 8 cm of intramalleolar distance is normal throughout most of childhood.

Lower Limb Rotation

Rotational deformity (foot progression angle) is assessed by first observing the child walking. The other assessments (hip rotation, tibial rotation, and foot shape) are made with the child in the prone position. Prone examination of infants or young children is typically performed with the child on the mother's lap; for older children, the examination table is used (Figure 6).

Foot Progression Angle

The foot progression angle is assessed by watching the child walk. The average amount of intoeing or outtoeing

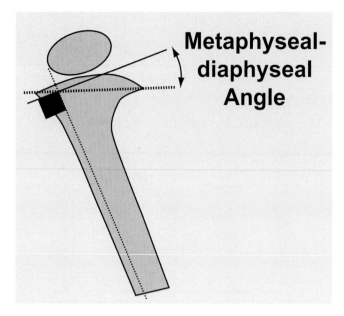

Figure 5 Schematic representation showing that the metaphyseal-diaphyseal angle is formed by relating the axis of the tibia with a line drawn through the edges of the metaphysis.

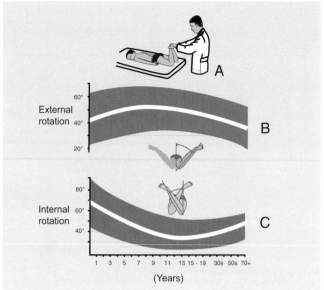

Figure 7 **A,** Schematic representation showing how to assess hip rotation in children. The child should be examined in the prone position. The legs should be rotated symmetrically to their maximum internal and external rotation. No force should be applied. Hip rotation is normally symmetric. Charts showing how internal rotation increases in early childhood and then declines with age **(B)**; external rotation is greatest at birth and declines over the first decade of life **(C)**.

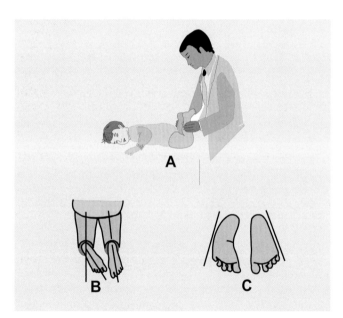

Figure 6 Schematic representation showing how to assess thigh foot angle and metatarsus adductus in children. The child should be examined in the prone position **(A)** and the relationship of the axis of the thigh and foot should be noted **(B)** to assess tibial rotation. Then the angle formed to show the thigh-foot angle should be estimated or measured. The shape of the sole of the foot should also be observed. Normally, the lateral border of the foot is straight. A convex lateral border is seen in patients with metatarsus adductus **(C)**.

of each foot should be estimated. Slight intoeing to approximately 5° of intoeing is within the normal range.

Hip Rotation

With the child's knees flexed to a right angle, both legs are rotated to a degree that is comfortable, and the amount of internal and external rotation is estimated. It is important that orthopaedists are aware of the normal developmental pattern of hip rotation (Figure 7). External rotation is most pronounced in early infancy and declines throughout childhood. This pattern accounts for the external rotation that is typically observed when the infant first starts to stand. Internal rotation gradually increases and peaks during mid-childhood. Internal rotation is approximately 10° greater in girls, which accounts for the femoral antetorsion syndrome that is most pronounced in mid-childhood and more common in girls. Hip rotation is normally symmetric. Asymmetric rotation may indicate the presence of hip pathology. Asymmetric hip rotation should be evaluated by a clinical examination and radiographic screening of the hips.

Tibial Rotation

The axis of the thigh and the foot should be compared to measure the thigh-foot angle. Because the tibia externally rotates with growth, internal tibial torsion resolves with time; however, external tibial torsion often increases with growth (Figure 8).

Foot Shape

Forefoot adduction is assessed by observation. If the forefoot is adducted, severity and flexibility should be determined. To assess flexibility, the forefoot is gently abducted with one hand, while stabilizing the hindfoot with the other. Most deformities are flexible.

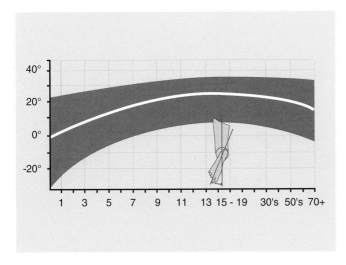

Figure 8 The tibial rotation chart shows the thigh-foot angle by age with mean values shown by the white line and the normal range in the shaded area. Note that the thigh-foot angle externally rotates with age.

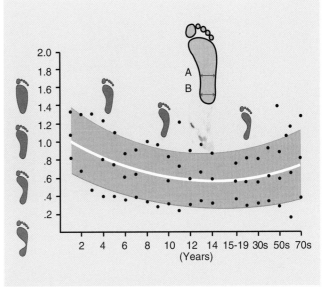

Figure 9 The longitudinal arch development chart shows normal values for the longitudinal arch through life. The mean value for each age is shown by the white line, with the normal range shown in the shaded area. Note that the arch develops over the first decade and that the range of normal is very wide.

Arch Development

Flattening of the longitudinal arch is another feature common in the growing infant and child. The longitudinal arch of the infant is obscured by plantar fat and appears flat. The arch develops in most children over the first decade of life (Figure 9) because of a reduction in plantar fat, increasing strength of the foot musculature, and normal reduction of joint laxity that occurs with growth. About 20% of individuals never develop an arch and live without disability with a flexible flatfoot.

Pathologic flatfeet are diagnosed by assessing flexibility. Stiff flatfeet are pathologic. This stiffness is usually the result of a contracture of the triceps or a tarsal coalition causing a reduction of subtalar motion. In pathologic flatfeet, the foot may show a persistence of loss of the arch when the foot is unweighted. In older children, these feet are often painful. Flexible flatfeet are a normal variation in adults and do not cause disability, as has been shown in military and civilian studies. The treatment of asymptomatic flexible flatfeet with inserts or shoe modifications is ineffective and unnecessary.

Motor Development

The acquisition of motor skills occurs with a wide range of variation in normal infants. Motor development should be assessed during the screening examination, and the history as given by the parents about these skills should be confirmed. Specifically, it should be determined whether the infant has head control, sitting balance, and the ability to walk and run. It should also be determined whether limb use and gait are symmetric. Comparisons with normal range values should be made when uncertainty arises. Infants with cerebral palsy who have mild hemiplegia may be first thought to have a rotational problem.

Gait Development

The development of mature gait occurs throughout the first several years of childhood, with the major characteristics achieved by 3 years and all elements of adult gait present by 7 years of age. Some variables in gait pattern are not uncommon in toddlers. However, consistently abnormal patterns, such as toe walking, abductor lurch, and knee flexion may be signs of an underlying disorder.

Clinical Conditions
Physiologic Bowing

Physiologic bowing is common and benign. Bowing is typically symmetric, involves both the femur and tibia, and is usually most prominent in toddlers. It usually resolves by 2 years of age. In children with physiologic bowing, the screening examination is typically normal and a family history is absent, in which instance radiographs are not necessary. If the deformity has not resolved by the age 2 years, an AP radiograph of the lower limbs should be obtained. This provides documentation of the severity of the bowing, permits measurement of the metaphyseal-diaphyseal angle, and allows evaluation for conditions such as rickets or bony dysplasia. No treatment is indicated for physiologic bowing.

Tibia Vara

Tibia vara or Blount disease is an idiopathic mechanical osteochondral dysplasia of the posteromedial aspect of the proximal tibial physis. Tibia vara is becoming increasingly common, possibly as a result of the childhood

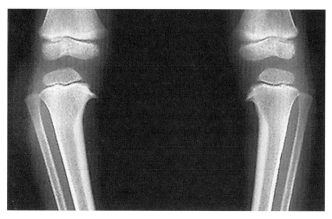

Figure 10 Radiograph of a 2-year-old child with bilateral mild infantile tibia vara. Note the beaking of the proximal medial tibial metaphysis.

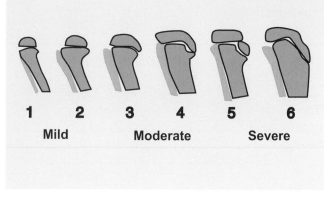

Figure 11 The Langenskiöld classification system categorizes tibia vara as mild (stages 1 and 2), moderate (stages 3 and 4), or severe (stages 5 and 6).

obesity epidemic in North America. Risk factors include obesity, African-American ethnicity, and certain geographic locations (such as residence in the southeastern United States). The onset of tibia vara commonly occurs in infancy, in which instance the disorder is usually bilateral and becomes apparent at 2 years of age. Some instances of infantile tibia vara resolve spontaneously. Juvenile or adolescent onset, which is less common, has a slightly different clinical presentation and is often unilateral and progressive. The natural history of tibia vara is poor, with progressively increasing deformity during childhood causing focal tibial vara, joint deformity, limb shortening, knee stiffness, gait disturbances, osteoarthritis, and pain.

A diagnosis of tibia vara is made by demonstrating the classic radiographic features (Figure 10). Early diagnosis is suggested by increasing varus after 2 years of age or a metaphyseal-diaphyseal angle greater than 16°. When uncertainty exits, the infant should be observed periodically until the diagnosis is clear. Treatment should be delayed until the diagnosis is established. Tibia vara is graded as mild, moderate, or severe by comparing the child's radiographs with established standards (Figure 11).

The effectiveness of bracing for mild tibia vara (Langenskiöld stages 1 and 2) is uncertain because mild tibia vara may resolve spontaneously. No prospective study has demonstrated the effectiveness of brace treatment in this patient population. Because of the poor prognosis of tibia vara, most pediatric orthopaedists elect to treat tibia vara with a long-leg orthotic device despite the lack of proof of effectiveness. This orthotic device is designed to reduce the loading on the proximal medial tibia. The design features include a fixed nonarticulated knee, an incorporated valgus stress, and a wearing regimen that includes day and night use. Each day, the child is allowed several hours out of the brace for bathing and for non–weight-bearing play. Brace treatment is contin-

ued until the deformity is corrected or until surgical correction becomes necessary.

Moderate tibia vara (Langenskiöld stages 3 and 4) is an indication for surgical correction. When possible, surgical correction should be done before the age of 4 years with a proximal tibial external rotational valgus osteotomy. In older children, MRI is recommended to determine the status of the proximal tibial physis. The resection of any physeal bar, stapling of the medial side, and osteotomy are treatment options.

Patients with severe tibia vara (Langenskiöld stages 5 and 6) present with deformity of the proximal tibial articular surface. The extent of articular deformity and the status of the proximal tibial physis should be assessed using MRI. Correction may require an elevation of the depressed subchondral bone to reduce the articular deformity in addition to an alignment osteotomy. Associated deformity of the distal femur may be present. Severe deformity and extreme obesity make treatment of tibia vara a challenge. The use of external fixation is often most effective.

Focal Fibrocartilaginous Dysplasia

Focal fibrocartilaginous dysplasia is a rare idiopathic deformity that causes a characteristic sclerotic concave defect of long bones filled with fibrocartilage. The most common site is the proximal medial tibia that causes a varus deformity. About half of the instances of focal fibrocartilaginous dysplasia resolve spontaneously. Management typically consists of observation and rarely osteotomy.

Familial Rickets and Skeletal Dysplasia Deformity

Familial rickets and skeletal dysplasia cause a generalized varus or valgus deformity. Because the underlying disease is not curable, and to reduce the likelihood of recurrence, correction should be delayed until close to the end of growth. Correction may require a multilevel osteotomy to establish an acceptable mechanical axis.

Genu Valgum

Nondisplaced fractures of the proximal tibial metaphysis in early childhood may cause overgrowth of the tibia, with a resulting valgus deformity of the upper tibia. Because this deformity is not preventable, the family of the child should be warned of this possible complication and assured that it can be effectively treated should it occur. The family should also be advised that the deformity usually resolves over a period of years without treatment; if it does not resolve, it can be surgically corrected in late childhood. Providing this information to the family in advance is very helpful in minimizing anxiety.

Severe physiologic knock-knee deformity is most common in obese girls in late childhood. The intramalleolar distance in these patients is greater than 8 to 10 cm, and slight asymmetry is common. The cause of this deformity is unknown, and the clinical course variable. The deformity may increase until growth is complete. The condition may aggravate patellofemoral instability and knee pain. The primary concern is usually the unsightly appearance.

Management of idiopathic genu valgum is controversial. Most patients are managed by observing the deformity over a period of 12 to 24 months. If the deformity is severe and causes disability, or is especially unsightly, it should be corrected by performing a physiodesis of the distal medial femoral physis using staples or plates. Patients should be followed up at 6-month intervals to avoid overcorrection. If correction occurs before maturity, the staples should be removed or the epiphysiodesis should be completed to prevent overcorrection.

If the deformity is severe and the patient presents close to the end of growth, correction of the tibia may also be necessary. A good option if the child is approaching skeletal maturity is to perform a bone block epiphysiodesis without drilling.

Posteromedial Tibial Bowing

Posteromedial tibial bowing is a congenital, idiopathic, unilateral deformity characterized by tibial bowing, shortening, and a calcaneal deformity of the foot. The calcaneal deformity always resolves spontaneously. The bowing improves spontaneously to a degree that is usually acceptable. Tibial shortening increases with growth, often to 3 to 5 cm by the end of growth. If the shortening is unacceptable, mild deformity should be corrected with a contralateral timed tibial epiphysiodesis. If the deformity is more severe, tibial lengthening may be indicated. During lengthening, any residual angulation can also be corrected.

Anterior Tibial Bowing

Anterior tibial bowing usually is associated with other deformities such as fibular hemimelia, and it often is not severe enough to require correction.

Anterolateral Tibial Bowing

Anterolateral tibial bowing is part of the spectrum of congenital pseudarthrosis of the tibia. The bowing may progress to fracture and nonunion. Neurofibromatosis is present in about half of the patients with anterolateral tibial bowing. It is managed by protection with a long-leg orthotic device to reduce the risk of fracture. Osteotomy and prophylactic grafting should be avoided in this patient population.

Rotational Conditions

Intoeing and outtoeing are common clinical conditions in infants and children. These rotational conditions typically concern the family, but they usually resolve spontaneously. Traditionally, management has been focused on intoeing. Data show that external rotational deformities are far more likely to cause disability than outtoeing. There are several reasons for this. First, both the tibia and femur externally rotate with growth, causing external torsion to increase during growth; conversely, internal rotation nearly always corrects before maturity. Second, external tibial torsion is likely to aggravate patellofemoral malalignment and be a cause of knee pain. External tibial torsion has been shown to be associated with Osgood-Schlatter disease and osteochondritis dissecans. Femoral retrotorsion has been associated with slipped capital femoral epiphysis and osteoarthritis of the hip and knee. In contrast, femoral antetorsion has not been found to be associated with osteoarthritis of the hip. Third, an external rotational deformity may degrade physical performance. Slight intoeing does not adversely affect athletic performance.

Metatarsus Adductus

Metatarsus adductus is usually the result of intrauterine position. As with other positional deformities, the condition resolves spontaneously. Ninety percent of flexible metatarsus adductus deformities resolve before the age of 5 years, and the remaining 10% of deformities resolve by the end of growth. Nonresolving metatarsus adductus, sometimes referred to as metatarsus varus, is rare but does not appear to cause disability in the adult.

Metatarsus adductus should be managed by observation. If the family is anxious about the deformity, it is recommended that pediatric orthopaedists consider photographically documenting the severity or make a copy of the sole of the foot on a copy machine. This documentation provides a record to show the family the improvement when the child is seen in follow-up. Although special shoes, exercises, braces, and other devices are commonly used to treat metatarsus adductus, this is a self-resolving condition that may take a few years to correct naturally. If the deformity is severe or stiff, long-leg bracing or casts are the most effective management.

Table 2 | Guidelines for Management of Family Expectations

Make an accurate diagnosis	An accurate diagnosis together with an understanding the natural history makes it possible to predict future outcomes.
Warn families about common complications and expected natural history	Advising the family in advance that a proximal tibial fracture may cause a knock-knee deformity or that an anterolateral bowed tibia may fracture can convert a potentially awkward outcome into one that enhances the standing of the pediatric orthopaedist with the family. This confidence enables orthopaedists to more effectively manage the ensuing problem. Advising families that intoeing will resolve but outtoeing may worsen is important information. When the child follows a pattern as predicted by the orthopaedist, the orthopaedist-parent relationship is enhanced.
Give the family reassurance	In this era of Internet families who are exposed to so much misinformation, receiving reliable information from an orthopaedist that the family trusts is especially important.
Avoid unnecessary treatment	It has been said that the best results in orthopaedics come from the vigorous treatment of conditions that resolve spontaneously. This approach, however, is unacceptable because it hurts the child. Treating the child to satisfy the family is inappropriate. It is the responsibility of orthopaedists to do what is best for the child, not what the family may wish.
Be the advocate for the child	Unnecessary or ineffective orthopaedic treatments are not benign. These treatments have been found to have an impact on the child. The experience of undergoing a pediatric orthopaedic intervention, when remembered by adults, has been shown to adversely impact self-esteem (Figure 12). In addition, recommending unnecessary treatment, which is expensive for the family and society, is poor medical practice.

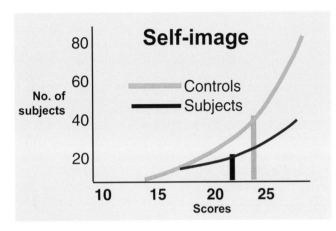

Figure 12 The orthopaedic treatment and self-image chart compares adult controls with subjects who underwent various orthopaedic treatments during childhood. Self-images scores were reduced in the treated subjects.

Internal Tibial Torsion

Internal tibial torsion is the most common cause of intoeing and is usually seen in toddlers. The thigh-foot angle is medially rotated in patients with internal tibial torsion, and the condition is commonly bilateral. Unilateral deformity is most common on the left side. Observation is the recommended management. Bracing, shoe modifications, or orthotic devices do not change the natural history of internal tibial torsion. The family should be advised that the intoeing will resolve over a period of several years.

Femoral Antetorsion

Femoral antetorsion usually develops in early childhood. It is most common in girls, it is symmetric, and it causes the typical W sitting position, inward facing patella, and an awkward running style. Femoral antetorsion is diagnosed in patients with internal rotation greater than 70° and reduced external rotation. The severity of femoral antetorsion is considered mild if internal rotation is between 70° to 80°, moderate if it is between 80° and 90°, and severe if it is greater than 90°. The intoeing caused by femoral antetorsion is usually most severe in patients between 4 and 7 years of age, after which it typically improves. The measuring of anteversion using diagnostic imaging is not helpful in guiding treatment in this patient population unless surgical correction is planned.

Shoe modifications, inserts, braces, physical therapy, sitting restrictions, or other nonsurgical measures are not helpful in treating patients with femoral antetorsion and are therefore best avoided. Surgical correction is rarely required and indicated only if the deformity is severe, disabling, and present in a child older than 10 years. Correction using an intertrochanteric femoral osteotomy with about 45° of outward rotation is recommended. The intertrochanteric level is recommended because the surgical scar is less noticeable, cancellous bone promotes rapid union, fixation is most simple, and the proximal site is most forgiving of any loss of correction.

External Tibial Torsion

External tibial torsion most likely requires surgical correction. The deformity may be bilateral; if unilateral, it is most likely to involve the right side. The deformity often increases with growth and is often associated with knee problems and functional disability. When external tibial torsion is severe (the patient has a thigh-foot angle greater than 40°) surgical correction should be done using a supramalleolar rotational osteotomy. The fibula should be divided obliquely if the tibial deformity is severe, and the tibia should be fixed with a small plate or crossed pins. Whenever possible, correction in the proximal tibia should be avoided because complications at this level are common.

Complex Rotational Deformity
Rotational deformity often occurs at more than one level. Femoral antetorsion and internal tibial torsion may coexist and cause severe intoeing. This combination is self-resolving and seldom requires treatment. External tibial torsion and femoral retrotorsion may coexist, compounding the severity of outtoeing. This double-level deformity reduces the threshold for performing a tibial osteotomy. The combination of external tibial torsion, pes valgus, and obesity is another syndrome in which each component aggravates the others. Correction may require a tibial rotational osteotomy, calcaneal lengthening, and heel-cord lengthening.

Torsional Malalignment Syndrome
Torsional malalignment syndrome, sometimes referred to as the miserable malalignment, consists of a combination of femoral antetorsion and external tibial torsion. The foot progression angle is normal, but the patellae are inwardly rotated. Knee pain is common. Management of torsional malalignment syndrome is difficult. Correction of severe deformity requires a double level osteotomy. Correction at the intertrochanteric and supramalleolar levels is recommended because of the improved safety of this procedure. Other pediatric orthopaedists recommend correction using osteotomies just above and below the knee. Although this approach makes anatomic sense, proximal tibial osteotomies post the greatest risk of extremity osteotomies. In addition, peroneal nerve palsy and compartment syndromes after proximal tibial osteotomy are not uncommon.

Managing Family Expectations
One of the most challenging aspects of treating children with motor development problems, such as congenital pseudarthrosis of the tibia or advanced tibia vara, is managing family expectations. Managing these expectations is made easier by following general principles (Table 2 and Figure 12).

Summary
Treating common developmental problems in children is challenging because motor development disorders include some of the most difficult conditions to treat. It is imperative, therefore, that pediatric orthopaedists establish an accurate diagnosis; to do so, an understanding of natural history and thoughtful, child-oriented management is required.

Annotated Bibliography
Evaluation
Hogan MT, Staheli LT: Arch height and lower limb pain: An adult civilian study. *Foot Ankle Int* 2002;23:43-47.

   The relationship of arch height and foot pain were studied in 102 civilian adult grocery store workers. Three were excluded because of foot pathology. In the remaining subjects, arch configuration was assessed and an algorithm that generates lower limb, foot and ankle, and shoe comfort scores was used. No relationship was found between arch index and lower limb disability. These findings support previous military studies showing that flexible flatfoot in adults is not a source of disability.

Clinical Conditions
Ferrick MR, Birch JG, Albright M: Correction of non-Blount's angular knee deformity by permanent hemi-epiphyseodesis. *J Pediatr Orthop* 2004;24:397-402.

   In this retrospective study, 75 patients (125 knee deformities) were treated using hemiepiphysiodesis. Deformity was idopathic in 38 patients, and 37 had etiologies other than tibia vara. In 106 of the knee deformities, correction was satisfactory; in 15, the procedure was performed too late to be effective, and 4 failures occurred because of technical problems. Fifteen knees in 11 patients were overcorrected. The authors concluded that the procedure is simple and effective with few complications. Follow-up is essential to prevent overcorrection.

Rotational Conditions
Bruce WD, Stevens PM: Surgical correction of miserable malalignment syndrome. *J Pediatr Orthop* 2004;24:392-396.

   This is a retrospective study of 14 patients (27 limbs) who were treated with femoral and tibial rotational osteotomies for femoral antetorsion, external tibial torsion, and knee pain. Follow-up ranged from 2 to 12 years. All patients experienced pain relief, and no persistent complications were reported.

Lincoln TL, Suen PW: Common rotational variations in children. *J Am Acad Orthop Surg* 2003;11:312-320.

   The authors studied current treatments for rotational variations and torticollis in children and indicated that most of these conditions resolve spontaneously. They stressed the need for a careful examination and exclusion of more serious disorders, such as malformations, inflammations, and neurologic problems.

Classic Bibliography

Blount WP: Tibia vara: Osteochondrosis deformans tibiae. *J Bone Joint Surg* 1937;19:1-29.

Choi IH, Kim CJ, Cho TJ, et al: Focal fibrocartilaginous dysplasia of long bones: Report of eight additional cases and literature review. *J Pediatr Orthop* 2000;20:421-427.

Delgado ED, Schoenecker PL, Rich MM, Capelli AM: Treatment of severe torsional malalignment syndrome. *J Pediatr Orthop* 1996;16:484-488.

Doyle BS, Volk AG, Smith CF, et al: Infantile Blount disease: Long-term follow-up of surgically treated patients at skeletal maturity. *J Pediatr Orthop* 1996;16:469-476.

Eckhoff DG, Kramer RC, Alongi CA, VanGerven DP: Femoral anteversion and arthritis of the knee. *J Pediatr Orthop* 1994;14:608-610.

Fraser RK, Dickens DR, Cole WG: Medial physeal stapling for primary and secondary genu valgum in late childhood and adolescence. *J Bone Joint Surg Br* 1995;77:733-735.

Fuchs R, Staheli LT: Sprinting and intoeing. *J Pediatr Orthop* 1996;16:489-491.

Harris RI, Beath T: Etiology of peroneal spastic flat foot. *J Bone Joint Surg Br* 1948;30:624-634.

Harris RI, Beath T: Hypermobile flat-foot with short tendo Achilles. *J Bone Joint Surg Am* 1948;30:116-140.

Heath CH, Staheli LT: Normal limits of knee angle in white children: Genu varum and genu valgum. *J Pediatr Orthop* 1993;13:259-262.

Langenskiöld A, Riska EB: Tibia vara (osteochondrosis deformans tibiae): A survey of seventy-one cases. *J Bone Joint Surg Am* 1964;46:1405-1420.

Staheli LT, Corbett M, Wyss C, et al: Lower-extremity rotational problems in children: Normal values to guide management. *J Bone Joint Surg Am* 1985;67:39-47.

Stevens PM, Maguire M, Dales MD, Robins AJ: Physeal stapling for idiopathic genu valgum. *J Pediatr Orthop* 1999;19:645-649.

Sutherland D, Olshen R, Cooper L, Woo S: The development of mature gait. *J Bone Joint Surg Am* 1980;62:336.

Wenger DR, Mauldin D, Speck G, et al: Corrective shoes and inserts as treatment for flexible flatfoot in infants and children. *J Bone Joint Surg Am* 1989;71:800-810.

Chapter 2

The Limping Child

Mohammad Diab, MD

Introduction

The evaluation of the limping child need not be a diagnostic "black box". It requires a thorough history and physical examination, which may be supplemented by laboratory and diagnostic imaging studies. The condition may be classified according to patient age and urgency. Different causes of limping occur with varying frequencies in the following three age groups: infant/toddler (age, younger than 3 years), child (age, 3 to 10 years), and adolescent (older than 10 years) (Table 1). Some disturbances of gait producing a limp are characteristic of certain ages (for example, limping associated with slipped capital femoral epiphysis in adolescents), whereas others are broadly distributed throughout all of the age groups (for example, limping associated with fracture). The various etiologies may be classified as those that require urgent treatment (such as hip pyarthritis) and those that can be managed electively (such as developmental dysplasia of the hip) (Table 2).

Disturbance of gait producing a limp may result from pain, weakness or other neuromuscular imbalance, or deformity. A painful or antalgic gait is defined by a shortened stance phase, which in extreme instances is manifested by a refusal of the patient to walk. Hip deformities producing a limp commonly result in a Trendelenburg gait, which is a shift of the body over the affected hip to reduce the moment arm exerted on weak abductor muscles. In patients with mild deformities, the limp may be apparent only after several cycles and may give way to pain as inflammation and/or muscle fatigue develops. Pain over the abductors or trochanter may be distinguished by its more lateral location from pain caused by hip disorders, which is typically anterior in the region of the groin.

The physical examination should be performed with the patient in the supine and then the prone position. The supine position may show hip obligate lateral rotation with flexion as occurs in patients with slipped capital femoral epiphysis. The prone position has the distinct advantage of allowing uncoupling of the knee from the hip, which may masquerade one for the other. In the su-

pine position, moving the knee requires flexion of the hip, which makes it difficult at times to determine which joint is the offender. In addition, as in the examination for torsion, the prone position allows simultaneous comparison of hip rotation (especially medial), which is the most sensitive to disease. The prone position will also reveal a hip flexion contracture that may be concealed by lumbar hyperlordosis without the physician manipulating the patient.

Only the most common causes of limp are discussed in this chapter. Studies on the limping child show that the cause is not always identified and that no final diagnosis is made in up to 25% of patients.

Transient Synovitis

Although the cause of transient synovitis is uncertain, it may be thought of as a reactive arthritis that most often affects the hip. Patients with transient synovitis frequently have a history of antecedent infection, and the condition occurs most frequently in infants or young children (age range, 3 to 10 years). Transient synovitis is characterized by an antalgic gait or refusal to walk, normal temperature to low fever, reduced range of motion of the hip, and normal to mildly elevated serologic markers of inflammation. Ultrasound evaluation typically shows a nonechogenic effusion. Treatment consists of symptomatic care, including activity modification and nonsteroidal anti-inflammatory agents. In most patients, symptoms and signs resolve over 1 to 3 days without sequelae.

Occasionally, a child may have transient synovitis with a prolonged duration, which may be referred to as reactive arthritis, a joint manifestation of a remote illness. For example, poststreptococcal reactive arthritis may persist for 1 to 3 weeks, again with mild elevation of inflammatory markers and no long-term sequelae. Reactive arthritis differs from septic arthritis in that the joint is not directly inoculated and differs from rheumatoid and seronegative arthritis in that it typically lasts less than 6 weeks.

Table 1 | Diagnosis of the Limping Child by Age

Infant/Toddler (younger than 3 years)
Nonpainful gait
Developmental dysplasia of the hip
Congenital limb deficiencies
Neuromuscular abnormalities
Painful gait
Toddler fracture
Osteomyelitis/septic arthritis
Miscellaneous infection
Transient synovitis
Reactive arthritis
Juvenile rheumatoid arthritis

Child (3 to 10 years of age)
Nonpainful gait
Developmental dysplasia of the hip
Congenital lower limb disorders
Painful gait
Legg-Calvé-Perthes disease
Osteomyelitis/septic arthritis
Transient synovitis
Stress fractures
Tumors (benign, malignant in older children)
Osteochondrosis
Osgood-Schlatter disease
Kohler's disease (osteochondrosis of the navicular bone)
Osteochondritis dissecans (knee, ankle)

Adolescent (older than 10 years)
Slipped capital femoral epiphysis
Legg-Calvé-Perthes disease osteonecrosis
Juvenile rheumatoid arthritis
Osteomyelitis/septic arthritis
Stress fractures
Overuse syndromes
Osteochondrosis (knee, ankle)
Benign or malignant tumors–especially if associated with pain at night or at rest

Table 2 | Triage of Limping Pediatric Patients*

Urgent	Elective
Hip pyarthritis	Transient synovitis of the hip
Osteomyelitis	Developmental dysplasia of the hip
Diskitis	Legg-Calvé-Perthes disease
Slipped capital femoral epiphysis	Chondrolysis of the hip
Toddler fracture	Rheumatoid arthritis
Leukemia	Osteoid osteoma
	Neuromuscular disease
	Discoid lateral meniscus
	Osteochondritis dissecans
	Lower limb-length discrepancy
	Tarsal coalition
	Overuse apophysitis

The triage of a limping child may be aided by dividing the cause into urgent and elective. Elective conditions may be referred to a specialist after the urgent causes are ruled out.

Infection

Pyarthritis

Infection of the hip may occur directly or secondarily from the proximal femoral metaphysis, which is intra-articular. It may be regarded as a surgical emergency, based on investigative evidence of irreversible cartilage damage after 6 hours of exposure to pus, or as an urgent condition, based on empiric clinical evidence of secondary arthritis in patients who undergo surgical treatment more than 72 hours after onset. The independent predictors that have been proposed to aid in the diagnosis of hip pyarthritis are listed in Table 3.

The probability of hip pyarthritis is greater than 90% if four of these predictors are present, approximately 75% if three predictors are present, 35% if two predictors are present, approximately 10% if one predictor is present, and 2% if no predictors are present. In addition to these diagnostic predictors, the C-reactive protein level is used to help determine the diagnosis of pyarthritis in children. C-reactive protein level has been shown to be a better independent predictor of pyarthritis in children than erythrocyte sedimentation rate. The negative predictive value of C-reactive protein level (< 10 mg/L) is 87%, whereas the positive predictive value is approximately 50%.

For patients with hip pyarthritis, a screening radiograph is obtained to look for indirect evidence of effusion (increased medial joint width) and to rule out other causes of limp, particularly osseous causes, such as osteomyelitis or fracture. Ultrasound will typically show evidence of a hip effusion, which may be distinguished from that seen in patients with transient synovitis by its echogenic pattern. A joint aspiration is essential when hip pyarthritis cannot be distinguished from transient synovitis, other types of arthritis, or osteomyelitis.

Transient synovitis is a diagnosis of exclusion and must be distinguished from septic hip arthritis. Patients with transient synovitis typically do not appear to be systemically ill, they may be able to walk, fever does not exceed 38.5°C, white blood cell count is below 12,000/mm³, erythrocyte sedimentation rate does not exceed 40 mm/h, C-reactive protein level does not exceed 20 mg/L, and improvement occurs within 36 hours. Failure to recognize and treat a septic hip can result in permanent damage to the hip; therefore, if there is any doubt regarding the diagnosis, diagnostic hip aspiration with blood cell count and bacteriologic cultures should be performed.

Table 3 | Independent Predictors That May Be Used in the Diagnosis of Hip Infection

Predictor	Probability of Hip Infection
Refusal to bear weight	0 predictors: 2%
Fever greater than 38.5°C	1 predictor: 10%
White blood cell count greater than 12,000 cells/mm^3	2 predictors: 35%
Erythrocyte sedimentation rate greater than 40 mm/hr	3 predictors: 75% 4 predictors: > 90%
C-reactive protein level < 10 mg/L	Negative predictive value: 87% Positive predictive value: 50%

Pyarthritis is characterized by a synovial white blood cell count of greater than 50,000/mm^3 with more than 75% polymorphonuclear leukocytes. In patients with transient synovitis, synovial white blood cell count is generally less than 15,000/mm^3 with less than 15% polymorphonuclear leukocytes. Inflammatory conditions such as rheumatoid arthritis can span the intervening spectrum. Gram stain and culture are positive in approximately 50% of patients. The most common infecting organisms are *Staphylococcus aureus*, *Streptococcus pneumoniae* and group B (neonates), and *Kingella kingae*.

Treatment of hip pyarthritis involves incision and drainage, followed by antibiotics. A drain is placed, which is removed based on response. Antibiotics are administered intravenously (cefazolin 50 to 150 mg/kg/day) until good clinical and laboratory response is achieved. The clinical response is measured by fever, pain, and ability of the patient to bear weight. Laboratory response is measured in the early period by C-reactive protein level. Absence of improvement after 72 hours necessitates a change of management, including additional workup to assess the patient for other sources of infection (extra-articular extension of infection) and/or repeat incision and drainage. A compliant patient with normal gastrointestinal absorption may receive oral antibiotics (cephalexin 50 to 150 mg/kg/day) once afebrile and reasonably comfortable, and once the C-reactive protein level has normalized (< 1 mg/L). Oral antibiotics may be terminated once the erythrocyte sedimentation rate has normalized (< 20 mm/hr). Both C-reactive protein level and erythrocyte sedimentation rate are more reliable than white blood cell count, which shows considerable variability in this patient population.

Osteomyelitis

The reported incidence of osteomyelitis is approximately 1 in 5,000 children younger than 13 years. Forty percent of all instances of osteomyelitis in children involve the tibia, followed by the femur (20%) and the calcaneus (10%). Boys are affected twice as frequently as girls. Decreased limb use and pain with palpation are the most common presenting signs (80% of patients), followed by swelling (60%) and fever (40%). Proximal femoral osteomyelitis may be difficult to distinguish from hip pyarthritis. In such instances, an ultrasound evaluation of the hip is a useful diagnostic aid because the absence of an effusion makes a diagnosis of hip pyarthritis unlikely. Occasionally, the intra-articular location of the femoral neck may link proximal femoral osteomyelitis with hip pyarthritis.

Early in the course of osteomyelitis, radiographs may be normal because osseous changes do not become apparent for 7 to 10 days. Technetium Tc 99m-labeled bone scanning is highly sensitive (> 90%) and can show abnormal tracer uptake within 24 hours, suggesting the diagnosis of osteomyelitis. Reduced uptake ("cold" bone scan) indicates a more serious infection than increased uptake ("hot" bone scan) because it indicates the presence of osteonecrosis, and therefore reduced antibiotic vascular access. Blood cultures are positive in 50% of patients, whereas needle aspiration of the affected bone will yield organisms in 80% of patients. The site of aspiration may be localized by the physical examination, or by bone scanning in patients whose radiographs are negative. Aspiration should proceed slowly to allow the distinction of a subperiosteal abscess from an osseous abscess. The most common infecting organism overall in all age groups with osteomyelitis is *S aureus* (80%), with *Streptococcus* and gram-negative infections being prominent in infancy.

Visible radiographic change, such as an abscess ("hole in bone"), often indicates the need for surgical débridement, followed by antibiotics. In the absence of radiographic changes, and after surgical débridement, the protocol for antibiotic therapy resembles that for hip pyarthritis. Failure of treatment is associated with incomplete débridement and polymicrobial infection. Additional details on the diagnosis and management of osteomyelitis are found in chapter 6.

Diskitis

Diskitis presents as a triad of pain, fever, and reduced intervertebral disk height on spinal radiograph. Pain in the infant/toddler typically manifests as refusal to walk; the child may report vague abdominal pain, and often it is not until adolescence that the process can be localized to the back. Access to the intervertebral disk occurs through vascular channels that traverse the ring epiphyses in the immature skeleton. As with osteomyelitis, radiographic changes take 1 to 2 weeks to become apparent, whereas scintigraphy or MRI will show the disease process earlier. Treatment consists of antibiotic therapy as described for patients with osteomyelitis. Bracing was recommended in the past and may help alleviate symptoms, but there is no high-level evidence that bracing offers benefits over antibiotic therapy alone (see chapter 6).

Hip

Developmental Dysplasia of the Hip

In the infant/toddler or young child, developmental dysplasia of the hip with dislocation produces a painless waddling limp associated with lumbar hyperlordosis if it is bilateral or a short leg, Trendelenburg gait if it is unilateral. Abductor weakness caused by proximal migration of the dislocated hip produces this Trendelenburg gait as the body shifts laterally toward the affected limb during stance phase. On physical examination, an adductor contracture of the affected hip is often observed, and in some patients a dislocatable hip can be detected using the Barlow maneuver and a reducible hip can be detected using the Ortolani maneuver. In addition, shortening of the affected limb (Galeazzi or Allis sign) and asymmetry of groin and thigh skin folds may be present. The older child and adolescent may present with both a Trendelenburg gait and an antalgic gait as a result of early degenerative changes or a labral tear. Radiographs of the pelvis will typically show dislocation and/or acetabular dysplasia with or without secondary femoral head changes. Treatment varies according to age and the type of dysplasia; the ultimate goal of treatment is to achieve a supple and concentrically reduced hip.

Legg-Calvé-Perthes Disease

Legg-Calvé-Perthes disease represents ischemia of the proximal femoral epiphysis in children. Four radiographic stages of Legg-Calvé-Perthes disease have been described: ischemia, collapse and fragmentation, reconstitution, and remodelling with residual deformity. In the ischemic stage, the child presents with a painful limp. This often evolves into a painless limp associated with hip stiffness. The end stage is characterized by coxa brevis (short neck) caused by premature closure of the proximal femoral physis, relative overgrowth of the greater trochanter, caput planum (flat head) caused by collapse, and caput magnum (large head) caused by swelling of the epiphysis during reperfusion and recovery. The shortened neck and high greater trochanter disadvantage the hip abductors and produce a Trendelenburg gait. The flat and large head eventually leads to osteoarthritis, which is determined by the degree of femoral head asphericity and hip incongruity. Thus, the limp that characterizes Legg-Calvé-Perthes disease is initially the result at the outset of pain, then the result of deformity and associated weakness, and finally the result of both.

The typical clinical presentation of a pediatric patient with Legg-Calvé-Perthes disease is a 4- to 8-year-old Caucasian boy (Legg-Calvé-Perthes disease is more common in boys than girls), who may be small for his age and hyperactive, with hip stiffness and a limp. Workup should include radiographs of the hips, which may be negative initially in the ischemic stage. Eventu-

ally, however, the radiographic stages will progress from a small epiphysis with increased density relative to the opposite side to a fragmented and reossifying epiphysis with variable degrees of flattening. The subchondral fracture that heralds the onset of fragmentation may occasionally be present. MRI and technetium bone scanning may show changes in the proximal femoral epiphysis at the outset of the disease. However, current treatment guidelines are based primarily on the age of the patient and radiographic grade. As a result, imaging modalities that allow an earlier diagnosis do not as yet influence surgical management. More details on the management of Legg-Calvé-Perthes disease are presented in chapter 13.

Slipped Capital Femoral Epiphysis

Slipped capital femoral epiphysis occurs when weakness at the capital femoral physis results in displacement of the proximal metaphysis and the remainder of the femur into extension to produce an apex anterior and lateral deformity. The epiphysis, which is retained in the acetabulum, assumes a relatively posterior and inferior position. In chronic slips, patients will present with an antalgic limp associated with external rotation of the affected limb. Slipped capital femoral epiphysis is the most common disorder of the hip in adolescents; it affects overweight, Pacific Islanders more than African Americans, African Americans more than Caucasians, Caucasians more than Asians, and boys more than girls. Pain referred to the knee is a common presenting complaint in patients with slipped capital femoral epiphysis. The apex anterior deformity abuts the acetabulum with hip flexion, forcing obligate lateral rotation as the femoral neck rolls along the acetabular rim. Thus, there is loss of medial rotation of the hip as well as femoroacetabular impingement, which may lead to labral tear, acetabular articular injury, and worsening femoral neck deformity. In patients with the severe slipped capital femoral epiphysis, the greater trochanter is displaced proximally, which leads to hip abductor weakness and a Trendelenburg gait. Premature fusion of the proximal femoral physis, resulting from the disease or its surgical treatment, produces a short limb.

Although the clinical presentation of patients with slipped capital femoral epiphysis is predictable, it continues to be a diagnostic challenge, has the longest duration of symptoms before diagnosis, and is the most commonly missed serious cause of limp. Additional workup for patients with suspected slipped capital femoral epiphysis should include AP and lateral radiographs of the hips, which will typically show physeal widening, slip of the epiphysis, signs of remodelling, and secondary osseous damage in patients with long-term disease. When radiographs are equivocal (the patient is in the "preslip" phase), technetium bone scanning or MRI is helpful.

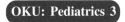

Treatment for slipped capital femoral epiphysis includes screw fixation, with or without reduction (either closed or open). Patients with long-term slipped capital femoral epiphysis who have severe deformity and significant impingement may benefit from labral repair, débridement, and/or realignment osteotomy. Details of treatment for slipped capital femoral epiphysis are covered in chapter 13.

Chondrolysis of the Hip

Idiopathic chondrolysis of the hip is an obscure condition that is characterized by a limp associated with stiffness of the hip. The female to male ratio is 5:1, and 5% of patients with idiopathic chondrolysis of the hip are affected bilaterally. The average age at presentation is 12.5 years for girls and 14.8 years for boys. Early reports suggested an increased prevalence in African Americans, but this has not been substantiated by later reports. The range of time to diagnosis is 1 to 18 months, which reflects the unfamiliar nature of this condition to most clinicians. Patients with idiopathic chondrolysis of the hip typically have no history of an antecedent event, no fever, and no other constitutional symptoms or signs. Laboratory test results are often normal, with the exception of the erythrocyte sedimentation rate, which may be elevated in approximately 10% of patients. The radiographic features include reduction of joint width (the pathognomonic finding) and subchondral blurring in the early stages of the disease, followed by protrusio acetabuli, premature physeal obliteration, and marginal osteophytes in the later stages. Surgical findings include nonspecific inflammatory changes in capsule, synovia and synovial membrane, and cartilage loss. No single treatment has been shown to affect the natural history of the disease, including anti-inflammatory medications, immobilization, range-of-motion exercises, intra-articular injection of corticosteroid, and soft-tissue release such as capsulectomy. Approximately half of all patients experience complete but painless ankylosis of the hip.

Chondrolysis of the hip also may be seen in patients with slipped capital femoral epiphysis, either as a result of the primary disease or its treatment (particularly in those who have undergone subtrochanteric realignment osteotomy).

Toddler Fracture

A toddler fracture is a low-energy, nondisplaced, or minimally displaced fracture of the lower limb that causes an antalgic limp or refusal to bear weight. There is often no swelling nor any focal tenderness. The term has been applied historically to a fracture of the tibial shaft, but may be expanded to any fracture of the lower limb with the typical presentation (for example, a fracture of the calcaneus). The nondisplaced fracture may be diagnosed on radiographs 7 to 10 days after injury at which time evidence of periosteal elevation will be apparent. Bone scanning may be used to assess acute fractures, especially during a workup to exclude other causes of limp such as infection. Treatment usually consists of the use of a weight-bearing cast for 3 to 4 weeks.

Rheumatoid Arthritis

Patients with Still's disease (systemic juvenile rheumatoid arthritis) are systemically ill with visceral involvement, but this condition does not pose a significant diagnostic dilemma. The polyarthric form of the disease has a bimodal age distribution (in infants and adolescents), affects multiple small and large joints, and is significantly disabling. Patients have widespread musculoskeletal disease and require multiple orthopaedic interventions. They have joint swelling, stiffness and deformity, gracile bones, and limited physical capacity, and often must be confined to wheelchairs as adults. Pauciarthric rheumatoid arthritis, defined as painless swelling lasting longer than 3 weeks and involving up to five joints, first presents in infants or girls more frequently than in boys. Pauciarthric rheumatoid arthritis of a single joint in the lower limb, most frequently the knee followed by the ankle and subtalar joints, may produce a limp. Unlike children with polyarthric rheumatoid arthritis, children with pauciarthric rheumatoid arthritis may present with a mismatch between symptoms and signs; for example, a systemically calm infant may present with a warm and swollen knee. Unlike children with pyarthritis, children with pauciarthric rheumatoid arthritis typically have less pain and appear less distressed.

Perhaps the greatest challenge in making the initial diagnosis of rheumatoid arthritis is posed by the considerable variability of its presentation. Patients with rheumatoid arthritis often have a history that betrays chronicity in contradistinction to patients with pyarthritis. The history also may reveal a temporal pattern, especially the classic symptom of morning stiffness. Evaluation should include aspiration and synovial analysis, as well as serologic analysis to determine erythrocyte sedimentation rate and test for the presence of antinuclear antigen, which is present in 50% or more of patients with the pauciarthric form of rheumatoid arthritis. It is essential to establish the diagnosis because iritis in this patient population may lead to blindness. All patients with rheumatoid arthritis should have, therefore, a prompt referral to an ophthalmologist. Nonsurgical treatment consists of medications, including nonsteroidal anti-inflammatory agents, slow-reacting remittives and cytotoxic drugs, and articular steroid injection. Surgical treatment, which is most commonly required for patients with the polyarthric form of rheumatoid arthritis, can include synovectomy, contracture release, osteotomy, and limb equalization. End-stage disease may require joint ablation (typically arthroplasty, but occasionally arthrodesis).

Tumor

Leukemia

Leukemia is the most common cancer of childhood. A hallmark of leukemia is migratory bone pain. Acute lymphoblastic leukemia, the most common form of the disease, presents in the infant or young child, approximately 20% of whom have musculoskeletal complaints, and approximately 10% of whom have an initial presentation of limp. Key features of the diagnosis include physical evidence of systemic disease, such as fever, easy bruising, lymphadenopathy, and signs of anemia, as well as laboratory abnormalities, such as elevated erythrocyte sedimentation rate, thrombocytopenia or anemia, and increased lymphoblasts on peripheral smear. Radiographs may show characteristic transverse radiolucent metaphyseal bands (leukemia lines), although changes are nonspecific and may be interpreted as disuse osteopenia. The diagnosis is established by bone marrow biopsy.

Osteoid Osteoma

Osteoid osteoma is a benign neoplasm that affects children and/or adolescents. One half of instances of osteoid osteoma involve the femur and tibia, most frequently the proximal femur. The classic presentation includes night pain that is relieved by nonsteroidal anti-inflammatory agents. Variability in presentation accounts for significant delay in diagnosis, with 75% of patients diagnosed from 6 months to 2 years after the onset of symptoms. Workup includes radiographs, which may show evidence of sclerosis surrounding a radiodense nidus. Bone scanning will typically show focal, intense, increased tracer uptake. CT or MRI is useful for anatomic characterization of the neoplasm in anticipation of surgical excision.

Neuromuscular Disease

Pregnancy, birth history, and developmental history may lead to the diagnosis of one of many possible underlying neuromuscular disorders, such as spastic cerebral palsy, muscular dystrophy, peripheral neuropathy, spinal dysraphism, spinal muscular atrophy, or ataxia. The most common neuromuscular cause of limp in a child is spastic hemiplegic cerebral palsy. Patients with this disorder typically present with toe walking between 12 and 18 months of age. A history of motor delay and early hand dominance are supported by clinical findings of increased gastrocnemius-soleus muscle tone and upper motor neuron signs. Walking deficits or abnormal gait may be elicited by stress testing, as in asking the patient to run, which also may help assess upper limb posturing.

Children with Duchenne muscular dystrophy are typically 2 to 3 years of age at first diagnosis and male. The limp is a result of proximal muscle weakness and is characterized by mild ankle equinus as the child tries to keep the joint reaction forces anterior to the knee and posterior to the hip, and a Trendelenburg gait with lumbar hyperlordosis. Proximal muscle weakness produces this gait pattern and the Gower's sign (the patient uses the upper limbs to "walk up" the lower limbs when rising from a seated position to standing). Elevation of the serum creatinine phosphokinase level supports the diagnosis of Duchenne muscular dystrophy.

Knee

Discoid Meniscus

Although rare, this is the most common meniscal derangement in childhood, with an incidence of approximately 1% to 15% (in Japanese and Korean children). More than 99% of patients with this disorder have lateral discoid meniscus. Most patients with discoid meniscus present in the third or fourth decade of life. In childhood, patients often initially present with snapping or clunking of the knee with motion or a painless limp. These symptoms do not typically cause pain until late in the first decade of life or adolescence, at which time a painful limp and effusion may become evident. Symptoms and signs include pain, effusion, and snapping, which are caused by a tear or instability of the meniscus. Bilateral discoid meniscus occurs in approximately 10% of patients. Three types of discoid meniscus have been distinguished: complete, incomplete, and Wrisberg variant (highly unstable meniscus remnant). Radiographs may show increased lateral joint width in this patient population. MRI can aid in the characterization of the type of discoid meniscus in addition to showing associated tears.

Observation is recommended for the asymptomatic child with discoid meniscus. Occasionally, total meniscectomy is the only reasonable option (for patients with the Wrisberg variant that cannot be repaired). Although some studies have shown acceptable results in young adults who underwent this procedure as children, others have shown poor long-term results, particularly in regard to pain and stiffness from premature osteoarthritis.

Osteochondritis Dissecans

The term "osteochondritis dissecans" was coined by Koenig to describe dissection of bone and cartilage off the articular end of a long bone. This condition most commonly affects the knee (the lateral aspect of the medial femoral condyle in 70% of patients, the lateral femoral condyle in 20%, and the patella in 10%) followed by the trochlea of the talus. Bilaterality occurs in approximately 20% of patients. The male to female ratio is 1.5:1. The cause of osteochondritis dissecans is unknown, but articular trauma and subchondral ischemia are believed to be contributing factors. Patients typically present with a painful limp with or without effusion and mechanical signs. Four types of osteochondritis dissecans have been identified: the overlying cartilage is intact, the overlying cartilage is partially broken and produces a hinged lesion, the overlying cartilage is completely broken and produces a free but located lesion, and a completely displaced lesion that produces a mobile body. The factors associated with a good prognosis in patients with osteochondritis dissecans are listed in Table 4.

The treatment of osteochondritis dissecans is controversial. Intact lesions may be treated symptomatically with or without activity modification or immobilization. In one multicenter study, no treatment effect was demonstrated when comparing various nonsurgical methods and with drilling of stable nondissected lesions (to disrupt the sclerotic margin and stimulate new bone ingrowth), despite the fact that the latter is widely performed. For hinged and free but located lesions (dissection evident on imaging or during surgery), the bed may be curetted with or without bone grafting, and the lesion is fixed to aid healing and avoid dislodgement. Mobile bodies may be returned and fixed to their donor sites if they are acute, fit well, and have sufficient bone remaining to heal. If the mobile bodies are longstanding, they usually do not fit because they have been rounded and smoothed by the joint, and they have lost their osseous base. Such mobile bodies are removed, and the base may be treated by various reconstructive methods, including microfracture, osteochondral grafting, and chondrocytes transplantation. Sufficient long-term follow-up data are not yet available to determine which of these reconstructive techniques is more effective.

Despite the recognition of favorable criteria, and despite rapid evolution and innovation in surgical treatment techniques, overall outcome is guarded, with significant long-term sequelae reported in approximately 25% of patients. For more information on osteochondritis dissecans and other conditions of the knee, see chapter 16.

Lower Limb-Length Discrepancy

Lower limb-length discrepancy manifests clinically as a painless limp. Children will use toe walking to compensate for the shorter limb when the discrepancy is approximately 5%. Other compensatory gait patterns include increased hip and knee flexion in the longer limb, circumduction of the long leg, and vaulting over the long leg. The first step in the evaluation of a patient with lower limb-length discrepancy is to distinguish a relative lower limb hemihypertrophy from hemihypotrophy. Both hemihypertrophy and hemihypotrophy may be idiopathic.

Table 4	Factors Associated With Good Prognosis in Patients With Osteochondritis Dissecans
Typical location on the lateral aspect of the medial femoral condyle
Young age (preadolescence better than skeletally immature adolescent; skeletally immature better than mature)
Small lesion (< 20 mm)
No effusion
No dissection on imaging

As a rule, hemihypertrophy has a unifying vascular etiology with subsequent limb overgrowth; vascular malformations are a common cause. Trauma and conditions such as rheumatoid arthritis may lead to hemihypertrophy by means of increased blood flow and subsequent limb overgrowth. In patients with true hemihypertrophy who have upper and lower limb asymmetry as well as facial asymmetry, the workup should include an abdominal ultrasound to rule out Wilms' tumor or other lesions that may produce shunting of blood to the affected limb. Causes of hemihypotrophy may be classified as congenital, including bone deficiency syndromes, or acquired, including trauma and infection, which may lead to growth plate injury; rheumatoid arthritis, which may produce premature physeal closure, and neuromuscular disease, which can result in limb underdevelopment.

The diagnosis of lower limb-length discrepancy usually is established by physical examination. The most accurate method of diagnosis has been to place blocks under the shorter limb to level the pelvis. Radiographs are indicated to identify a pathologic cause of the limb-length discrepancy and to guide treatment for children who will not stand. After identification of the primary cause, the general principles of management of lower limb-length discrepancy may be followed, which include serial physical and radiographic examination, estimation of discrepancy at skeletal maturity, and intervention if a significant discrepancy of ≥ 1 inch or 5% difference is predicted. For more information on limb discrepancy, see chapter 15.

Tarsal Coalition

Patients with tarsal coalition typically present with a painful limp that is associated with restricted range of motion and variable flattening of the foot. The incidence of tarsal coalition is unknown because most patients are asymptomatic, but it has been estimated to be 1% to 5%. The two most common forms are talocalcaneal coalition, which typically occurs in the first part of the second decade of life, and calcaneonavicular coalition, which typically occurs slightly earlier. The incidence of more than one coalition is 10% to 20%, and bilaterality occurs in approximately 50% of patients. Onset of symptoms usually coincides with transformation of the coalition from cartilage to bone. Workup should include anterolateral and lateral radiographs to evaluate foot shape and secondary signs (such as elongation of the anterior process of the calcaneus, the so-called "anteater nose" sign), Harris axial radiographs to evaluate the subtalar joint, and oblique radiographs to assess for a calcaneonavicular coalition. CT is useful to determine the extent of the tarsal coalition, which aids in surgical decision making, and to determine whether additional coalition is present.

Nonsurgical management of tarsal coalition consists of nonsteroidal anti-inflammatory agents, activity modification, and immobilization in a below-the-knee walking cast for 6 weeks. If patients do not respond favorably to nonsurgical management, then surgical treatment is a reasonable treatment option. Resection is reserved for tarsal coalitions involving less than 50% of the subtalar joint and when there is no significant associated foot deformity (defined by one study as ≤ 15° hindfoot valgus) and for calcaneonavicular coalitions. Osteotomy may be added to restore foot shape and improve outcome of resection (calcaneal lengthening with talocalcaneal resection). Arthrodesis is reserved for large coalitions, significant degenerative arthritis, and failed resections. Overall outcomes are better for calcaneonavicular coalitions than for talocalcaneal coalitions.

Overuse Apophysitis

Overuse apophysitis as a cause of painful limp is thought to be caused by rapid growth, increasing body weight, and increased stress on the apophysis as a result of participation in high-level athletic activities. The most common site of overuse apophysitis is the knee, followed by the heel. Repetitive trauma to the tibial apophysis exerted through the patellar ligament results in Osgood-Schlatter disease, and repetitive trauma to the calcaneal apophysis by the Achilles tendon results in Sever's disease. Physical examination is usually diagnostic, with the identification of clear focal pain and swelling over the affected apophysis. The inflammatory signs are much less dramatic than with infection, tumors, or fractures, which are considered in the differential diagnosis. Additional radiographs are necessary only in the rare instances of diagnostic uncertainty. In fact, radiographs are best avoided because they may be a cause of alarm to the inexperienced physician and to the patient. Treatment begins by educating and reassuring the family that the condition is benign. This should be followed by symptomatic care, with nonsteroidal anti-inflammatory agents and activity modification as needed. Stretching exercises to decrease traction on the affected apophysis can be helpful, as can heel lift exercises to relax the Achilles tendon. Short-term immobilization is a treatment of last resort (see chapter 18).

Annotated Bibliography

Kocher MS, Mandiga R, Zurakowski D, Barnewolt C, Kasser JR: Validation of a clinical prediction rule for the differentiation between septic arthritis and transient synovitis of the hip in children. *J Bone Joint Surg Am* 2004;86:1629-1635.

This study is a follow-up to an index study in 1999 of 51 patients with septic arthritis and 103 patients with transient synovitis. Four independent predictors were identified: history of fever, refusal to bear weight, erythrocyte sedimentation rate greater than 40 mm/hr, and leukocyte count greater than 12,000 cells/mm^3. The authors found that the predicted probability of septic arthritis was 9.5% for patients with one predictor, 35% for those with two predictors, 73% for those with three predictors, and 93% for those with four predictors.

Levine MJ, McGuire KJ, McGowan KL, Flynn JM: Assessment of the test characteristics of C-reactive protein for septic arthritis in children. *J Pediatr Orthop* 2003;23: 373-377.

The authors of this study assessed 133 children who had C-reactive protein levels determined within 24 hours of presentation. They reported that 39 (29%) had a positive joint aspirate for septic arthritis (defined as > 50,000 cells/mm^3 with > 75% polymorphic neutrophils). For both C-reactive protein level and erythrocyte sedimentation rate, they found that the negative predictive value was better than positive predictive value. Specifically, a C-reactive protein level less than 10 mg/L had a negative predictive value of 87%, and an erythrocyte sedimentation rate less than 25 mm/hr had a negative predictive value of 85%, where as a C-reactive protein level greater than 10 mg/L had a positive predictive value of 34%, and an erythrocyte sedimentation rate greater than 25 mm/hr had a positive predictive value of 35%. These latter findings contribute data on the most useful laboratory test for septic arthritis, C-reactive protein level, to the four predictors listed above.

Skaggs DL, Roy AK, Vitale MG, et al: Quality of evaluation and management of children requiring timely orthopaedic surgery before admission to a tertiary pediatric facility. *J Pediatr Orthop* 2002;22:265-267.

The authors of this study assessed 372 patients who underwent "timely" surgery for fracture, infection, slipped capital femoral epiphysis, or compartment syndrome; 142 children had initial treatment at a nontertiary care center, of whom 44 (31%) had a misdiagnosis or a greater than 48-hour delay in appropriate treatment. Of these 142 children, 31 (22%) had fractures and/or dislocations and 9 (6.5%) had slipped capital femoral epiphysis. The data illustrate the difficulty in diagnosis of these two conditions for the primary care provider.

Classic Bibliography

Fernandez M, Carol CL, Baker CJ: Discitis and vertebral osteomyelitis in children: An 18 year review. *Pediatrics* 2000;105:1299-1304.

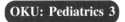
Fischer SU, Beattie TF: The limping child: Epidemiology, assessment and outcome. *J Bone Joint Surg Br* 1999; 81:1029-1034.

Freiberger RH, Loitman BS, Helpern M, Thompson TG: Osteoid osteoma: A report of 80 cases. *AJR Am J Roentgenol* 1959;82:194-211.

Hefti F, Beguiristain J, Krauspe R, et al: Osteochondritis dissecans: A multicenter study of the European Pediatric Orthopedic Society. *J Pediatr Orthop B* 1999;8:231-245.

Hughes AW: Idiopathic chondrolysis of the hip: A case report and review of the literature. *Ann Rheum Dis* 1985;44:268-272.

John SD, Moorthy CS, Swischuk LE: Expanding the concept of the toddler's fracture. *Radiographics* 1997;17: 367-376.

Karwowska A, Davies HD, Jadavji T: Epidemiology and outcome of osteomyelitis in the era of intravenous-oral therapy. *Pediatr Infect Dis J* 1998;17:1021-1026.

Kocher MS, Mandiga R, Zurakowski D, Barnewolt C, Kasser JR: Validation of a clinical prediction rule for the differentiation between septic arthritis and transient synovitis of the hip in children. *J Bone Joint Surg Br* 1999;81:1029-1034.

Kumai T, Takakura Y, Akiyama K, Higashiyama I, Tamai S: Histopathological study of nonossoeus tarsal coalition. *Foot Ankle Int* 1998;19:525-531.

Lovett RW, Morse JL: A transient or ephemeral form of hip disease. *Boston Med Surg J* 1892;127:161.

McDonald R: Sudden acute limp in children: Some causes of a common symptom. *Clin Pediatr (Phila)* 1967; 6:571-575.

Neuschwander DC: Discoid meniscus. *Op Tech Orthop B* 1995;5:78-87.

Song KM, Halliday SE, Little DG: The effect of limb-length discrepancy on gait. *J Bone Joint Surg Am* 1997; 79:1690-1698.

Terjesen T, Osthus P: Ultrasound in the diagnosis and follow-up of transient synovitis of the hip. *J Pediatr Orthop* 1991;11:608-613.

Tong CW, Griffith JE, Lam TP, Cheng JC: The conservative management of acute pyogenic iliopsoas abscess in children. *J Bone Joint Surg Br* 1998;80:83-85.

Tuten HR, Gabos PG, Kumar SJ: The limping child: a manifestation of acute leukemia. *J Pediatr Orthop* 1998; 18:625-629.

Chapter 3

Overuse Injuries in Pediatric and Adolescent Athletes

Kevin Shea, MD

Ronald P. Pfeiffer, EdD, LAT, ATC

Peter J. Apel, MD

Epidemiology

In the United States, approximately 30 million preadolescents and adolescents participate in organized sports. Although sports participation has numerous health benefits for young athletes, it also entails risk of injury. A recent survey of 11,840 children (age 5 to 17 years) participating in sports or recreational activities estimated that 4,379,000 injuries occur annually, with 1,363,000 of these injuries classified as serious (requiring hospitalization, surgical treatment, missed school, or half a day or more of bed rest). Based on these data, sports injuries were estimated to account for 36% of all injuries reported for this age group. It is important to note that these data also included non–sports-related injuries, such as those sustained on playground equipment and skateboards. A study of children age 7 to 13 years involved in community-organized baseball, softball, soccer, and football was conducted over two playing seasons. Injury rates in injuries per 100 athlete-exposures were 1.7 for baseball, 1.0 for softball, 2.1 for soccer, and 1.5 for football. Football had the highest frequency of injuries per team per season (14.0) when compared with baseball (3.0) and softball (2.0). Contusions were the most common injury and, except for softball, the odds of being injured were higher during games than practice.

For adult and youth populations, sports-injury research has placed more emphasis on traumatic injuries than overuse injuries. Overuse injuries, although a separate category of injuries, represents a large proportion of overall injuries. Several factors have been described that contribute to overuse injury, including intense training programs and vulnerable anatomic regions in young athletes (growth cartilage at the physis, joint surface, and apophysis). Although many of these injuries do not result in long-term disability, these injuries can have psychologic and social affects on injured athletes.

Gender Differences in Sports Injuries

In sports that involve planting, jumping, and directional change activities, adult females have higher rates of knee injuries than males. Most studies reporting knee injuries among athletes have evaluated skeletally mature patients, although some recent studies have focused on skeletally immature athletes. No differences in injury rates between genders were noted in a study of youth soccer participants, but the specific incidences of knee injuries were not reported. The American Academy of Pediatrics (AAP) reported a male-to-female overall injury rate ratio of 1:2 in youth soccer, assuming similar risk exposure. A recent study of approximately 6 million injury claims from a single insurance company providing coverage for youth soccer leagues revealed a higher ratio of knee and anterior cruciate ligament injuries in female youth soccer players when compared with males age 12 through 15 years. These studies have focused on traumatic rather than overuse injuries, making it difficult to assess gender patterns for overuse injuries in young athletes. Future research will need to focus on factors that lead to significantly higher injury rates in young female athletes compared with their male peers.

Unique Anatomy and Implications for Injury

Differences in the anatomy of young athletes should be considered when evaluating overuse injuries. In particular, young athletes have unique anatomy because of the physis, apophysis, and epiphysis, which are prone to overuse injuries. In addition to anatomic considerations, sports medicine practitioners must have an understanding of the process of puberty when treating pediatric and adolescent athletes. Aside from the obvious body mass differences between children and adults, anatomic differences are also present within the musculoskeletal system. American children begin their growth spurt at age 11 years for boys and 9 years for girls, with peak height velocity occurring at 13.5 years for boys and 11.5 years for girls. Puberty involves profound changes in children, both physically and psychologically. Growth during puberty accounts for 17% to 18% of the final height for boys and 17% for girls, with boys doubling their total muscle mass between the ages of 10 and 17 years.

The Physis

The physis contributes to longitudinal growth of the bone and is susceptible to both traumatic and overuse injuries in young athletes. The region of greatest risk for injury is the area between the hypertrophic cells and region of calcification. Physeal fractures are caused by an array of mechanisms that can be acute and chronic in nature. Although traumatic injury to the physis may produce more dramatic growth disturbances, overuse injury can also lead to deformity and other problems. Examples of physeal overuse injury include proximal humeral physis injuries in little league pitchers and physeal changes that can occur in the distal radius of gymnasts. A recent study also demonstrated physeal injury in the knee in running athletes, with evidence of widening on radiographs, as well as notable signal changes on MRI scans. These injuries are also seen around the ankle, especially the distal fibular region.

The Apophysis

The apophysis is anatomically similar to the epiphysis and represents the attachment site for tendon to bone. The apophyses are under constant tension during puberty. As bone growth accelerates, it has been suggested that tension can increase even more as the musculotendinous system falls behind the skeletal system in rate of growth. The mechanisms of apophyseal injuries are similar to those causing muscle strains in adults. Apophysitis can also result from overuse and may worsen during periods of rapid growth associated with puberty. Areas commonly involved include the tibial tubercle, calcaneus, medial distal humerus (epicondyle), base of the fifth metatarsal, iliac crest, ischial tuberosity, distal patella, and tarsal navicular.

The Epiphysis

The epiphysis is another region that appears prone to overuse injury in young athletes. Osteochondritis dissecans can involve both the articular cartilage and subchondral epiphyseal bone. In children, the regions most vulnerable to this type of injury are the elbow, knee, and ankle. The etiology of osteochondritis dissecans remains undetermined, although it is likely multifactorial, involving trauma, ischemia, genetics, and other causes. Skeletally immature gymnasts are also prone to develop epiphyseal deformity in the distal radius, probably secondary to the high compressive loads on the upper extremity that occur during normal gymnastic activity.

Special Issues in Young Athletes

Although research on overuse injuries in young athletes is limited, it is widely believed that overuse injuries are commonplace in young athletes. Several factors are thought to contribute to this trend. More young athletes are participating in sports and recreational activities,

Table 1	Issues for Evaluating Young Athletes
Does the athlete compete in multiple sports at one time?
Does the athlete have adequate rest during the season?
Has the athlete chosen to focus on one sport year round, which includes participation with traveling teams and in special training camps?
Does the family hope or expect their child to continue the athletic career to obtain a college scholarship or participate in professional competition?
Are the parents involved appropriately in encouraging their child's participation in sports?

and many of these athletes are participating in multiple sports year-round or focusing on one sport continuously. Many parents are involved in the athletic pursuits of their children. In most instances, parents can make a positive contribution to their children's sport participation. In some instances, however, parents may be involved at a level that is detrimental to the young athlete, and this needs to be considered when treating these patients.

The AAP has outlined guidelines related to sport participation for young athletes. This information is readily available to parents, coaches, and physicians on the AAP Website (http://www.aap.org). The AAP recommends that athletes play sports for enjoyment, to improve self-esteem, and to improve athletic skills. If these are not priorities in youth sports, then participation in sports potentially is harmful because it can decrease self-esteem, diminish athletic skills, and discourage additional participation in sports. The issues that should be considered when evaluating young athletes for overuse injuries are listed in Table 1.

For many overuse injuries, the intensity, duration, and magnitude of training need to be considered, and modifications may be necessary to treat and prevent these injuries. Along with the young athlete, many parents and coaches will require education about training errors that lead to overuse injuries or burnout.

Approximately half of sports injuries in children are overuse injuries. Studies have suggested similar injury rates for both genders. In older athletes, females have a higher incidence of stress fractures and patellofemoral pain.

Appropriate shoe type, especially for athletes participating in running-based and endurance sports, is important. Proper coaching techniques are also important, particularly for throwing athletes. The use of proper mechanics for throwing in baseball and football are essential; in many regions, coaches specialize in teaching these mechanics. Physicians have the opportunity to educate coaches, parents, and athletic trainers about appropriate training techniques to reduce the incidence of

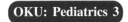
Table 2	Prevention of Overuse Injuries in Pediatric and Adolescent Athletes

Preparticipation Examinations
   Screening by a physician can identify risk factors for injury and provide an opportunity to develop specific recommendations for addressing them.

Proper Adult Supervision and Coaching
   Leagues and parents should ensure that coaches have the resources to become educated about recognizing and preventing overuse injuries common in their sport and that athletes are properly supervised.

Training Programs That Emphasize General Fitness and Avoid Excessive Training Volumes
   Although individual situations vary, the 10% rule—limiting increases in training frequency, intensity, and duration to no more than 10% per week—serves as a general guide. Periodization of training, which systematically varies training volume and incorporates scheduled rest periods, should also be considered.

Delaying Sport Specialization
   Allow children to experiment with different activities to develop a variety of skills and interests.

Careful Monitoring of Training for Children Undergoing Growth Spurts
   It might be appropriate to modify training during this time period because of the growth-related factors that can lead to injury.

(Adapted with permission from DiFiori JP: Overuse injuries in young athletes: An overview. Athletic Therapy Today 2002;7:25-29.)

overuse injuries. Physicians can provide education that encourages young athletes to avoid specialization at too young an age, or to encourage athletes to alternate sports during consecutive seasons, to reduce the risk of overuse injury. Prevention must be a priority for everyone involved in athletic activities. This is particularly true for overuse injuries because as many as 50% may be preventable. Table 2 lists guidelines to help prevent overuse injuries in pediatric and adolescent athletes.

Overuse injuries occur when activity levels exceed the body's ability to recover. Contributing to overuse injuries is the fact that young athletes undergo periods of accelerated long bone growth, typically between the ages of 6 and 14 years, resulting in length increases by a factor of 1.4. The associated soft tissues (muscles, tendons, and apophyses) may not immediately adapt to these sudden changes in limb length. Therefore, children undergoing rapid growth may experience increased tension within these associated soft tissues. Unlike adults in whom tendinosis is a common overuse injury, skeletally immature athletes may be more likely to have overuse syndromes associated with pain in apophyseal regions. When tendinosis occurs in young patients, it can be treated in a manner similar to that for adults. Common sites for apophysitis are shown in Table 3. Apophysitis tends to be self-limiting and usually resolves with maturation of the apophyses. Activity modification may be necessary along with local measures such as stretching, icing before and after athletic activity, and intermittent nonsteroidal anti-inflammatory use.

Osgood-Schlatter Disease

Osgood-Schlatter disease is characterized by pain, tenderness, and localized swelling of the tibial tubercle. The diagnosis is made based on clinical examination. In some patients, radiography may be necessary to confirm the absence of other potentially more serious condi-

Table 3	Common Anatomic Sites for Apophysitis

Tibial tubercle (Osgood-Schlatter disease)
Calcaneus (Sever disease)
Medial distal humerus (Little Leaguer's elbow)
Iliac crest
Base of fifth metatarsal (Iselin disease)

tions. Treatment of Osgood-Schlatter disease includes reduced activity, application of ice before and after activity, and stretching of the quadriceps and hamstring muscles. Nonsteroidal anti-inflammatory drugs (NSAIDs) may be prescribed for intermittent use unless contraindicated; long-term use of NSAIDs should be discouraged. Knee sleeves and knee straps may be helpful, although it is difficult to predict which patients will respond to these devices. In contact sports or in sports played on a hard court surface, it may be helpful for athletes to wear padded knee sleeves to protect the tibial tubercle from direct contusions, which can significantly aggravate symptoms.

Sever's Disease

Sever's disease, also known as calcaneal apophysitis, is characterized by pain in the area of the calcaneal apophysis. Associated with running and jumping sports, Sever's disease occurs frequently before or during peak growth in both genders. The diagnosis can be based on physical findings, including a positive squeeze test in association with a tight Achilles tendon as well as pain over the calcaneal apophysis. Treatment includes activity modification, Achilles tendon stretching, and icing before and after athletic activity.

In skeletally immature soccer players, Sever's disease commonly occurs. This repetitive traction injury to the calcaneal apophysis is attributable to long periods of running in cleated shoes without adequate heel cushion or arch support. Once identified, this overuse injury can be treated by reducing the amount of running and impact demands, improving calf flexibility, and using a heel pad or heel cup in the soccer shoe.

Little Leaguer's Elbow and Shoulder

Little leaguer's elbow is traditionally associated with medial elbow pain, but young athletes can also develop pathology in the medial or lateral regions of the elbow. The medial elbow is subject to significant traction and valgus loading during the early and late cocking phases of the overhand throw. Pain over the medial elbow is a form of apophysitis that is related to valgus overload and stress on the medial joint capsule, ligaments, and medial epicondyle or apophyseal region. Pain over the lateral elbow region in throwers is associated with compressive forces related to the late cocking and early acceleration phases of the overhand throw. Specific damage may involve osteochondritis of the radial head, capitellum, or both.

Overuse injury of the shoulder region can also occur in young athletes with an open physis. The proximal humeral physis is prone to overuse, which may also be related to the torsional stress on the physis during cocking and early acceleration phases of the overhand throw. Radiographs may demonstrate widening of the physis and/or subtle changes in the surrounding bone.

Management of shoulder and elbow overuse injuries consists of rest for the throwing arm. This may be accomplished by reducing the number of pitches thrown, switching to another position that requires less throwing, and in patients with severe injuries, cessation of all throwing activities. In most instances, baseball/softball athletes can continue athletic participation, although perhaps in a new position that requires less throwing. Limiting the number of innings per game and pitches thrown per week is an effective method for reducing elbow and shoulder injuries in young pitchers. Guidelines proposed by the AAP are summarized in Table 4. Consideration should also be given to the athlete's age and the type of pitch being thrown. Certain pitches place greater stress on the anatomic components of the arm; for example, USA Baseball recommends that children younger than 14 years should not be taught to throw a curve ball.

Iselin's Apophysitis

Iselin's apophysitis involves the insertion of the peroneus brevis tendon at the proximal tuberosity of the fifth metatarsal. The apophysis becomes inflamed by excessive stress from foot inversion associated with sporting activities that involve running and cutting, which results in a traction apophysitis. Symptoms of Iselin's apophysitis include pain at the tubercle that can be reproduced by resisting eversion. The treatment for this condition typi-

Table 4 | AAP Position Statement Guidelines for Reducing Elbow and Shoulder Injuries in Young Pitchers

Participation should be limited to three or four innings per game

Fewer than 90 pitches should be thrown per outing

Pitch count should be held to less than 200 pitches per week

Mandatory rest periods should be taken between pitching appearances

Reproduced with permission from the American Academy of Pediatrics, Elk Grove Village, IL.)

cally involves application of ice and pain management with NSAIDs in conjunction with ankle resistive exercises to improve peroneal strength. A short period of casting may also be helpful in some patients.

Pelvic Apophysitis

Apophysitis of the pelvis, specifically when it involves either the iliac crest or the ischial tuberosity, typically occurs in active adolescent patients between the ages of 8 and 15 years. In patients with iliac apophysitis, pain usually occurs bilaterally on trunk rotation in the absence of any history of crest contusion. Osteomyelitis, Legg-Calvé-Perthes disease, and slipped capital femoral epiphysis or other pelvis disorders should be ruled out in this patient population. With ischial apophysitis, the pain is typically localized to the ischial tuberosity. Although many patients will present with an insidious onset of symptoms, some will recall a distinct injury event that led to the development of symptoms. If the patient reports a popping or tearing sensation in the region of the tuberosity, the presence of an avulsion must be considered. Treatment of pelvic apophysitis is conservative and includes rest, ice, and NSAIDs, and flexibility and strengthening exercises.

Stress Fractures

Although stress fractures occasionally occur in prepubescent pediatric athletes, they are more common in adolescent or high-school–age athletes. Sports that require significant running, such as cross country, soccer, and basketball, seem to pose a higher risk for these types of injuries. Stress fractures are thought to occur with repetitive stresses below the bone failure threshold, but they occur at a rate that does not allow for adequate bone remodeling and response to stress.

Locations include the lumbar spine, pelvis, femoral neck or shaft, patella, tibia, medial malleolus, talus, tarsals, metatarsals, and sesamoids. As in adult patients, the tibia is the most common location for stress fractures in skeletally immature patients. Although stress fractures are more common in the lower extremities, rare instances of upper extremity stress fractures in young patients who participate in throwing sports and gymnastics have been reported.

Stress fractures in both male and female athletes may be associated with osteopenia or osteoporosis, especially in athletes who participate in endurance activities. Athletes with recurrent stress fractures and females with a history of amenorrhea or menstrual irregularities may need formal evaluation for management of underlying endocrine and/or bone metabolic disorders.

Patients with stress fractures typically present with localized pain that has developed in an insidious manner. Palpation of the involved region may demonstrate local tenderness and swelling. The diagnosis is typically made from clinical examination, radiographs, and other imaging modalities including bone scanning and MRI. Most of these injuries can be treated with activity modification that is sufficient to allow for bone healing. Many stress fractures can be prevented with appropriate training methods because many of these injuries are thought to occur as a result of training errors. For running sports, activity modification may include decreased mileage or practice time. Athletes may consider replacing running for conditioning with weight training, exercise bike training, swimming, or a pool-based unweighted running program. These types of training modifications will allow patients to maintain aerobic conditioning, while allowing for healing of the stress fracture. In patients with severe stress fractures, complete rest may be necessary.

Femoral neck stress fractures rarely occur in younger patients, although several recent reports have documented this entity in skeletally immature patients. Patients typically present with groin or anterior thigh pain, and specific areas of tenderness may not be identified on physical examination. Plain radiography may not identify the lesion, in which instance bone scanning or MRI may be necessary. Femoral neck stress fractures must be treated with great care because a displaced femoral neck fracture can lead to osteonecrosis. The risk of displacement may be higher in tension side than compression side fractures. Tension side fractures may require prophylactic surgery to prevent fracture progression and/or displacement of the fracture. Some tibial stress fracture patterns may also have a higher risk of serious complications, such as delayed healing or progression to a complete fracture. These injuries typically involve the anterior cortex of the tibia and may require management such as activity modification and ultrasound or other stimulation methods. In patients who do not respond to nonsurgical treatment, intramedullary nailing may be necessary.

Back Injuries in Young Athletes

Back injuries in young athletes are common, especially among those who participate in running sports and gymnastics. A recent study reported a 14% incidence of sports-related back pain in pediatric and adolescent soccer players. Although back pain in pediatric patients can be associated with significant underlying pathology such as diskitis, osteomyelitis, and tumors, many young athletes may have back pain that is not associated with these serious conditions. In contrast to adults, disk pathology is relatively rare in young athletes. (More detailed information on specific spinal conditions appears in the spine section of this book.)

Spondylolysis occurs in approximately 6% of the population by the age of 6 years, and it is probably more common in young athletes involved in diving, gymnastics, and dance. Interior linemen and wrestlers may also have a higher risk of developing this condition. Repetitive hyperextension of the lumbar spine may predispose athletes to this type of injury. Spondylolysis can be associated with a stress fracture and with an elongated but intact pars. In certain patients, spondylolysis can progress to spondylolisthesis.

Patients with spondylolysis typically present with low back pain. Patients with more severe spondylolysis may also have tight hamstrings and altered gait. Plain radiographs may not always show evidence of a spondylolysis, but they will show evidence of a spondylolisthesis. In patients with normal radiographs, bone scanning with CT and single photon emission CT may be necessary to make the diagnosis. The indications for MRI in the evaluation of spondylolysis are unclear. A recent study used MRI to identify patients with spondylolysis that was initially not detected using CT. Patients with spondylolysis are treated initially with activity modifications and bracing when pain is severe or does not respond to activity modification. A recent case series study suggested that young soccer players with spondylolysis responded well to a 3-month rest period away from soccer. In patients with a spondylolisthesis, referral to a pediatric spine surgeon is appropriate to determine the best course of treatment.

Foot and Ankle Injuries

Recent studies have suggested a higher incidence of overuse injuries of the foot and ankle in adolescent athletes than was previously reported. Adolescent athletes in high-mileage running sports seem to be prone to numerous foot and ankle problems, including fasciitis, calcaneal osteochondritis, tendinosis, and stress reactions. Proper training methods, which include appropriate shoe selection and replacement, monitoring weekly mileage and workout intensity, and the selection of appropriate running surfaces may help reduce the risks of these injuries. Feedback to coaches and parents can reduce the incidence and severity of these injuries.

Strength Training and Injury Prevention

Although there has been historical bias against weight training in children, several studies have demonstrated

Table 5 | AAP Recommendations for Pediatric and Adolescent Weight Training

Strength-training programs for preadolescents and adolescents can be safe and effective if proper resistance-training techniques and safety precautions are followed.

Preadolescents and adolescents should avoid competitive weight lifting, power lifting, body building, and maximal lifts until they reach physical and skeletal maturity.

When pediatricians are asked to recommend or evaluate strength-training programs for children and adolescents, the following issues should be considered:

Before beginning a formal strength-training program, a medical evaluation should be performed by a pediatrician. If indicated, a referral may be made to a sports medicine physician who is familiar with various strength-training methods as well as risks and benefits in preadolescents and adolescents.

Aerobic conditioning should be coupled with resistance training if general health benefits are the goal.

Strength-training programs should include a warm-up and cool-down component.

Specific strength-training exercises should be learned initially with no load (resistance). Once the exercise skill has been mastered, incremental loads can be added.

Progressive resistance exercise requires successful completion of 8 to 15 repetitions in good form before increasing weight or resistance.

A general strengthening program should address all major muscle groups and exercise through the complete range of motion.

Any sign of injury or illness from strength training should be evaluated before continuing the exercise in question.

(Reproduced with permission from the American Academy of Pediatrics, Elk Grove Village, IL.)

positive effects of weight training in young athletes. Properly structured, supervised strength training can produce strength gains in young children with a low risk of injury. The mechanism of strength gain in the prepubescent age group is thought to be neurologic in that the training improves muscle-activation capabilities. Under appropriate training conditions, increases in muscle mass are not expected until children pass through adolescence.

Studies that have evaluated the link between injury prevention and strength training suggest a reduced risk of injury secondary to strength training. Most of these studies have focused on traumatic injuries and have research design limitations, but the findings suggest some beneficial effects on the reduction of overuse injury as well. In an 8-year study, a preseason, total-body conditioning program that included weight training revealed a significant reduction in both the number and severity of knee injuries in varsity high school football players. Another study investigated the effects of diversified variable resistance isokinetic and isotonic exercises on the incidence of injury in a cohort of high school male and female athletes involved in basketball, gymnastics, volleyball, wrestling, and football. A time-loss injury resulted in removal from athletic practice or activity or a subsequent missed practice or competitive event. One group completed the weight-training program only during the preseason and competitive season, whereas a second group completed a year-round conditioning program, and a third (control) group did not use weight training during the off-season and was limited to weight training once per week or less during the competitive season. The combined weight-training groups had an overall injury rate of 26.2%, whereas the control group had an injury rate of 72.4%.

More recent findings also support the premise that resistance training may lower both overall injury rates and the rate of injury to specific joints such as the knee. In one study, 42 of 300 female soccer players age 14 to 18 years participated in a 7-week preseason conditioning program that included cardiovascular conditioning, plyometric training, sport-cord drills, strength training, flexibility exercises, and acceleration training. Over the following year, the injuries that were severe enough to cause the athlete to miss either a competitive event or athletic practice were monitored. The trained group had a significantly lower incidence of overall injury (14.3%) than the control group (33.7%). All injuries involved the lower extremities, with most occurring at the knee and ankle. Anterior cruciate ligament injury rates were not significantly different between the groups, but a trend toward fewer injuries in the treatment group was noted. The treatment group had one anterior cruciate ligament injury, representing 2.4% of the total injuries; the control group had eight anterior cruciate ligament injuries, representing 3.1% of the total injuries. The lack of a significant difference may have resulted from the small sample size of this study rather than the lack of a training effect.

The effectiveness of a preseason conditioning program in reducing knee injuries was assessed in a large-scale study of high school female soccer, basketball, or volleyball athletes. The female teams were divided into training and control groups; a male athlete control group was also included for comparison. The intervention program included strength training with weights and plyometric training. In one athletic season, the incidence of knee injuries was 0.12% in the training group and 0.43% in the untrained group (the incidence of knee injuries in the untrained group was 3.6 times

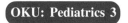

higher than in the trained counterparts). The incidence of knee injuries in the male athletes was 0.09%; thus, the incidence of knee injuries in untrained females was 4.8 times higher than in males.

Strength Training Guidelines

The decision to include some form of strength training in the overall activity program of pediatric and adolescent athletes should be based on the availability of proper equipment, instruction in lifting techniques, and supervision. Personnel should be trained in currently accepted practices with respect to both the design and implementation of age-appropriate resistance training programs. Preventing training-related injuries is of the utmost importance, and prevention is best accomplished by incorporating the principles of periodization, which include varying the volume and intensity of training throughout the year in an effort to maximize benefits while avoiding overtraining. Whenever possible, personnel providing instruction and supervision in resistance training should have received specialized, formal instruction by organizations such as the National Strength and Conditioning Association (NSCA) or the National Athletic Trainers' Association. Credentials indicating expertise in exercise prescription include Certified Strength and Conditioning Specialist, granted by the NSCA and Certified Athletic Trainer, granted by the National Athletic Trainers' Association. Personnel without these credentials should at least have a bachelor's or advanced degree in a field such as physical education, exercise or movement science, or kinesiology.

Position and Policy Statements

Two major professional organizations, the AAP (Table 5) and the NSCA (http://www.nsca-lift.org/Publications/posstatements.shtml#Youth/), have published position and/or policy statements on resistance training for pediatric and adolescent athletes. Although a complete list of the details of these statements is beyond the scope of this chapter, these documents may be obtained and reviewed at the Websites of these organizations. Making copies of these statements available for parents, coaches, and youth sports organizations is useful when asked to provide recommendations regarding the efficacy of resistive-exercise programs for pediatric and adolescent athletes.

Annotated Bibliography

Epidemiology

Hogan KA, Gross RH: Overuse injuries in pediatric athletes. *Orthop Clin North Am* 2003;34:405-415.

This article presents a comprehensive review of the recent literature on pediatric overuse injuries.

Radelet MA, Lephart SM, Rubinstein EN, Myers JB: Survey of the injury rate for children in community sports. *Pediatrics* 2002;110:E28.

The authors of this prospective study evaluated the baseline injury rate for 7- to 13-year-old children who participated in community organized baseball, softball, soccer, and football. Educational strategies to reduce injury for those that work in youth sports and safety guidelines for youth sports are also discussed.

Gender Differences in Sports Injuries

Shea KG, Pfeiffer R, Wang JH, Curtin M, Apel PJ: Anterior cruciate ligament injury in pediatric and adolescent soccer players: An analysis of insurance data. *J Pediatr Orthop* 2004;24:623-628.

The authors of this study found that pediatric and adolescent female athletes have a significantly higher rate of knee and anterior cruciate ligament injuries compared with male athletes. These findings are similar to those of adult athletes with anterior cruciate ligament injuries.

Special Issues in Young Athletes

Adirim TA, Cheng TL: Overview of injuries in the young athlete. *Sports Med* 2003;33:75-81.

A review of the recent literature on injuries in young athletes and recommendations to reduce injuries is presented.

Bettin D, Pankalla T, Bohm H, Fuchs S: Hip pain related to femoral neck stress fracture in a 12-year-old boy performing intensive soccer playing activities: A case report. *Int J Sports Med* 2003;24:593-596.

This article presents a case report of a young athlete with hip pain related to a femoral neck stress fracture.

El Rassi G, Takemitsu M, Woratanarat P, Shah SA: Lumbar spondylolysis in pediatric and adolescent soccer players. *Am J Sports Med* 2005;33:1688-1693.

Results from this study showed that youth soccer players with symptomatic spondylolysis responded well to a 3-month period of rest.

Fallon KE, Fricker PA: Stress fracture of the clavicle in a young female gymnast. *Br J Sports Med* 2001;35:448-449.

This article presents a case report of a young female gymnast with a stress fracture of the clavicle.

Hawkins D, Metheny J: Overuse injuries in youth sports: Biomechanical considerations. *Med Sci Sports Exerc* 2001;33:1701-1707.

This article provides a biomechanical perspective on sports injuries in young athletes. Basic tissue and gross movement mechanical principles are used to identify growth, morphologic, and movement factors that may predispose a child to an overuse injury.

Kennedy JG, Knowles B, Dolan M, Bohne W: Foot and ankle injuries in the adolescent runner. *Curr Opin Pediatr* 2005;17:34-42.

A review of the increasing incidence of overuse foot and ankle injuries in the adolescent athlete and factors that contribute to these injuries is presented.

Klingele KE, Kocher MS: Little league elbow: Valgus overload injury in the paediatric athlete. *Sports Med* 2002;32:1005-1015.

This article describes the clinical presentations, mechanics, and treatment options for elbow injuries in young throwing athletes.

Lehman RA Jr, Shah SA: Tension-sided femoral neck stress fracture in a skeletally immature patient: A case report. *J Bone Joint Surg Am* 2004;86-A:1292-1295.

This case report describes the presentation and treatment of a rare tension-sided stress fracture of the femoral neck in an adolescent patient.

Maezawa K, Nozawa M, Sugimoto M, Sano M, Shitoto K, Kurosawa H: Stress fractures of the femoral neck in child with open capital femoral epiphysis. *J Pediatr Orthop B* 2004;13:407-411.

This article describes the presentation and treatment of a stress fracture of the femoral neck in a 5-year-old girl and a 12-year-old boy.

Varner KE, Younas SA, Lintner DM, Marymont JV: Chronic anterior midtibial stress fractures in athletes treated with reamed intramedullary nailing. *Am J Sports Med* 2005;33:1071-1076.

In this small case study, the outcomes of patients with anterior cortex tibial stress fractures were reviewed. Patients did not respond to nonsurgical treatment and were treated with intramedullary nailing. This treatment resulted in a low complication rate and a high rate of return to participation in sport activities.

Strength Training and Injury Prevention

Bernhardt DT, Gomez J, Johnson MD, et al: Strength training by children and adolescents. *Pediatrics* 2001;107: 1470-1472.

The article outlines current information on the risks and benefits of strength training for children and adolescents.

Classic Bibliography

Abbassi V: Growth and normal puberty. *Pediatrics* 1998; 102:507-511.

Arendt E, Dick R: Knee injury patterns among men and women in collegiate basketball and soccer: NCAA data and review of literature. *Am J Sports Med* 1995;23:694-701.

Barrow GW, Saha S: Menstrual irregularity and stress fractures in collegiate female distance runners. *Am J Sports Med* 1988;16:209-216.

Bijur PE, Trumble A, Harel Y, Overpeck MD, Jones D, Scheidt PC: Sports and recreation injuries in us children and adolescents. *Arch Pediatr Adolesc Med* 1995;149: 1009-1016.

Biondino CR: Anterior cruciate ligament injuries in female athletes. *Conn Med* 1999;63:657-660.

Boden BP, Osbahr DC: High-risk stress fractures: Evaluation and treatment. *J Am Acad Orthop Surg* 2000;8: 344-353.

Brukner P, Fanton G: Bergman AG, Beaulieu C, Matheson GO: Bilateral stress fractures of the anterior part of the tibial cortex: A case report. *J Bone Joint Surg Am* 2000;82:213-218.

Busch M: Sports medicine, in Morrissy RT, Weinstein SL (eds): *Lovell & Winter's Pediatric Orthopaedics*. Philadelphia, PA, Lippincott-Raven, 1996.

Cahill BR, Griffith EH: Effect of preseason conditioning on the incidence and severity of high school football knee injuries. *Am J Sports Med* 1978;6:180-184.

Caine D, Cochrane B, Caine C, Zemper E: An epidemiologic investigation of injuries affecting young competitive female gymnasts. *Am J Sports Med* 1989;17:811-820.

Canale ST, Williams KD: Iselin's disease. *J Pediatr Orthop* 1992;12:90-93.

Coady CM, Micheli LJ: Stress fractures in the pediatric athlete. *Clin Sports Med* 1997;16:225-238.

Current comment from the American College Of Sports Medicine: August 1993. The prevention of sport injuries of children and adolescents. *Med Sci Sports Exerc* 1993; 25:1-7.

Dalton SE: Overuse injuries in adolescent athletes. *Sports Med* 1992;13:58-70.

DiFiori J: Overuse injuries in children and adolescents. *Phys Sportsmed* 1999;27.

Faigenbaum A, Kraemer W, Cahill B, et al: Youth resistance training: Position statement paper and literature. *Strength Cond* 1996;18:62-75.

Federico DJ, Lynch JK, Jokl P: Osteochondritis dissecans of the knee: A historical review of etiology and treatment. *Arthroscopy* 1990;6:190-197.

Gray J, Taunton JE, McKenzie DC, Clement DB, McConkey JP, Davidson RG: A survey of injuries to the anterior cruciate ligament of the knee in female basketball players. *Int J Sports Med* 1985;6:314-316.

Griffin LY, Agel J, Albohm MJ, et al: Noncontact anterior cruciate ligament injuries: Risk factors and prevention strategies. *J Am Acad Orthop Surg* 2000;8:141-150.

Hajek MR, Noble HB: Stress fractures of the femoral neck in joggers: Case reports and review of the literature. *Am J Sports Med* 1982;10:112-116.

Harmon KG, Ireland ML: Gender differences in noncontact anterior cruciate ligament injuries. *Clin Sports Med* 2000;19:287-302.

Heidt RS Jr, Sweeterman LM, Carlonas RL, Traub JA, Tekulve FX: Avoidance of soccer injuries with preseason conditioning. *Am J Sports Med* 2000;28:659-662.

Hejna W, Rosenberg A, Buturusis D, Krieger A: The prevention of sports injuries in high school students through strength training. *NSCA Journal* 1982;4:28-31.

Hergenroeder AC: Prevention of sports injuries. *Pediatrics* 1998;101:1057-1063.

Injuries in Youth Soccer: A subject review. American Academy of Pediatrics: Committee on Sports Medicine and Fitness. *Pediatrics* 2000;105:659-661.

Kraemer W, Fry A, Frykman P, Conroy B, Hoffman J: Resistance training and youth. *Ped Exerc Sci* 1989;1:336-350.

Lokiec F, Wientroub S: Calcaneal osteochondritis: A new overuse injury. *J Pediatr Orthop B* 1998;7:243-245.

Madden CC, Mellion MB: Sever's disease and other causes of heel pain in adolescents. *Am Fam Physician* 1996;54:1995-2000.

Micheli LJ: Back injuries in gymnastics. *Clin Sports Med* 1985;4:85-93.

Mubarak SJ, Carroll NC: Familial osteochondritis dissecans of the knee. *Clin Orthop Relat Res* 1979;140:131-136.

Mubarak S, Carroll NC: Juvenile osteochondritis dissecans of the knee: etiology. *Clin Orthop Relat Res* 1981;157:200-211.

Omey ML, Micheli LJ: Foot and ankle problems in the young athlete. *Med Sci Sports Exerc* 1999;31:S470-S486.

Ozmun JC, Mikesky AE, Surburg PR: Neuromuscular adaptations following prepubescent strength training. *Med Sci Sports Exerc* 1994;26:510-514.

Pappas AM: Osteochondroses: Diseases of the growth centers. *Phys Sportsmed* 1989;17:51-62.

Pfeiffer R, Francis R: Effects of strength training on muscle development in prepubescent, pubescent and postpubescent males. *Phys Sportsmed* 1986;14:134-143.

Ralston BM, Williams JS, Bach BR, Bush-Joseph CA, Knopp WD: Osteochondritis dissecans of the knee. *Phys Sportsmed* 1996;24.

Ramsay JA, Blimkie CJ, Smith K, Garner S, Macdougall JD, Sale DG: Strength training effects in prepubescent boys. *Med Sci Sports Exerc* 1990;22:605-614.

Schmidt-Olsen S, Jorgensen U, Kaalund S, Sorensen J: Injuries among young soccer players. *Am J Sports Med* 1991;19:273-275.

Sewall L, Micheli L: Strength training for children. *J Pediatr Orthop* 1986;6:143-146.

Stone M, O'Bryant H, Garhammer JA: Hypothetical model for strength training. *J Sports Med Phys Fitness* 1981;21:342-351.

Teitz CC, Hu SS, Arendt EA: The female athlete: Evaluation and treatment of sports-related problems. *J Am Acad Orthop Surg* 1997;5:87-96.

Voss LA, Fadale PD, Hulstyn MJ: Exercise-induced loss of bone density in athletes. *J Am Acad Orthop Surg* 1998;6:349-357.

Walker RN, Green NE, Spindler KP: Stress fractures in skeletally immature patients. *J Pediatr Orthop* 1996;16:578-584.

Watkins J, Peabody P: Sports injuries in children and adolescents treated at a sports injury clinic. *J Sports Med Phys Fitness* 1996;36:43-48.

Weltman A, Janney C, Rians CB, et al: The effects of hydraulic resistance strength training in pre-pubertal males. *Med Sci Sports Exerc* 1986;18:629-638.

Yamane T, Yoshida T, Mimatsu K: Early diagnosis of lumbar spondylolysis by MRI. *J Bone Joint Surg Br* 1993;75:764-768.

Zelisko JA, Noble HB, Porter M: A comparison of men's and women's professional basketball injuries. *Am J Sports Med* 1982;10:297-299.

Chapter 4

Assessing and Treating Musculoskeletal Pain in Children

Corrie T. M. Anderson, MD

Introduction

Pain has been identified as the fifth vital sign by the Joint Commission on Accreditation of Healthcare Organizations (JCAHO) to underscore the importance of pain management in children. This chapter reviews the management of acute pain after injury or surgical procedures. Assessment of patients with chronic pain is also reviewed. Treatment using pharmacologic and nonpharmacologic methods for acute and chronic pain are discussed along with several specific pain conditions.

Musculoskeletal Pain and Musculoskeletal Pain Management

Assessing Pain

Transmission and perception of pain involves a complicated set of neuronal cellular receptors, molecules, and neuronal pathways that ends with the subjective interpretation of the experience at the cortical level (Figure 1). Numerous studies over the past two decades have demonstrated that children of all ages feel pain. Although some aspects of pain in the neonate and young infants (and in some adults) may be subcortical or reflexive, it is assumed that nonverbal children experience pain, can suffer the untoward sequelae of unrelieved pain, and are subject to the beneficial protective aspects of pain. For a list of pain term definitions, see Table 1.

Periodic monitoring and documenting of pain scores has become a parameter critically evaluated by JCAHO. A standard set of age-appropriate, pain-assessment tools is important for assessing and treating pediatric patients with pain. Pain assessment measures may be classified as behavioral, physiologic, or self-reported. Behavioral measures use displays of distress (grimaces, cries, and protective guarding gestures). Physiologic measures quantify a child's level of distress by changes in blood pressure, heart rate, and pupil size. Self-report tools are considered the most reliable and accurate measures and include descriptive words, numerical ratings, and drawings to express the quantity and quality of a patient's pain. Both physiologic and behavioral methods of pain evaluation should be used in young children. Four pain assessment scales can be used: the Modified Infant Pain Scale; the Face, Legs, Activity, Cry, and Consolability Behavioral Pain Assessment Scale (Table 2); the Wong-Baker Faces Scale; and the Numerical Rating Scale.

Wide variation in the accuracy of parental or nurse estimation of a patient's pain can exist, and although it is important and now mandatory to have pain assessment and treatment, attempts to reach a specific pain score could result in respiratory or cardiovascular problems. Some patients will be comfortable with a pain score of 5 out of 10 and other patients who are visibly somnolent may report that their pain score is 10 out of 10. If appropriate, it should be determined directly from the patient which pain score they would like to use. This can preclude excessive sedation or worse, respiratory arrest. The addition of other medication adjuncts or nonpharmacologic therapies may provide safe relief.

Treating Pain

Nonpharmacologic Therapies

All children benefit from psychological support during painful or frightening situations. Favorite toys, recordings of familiar sounds, and parental presence have been found to decrease anxiety and agitation. Psychological treatment of pain has been an effective adjunct or alternate therapy to pharmacologic modalities of pain management. Patient preparation is perhaps the most widely used psychological intervention. Desensitization can help a child cope with medical and surgical procedures. Distribution of information, including a description of the procedure in age-appropriate language, helps to allay fears. Examples include handling the oxygen mask to be used during the induction of anesthesia or performing the proposed and feared procedure on a doll. Positive reinforcement following an encounter can be enacted by all members of the medical team using tangible rewards such as stickers, badges, or rewards of time and attention. Uncooperative behavior should never be punished.

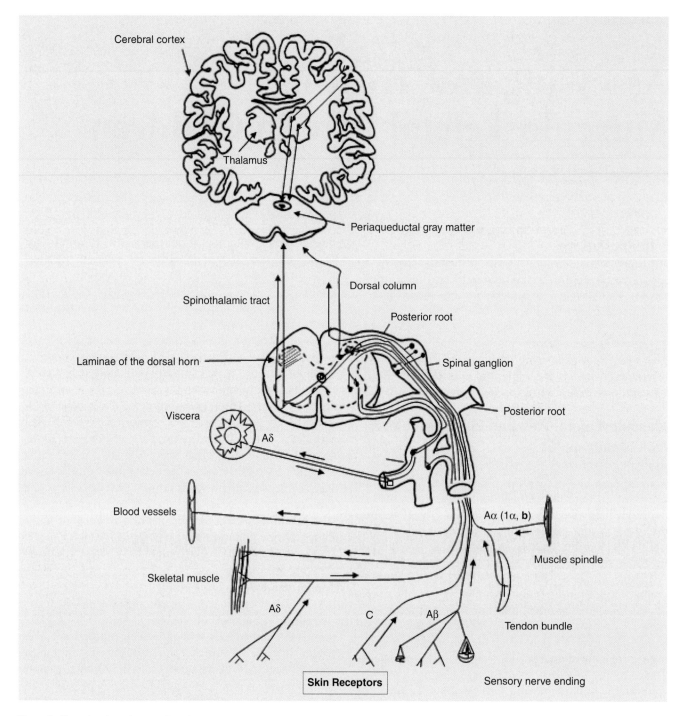

Figure 1 Illustration shows the ascending pain pathways.

Pharmacologic Pain Treatment Strategies

Pain is easier to prevent than to treat. Preemptive analgesia is conceptually a method of prevention before pain starts. Several recent studies have demonstrated the effectiveness of preemptive analgesia that limits nociceptive transmission and may prevent central sensitization or "wind-up" and chronic pain. Administration of local anesthetics, nonsteroidal anti-inflammatory drugs (NSAIDs), or opioids is protective. It is important to note that more than 70% of the drugs listed in the *Physician's Desk Reference* do not have labeling for children. Table 3 lists several methods for treating acute pain in children. The advantages and disadvantages of each method are noted.

Acetaminophen

Acetaminophen is used for treating mild pain or fevers and often used in combination with other analgesics. It provides an opioid-sparing effect. Overdose can cause liver failure and death, and overdose is a risk in patients with liver disease, renal dysfunction, or low intravascular volume. The oral dose used to treat fevers is 0 to 15 mg/kg. For children with mild pain the dose is 20 to 40 mg/kg rectally, followed by 15 to 20 mg/kg every 6 to 8 hours.

Table 1 | Pain Terms

Allodynia: Lowered threshold; pain resulting from a stimulus that does not normally provoke pain

Analgesia: Absence of pain in response to stimulation that would normally be painful

Anesthesia dolorosa: Pain in an area or region that is anesthetic

Causalgia: A syndrome of sustained burning pain, allodynia, and hyperpathia after a traumatic nerve lesion, often combined with vasomotor and sudomotor dysfunction and later trophic changes

Central pain: Pain initiated or caused by a primary lesion or dysfunction in the central nervous system

Dysesthesia: An unpleasant abnormal sensation, either spontaneous or evoked

Hyperalgesia: An increased response to a stimulus that is normally painful

Hypoalgesia: Diminished pain in response to a normally painful stimulus

Hyperpathia: Raised threshold; stimulus and response mode may be the increased response: same or different

Hypoesthesia: Decreased sensitivity to stimulation, excluding the special senses

Neuropathic pain: Pain initiated or caused by a primary lesion or dysfunction in the nervous system

Neuralgia: Pain in the distribution of a nerve or nerves

(Adapted with permission from Merskey H, Bogduk (eds): Classification of Chronic Pain: Descriptions of Chronic Pain Syndromes and Definitions of Pain Terms, ed 2. Seattle, WA, International Association for the Study of Pain, 1994, pp 209-214.)

Nonsteroidal Anti-inflammatory Drugs

NSAIDs are used to treat mild to moderate pain and provide an opioid-sparing effect (Table 4). They act by reducing prostaglandins and leukotrienes through inhibition of cyclooxygenase synthetase (COX) types 1 and 2. Adverse effects include liver toxicity, water retention, reversible platelet dysfunction, hyperkalemia, increased blood pressure, renal dysfunction, and gastrointestinal hemorrhage. Ketorolac, a widely used NSAID, is the only parenteral NSAID available in the United States. Recommended dosing of ketorolac is 0.25 mg/kg up to 0.5 mg/kg every 6 hours. For children, ketorolac has comparable analgesic effects, fewer adverse effects, and decreased medication needs when compared with opioids used for minor surgical procedures. For children younger than 1 year, this drug should be administered cautiously.

Multiple animal studies have demonstrated a deleterious effect on bone healing when animals were given COX inhibitors. Nevertheless, there are no well-controlled human studies demonstrating unequivocally that there is poor bone healing in patients taking these drugs. Until further studies clearly delineate the risks, personal preference will dictate prescriptive practices.

Concerns about bleeding and the other adverse effects associated with the less-selective NSAIDs led to trials of celecoxib, rofecoxib, and valdecoxib (COX-2 inhibitors). The enthusiasm for COX-2 inhibitors has waned with reports of increased cardiovascular complications in adult patients. Two of the drugs, rofecoxib and valdecoxib, have been voluntarily withdrawn from the marketplace.

Opioids

Opioid binding leads to hyperpolarization of the neuron. The resulting inhibition or suppression of neuronal activity is why the patient experiences less pain when taking opioids. Hepatic enzyme immaturity, reduced renal function, higher volume of drug distribution, and low drug

Table 2 | The Face, Legs, Activity, Cry, and Consolability Behavioral Pain Assessment Scale

	Scoring		
Categories	**0**	**1**	**2**
Face	No particular expression or smile	Occasional grimace or frown, withdrawn, disinterested	Frequent to constant quivering chin, clenched jaw
Legs	Normal position or relaxed	Uneasy, restless, tense	Kicking, or legs drawn up
Activity	Lying quietly, normal position, moves easily	Squirming, shifting back and forth, tense	Arched, rigid or jerking
Cry	No cry (awake or asleep)	Moans or whimpers; occasional complaint	Crying steadily, screams or sobs, frequent complaints
Consolability	Content, relaxed	Reassured by occasional touching, hugging, or being talked to, distractible	Difficulty to console or comfort

Each of the five categories is scored from 0 to 2, resulting in a total score between 0 and 10. (Copyright © 2002, The Regents of the University of Michigan. Reproduced with permission.) .

Table 3 | Methods of Acute Pain Treatment for Pediatric Patients

Method	Advantages	Disadvantages	Procedure
Continuous intravenous	More stable plasma levels No peaks and valleys Appropriate for all ages Less labor intensive	Equipment costs Careful titration required No patient control possible	All except for very short procedures Major reconstruction Nephrectomy
Patient-controlled anesthesia	Exquisite patient control Safe Enhances nursing time Good for episodic pain	Pump costs Requires patient cooperation Not useful in patients younger than 4 years	All procedures for which age is not a concern and hospital stay is sufficiently long
Opioid boluses	Good for episodic pain Less costly for short stays Can be used for all ages	Unstable plasma levels if dosing interval is not appropriate Expensive if hospital stay is long	All procedures
Peripheral nerve block (brachial plexus or femoral nerve)	Very effective Inexpensive Requires little training Preemptive analgesia	Short duration Vascular injection Nerve damage	Upper extremity surgery Femoral fractures and lower limb surgery
Caudal (one shot)	Effective Inexpensive Requires little training Lowers anesthetic requirement if done at beginning of surgery	Vascular injection Intraosseous injection Nerve damage, epidural hematoma Bowel or bladder perforation Dural puncture Postdural puncture headache	Good for any procedure below the clavicle
Epidural (caudal or lumbar)	Constant level of analgesia Safe Enhances nursing time Muscle relaxation with concentrated local anesthetics or patients can ambulate with dilute epidural solutions	Lumbar approach is technically difficult in children Nerve damage Epidural hematoma Bowel or bladder perforation Dural puncture Postdural puncture headache Vascular injection	Good for any procedure below the clavicle Revascularization Thoracic, major lower extremity repair/osteotomies
Wound infiltration	Constant level of analgesia Safe Enhances nursing time Technically easy Requires little training Requires no special equipment Localized effects	Visceral pain will not be treated Higher local anesthetic absorption Fewer attachments (pumps/poles)	Procedures in which somatic pain is most severe
Topical	Safe Effective Technically easy Requires no special equipment Localized effects	Vasoconstriction at site Methemoglobinemia in high doses Limited availability in some hospitals	Intravenous placement Skin grafting

clearance all play a role in causing infants younger than 6 months to be more sensitive to the effects of opioids. Because of interindividual variability in drug metabolism and sensitivity, drugs must be titrated to effect. All opioids will cause a similar degree of respiratory depression at equal analgesic doses. It is important to use an opioid conversion table when switching opioids and to reduce the dose by 25% to 30% because of incomplete cross-tolerance between opioids (Table 5).

Opioids can be administered to a child through multiple routes, including orally, rectally, intranasally, trans-dermally, sublingually, intramuscularly, and intravenously. For younger children, elixirs are well tolerated. Common oral opioid preparations include codeine and oxycodone. Both of these drugs can be given to children to treat postoperative and procedural pain. The weaker of the two agents, codeine, is useful for mild pain. Oxycodone is prescribed for moderate to severe pain. Recommended doses of codeine range from 0.5 to 1 mg/kg every 4 hours. Approximately 10% of the pediatric population is insensitive to codeine. They have a decreased ability to convert codeine to morphine because they lack

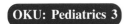

Table 4 | NSAIDs for the Treatment of Moderate Pain

Medication	Dose	Route	Dosing Interval
Ibuprofen	10 mg/kg	Oral	Every 6 to 8 hours
Naproxen	5 to 7 mg/kg	Oral	Every 8 to 12 hours
Acetaminophen	10 to 15 mg/kg	Oral	Every 4 to 6 hours
	20 to 40 mg/kg for first dose; 15 to 20 mg/kg thereafter	Rectal	Every 4 to 6 hours
Ketorolac	0.5 mg/kg	Intravenous	Every 6 to 8 hours
	15 to 30 mg/kg not to exceed 5 days or 120 mg/kg/day	Oral	Every 6 hours
Celecoxib	2 to 4 mg/kg	Oral	Every 12 hours

Doses are for patients who weigh less than 60 kg; The hospital pharmacist or pain service should be consulted for dosing in children younger than 1 year

Table 5 | Opioid Narcotics Used in Pediatric Pain Management

Opiate	Equipotent		Bioavailability	Comments
	Oral Dose	**Intravenous Dose**		
Morphine	0.3 mg/kg every 3 to 4 hours	0.1 mg/kg every 3 to 4 hours	20% to 40%	Poor absorption from stomach Seizures in newborns Histamine release Consider giving every 2 hours
Methadone	0.2 mg/kg every 6 to 12 hours	0.1 mg/kg every 6 to 12 hours	80%	Administered intravenously, subcutaneously, or intramuscularly Long half-life requires titration and possible dose reduction when switching from an intravenous agent
Fentanyl	Not recommended	0.001 mg/kg every 5 minutes to every 1 hour	NA	Ideal for procedural pain and bradycardia Chest wall rigidity (treat with naloxone or muscle relaxant)
Nalbuphine	0.3 mg/kg every 2 to 4 hours	0.1 mg/kg every 4 hours	20% to 30%	Kappa agonist and mu antagonist Less dysphoria than with other mixed agonists Can antagonize ventilatory depressant effects of opiate agonist while maintaining analgesia
Codeine	0.5 to 1.0 mg/kg every 3 to 4 hours	NA	40% to 70%	Oral administration only 10% of population cannot metabolize codeine into active form of morphine
Oxycodone	0.1 mg/kg every 3 to 4 hours	NA	60% to 80%	Oral administration only
Hydrocodone	0.1 mg/kg every 3 to 4 hours	NA	60% to 80%	Oral administration only

All opioid agonists can cause urinary retention, inappropriate secretion of antidiuretic pruritus hormone, dysphoria, euphoria, sleep disturbances, and dry mouth; NA = not applicable

function in one or more of the cytochrome P450 isoenzymes that are involved with codeine metabolism. The most typical isoenzyme is CYP-2D6. In addition, the propensity for codeine to cause constipation and to be nauseating has led pediatric pain clinicians to use other agents such as hydrocodone, oxycodone, or morphine.

Vicodin (Abbott Laboratories, Abbott Park, IL) and Lortab (UCB Pharmaceuticals, Smyrna, GA), then Tylox (Ortho-McNeil Pharmaceuticals, Raritan, NJ), and Percocet (Endo Laboratories, Chadds Ford, PA) have hydrocodone and oxycodone as their active ingredients, respectively. The pharmacokinetics of oxycodone is extremely variable, so it must be titrated to effect. Oxycodone is manufactured in multiple forms, including a sustained release formulation (OxyContin, Purdue Pharmaceuticals, Stamford, CT). When used alone or combined with acetaminophen it is effective in treating mild to severe pain. Typical doses for oxycodone are 0.1 to 0.2 mg/kg every 4 hours. Because the liver metabolizes oxycodone to morphine, care must be taken when prescribing this drug to patients with any degree of liver disease. The lack of metabolism of codeine in some patient populations mentioned above has not been reported with oxycodone.

Hydrocodone is not as potent as morphine; therefore, it is useful for treating only mild to moderate pain. Doses of 0.05 to 0.1 mg/kg are suggested as starting doses. An elixir is available in some geographic locations.

Morphine is the prototypical opioid. It has multiple formulations, including parenteral, liquid, and sustained-release preparations. It can be given safely to children of all ages starting with premature neonates. Its relatively short half-life (3 to 4 hours) dictates that morphine can be administered every 2 to 3 hours to minimize pain. Targeted intravenous infusions at 10 to 30 μg/kg/hr in infants are tolerated well, but must be accompanied by cardiopulmonary monitoring and oximetry. For older children, analgesics administered through patient-controlled analgesia (PCA) pumps increase nursing efficiency and patient satisfaction.

Meperidine (Demerol, Sanofi-Aventis, Bridgewater, NJ) is an opioid agonist that has been administered for moderate to severe pain and for shivering. It has been combined with Phenergan (Wyeth Pharmaceuticals, Philadelphia, PA) and thorazine (known as DPT) and has been given parenterally as a sedative cocktail. Meperidine is metabolized in the liver to an active metabolite, normeperidine. This metabolite has a long half-life (14 to 21 hours in normal individuals).

Methadone is a synthetic form of morphine that has excellent mucosal absorption. It is inexpensive, rapidly acting, and it has no known active metabolites other than morphine. If a patient has chronic severe pain or if expensive computer-controlled pumps are not available, methadone is ideal because of its prolonged half-life (6 to 36 hours). Additionally, methadone inhibits the effects of excitable amino acids at the N-methyl-aspartate receptors, which is a benefit in the treatment of neuropathic pain or chronic pain. Methadone is available as an elixir, as an injectable, or in tablet form. A pharmacist or pain expert should be consulted if dosing adjustments need to be made.

Fentanyl (Janssen Pharmaceutica Products, Titusville, NJ) is a shorter-acting (duration action, 30 to 45 minutes), more potent opioid (70 to 100 times stronger) than morphine that can be administered intravenously or through skin with a patch. Fentanyl is popular for short, painful procedures such as bone setting or wound suturing. Fentanyl given intravenously has a rapid onset (2 to 3 minutes) and limited cardiovascular effects. For acute pain, incremental doses of 1 to 3 μg/kg

of fentanyl every 5 minutes can be given safely if the appropriate monitoring and resuscitation equipment is available. Physicians should be aware that there is increased risk of respiratory failure if other depressant agents such as Ativan (Wyeth Pharmaceuticals) are administered concomitantly. The use of fentanyl patches is not advised in children younger than 2 years.

Nalbuphine (Nalbain, Endo Laboratories) is a mixed agonist-antagonist that is structurally related to naloxone and oxymorphine. The partial-agonists and the agonists-antagonists are able to relieve the pain associated with acute or chronic painful perturbations. As with the pure agonists, these agents can be administered through a variety of routes. Absent from the partial-agonist and agonist-antagonist preparations is the euphoria that is associated with the pure agonists. It has been suggested that the mood elevation associated with the pure agonists is directly responsible for their abuse; therefore, a potential benefit of the agonists-antagonists is the absence of this effect. Additionally, the incidence of other adverse effects associated with the administration of morphine-like drugs appears to be less frequent with the agonist-antagonists. Nalbuphine is highly lipophilic and is equipotent to morphine. The respiratory depression associated with pure agonists such as morphine can be reversed with nalbuphine and other agonists-antagonists without reversing pain relief.

Patient-Controlled Analgesia

The continuous infusion of analgesics or the administration of analgesic agents on a fixed time schedule fails to account for the variable nature of pain intensity, the inherent biologic differences in patients, and the fluid psychological states of the pediatric patient. Fixed dosing negates the ability to respond to individual analgesic needs. Studies in adults demonstrate that the amount of pain medication required to achieve effective pain relief varies greatly among individuals; that small discrete doses of pain medication, given frequently, help maintain plasma drug levels better than as needed or around-the-clock intramuscular injections; and that pharmacokinetic variables such as volume of distribution and elimination do not correlate with pain medication dosing requirements.

A more rational approach to pain treatment is to use the concept of PCA, which represents any methodology that allows a patient to receive on-demand analgesia in amounts that will control their pain. Pediatric patients commonly use a PCA pump for postoperative pain control (Table 6). The route of administration is typically intravenous; however, drugs can also be given subcutaneously, transdermally, epidurally, or through a properly placed nerve catheter using a PCA pump. A patient must understand how to use a PCA pump and want to control their own analgesia and have the ability to phys-

Table 6 | Common Intravenous PCA Dosing

Drug	Demand Dose	Continuous (basal)	Hourly Maximum	Lockout
Morphine	10 to 20 µg/kg	0 to 20 µg/kg/h	100 µg/kg	6 to 8 minutes
Hydromorphone	3 to 5 µg/kg	0 to 5 µg/kg/h	20 µg/kg	6 to 8 minutes
Fentanyl	0.25 to 0.5 µg/kg	0.15 µg/kg/h	1 µg/kg	6 to 8 minutes
Nalbuphine	10 to 20 µg/kg	0 to 20 µg/kg/h	100 µg/kg	6 to 8 minutes

ically activate the pump. A child as young as 3 years, 9 months reportedly is able to use a PCA pump properly.

Regional Anesthesia and Analgesia

The administration of opioids, either alone or in combination with local anesthetics via the caudal, epidural, or spinal routes, has been shown to bring about striking postoperative analgesia for patients undergoing cardiac, abdominal, orthopaedic, and maxillofacial surgery. The close proximity of the opioid receptors in the spinal cord to the subarachnoid space and the epidural space allows for the administration of much smaller doses of drug to achieve the same analgesic effect. The advantage of intrathecal or spinal opioids used alone is that they can produce profound analgesia while preserving motor function, touch, and hemodynamic stability. Nausea, vomiting, decreased gastrointestinal motility, urinary retention, respiratory depression, and pruritus all occur with neuraxial opioid administration. Respiratory depression can occur with intrathecal morphine and can be minimized by using highly lipophilic and short-acting opioids such as fentanyl and sufentanil while avoiding parenterally administered opioids. The caudal approach to the administration of local anesthetics and opioids has become popular for pediatric outpatient pain treatment. Performing a caudal block at the beginning of surgery, if time permits, generally reduces the need for other analgesics or anesthetics, leading to a shorter wake-up time.

Bupivacaine and lidocaine are the major local anesthetics used to perform caudal anesthesia. Several concentrations of bupivacaine have been investigated, and more concentrated solutions appear to provide no advantage over the 0.125% solution. The benefit of the more dilute solution is that there is less motor block. This may be significant if patient discharge is dependent on ambulation.

Regional anesthesia alone or in conjunction with general anesthesia has been documented to create a reduction in the hormonal stress response, which is three to five times greater in neonates compared with adults. Studies have also demonstrated less phantom limb pain after amputations, better postoperative pain scores, and prolonged reduction in pain scores up to 10 days after surgery. A variety of other regional anesthetic blocks have been performed successfully in ambulatory patients, including blockade of the stellate ganglion, brachial plexus, celiac plexus, sciatic nerve, femoral nerve, the ilioinguinal and iliohypogastric nerves, and fascia iliaca.

The need for a reliable topical anesthetic agent for use in pediatric patients is important. Several studies have investigated the efficacy of a eutectic mixture of lidocaine-prilocaine, EMLA (AstraZeneca, Wilmington, DE), applied to the skin of outpatients for venous cannulation. Researchers have found this mixture effective in reducing pain associated with venous catheterization.

Chronic Pain and Chronic Pain Management

The International Association for the Study of Pain defines chronic pain as pain without apparent biologic value that has persisted beyond the normal tissue healing time. Recent studies have found that the incidence of chronic musculoskeletal pain in the pediatric population is 5% to 30% and includes growing pains, overuse injury syndrome, back pain, and limb pain. It is important for physicians to recognize that both acute and chronic pain states can exist in the same patient. For example, a patient with Ewing's sarcoma may have persistent bone pain that is exacerbated by a fracture, thus causing acute discomfort overlaid on a chronic pain profile.

Given the complexity and wide variety of chronic musculoskeletal abnormalities, it is important for examining physicians to refer the patient to the appropriate pain specialist for evaluation and treatment if the chronic pain is causing functional disability and is of concern to the physician or family. Myofascial pain syndrome, fibromyalgia, phantom pain, and reflex sympathetic dystrophy are all chronic pain syndromes that are likely to be encountered in a busy practice.

The initial assessment of the patient with chronic pain should include a careful history and a detailed physical examination. If the patient is verbal, it is best to obtain the history directly from the patient. Often a parent will speak for the child or interrupt the child while the history is being obtained; therefore, the parent may need to wait outside the examination room. The history should include the child's birth history, developmental history, family and social history, list of hospitalizations,

Table 7	Differential Diagnosis Categories for Chronic Musculoskeletal Pain
Infectious disease
Inflammatory condition
Hematologic disorder
Rheumatologic disorder (collagen vascular)
Neoplasm
Psychogenic condition
Trauma
Metabolic disorder

Table 8	Methods and Drugs Used in Chronic Pain Management
Ablative neurosurgery
Acupuncture/acupressure
α-adrenergic blocking agents
Anticonvulsants
Antidepressants
Anxiolytics
Biofeedback
Bisphosphonates
Cognitive behavioral interventions
Family therapy
Massage
Miscellaneous agents (octreotide, calcitonin)
Muscle relaxants (baclofen/Valium)
N-methyl-D-aspartate receptor antagonists (ketamine)
NSAIDs
Opioids
Physical and occupational therapy
Psychostimulants
Regional analgesia/anesthesia
Spinal cord implants
Steroids
Topical agents (lidocaine/capsaicin creme)

and drug, alcohol, and sexual history. A relevant pain history must record pain location, intensity, quality, character, factors exacerbating or ameliorating the pain, associated symptoms, and timing of the pain. Anxiety, insomnia, obsession, depression, peer interactions, and information on pending litigation are stressors that can be significant and must be investigated. A recent change in the family or patient's social environment such as the hospitalization or death of a family member, a change in school, addition of a new child, or a divorce may influence pain behavior. Patients with chronic pain who have seen multiple specialists may be taking a wide variety of medications. Chronic pain in children has at times been a surrogate for child abuse or Munchausen syndrome by proxy.

A complete physical examination should be performed. The vital signs, including a pain score, are important to record at every encounter. Careful attention should be paid to the child's general appearance, posture, muscle tone, coordination, and strength. The facial reactions should be assessed for concordance with the expressed amount of pain; abnormal skin temperature and coloration should be assessed as well. Limb girth should be measured for evidence of disuse atrophy.

Laboratory studies such as blood count, erythrocyte sedimentation rates, C-reactive protein level, or rheumatologic studies should be considered if inflammation is evident. Diagnostic imaging studies can be specific (such as radiographs and MRI) or nonspecific (such as bone scanning or scintigraphy). Laboratory and imaging studies should be done to evaluate the differential diagnosis rather than as routine screening. The list of possible differential diagnoses is large, but falls into several categories (Table 7).

In the setting of chronic pain, studies have often been performed and repetition is not usually necessary. The cost of time and money to evaluate chronic pain can be considerable.

The patient and the family should be educated about pain, made aware of its subjective nature, and introduced to a multidisciplinary or interdisciplinary approach to chronic pain management, including consulta-

tion with anesthesiologists with specialization in pain management, physical therapists, psychologists, and psychiatrists (Table 8). Ultimately, the family psychodynamics may need to be explored to improve the patient's outlook. Psychologists and psychiatrists are better equipped to deal with problems associated with chronic pain such as depression, obsession, and somatization. Referral to a pain management specialist or pain management center that uses a multidisciplinary approach in the treatment of a child's chronic pain will offer the patient and the family a wider variety of therapeutic options.

Fibromyalgia and Myofascial Pain Syndrome

Two common pain syndromes involving the musculoskeletal system are fibromyalgia syndrome and myofascial pain syndrome. The terms "fibromyalgia" and "myofascial pain" are often incorrectly interchanged. Fibromyalgia syndrome is characterized by chronic pain, multiple tender points located in muscles and other soft tissues, stiffness, and hyperalgesia that involves the entire body. The etiology of fibromyalgia syndrome is unknown. The prevalence of this disease in the general population is estimated to be between 0.5% and 5%. It appears to have a higher rate of occurrence in patients with diabetes and irritable bowel syndrome. The syndrome has been reported to have an incidence as high

Table 9 | Clinical Characteristics of Fibromyalgia and Myofascial Pain

Clinical Characteristics	Fibromyalgia	Myofascial Pain
Musculoskeletal pain	Localized, regionalized	Generalized
Muscle spasms	Common	Uncommon
Trigger points	Localized, regionalized	Rare
Tender points	Uncommon	Multiple, generalized axial
Taut band	Uncommon	Multiple generalized
Fatigue	Uncommon	Common
Sleep	Nonrestorative	Nonrestorative
Headaches	Localized	Generalized
Referred pain	Common	Uncommon
Paresthesias	Regionalized	Generalized
Irritable bowel	Uncommon	Common

(Adapted with permission from Knobler RL (ed): Contemporary Approaches to Managing Pain: Emerging Concepts in Myofascial Pain. Princeton, NJ, Professional Postgraduate Services, 1998.)

as 6.2% in school-age children, with an average age at diagnosis of 13 to 15 years. Fibromyalgia syndrome is more common in female patients in both the adult and pediatric populations, with the diagnosis of fibromyalgia syndrome being made about three to seven times more frequently in female than male children. The disease is rare in African-American children. The American College of Rheumatology has developed two criteria for the diagnosis of fibromyalgia in adults. First, a patient must have widespread pain involving both sides of the body above and below the waist for a minimum of 3 months. Second, the pain must be present in at least 11 of 18 designated tender points when palpated. In children, the positive test criteria for fibromyalgia syndrome require that pain must be present in only 5 of 11 designated tender points when palpated.

Fibromyalgia syndrome can cause significant physical and psychological impairment and affects the quality of life because of the functional disability that it causes. Pain along with sleep disturbances are prominent clinical manifestations of this disease. Patients with fibromyalgia can have a range of other associated symptoms that include but are not limited to headache, fatigue, depression, anxiety joint pain, soft-tissue tenderness, jaw pain, and paresthesias. Several diseases and symptoms are associated with or should be considered in the differential diagnosis of fibromyalgia syndrome, including growing pains, chronic fatigue syndrome, restless leg syndrome, temporomandibular joint dysfunction, thyroid disease, inflammatory bowel disease, anterior chest wall syndrome, depression, and dysautonomia. Approximately 20% of patients with irritable bowel syndrome have fibromyalgia syndrome.

Fibromyalgia syndrome has no known cure. Low-dose antidepressants, NSAIDs, opioids, muscle relaxants, and sedatives have had limited success in clinical trials for the treatment of fibromyalgia syndrome. The

US Federal Drug Administration has placed a warning on all antidepressants that there is an increased risk of suicidal ideation in adolescent patients with major depressive disorder who take antidepressants.

Symptomatic or palliative therapy should be directed at pain relief, improved physical conditioning, and restoration of sleep. The multifaceted nature of the disease necessitates a multidisciplinary team. A complementary educational program for the patient and parent offers the best opportunity for relief of this disease.

Myofascial pain syndrome is a disorder that can affect any skeletal muscle or group of skeletal muscles in the body. Although myofascial pain is common in the general adult population, the prevalence in the pediatric population is unknown. It can occur in infants and small children. In contrast to fibromyalgia syndrome, myofascial pain syndrome is characterized by trigger points that are localized (Table 9). When the trigger points are palpated, they feel like nodules within the muscle. There are four classic features of myofascial pain syndrome: (1) taut bands of muscle that are palpable, (2) a localized tenderness within the taut band, (3) pressure on a trigger point within the taut band causes a reproducible pattern of referred pain, and (4) a positive sign is present when pressure is applied to the tender area. Pain from trigger points is dull in character and is persistent. Patients with myofascial pain syndrome may experience tightness, stiffness, muscle atrophy, and muscle weakness. Trigger points begin as taut bands in muscles, which are usually asymptomatic but can become painful trigger points with the onset of psychological stress, muscle tension, poor posture, or acute trauma. There are both major and minor criteria for the diagnosis of myofascial pain syndrome.

Myofascial pain syndrome is not a fatal disease and is found equally in both men and women. Myofascial pain syndrome may arise from abnormalities in the mo-

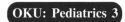

Table 10 | Diagnostic Criteria for Complex Regional Pain Syndrome

Clinical
  Positive sensory abnormalities
    Spontaneous pain
    Mechanical hyperalgesia
    Thermal hyperalgesia
    Deep somatic hyperalgesia
  Vascular abnormalities
    Vasodilation
    Vasoconstriction
    Skin temperature asymmetries
    Skin color changes
  Edema
    Sweating abnormalities
    Swelling
    Hyperhidrosis
    Hypohidrosis
  Motor and trophic changes
    Motor weakness
    Tremor
    Dystonia
    Coordination deficits
    Nail and hair changes
    Skin atrophy
    Joint stiffness
    Soft-tissue changes

Interpretation
  For clinical use
    Three or more symptoms from each category and two or more
      signs from each category (sensitivity, 0.85; specificity, 0.60)
  For research use
    Four symptoms from each category and two or more signs from
      each category (sensitivity, 0.70; specificity, 0.96)

tor end plates of muscles in the disease area. It is thought that the low-threshold, afferent mechanoreceptors associated with the affected muscle are sensitized and send pain signals to the central nervous system.

Because the differential diagnosis for myofascial pain syndrome includes hypothyroidism, hypoglycemia, infection, and fibromyalgia syndrome, a complete history and physical examination are important. The character of the patient's pain must be determined as well as the onset of the pain and its modulating factors that either suppress the pain or increase it.

Although no treatment has been fully validated, the most commonly used treatment for myofascial pain syndrome is the injection of trigger points. The type of local anesthetic used does not appear to matter. There are no well-controlled trials showing a greater benefit of lidocaine over bupivacaine. Water, saline, and botulinum toxin have been effective treatments in some patients with myofascial pain syndrome. Insertion of a needle without the injection, a practice called "dry needling", has also been used as a treatment. Spraying the muscle

with a vapor coolant spray and then stretching has also been reported. Other therapies include transcutaneous electrical nerve stimulation, acupuncture, massage, and biofeedback.

Complex Regional Pain Syndrome

Complex regional pain syndrome is characterized by the feeling of pins and needles, burning, tingling, and severe pain out of proportion to the inciting injury occurring in an extremity. Other associated symptoms include autonomic and motor changes such as cyanosis, edema, mottling, temperature sensitivity, and hyperalgesia; hence, the label of neuropathic pain (Table 10). Through increased educational efforts, neuropathic pain in children is becoming a more recognized clinical entity. The incidence of neuropathic pain in children is unknown because of its underdiagnosis, but it is an unusual diagnosis in pediatrics. Orthopaedic physicians are increasingly being asked to diagnose and to treat patients with neuropathic pain. Unfortunately, neuropathic pain can have significant morbidity. Delay in diagnosis and treatment can result in a more difficult condition to remedy.

There are a number of different types of neuropathic pain, two of which have special interest to anyone caring for children. Complex regional pain syndrome and causalgia are major subtypes of a constellation of chronic painful disorders of the autonomic nervous system. Thus, each is a form of neuropathic pain. Both complex regional pain syndrome and causalgia have been described in children and in adults. These disorders were first described in Civil War era soldiers with traumatic limb injuries. A history of musculoskeletal trauma is usually linked to these chronic pain states. Posttraumatic pain syndrome, posttraumatic spreading neuralgia, reflex neurovascular dystrophy, and minor causalgia are just a few terms used to describe complex regional pain syndrome.

Of the numerous therapies used in the treatment of complex regional pain syndrome, sympathetic blockade has been successful in a subset of patients with complex regional pain syndrome, which once led to the notion that complex regional pain syndrome was a sympathetically maintained pain state. Further work, however, has shown that patients may have sympathetically independent pain but still have the clinical features of complex regional pain syndrome or causalgia. Causalgia is a pain disorder in which a major nerve has been traumatized. Unfortunately, the clinical manifestations that distinguished complex regional pain syndrome and causalgia are not easily separated. This led the International Association for the Study of Pain to attempt to clarify the nomenclature of these diseases. Complex regional pain syndrome type I and type II are now used to refer to complex regional pain syndrome and causalgia, respectively. Patients with either type of pain may or may not have sympathetically maintained pain.

The underlying pathophysiology of the disease has not been fully elucidated. There may be a genetic linkage for patients at risk for the disease. An association with HLA-DR13 has been demonstrated. The most common etiology of complex regional pain syndrome type I is trauma to a distal extremity. A sprain, fracture strain, tight cast, or limb surgery can precipitate the complex regional pain syndrome type I. Complex regional pain syndrome type II occurs after major nerve trauma such as a brachial plexopathy, stroke, or surgery on a nerve. The pain associated with complex regional pain syndrome type II is not limited to the distribution of the injured nerve. Burning pain, allodynia, hyperalgesia, and edema are clinical features of both complex regional pain syndrome type I and type II. Other clinical signs include spontaneous pain not coinciding with a nerve distribution, skin color changes, swelling, hyperhidrosis, hypohidrosis, motor weakness, tremors, dystonia, nail changes, joint stiffness, and soft-tissue changes such as edema.

Complex regional pain syndrome is associated with major debilitation and alteration in lifestyle. Although complex regional pain syndrome is not fatal, patients commonly have suicidal ideation and major psychological disruptions because of the unrelenting pain. Patients of all ages can be afflicted with complex regional pain syndrome. The highest incidence in the pediatric population occurs during the adolescent years (mean age, 12 to 13 years). Women appear to be most commonly affected; 60% to 80% of patients diagnosed are women. In addition to the symptoms already noted, complex regional pain syndrome can lead to bone demineralization, asymmetric limb temperature, sudomotor changes, and trophic skin changes.

Other diseases that can mimic complex regional pain syndrome include inflammatory diseases such as tendinitis and bursitis, myofascial pain syndrome, Raynaud's disease, Raynaud's phenomenon, deep venous thrombosis, cellulitis, vascular insufficiency, lymphedema, erythromelalgia, and posttraumatic nerve injury from surgery or trauma in which pain is in the distribution of the nerve.

The patient's history should be detailed and include queries about trauma, symptoms, psychological stress, the character and distribution of the pain, and other sensations such as allodynia, tenderness, and hyperpathia. On physical examination, attention should be paid to the assessment of autonomic changes such as cyanosis, muscle weakness, edema, hyperhidrosis, and hypohidrosis. The laboratory tests that have been used in this patient population include thermography, electromyography, Doppler flow studies, diagnostic imaging studies (including plain radiography and MRI), scintigraphy scans to assess bone metabolism, temperature de-

termination, psychological testing, sweat test, and sympathetic blockade.

Once the diagnosis of complex regional pain syndrome has been made, a treatment scheme can be proposed. The therapeutic management of complex regional pain syndrome type I and type II has had varied success, however, because of the heterogeneity of the patient population and the insufficient number of well-controlled clinical trials in children. Peripheral and central nerve blocks; neuromodulation (with spinal cord stimulation, transcutaneous electrical nerve stimulation, or drug therapy); a variety of intravenous agents, including bretylium, ketamine, and systemic alpha-adrenergic drugs; and sympathetic nerve blocks all have been reported to be effective in the treatment of complex regional pain syndrome. A consensus report on the treatment of complex regional pain syndrome generated by a number of the world's experts on complex regional pain syndrome in adults and children promotes a systematic approach to therapy that is focused on the restoration of functionality through desensitization, increased mobility, and social support. Aggressive and immediate patient education and physical therapy are regarded as imperative. These treatments can be instituted even before referring these patients to a specialist.

Phantom Pain

Within the spectrum of patients seen by orthopaedists, patients with phantom sensation or phantom pain can be the most troubling. Phantom pain or phantom sensation reflects the feeling that the appendage is still present after it has been removed. The pain these patients endure is difficult to manage, and the conditions under which the pain has occurred are usually dire or, at the least, distressing. Deafferentation pain or anesthesia dolorosa are other terms that have been used to describe this type of chronic pain. The incidence of phantom limb pain in adults has been reported to range from 60% to 80%. Phantom limb pain in children appears to have a different clinical course than in adults. The etiology of the disease leading to amputation and the presence and quality of pain in the affected area prior to amputation appear to influence the postamputation pain. Pain associated with amputation decreases more frequently with time in children than adults. The onset of the pain is typically 1 week after the amputation. Because patients with a congenital absence of a limb and children younger than 6 years rarely have phantom pain, the development of the central nervous system may have a role in the evolution of the disease.

Pretreatment with a number of agents has impacted the frequency of phantom limb and phantom stump pain. One study demonstrated the effectiveness of epidural local anesthetics plus an opioid administered 3 days prior to amputation compared with the administration of intravenous opioids. In another attempt to diminish phantom pain, a double-blind, randomized trial showed that gabapentin, an anticonvulsant, was effective in the treatment of phantom limb pain in adults. Gabapentin has been successfully used to treat phantom pain in children. Acupuncture, trigger point injections, transcutaneous electrical nerve stimulation, and surgery along with a variety of medications have been used for the treatment of phantom pain. Pharmacologic treatment with low-dose amitriptyline, carbamazepine, or opioids has generated anecdotal reports of success. With sleep disturbance being one of the biggest problems for patients with chronic pain, a small dose of an antidepressant before bedtime has the effect of aiding sleep and reducing the pain. Generally, 10 to 25 mg of amitriptyline 1 to 2 hours before bedtime has been effective in restoring sleep.

Summary

Pain and suffering affects children and alters the dynamics of the family and their relationship to health care providers. In the past, there has been an inadequate knowledge base about the physiologic, behavioral, and biochemical differences of pediatric patients in their response to pain and pain management. Archaic ideas about addiction, the inability of children to verbalize their distress, and the inability of caregivers to understand that distress have delayed the application of many treatment modalities that have been found to be useful in adult patients with pain. The modern treatment of pain in children uses both pharmacologic and nonpharmacologic means to reduce suffering. The use of multidisciplinary pain services in the management of pain is leading to dramatic improvements in pediatric pain care.

Annotated Bibliography

Musculoskeletal Pain and Musculoskeletal Pain Management

Berde CB, Sethna NF: Analgesics for the treatment of pain in children. *N Engl J Med* 2002;347(14):1094-1103.

Two of the leading experts in pediatric pain management provide a well-referenced article covering several developmental aspects of pain and all of the major analgesics used for the treatment of pain in children.

Fitzgerald M: The development of nociceptive circuits. *Nat Rev Neurosci* 2005;6(7):507-520.

The author provides a concise discussion of the development of excitatory and inhibitory pain pathways in newborns that supports the existence of pain in infants.

Gajraj NM: The effect of cyclooxygenase-2 inhibitors on bone healing. *Reg Anesth Pain Med* 2003;28(5):456-465.

The author reviews the current animal and human data on COX-2 inhibitors and compares drugs, doses, and animal mod-

els. The author concludes that there are no human data to indicate that COX-2 agents have a negative effect on bone healing.

Lönnqvist PA, Morton NS: Postoperative analgesia in infants and children. *Br J Anaesth* 2005;95:59-68.

The authors of this review article provide an update on the recent advances in the postoperative care of pediatric patients. The safety of regional anesthesia in children and the use of ultrasound in the performance of conduction blockade are discussed.

Pokela ML, Anttila E, Seppala T, Olkkola KT: Marked variation in oxycodone pharmacokinetics in infants. *Paediatr Anaesth* 2005;15(7):560-565.

Children age 0 to 6 months who were undergoing surgical interventions were administered oxycodone so that a pharmacokinetic profile of this drug in young children could be determined. The authors concluded that the half-life and clearance of oxycodone varies greatly in this age group and recommend that the drug should be carefully titrated to maximize safety and minimize adverse effects.

Chronic Pain and Chronic Pain Management

Berde CB, Lebel A: Complex regional pain syndromes in children and adolescents. *Anesthesiology* 2005;102:252-255.

The authors review complex regional pain syndrome in pediatric patients and comment on the use of continuous peripheral nerve catheters for its treatment.

Graboski CL, Gray DS, Burnham RS: Botulinum toxin A versus bupivacaine trigger point injections for the treatment of myofascial pain syndrome: A randomised double blind crossover study. *Pain* 2005;118(1-2):170-175.

In this study, botulinum toxin A was compared with bupivacaine trigger point injections for the treatment of patients with myofascial pain syndrome. The authors found no difference in the effectiveness of the treatments, but the greater cost of the botulinum toxin A preparation led them to conclude that bupivacaine was a better agent for treatment.

King S: Assessment and management of somatoform pain disorders, in: Schechter NL, Berde CB, Yaster M (eds): *Pain in Infants, Children, and Adolescents*. Philadelphia, PA, Lippincott Williams & Wilkins, 2003, pp 293-302.

The author discusses the epidemiology of somatic pain disorders as well as the assessment and treatment of these disorders in the pediatric population.

Raja SN, Grabow TS: Complex regional pain syndrome: I. Reflex sympathetic dystrophy. *Anesthesiology* 2002; 96(5):1254-1260.

In this review article, the authors thoroughly detail the pathophysiologic mechanisms of complex regional pain syndrome type 1 and type 2.

Thomas CR, Brazeal BA, Rosenberg L, Robert RS, Blakeney PE, Meyer WJ: Phantom limb pain in pediatric burn survivors. *Burns* 2003;29:139-142.

In this retrospective study, the authors reviewed the medical charts of severely burned patients who underwent limb amputation. Over a 30-year period, they found that 227 children had amputations, but only 39 children required major limb amputation, 34 of whom met the criteria to be analyzed further (death or severe brain injury). The authors found that opioid and antidepressant drugs were commonly used for treatment and that electrical injury before amputation placed patients at a greater risk for phantom limb pain.

Classic Bibliography

Bach S, Noreng MF, Tjellden NU: Phantom limb pain in amputees during the first 12 months following limb amputation, after preoperative lumbar epidural blockade. *Pain* 1988;33:297-301.

Dubois RN, Abramson SB, Crofford L, et al: Cyclooxygenase in biology and disease. *FASEB J* 1998;12:1063-1073.

Hong CZ, Simons DG: Pathophysiologic and electrophysiologic mechanisms of myofascial trigger points. *Arch Phys Med Rehabil* 1998;79(7):863-872.

Joint Commission on Accreditation of Health Care Organizations: *Standards for Pain Assessment and Treatment: Comprehensive Accreditations Manual for Ambulatory Care, Behavioral Health Care, Health Care Networks, Home Care Hospitals, and Long-Term Care.* Oakbrook, IL, Joint Commission on Accreditation of Health Care Organizations, 1999.

Krane EJ, Heller LB: The prevalence of phantom sensation and pain in pediatric amputees. *J Pain Symptom Manage* 1995;10:21-29.

McGrath PA: *Pain in Children: Nature, Assessment, and Treatment.* New York, NY, Guilford Publications, 1990.

Merskey H: Bogduk (eds): *Classification of Chronic Pain: Descriptions of Chronic Pain Syndromes and Definitions of Pain Terms*, ed 2. Seattle, WA, International Association for the Study of Pain, 1994.

Murray CS, Cohen A, Perkins T, Davidson JE, Sills JA: Morbidity in reflex sympathetic dystrophy. *Arch Dis Child* 2000;82:231-233.

Rosow C: Agonist-antagonist opioids: Theory and clinical practice. *Can J Anaesth* 1989;36(3 pt 2):S5-S8.

Ross AK, Eck JB, Tobias JD: Pediatric regional anesthesia: Beyond the caudal. *Anesth Analg* 2000;91(1):16-26.

Stanton-Hicks M, Baron R, Boas R, et al: Complex regional pain syndromes: Guidelines for therapy. *Clin J Pain* 1998;14:155-166.

van Hilten JJ, van de Beek WJ, Roep BO: Multifocal or generalized tonic dystonia of complex regional pain syndrome: A distinct clinical entity associated with HLA-DR13. *Ann Neurol* 2000;48:113-116.

Watcha MF, Ramirez-Ruiz M, White PF, Jones MB, Lagueruela RG, Terkonda RP: Perioperative effects of oral ketorolac and acetaminophen in children undergoing bilateral myringotomy. *Can J Anaesth* 1992;39(7):649-654.

Wilson: John T: An update on the therapeutic orphan. *Pediatrics* 1999;104:585-590.

Yunus MB, Masi AT: Juvenile primary fibromyalgia syndrome: A clinical study of thirty-three patients and matched normal controls. *Arthritis Rheum* 1985;28(2):138-145.

Chapter 5

Neck Conditions

Joseph G. Khoury, MD

James O. Sanders, MD

Introduction

Not all physicians are comfortable evaluating pediatric cervical spine injuries because these injuries are relatively rare, even in the busiest orthopaedic practices. On the rare occasion that pediatric patients with cervical spine injuries do present for evaluation, it is important for orthopaedists to be aware of the recent advances in diagnosing, understanding, and treating these disorders.

Trauma

Pediatric cervical spine injuries are less common than thoracic and lumbar injuries. Several recent large case series from level 1 trauma centers have improved the understanding of these injuries. Mortality rates as a result of pediatric cervical spine injuries range from 4% to 18%. Trauma caused by motor vehicle collision is the most common mechanism of injury for all age groups. Although young children are more likely to be injured in a motor vehicle collision than adults, the incidence of injury related to falls and dives increases in older children and sports-related injuries are more common in adolescents. Spinal injuries in young children (younger than 8 years) primarily occur in the upper three levels, whereas those in older children (9 years of age or older) begin to approximate adult patterns, with more subaxial injuries. Upper cervical spine (occiput through C4) injuries make up nearly two thirds of spinal injuries. Young patients more often have associated neurologic injuries, closed head injuries, and higher injury severity scores overall compared with older children. Because of the hypermobility of the spine, young children can also experience spinal cord injury without radiographic abnormality, the most likely mechanism of which is vascular disruption from differential spinal cord stretch and cord contusion.

Apart from AP and lateral radiographs, other radiographic views can be difficult to obtain in injured children. The radiographic evaluation of the cervical spine in injured children is challenging because of incomplete ossification and the presence of many growth centers. In a child who is alert, conversant, and has no neurologic deficits, no cervical tenderness, no painful distracting injury, and is not intoxicated, cervical spine radiographs are not necessary to exclude the presence of an injury. The odontoid view is very difficult to obtain in injured children and is rarely helpful. Likewise, recent studies have reported that flexion-extension views and oblique views add few relevant data in the assessment of a child with an acute injury. In one study that reviewed injuries in 51 children younger than 16 years, the odontoid view was not helpful in making the diagnosis in any patient younger than 8 years. The odontoid view aided in the diagnosis of a type III odontoid fracture in one patient between the ages of 9 and 16 years. In a similar study, the usefulness of flexion-extension radiographs in the acute trauma setting was assessed. In 224 patients with normal static examinations, flexion-extension radiographs contributed no useful information. The authors recommended omitting flexion-extension radiographs in children with a history of trauma and normal static examination of the cervical spine. In another study involving 109 children with blunt cervical spine trauma, the oblique radiograph did not contribute to the diagnostic accuracy of the standard AP and lateral radiographs in detecting the presence of cervical spine injury in children. If an upper cervical spine injury is suspected after reviewing standard AP and lateral radiographs, a CT scan should be obtained. Conversely, a CT scan in a patient with normal radiographs is unlikely to yield positive results. If an injury is suspected but not seen, the neck should be stabilized until an adequate physical examination can be performed. If flexion views are needed after the acute injury, then knowledge of normal radiographs can be helpful. However, MRI can be used to directly visualize soft-tissue injuries. The tectorial membrane is the critical structure that must be disrupted before significant instability occurs between the occiput and C2. MRI has been reported to have a sensitivity of 87% and a specificity of 100% for predicting instability at this level.

Several specific cervical spine injury mechanisms are preventable, as evidenced by the drastic reduction in

American football injuries with strict enforcement of no-spearing rules and Florida's success in reducing diving injuries with the Feet-First First-Time campaign. Trampolines were responsible for more than 6,500 cervical spine injuries in children in 1998, and paraplegia, quadriplegia, and death have been reported to occur as a result of trampoline-related injuries. As a result, support is growing for banning the use of trampolines by children. Although car seat restraints are effective in preventing bodily injury, their effectiveness has been called into question in preventing permanent spinal cord deficits and closed head injuries because these devices do not restrain the head and neck. Design modifications to restrict head movement during motor vehicle collisions may improve outcomes in young patients. In baseball, head-first sliding poses the greatest risk of injury to young athletes, and it is more dangerous than feet-first sliding. Although many athletic coaches assume that head-first sliding is faster than feet-first sliding, a recent study showed no difference between them. Helmet use among skiers and snowboarders is on the rise. In snow sports, participants have argued against the use of helmets, citing impaired peripheral vision and impaired hearing as factors that contribute to accidents and therefore cervical spine injury. However, a recent study showed that helmet use in skiers and snowboarders younger than 13 years does not increase the incidence of cervical spine injury and does reduce the incidence of head injury that requires investigation or treatment. The involvement of orthopaedists in promoting these protective measures can be crucial to their success.

Torticollis

Torticollis can be subdivided into torticollis of infancy (congenital torticollis) and acquired torticollis (Table 1). Paroxysmal torticollis in infancy is an additional type that does not necessarily have an associated congenital component. Acquired torticollis generally affects older children and consists of entities such as C1-C2 rotatory subluxation/fixation, Grisel's syndrome, posterior fossa tumors, and others.

Congenital torticollis generally presents within the first 3 months of life (by day 24 on average). Although the etiology remains elusive, a recent electron microscopy study examined the cellular makeup of tissue found in both the pseudotumor and in simple congenital muscular torticollis without pseudotumor. The ultrastructure of the pseudotumor consisted of many cell types, including myoblasts, fibroblasts, myofibroblasts, and other mesenchymal-like cells. In simple muscular torticollis without a pseudotumor, the collagen fibrils and fibrocytes were found to be arranged in tight parallel bundles, and the ultrastructure of those cells revealed decreased myofibrillae. Several epidemiologic studies

Table 1	Classification of Torticollis
Congenital (of infancy)	
Sternocleidomastoid tumor	
Muscular torticollis	
Postural torticollis	
Paroxysmal torticollis of infancy	
Acquired	
C1-C2 rotatory instability	
Grisel's syndrome	
Positioning	
Posterior fossa tumor	
Oculomotor	

have demonstrated a strong correlation between torticollis and breech/assisted delivery (including forceps and vacuum-assisted delivery) and other birth trauma. The incidence of breech presentation and cesarean section are also higher in children with congenital torticollis.

Congenital torticollis has been subdivided into three main categories: sternocleidomastoid tumor (42% to 55% incidence), muscular torticollis (30% to 34% incidence), and postural torticollis (11% to 22% incidence). The paroxysmal torticollis of infancy type has been linked to a calcium-channel mutation, strengthening the suspicion of a link between this condition and the migraine aura. The association between congenital torticollis and developmental dysplasia of the hip has been further investigated by two new studies, one of which involved ultrasound screening of all children with torticollis; the other was a retrospective review using radiography. The incidence of clinically important developmental dysplasia of the hip requiring treatment was 8.5% in the ultrasound study and 8% in the retrospective study, both of which are far lower than the 20% incidence that has often been cited.

Ultrasound has been used more extensively in recent years in the evaluation of patients with congenital torticollis. Different classification systems have been proposed using ultrasound examination of the involved muscle that describe the extent of fibrosis in the muscle, both in cross-sectional area and length. Studies have found a good correlation between the severity of fibrosis and the need for surgery. In addition, other studies have been able to apply clinical subgroupings to large groups of patients with congenital torticollis and thereby identify factors related to the prognosis. The degree of limitation of rotation of the neck on presentation has correlated with the success of nonsurgical treatment in several prospective studies. In addition, larger tumor, hip dysplasia, the presence of craniofacial asymmetry, and older age at presentation have all been shown to correlate with the need for surgical treatment. The presence of a pseudotumor as opposed to simple muscular torticollis and postural torticollis seems to decrease the likelihood that a therapeutic stretching program will be effective.

The cornerstone of initial treatment of all categories of congenital torticollis for children of any age is physical therapy, which generally consists of gentle supervised or unsupervised passive range of motion combined with altering the environment to encourage the child to look in the opposite direction and thus contribute to active range of motion. The success of nonsurgical treatment has been shown to correlate with the subgroup as well as the degree of loss of rotation on presentation, age at presentation, and a history of birth difficulties. Other reports have been less encouraging regarding the success of manual stretching. One study illustrated deteriorating results with physical therapy in successfully treating congenital torticollis in older age groups. In this study, no children presenting between the ages of 0 and 3 months required surgery, whereas 25% of those in the 3- to 6-month age group, 70% of those in the 6- to 18-month group, and 100% of all of those older than 18 months ultimately required surgery. In another study, 20 of 72 children with congenital torticollis (mean age, 19.5 months) ultimately required surgery.

A snapping or sudden sensation of giving way can be experienced by the treating physician, parent, or therapist while performing manual stretching on children with congenital torticollis. This has been reported to occur in 41 of 455 patients in one series. This study used ultrasound and found the snapping to correlate with a partial versus complete tear of the sternocleidomastoid muscle. At 3.5-year follow-up, no difference in the outcomes was reported in those who had experienced the snapping episode compared with those who had not, and there were no identifiable, long-term sequelae.

Surgical treatment is indicated when a patient has undergone at least 6 months of controlled manual stretching and has residual head tilt, deficits of passive rotation or lateral bending of more than 15°, or a tight band that is palpable in the muscle. Surgical outcomes have also been correlated to the age of the patient at the time of surgery, with 88% of patients having excellent results overall, which dropped to 63.6% in patients who were older than 10 years at the time of surgery. Many surgical treatments have been described, including unipolar, bipolar, and Z-lengthening techniques, with emphasis on preserving the contour of the neck and preventing recurrence. Postoperative management generally includes physiotherapy and/or bracing to help prevent recurrence. New surgical techniques have been described to improve correction while preserving the cosmetic appearance and protecting the spinal accessory nerve. One new surgical technique involves subperiosteal lengthening of the sternocleidomastoid muscle at its mastoid insertion and division of lower fibrotic bands. Minimal postoperative fibrosis and excellent cos-metic outcomes have been reported using this technique. Endoscopic release has also been described, with excellent long-term results reported in 85 patients. The endoscopic approach has been purported to provide improved visualization of the areas requiring release and better protection of the spinal accessory nerve. These newer surgical techniques, however, have not been studied in a controlled fashion with comparison to established techniques.

With the increasing effectiveness of the Back to Sleep campaign to prevent sudden infant death syndrome, plagiocephaly has become a more frequently encountered problem among physicians who treat torticollis. According to a recent prospective study of 200 normal infants who were followed from birth to 2 years of age, several factors contributed to the development of plagiocephaly: limited neck rotation, decreased activity level, and supine sleeping position. The study reported that the prevalence of plagiocephaly significantly increased between week 6 and month 4 and then gradually decreased until age 2 years. Plagiocephaly generally resolves without treatment by age 2 years. An early assessment of the range of motion for all infants and variation of the infant's head position during sleep is recommended.

With increased sensitivity of physicians and parents to plagiocephaly, the interest in cranial orthotic devices for the treatment of this deformity has gained more attention. A 2003 meta-analysis of cranial orthotic devices for plagiocephaly was conducted to determine whether patients with plagiocephaly have cognitive delays that can be attributed to the plagiocephaly and whether cranial orthotic devices can correct cranial asymmetry. Some evidence exists that decreased infantile movement caused by developmental delays may lead to plagiocephaly. Moreover, findings in the medical literature are mixed as to whether cranial orthotic devices can improve cranial symmetry. It is important to point out that cranial orthotic devices are contraindicated in patients with fused cranial sutures. One study emphasized counterpositional therapy in this patient population, including the use of foam wedges and sandbags to position the sleeping infant's head in such a way to avoid pressure on the flattened area of the skull. This study also emphasized aggressive early treatment of congenital muscular torticollis to prevent the resulting secondary changes of plagiocephaly.

When torticollis occurs in an older child or adolescent with no previous history of the disorder, the differential diagnosis varies from that for congenital torticollis. This entity has many different pseudonyms, including acute torticollis, nontraumatic torticollis, acquired torticollis, atlantoaxial rotatory fixation, or atlantoaxial rotatory subluxation. The latter two terms represent a radiographic (specifically dynamic CT) diagnosis and should be reserved for that situation. Acquired torticollis should be used as a general description until a specific diagnosis is established. Potential diagnoses are Grisel's syndrome (which is associated with an inflammatory process in the retropharyngeal venous plexus associated either with ear, nose, and throat surgery or infection in these locations), posterior fossa tumors, intraoperative positioning of the neck in rotation, and clavicle fractures. In patients with acute nontraumatic torticollis, a specific diagnosis often cannot be identified. Acquired torticollis has been described in association with clavicle fractures with the head and neck most often bent laterally toward and rotated away from the fractured clavicle. Often, this bending of the head and neck is in response to the pain of the fracture, but it may also be associated with true atlantoaxial rotatory displacement. If torticollis persists after the initial pain of the clavicle fracture has subsided, the diagnosis of atlantoaxial subluxation in association with a clavicle fracture should be considered.

The pathogenesis of otherwise idiopathic acquired torticollis is still unknown. A recent arthrography study revealed a tear in the atlantoaxial joint capsule on the dislocated side; evidence of healing was found with a repeat arthrography study after a period of immobilization. Previous theories have suggested an infolding of the synovium and/or capsule into the C1-C2 facet as a mechanism of injury, but there has been no evidence to support this. In one study, MRI was done within hours of presentation in a patient with acute atraumatic torticollis and an acute fluid-filled cleft was found in the C2-C3 uncovertebral joint, suggesting an acute rupture of the disk. A repeat MRI scan obtained 3 weeks after symptoms had resolved was completely normal. In another case report, evidence of avulsion of the apical and alar ligament on a dynamic CT scan was reported.

The diagnosis of C1-C2 rotatory subluxation/fixation has classically relied on dynamic CT as the diagnostic imaging gold standard. Recently, a classification system using dynamic CT was described in which the change and degree of rotation in each direction are recorded as stage 0 (no difference), stage 1 (< 15° difference, but C1 crosses the midline of C2), or stage 2 (< 15° difference, but C1 does not cross the midline of C2). In this study, the number of days the patient had symptoms before the diagnosis was made correlated with these stages: patients who were classified as stage 0 had 6.7 days of symptoms, those who were stage 1 had 8.6 days of symptoms, and those who were stage 2 had 20 days of symptoms. The intensity of symptoms and treatment also correlated with the stage. In another study, the reliability of dynamic CT interpretation has been called into question by comparing the intraobserver and interobserver reliability of dynamic CT scans in 18 patients with acute torticollis and 12 normal subjects. The authors reported poor and fair interobserver reliability in first and second examinations, respectively. The intraobserver reliabilities

were rated as poor, slight, moderate, and almost perfect for the four observers in this study, respectively. In another study, dynamic CT scans were obtained in 10 normal children with no evidence of instability on lateral flexion and extension radiographs. This study demonstrated between 74% and 85% loss of contact between the C1 and C2 facets on right and left rotation images. These scans were read by radiologists as showing rotatory subluxation in all instances. In another age-matched, controlled study of 33 consecutive patients with acute acquired torticollis, no statistically significant differences in the range of atlantoaxial rotation either toward or away from the deformity were reported when comparing the study group with the control group. Because the authors of this study could not demonstrate the presence of atlantoaxial rotatory subluxation or fixation in their entire series of 33 consecutive patients with acute torticollis, this suggests that the existence of the phenomenon itself is doubtful. They concluded that acquired torticollis is not necessarily a sign of pathology at the atlantoaxial joint and that it is not necessary to obtain CT scans in this group of patients at the time of presentation. In patients presenting with acquired torticollis who are neurologically normal within a reasonably short time frame, a trial of conservative treatment may therefore be undertaken without obtaining a CT scan. Three-dimensional reformations of CT scans may improve specificity and sensitivity for diagnostic and surgical planning.

The treatment of acquired torticollis is generally conservative, consisting of anti-inflammatory medications, muscle relaxants, soft or semirigid immobilization, and halter or halo traction, depending on the duration of symptoms before the diagnosis is made. For patients with symptoms lasting for more than 1 month before the initiation of treatment, reduction with halter or halo traction followed by 6 weeks of immobilization has been the classic recommendation. However, there have been several reports of recurrence after a 6-week period of immobilization, and several authors have recommended 3 months of immobilization for patients with a long duration of symptoms before presentation or a prolonged period of traction to obtain reduction. A longer period is required to obtain reduction in patients with a longer duration of symptoms. Some authors have recommended surgery for all patients with type III atlantoaxial rotatory subluxation because of the high rate of recurrence, even after 6 months of halo vest immobilization after reduction. Surgery generally consists of posterior fusion in patients who are neurologically intact. One case report described an anterior transoral release of both atlantoaxial joints, allowing reduction of a chronic fixed deformity in a quadriplegic patient followed by a posterior fusion with full neurologic recovery.

Surgical Techniques

C1-C2 fusions are generally performed to treat patients with congenital malformations, juvenile rheumatoid arthritis, or rotatory subluxation using Gallie or Brooks wiring techniques. Postoperative subaxial kyphosis has frequently been observed in this patient population, and occipitocervical arthrodesis to prevent this deformity has been advocated. A recent long-term follow-up study has shown that this phenomenon occurs in approximately one third of patients and can be expected to gradually resolve with time.

Various Diagnoses Associated With Cervical Spine Injuries

Klippel-Feil Syndrome

Klippel-Feil syndrome has traditionally been classified based on the patterns of intervertebral fusion. The classic physical findings of a short neck with limited motion and a low hairline are rarely helpful in making the diagnosis. More often, patients present for unrelated problems or neurologic symptoms, and the diagnosis is made incidentally on radiographic studies showing fusion of contiguous vertebral segments. Recent studies have reported several families with Klippel-Feil syndrome, the symptoms of which are similar among members of the family, but differ among families, suggesting genetic heterogeneity. Based on these data, four new classes of Klippel-Feil syndrome have been described in a comprehensive classification that addresses genetic heterogeneity. The incidence of neurologic symptoms ranges from 26% to 37% in recent series. Risk factors appear to be related to the presence of degenerative changes at the unfused levels, a narrow bony canal, and the frequency of occipitocervical anomalies rather than the number of mobile blocks or age. Flexion-extension MRI is currently the best modality for detecting spinal cord impingement. Cervical spondylosis or disk herniation are the most common findings in patients with symptoms and are not necessarily found clustered around the sites of fusion. In a study that reported 25-year experience in treating patients with Klippel-Feil syndrome, data from 57 patients were reviewed with respect to the incidence of scoliosis. Overall, 70% of patients developed scoliosis, with the average Cobb angle correlating with the type of Klippel-Feil syndrome.

Cerebral Palsy

Patients with cerebral palsy, particularly those with athetosis or dystonic types, may develop cervical spondylosis that can progress to myelopathy and/or instability. Atraumatic atlantoaxial instability has been reported in patients with spastic cerebral palsy.

Detecting myelopathy or other neurologic changes in patients with cerebral palsy can be difficult because of the baseline neurologic status, difficulty in cooperating with the physical examination, and poor verbal skills of the patient. If changes are suspected, the appropriate diagnostic studies such as CT and MRI can be difficult to perform and may even require general anesthesia. It is important that the treating physician is able to recognize the signs of cervical cord dysfunction in this patient population. Any significant alteration of muscle tone, especially spastic to hypotonic accompanied by torticollis, should indicate that a workup should be performed to rule out cervical myelopathy. (Although alteration of muscle tone from hypotonic to spastic represents a typical clinical scenario, muscle tone alteration from spastic to hypotonic is more commonly the result of myelopathy.) In addition, bradycardia, apnea, or any other acute change in respiratory status should prompt additional investigation.

Osteogenesis Imperfecta

Patients with osteogenesis imperfecta are known to develop basilar invagination. The exact incidence and significance of this finding is not known. In a recent study of 130 patients with osteogenesis imperfecta (85 with type I, 21 with type III, 24 with type IV), lateral radiographs were obtained for all patients to identify basilar invagination. Eight patients had suspected invagination on plain radiography that was confirmed with MRI. No children developed neurologic symptoms or signs. At an average 5-year follow-up, only one in seven patients had an increase in the degree of basilar invagination, but none had developed neurologic symptoms. The authors recommend the use of MRI in this patient population only if the screening radiographs suggest the possibility of basilar invagination; they emphasized their finding that neurologic symptoms are not present as often as expected. Surgical decompression and fusion is recommended only for those with neurologic changes and is not recommended for patients with MRI evidence of neural compression alone because it is poorly tolerated. Decompression frequently involves anterior surgery such as clival-odontoid-anterior arch resection combined with a posterior fusion. In patients with severe osteogenesis imperfecta, an open door maxillotomy may be required (Le Fort I osteotomy of the maxilla combined with a midline split of the soft palate and maxilla).

Juvenile Chronic Arthritis

Patients with juvenile chronic arthritis often have cervical spine involvement. In a recent large series from Finland, 159 patients with documented juvenile chronic arthritis were reviewed radiographically after the age of 18 years. The most common findings were apophyseal joint ankylosis (noted in 41% of patients), anterior atlantoaxial instability (noted in 17%), and atlantoaxial impaction (noted in 25%). In addition, the fourth cervical vertebra was found to be abnormally small in 26% of patients, all of whom tended to have earlier disease onset and short body stature.

Down Syndrome

It is well established that children with Down syndrome can have cervical instability. The incidence of atlanto-axial instability with an atlantodens interval greater than 5 mm ranges from 9% to 22%. More recently, occipitoatlantal instability has been recognized and discussed with more frequency, and an incidence of up to 60% has been reported. Many patients can have instability at both levels, but symptomatic instability is rare. It has been proposed that increased instability is related to ligamentous laxity in addition to an increased incidence of bony abnormalities, including os odontoideum, spina bifida occulta of C1, and persistence of synchondroses at many levels. Treatment guidelines, which are hotly debated, should be based on symptoms and the space available for the spinal cord. The governing body of the Special Olympics requires screening radiographs before athlete participation; however, the information from these radiographs is difficult to interpret because so many patients are asymptomatic. If neurologic symptoms develop, disease progression is slow, and there have been very few reported instances of catastrophic neurologic injury that were not preceded by a prolonged period of prodromal symptoms. Many surgical series have reported high complication rates, including intraoperative neurologic injury from sublaminar wiring and other instrumentation as well as a high rate of nonunion requiring prolonged immobilization after surgery. However, in recent series, results have improved dramatically with fusion rates of 96% and more patients experiencing excellent outcomes with the use of internal fixation. One recent study described premature subaxial degeneration and instability leading to myelopathy in young adults with trisomy 21, which emphasized that these patients need continued follow-up in adulthood.

22Q11.2 Deletion Syndrome

The 22Q11.2 deletion syndrome has been recognized to occur in 1 of 400 live births and has a 100% incidence of associated occipitocervical and upper cervical anomalies. The most common anomalies include platybasia (91% of patients), dysmorphic C1 (75% of patients), open posterior arch of C1 (59% of patients), and dysmorphic dens (58% of patients). Clinicians who treat pediatric patients with cervical spine conditions will likely encounter this diagnosis with increasing frequency in the future and should be familiar with its manifestations.

Cleft Lip and Palate

In a large retrospective study comparing the dental radiographs of children with cleft lip and palate anomalies and those of children without such anomalies, a statistically significant increased rate of cervical vertebral anomalies was reported in individuals with cleft lip and palate compared with those without cleft lip and palate. Specifically, 611 patients with three different cleft lip and palate subtypes (cleft palate only, bilateral cleft lip and palate, unilateral cleft lip and palate) were studied and compared with 264 children without cleft lip and palate. Vertebral anomalies (most commonly fusions and posterior arch deficiency) were found in 25.6% of the cleft palate only group, 16.3% of the bilateral cleft lip and palate group, and 11.1% of the unilateral cleft lip and palate group. In the group without cleft lip and palate, 9.1% had cervical vertebral anomalies. The differences were significant only between the cleft palate only group and the group without cleft lip and palate.

Tumors/Infection

Eosinophilic granuloma involving the spine is relatively common. In a recent case series of 26 children with eosinophilic granuloma of the spine confirmed using biopsy (44 involved vertebrae), 45% of lesions were found in the cervical spine, 32% were found in the thoracic spine, and 23% were found in the lumbar spine. Lesions were classified based on the severity of collapse and whether the collapse was symmetric or asymmetric. Spinal deformity occurred in four children (two of whom required fusion). No relationship between the need for surgery and the severity of collapse or symmetry of collapse was reported.

The frequency of tuberculous infection of the cervical spine has been increasing in certain regions of the world. Published case reports and series have begun to appear in the literature. Diagnosis is typically based on the presenting symptoms, which often consist of neck and arm pain, torticollis, and weakness in one or both arms. Treatment consists of an anterior approach to remove all infected material and bone and allow for reconstruction of the anterior column to restore alignment. In one series of 14 patients, 12 had complete recovery of neurologic symptoms, and 2 had marked improvement using an anterior approach. The kyphosis improved from an average of 21.6° to 2.5° at final follow-up.

Summary

With the expansion of the knowledge base in this area, orthopaedic surgeons are now better equipped to evaluate children with neck conditions. Children with potential neck injuries can now be evaluated and cleared or treated in a more streamlined and unambiguous manner. Additionally, the prognosis for various types of tor-

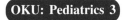
ticollis is now more predictable and the treatments are better defined. Specific advances in many neck conditions with associated cervical spine implications continue to be made.

Annotated Bibliography

Trauma

Cirak B, Ziegfeld S, Knight VM, Chang D, Avellino AM, Paidas CN: Spinal injuries in children. *J Pediatr Surg* 2004;39:607-612.

In this study, all children (N = 406; mean age, 9.48 years) presenting to a single level 1 pediatric trauma center over a period of 11 years were reviewed. The authors reported that motor vehicle collisions were responsible for most injuries (29%). Falls ranked highest for children 2 to 9 years of age and sports injuries ranked highest for those 10 to 14 years of age. The occiput through C4 ranked highest for injury level. The incidence of spinal cord injury without radiographic abnormality was 6% in this series.

Hernandez JA, Chupik C, Swischuk LE: Cervical spine trauma in children under 5 years: Productivity of CT. *Emerg Radiol* 2004;10:176-178.

The authors studied the yield of CT in the setting of normal cervical spine plain radiographs. Of 606 patients included in this series, 459 were cleared by examination and plain radiographs; 147 underwent CT to clear the cervical spine and 143 of these had normal examinations. Of the four patients with positive findings on CT, all had evidence of cervical spine injuries on the initial plain radiographs, indicating that the yield of CT in the setting of adequate normal plain radiography was low.

Kane SM, House HO, Overgaard KA: Head-first versus feet-first sliding: A comparison of speed from base to base. *Am J Sports Med* 2002;30:834-836.

This study was conducted to assess the assumption that head-first sliding in baseball is faster. Sixty players, ranging from Little League to college level, were evaluated sliding from first base into second base either head first or feet first and timed in their 40-yard sprint. No statistical difference was found in the speed between head-first and feet-first sliding at all levels of play.

Viccellio P, Simon H, Pressman BD, Shah MN, Mower WR, Hoffman JR: A prospective multicenter study of cervical spine injury in children. *Pediatrics* 2001;108:E20.

Although the National Emergency X-Radiography Utilization Study (NEXUS) instrument has been used in the adult injury setting to help determine whether radiographs should be obtained in trauma victims, its use has not been validated in the pediatric population. The authors performed a prospective, multicenter study to determine the reliability of the NEXUS criteria in the pediatric population, in which 3,065 patients younger than 18 years were enrolled. The NEXUS criteria for obtaining radiographs include midline cervical tenderness, in-

toxication, altered alertness, focal neurologic deficit, and presence of a painful distracting injury. The authors found that 19.7% of children were deemed low risk by the NEXUS instrument criteria, and none of these patients had a spinal cord injury or occult cervical injury. Thus, the NEXUS criteria were deemed useful in evaluating cervical spine injuries in children.

Zuckerbraun BS, Morrison K, Gaines B, Ford HR, Hackam DJ: Effect of age on cervical spine injuries in children after motor vehicle collisions: Effectiveness of restraint devices. *J Pediatr Surg* 2004;39:483-486.

In this study, the incidence of permanent spinal cord deficit was reported to be 57% in children age 8 years or younger versus 13% in children age 9 to 18 years despite the use of restraint devices. The incidence of closed head injury was 50% in children age 8 years or younger compared with 7% in children age 9 to 18 years in this same series despite the use of restraint devices. These findings suggest that the restraint devices are either inadequately or improperly used in younger patients.

Torticollis

Alanay A, Hicazi A, Acaroglu E, et al: Reliability and necessity of dynamic computerized tomography in diagnosis of atlantoaxial rotatory subluxation. *J Pediatr Orthop* 2002;22:763-765.

A collection of dynamic CT scans from 18 patients with acquired torticollis and 12 age- and gender-matched normal subjects were given to four experienced, blinded observers on two occasions spaced 1 month apart. The interobserver reliability for properly diagnosing atlantoaxial rotatory subluxation was –0.015 for the first evaluation and 0.327 for the second evaluation. The interobserver kappa coefficients ranged from –0.204 to 1.00. Of the 18 patients with acute torticollis, between 1 and 6 of them had the diagnosis confirmed by CT. In 3 of the 12 normal subjects, atlantoaxial rotatory subluxation was diagnosed by the observers.

Hicazi A, Acaroglu E, Alanay A, Yazici M, Surat A: Atlantoaxial rotatory fixation: Subluxation revisited. A computed tomographic analysis of acute torticollis in pediatric patients. *Spine* 2002;27:2771-2775.

The authors of this study compared 33 patients who had presented consecutively at one center with acquired torticollis with a group of 12 age-matched control subjects (with normal neck range of motion) who were undergoing cranial CT for unrelated reasons. In the study group, 18.2% of patients had a recent upper respiratory infection, 24.2% had a minor trauma, 3% (one patient) had middle-ear surgery, and 54.6% had no identifiable cause for the torticollis. All had spasm of the sternocleidomastoid muscle in opposition to the cock robin position. No instances of atlantoaxial rotatory subluxation or atlantoaxial rotatory fixation were found using dynamic CT. There was no statistical difference in the amount of rotation to either side in the study group or in the amount of rotation compared with the control group.

Hutchison BL, Hutchison LAD, Thompson JMD, Mitchel EA: Plagiocephaly and brachycephaly in the first two years of life: A prospective cohort study. *Pediatrics* 2004;114:970-979.

In this study, 200 normal infants recruited at birth and followed for 2 years were evaluated to determine the incidence and prevalence of plagiocephaly and identify related factors; 90.5% of these infants were successfully followed for 2 years. The prevalence of plagiocephaly increased to a maximum of 19.7% at 4 months of age and then decreased to 3.3% by 24 months of age without treatment. The authors reported that the factors related to the development of plagiocephaly included limited neck rotation, decreased activity level, and supine sleeping position. The authors recommended that pediatricians check neck range of motion during well baby examinations and encourage parents to vary the head position of the infant for sleeping while maintaining an overall supine position.

Lee SC, Lui TN, Lee ST: Atlantoaxial rotatory subluxation in skeletally immature patients. *Br J Neurosurg* 2002;16:154-157.

This is a report of six patients with Fielding type III atlantoaxial rotatory subluxation at a minimum 18-month follow-up. Delay in diagnosis ranged from 2 weeks to 5 months. All six patients experienced reduction after less than 2 weeks of traction (traction weight, 2 kg). Three of the first four patients experienced a recurrence despite halo vest immobilization. Two of these patients had a delay in diagnosis of 6 and 7 weeks, respectively. All three recurrences required posterior arthrodesis. The final two patients were treated with a posterior arthrodesis after reduction with excellent results.

McGuire KJ, Silber J, Flynn JM, Levine M, Dormans JP: Torticollis in children: Can dynamic computed tomography help determine severity and treatment? *J Pediatr Orthop* 2002;22:766-770.

In this retrospective review of 50 children (average age, 8.2 years) who presented with atlantoaxial rotatory subluxation and underwent dynamic CT, the amount of relative rotation was measured on CT and a staging system was developed. Stage 0 included patients with no lack of rotation; stage 1 included those with a lack of less than 15° of rotation, but in whom C1 crossed the midline of C2; stage 2 included those with a lack of less than 15° of rotation, but in whom C1 did not cross the midline of C2. The authors found that stage correlated with the time to diagnosis (6.7 days for stage 0, 8.6 days for stage 1, and 20 days for stage 2) as well as the intensity of treatment.

Surgical Techniques

Meyer NJ, Flately TJ, Dunn DD: Superiorly based laminoplasty in children: Average 6-8 year follow-up of 21 patients. *J Spinal Disord Tech* 2003;16:156-162.

Of 31 patients who underwent superiorly based laminoplasty, 21 who met the study criteria were available for follow-up. The average follow-up was 82 months (minimum, 18 months). The average laminoplasty covered 4.4 levels. The authors reported that there was no increase in preexisting deformity in 16 of 21 patients. Nonunion of the laminoplasty was identified in five patients. Laminoplasties were done in the cervical spine of three patients, one of whom developed kyphosis requiring fusion. The authors concluded that although laminoplasty does not eliminate spinal deformity, morbidity was less than with laminectomy and posterior elements are left in place if they are needed later for instrumentation or fusion mass.

Parisini P, Di Silverstre M, Greggi T, Bianchi G: C1-C2 posterior fusion in growing patients: Long-term follow-up. *Spine* 2003;28:566-572.

The authors studied 12 patients who underwent posterior C1-C2 fusion to analyze sagittal plane deformity (particularly subaxial kyphosis). The average patient age at the time of surgery was 10.9 years. Surgery was performed with the patients in a halo cast (after a period of traction for reduction) to maintain alignment, and postoperative halo casting was used for 7 to 9 weeks. At 7- to 13-year follow-up, the incidence of postoperative subaxial kyphosis was 33%. The symptoms of all patients were found to resolve with time, with final alignment of straight to lordotic.

Various Diagnoses Associated With Cervical Spine Injuries

Tsirikos AI, Chang WN, Shah SA, Miller R: Acquired atlantoaxial instability in children with spastic cerebral palsy. *J Pediatr Orthop* 2003;23:335-341.

In this retrospective review of three patients with severe spastic tetraplegia (mean age, 12.6 years), all three patients demonstrated atlantoaxial instability without a history of trauma. Symptoms at the time of presentation included changes in muscle tone, apnea, torticollis, or respiratory problems. One patient died as a result of an apneic episode while awaiting surgery, one refused surgery and experienced no improvement in neurologic status, and the third patient underwent decompression and fusion from the occiput to C2 and recovered all previous function.

Classic Bibliography

Baba H, Maezawa Y, Furusawa N, Chen Q, Imura S, Tomita K: The cervical spine in the Klippel-Feil syndrome: A report of 57 cases. *Int Orthop* 1995;19:204-208.

Buhs C, Cullen M, Klein M, Farmer D: The pediatric trauma c-spine: Is the "odontoid" view necessary? *J Pediatr Surg* 2000;35:994-997.

Cheng JCY, Tang SP, Chen TMK, Wong MWN, Wong EMC: The clinical presentation and outcome of treatment of congenital muscular torticollis in infants: A study of 1,086 cases. *J Pediatr Surg* 2000;35:1091-1096.

Clarke RA, Catalan G, Diwan AD, Kearsley JH: Heterogeneity in Klippel-Feil syndrome: A new classification. *Pediatr Radiol* 1998;28:967-974.

Davids JR, Wenger DR, Mubarak SJ: Congenital muscular torticollis: Sequela of intrauterine or perinatal compartment syndrome. *J Pediatr Orthop* 1993;13:141-147.

Demirbilek S, Atayurt HF: Congenital muscular torticollis and sternomastoid tumor: Results of nonoperative treatment. *J Pediatr Surg* 1999;34:549-551.

Lin JN, Chou ML: Ultrasonographic study of the sternocleidomastoid muscle in the management of congenital muscular torticollis. *J Pediatr Surg* 1997;32:1648-1651.

Phillips WA, Hensinger RN: The management of the rotatory atlanto-axial subluxation in children. *J Bone Joint Surg Am* 1989;71:664-668.

Ricchetti ET, States L, Hosalkar HS, et al: Radiographic study of the upper cervical spine in the 22Q11.2 deletion syndrome. *J Bone Joint Surg Am* 2004;86-A:1751-1760.

Rodgers WB, Coran DL, Kharrazi FD, Hall JE, Emans JB: Increasing lordosis of the occipitocervical junction after arthrodesis in young children: The occipitocervical crankshaft phenomenon. *J Pediatr Orthop* 1997;17:762-765.

Rouvreau P, Glorion C, Langlais J, Noury H, Pouliquen JC: Assessment and neurologic involvement of patients with cervical spine congenital synostosis as in Klippel-Feil syndrome: Study of 19 cases. *J Pediatr Orthop B* 1998;7:179-185.

Schultz KD, Petronio J, Haid RW, et al: Pediatric occipitocervical arthrodesis: A review of current options and early evaluation of rigid internal fixation techniques. *Pediatr Neurosurg* 2000;33:169-181.

Sun PP, Poffenbarger GJ, Durham S, Zimmerman RA: Spectrum of occipitoatlantoaxial injury in young children. *J Neurosurg* 2000;93:28-39.

Taggard DA, Menezes AH, Ryken TC: Treatment of down syndrome-associated craniovertebral junction abnormalities. *J Neurosurg* 2000;93:205-213.

Ulmer JL, Elster AD, Ginsberg LE, Williams DW: Klippel-Feil syndrome: CT and MR of acquired and congenital abnormalities of cervical spine and cord. *J Comput Assist Tomogr* 1993;17:215-224.

Chapter 6

Pediatric Orthopaedic Infections

Mininder S. Kocher, MD, MPH

Martin M. Dolan, MD

Jacob Weinberg, MD

Introduction

Pediatric orthopaedic infections can be challenging in terms of diagnosis and management. The differential diagnosis of musculoskeletal infection in children is varied and includes a range of infectious processes and other conditions. Children often present with similar symptoms, signs, and laboratory values. A timely and accurate diagnosis is essential for effective treatment. Management depends on the type and severity of infection, including both medical management with antibiotics and surgical management in specific patients.

Osteomyelitis

Osteomyelitis affects 1 in 5,000 children younger than 13 years. Infection usually occurs in the first decade of life. Boys are 2.5 times more commonly affected than girls. Before the era of antibiotics, the mortality rate associated with chronic osteomyelitis approached 50%. Modern treatment has decreased this mortality rate to less than 1%. Prompt diagnosis and intervention are guided by the patient's age, history, route of infection, and infecting organism.

Acute Hematogenous Osteomyelitis

Acute hematogenous osteomyelitis is the most commonly occurring type of osteomyelitis in children. The femur and tibia are the most frequently infected bones. Risk factors for acute hematogenous osteomyelitis include diabetes mellitus, hemoglobinopathies, chronic renal disease, rheumatoid arthritis, and immune compromise. Acute hematogenous osteomyelitis may be difficult to diagnose, but it is confirmed by imaging studies and cultures of the blood and bone.

Pathogenesis

Osteomyelitis is usually caused by the deposition of blood-borne organisms in the metaphysis. The capillary system in the metaphysis has a relatively slow flow. This allows organisms to migrate out of the vessel walls. The metaphyseal region has few reticuloendothelial cells available for phagocytosis. In the absence of purulence, this early stage of the disease is known as the cellulitic phase. Antibiotic treatment alone may control infection at this stage.

Purulence will form when osteomyelitis is untreated. The purulence can extend laterally through the porous metaphyseal cortex into the subperiosteal space, elevating the periosteum. As pressure increases under the periosteum, necrosis of bone occurs. Sequestrum is the loosely adherent dead bone that results from this process. Involucrum is new bone that forms with a limited vascular supply. Antibiotic accessibility is poor in this region; therefore, chronic osteomyelitis may result. If left untreated, the infection can travel down the diaphysis of the bone, leading to an ischemia of the entire bone. Each stage of this pathogenesis can be documented with diagnostic imaging studies.

Septic arthritis can be caused by osteomyelitis in regions where the metaphysis is intra-articular. In these regions, infection can exit the metaphysis and directly invade the adjacent joint. This process can occur in four locations: the proximal femur (hip), proximal humerus (shoulder), lateral distal tibia (ankle), radial neck (elbow).

Presentation

Presenting signs and symptoms of acute hematogenous osteomyelitis cover a broad spectrum. Some children present with malaise and low-grade fevers; others present with severe constitutional symptoms and high-grade fevers. Neonates with acute hematogenous osteomyelitis may have poor feeding and display irritability. They may also present with florid sepsis. In toddlers and young children, point tenderness can be localized in 50% of patients. Lower extremity involvement can lead to limping or refusal to walk. Joint motion may be limited because of local muscle spasms. Adolescents typically present with exquisite point tenderness. This tenderness occurs because adolescents have a thicker metaphyseal cortex associated with a dense fibrous periosteum, which results in a more contained infection. Furthermore, 30% to 50% of patients will have had a recent nonorthopaedic-related bacterial or viral infection. For

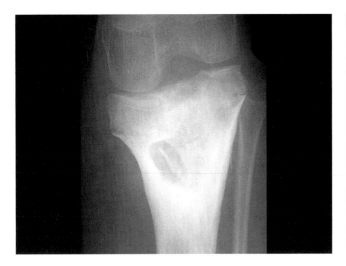

Figure 1 Radiograph demonstrating sequestrum of the proximal tibia associated with chronic osteomyelitis.

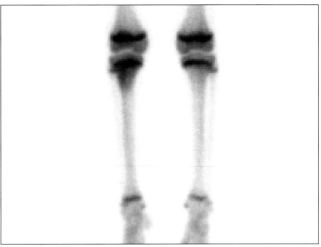

Figure 2 Bone scan demonstrating increased uptake in the patient's right proximal tibia from acute hematogenous osteomyelitis.

example, group A β-hemolytic streptococcal osteomyelitis can be associated with a varicella infection.

Any child suspected of having acute hematogenous osteomyelitis should undergo a thorough examination, including palpation of the affected bone and evaluation of adjacent joint range of motion. Gait should also be observed. Erythema and edema can be associated with subperiosteal abscess. Young children in particular should be assessed for hemodynamic stability. Diagnosing osteomyelitis in the pelvis or proximal femur is challenging. Patients typically have a limp associated with decreased hip range of motion. Local tenderness may be difficult to elicit.

The differential diagnosis of acute hematogenous osteomyelitis includes fracture, toxic synovitis, cellulitis, septic arthritis, thrombophlebitis, rheumatic fever, bone infarction, Gaucher's disease, and malignancy. Malignancies that can mimic osteomyelitis include osteosarcoma, Ewing's sarcoma, leukemia, neuroblastoma, and Wilms' tumor. Bone pain is the chief report in 18% of patients presenting with acute lymphocytic leukemia. Other orthopaedic conditions such as slipped capital femoral epiphysis and Legg-Calvé-Perthes disease should also be considered.

Laboratory Findings
The white blood cell count is elevated in only 25% of patients with acute hematogenous osteomyelitis; however, a left shift may be present. The erythrocyte sedimentation rate (ESR) is a nonspecific marker of inflammation and is elevated in 90% of patients with acute hematogenous osteomyelitis. The ESR rises slowly and peaks at 3 to 5 days. Once antibiotic therapy is initiated, ESR declines in 1 to 2 weeks. Neonates, children with sickle cell anemia, and children taking steroids may have a normal ESR in the presence of osteomyelitis.

C-reactive protein (CRP) is another acute phase reactant that can be used to diagnose acute hematogenous osteomyelitis. The plasma concentration of CRP can increase several hundredfold within 24 to 48 hours of the onset of infection. CRP levels are elevated in 98% of patients with acute hematogenous osteomyelitis and decline within 6 hours of the initiation of antimicrobial therapy. CRP levels may fall too quickly in patients with osteomyelitis to satisfy criteria for discontinuation of antibiotics.

Blood culture results are positive in only 30% to 36% of patients. Cultures taken directly from bone have a higher positive yield, ranging from 38% to 50%. Antimicrobial therapy should be guided by these results.

Diagnostic Imaging
Plain radiography can detect changes in the bone 7 to 14 days after the onset of infection. Periosteal elevation associated with purulent collections can be observed with radiography. Earlier changes are more subtle. Localized edema may displace muscle planes from the metaphysis and obliterate normal intermuscular fat planes. Untreated osteomyelitis associated with dense sequestered dead bone (Figure 1) and subperiosteal new bone formation can be observed radiographically.

Bone scanning may be more useful for localizing early infection when the physical examination is inconclusive. A whole body bone scan should be obtained to rule out multifocal osteomyelitis and possible malignancy. Technetium Tc 99m (^{99m}Tc) is the most accurate and readily available radioisotope for this purpose (Figure 2). The sensitivity of bone scanning is 89%, the specificity is 94%, and the overall accuracy is 92%. Decreased uptake on bone scanning is associated with devascularization of bone and subperiosteal abscess formation. This cold bone scanning is associated with more

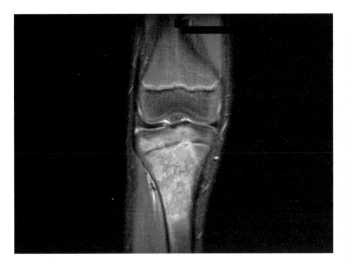

Figure 3 MRI scan demonstrating proximal tibial acute hematogenous osteomyelitis without abscess.

aggressive infection that possibly warrants surgical intervention. Bone scanning, however, carries a false-negative rate of 4% to 20% in early instances of osteomyelitis.

MRI is sensitive but not specific for detecting osteomyelitis as early as 3 to 5 days after disease onset. Edema in the bone marrow and soft tissue is easily visualized using MRI (Figure 3). Gadolinium may help define areas of necrosis. Decreased signal intensity is typically observed on T1-weighted images, and increased signal intensity is typically observed on T2-weighted images. Fracture or bone infarction may be difficult to distinguish from osteomyelitis on MRI scans.

CT and ultrasound may also be useful in the later stages of disease. CT is a quick and readily available diagnostic imaging modality. It can detect focal areas of bony destruction and areas of abscess formation. These changes, however, occur late in the disease course. Similarly, ultrasound can be used to detect a subperiosteal abscess. Sonographic findings include thickening of the periosteum, elevation of the periosteum, and swelling in the underlying muscle. In some patients, ultrasound may guide aspiration. Ultrasound may also be useful in differentiating a septic hip from osteomyelitis of the proximal femur.

Management

Children with suspected osteomyelitis should have the following blood tests performed: complete blood cell count with differential, ESR, CRP, and blood cultures. Radiographs of the involved bone should also be obtained. Bone scanning may help localize the infection. Ultrasound may be considered when infection is localized to the hip region. Hemodynamic status should be evaluated for potential admission to an intensive care unit.

Once the infection is localized, a bone aspiration should be performed. Disease in the spine or deep pelvis may require CT-guided aspiration. If pus is aspirated, the child should be admitted for surgical drainage. In the absence of purulence, the patient should be admitted for intravenous antibiotics and observation.

Staphylococcus aureus is the most common pathogen in acute hematogenous osteomyelitis, representing 60% to 90% of all instances. Other organisms include group A streptococcus and *Streptococcus pneumoniae*. Group B β-hemolytic streptococcus acute hematogenous osteomyelitis is typically associated with neonatal osteomyelitis. With the advent of the *Haemophilus influenzae* B vaccine, this common pathogen has been virtually eliminated as an agent of infection. In children with underlying diseases, more atypical organisms should be considered, such as *Salmonella*.

Parenteral antibiotics are required to prevent dissemination of disease and maximize bacteriocidal levels in the affected bone. Oral route antibiotics are highly dependent on intestinal absorption, renal clearance, and patient compliance. Neonates have poor intestinal absorption of antibiotics. In addition, 10% of infants and children do not respond to oral antibiotics and may need extended parenteral coverage. The preferred antibiotics for empiric *S aureus* coverage are oxacillin and cefazolin (Table 1). Children with allergies to these antibiotics can be covered with clindamycin or vancomycin. Methicillin-resistant *S aureus* (MRSA) is becoming more prevalent in pediatric musculoskeletal infections and poses treatment challenges because of the virulence of its infections. MRSA was first reported in the United States in 1961, 2 years after the introduction of methicillin. Since the late 1990s, US hospital facilities have experienced a steady increase in the number of nosocomial MRSA (N-MRSA) and community-associated MRSA (CA-MRSA) infections. Currently, 3% of all hospitalizations for infections are the result of MRSA. Osteomyelitis and septic arthritis are among the most common invasive infections caused by MRSA. MRSA bone and joint infections are typically more invasive and less responsive to treatment. Longer hospitalization, repeat surgical drainages, slower clinical and laboratory responses (ESR and CRP) to treatment, and complex infection (septic arthritis with associated osteomyelitis and intraosseous or pelvic abscess) can occur with MRSA. Most CA-MRSA organisms are not susceptible to treatment with β-lactam antimicrobials and erythromycin. Furthermore, it is imperative that appropriate antibiotic therapy is administered because delayed use of effective medication may lead to disability and death from severe illnesses such as empyema and necrotizing pneumonia. Obtaining a culture from the infection before initiating treatment is essential to identify possible MRSA infection. In addition, the possibility of MRSA infection should be considered in patients

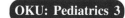
Table 1 | Initial Empiric Antibiotic Therapy for Septic Arthritis and Osteomyelitis

Patient Type	Probable Organism	Initial Antibiotic
Neonates	Group B streptococci, *S aureus*, or gram-negative bacilli	Oxacillin plus gentamicin or oxacillin plus cefotaxime or ceftriaxone (third-generation cephalosporin)
Infants and children younger than 4 years	*S aureus, Streptococcus pneumoniae*, group A streptococci (*Haemophilus influenza* if not vaccinated)	Oxacillin or nafcillin or clindamycin (penicillin resistance is becoming common for *S pneumoniae*) (Ampicillin/clavulanate if *H influenza* suspected)
If allergic to penicillin		Cefazolin
If allergic to penicillin and cephalosporins		Clindamycin or vancomycin
Children older than 4 years	*S aureus* (coagulase positive)	Nafcillin, cefazolin, clindamycin, ceftriaxione
Postoperative and nosicomial infections	MRSA and coagulase negative	Vancomycin (Many community-acquired MRSA infections are susceptible to clindamycin)
Shoe puncture	*Pseudomonas*	Aminoglycocides (gentamicin) and cefepime, cefotaxime, ciprofloxacin (best for adolescents)
Patients with sickle cell disease	*S aureus* or *Salmonella*	Oxacillin and cefotaxime

with osteomyelitis and septic arthritis that does not respond to conventional treatment. CA-MRSA can generally be treated with surgical drainage and/or various non–β-lactam antibiotics, including trimethoprim-sulfamethoxazole, minocycline, fluoroquinolones, vancomycin, linezolid, quinupristin-dalfopristin, and daptomycin. Vancomycin and clindamycin are often used for the treatment of MRSA infections; however, vancomycin should only be used in patients in whom severe infection and erythromycin-resistant MRSA isolates have been shown to induce resistance to clindamycin.

The child should be reevaluated 48 hours after admission. Discharge prerequisites include decreased pain, 24 hours of apyrexia, and improved range of motion. If the child is not improving clinically, MRI should be performed to rule out the presence of an abscess that might require drainage, and cultures should be assessed for appropriate antibiotic coverage.

The duration of treatment is based on the specific isolated organism and clinical response to treatment. A positive response includes a return to normal temperature and pulse, improvement in local symptoms, and an ability to tolerate and be rigorously compliant with oral medications. Cephalexin is the preferred oral agent for *S aureus* infection. Children younger than 5 years are at risk for neutropenia with the use of this agent. Extended treatment with oxacillin and clindamycin can result in elevated liver transaminase levels. The duration of parenteral antibiotics is 5 to 15 days in most patients. Previous studies have suggested that intravenous treatment until normalization of the CRP level and ongoing oral treatment until normalization of the ESR will decrease the duration of intravenous treatment and result

in a low rate of recurrence. The total course of antibiotics is usually 4 to 6 weeks. An evidence-based clinical practice guideline for the management of acute hematogenous osteomyelitis is shown in Figure 4.

Complications
Long-term complications of osteomyelitis include recurrent infection, limb-length discrepancy, joint deformity, and gait abnormality.

Special Circumstances
Neonate
Compared with older children, neonates are at increased risk for osteomyelitis because they have an immature host-defense mechanism and increased exposure to invasive procedures and disease processes in neonatal intensive care units. The humoral immune system of the infant is limited by maternal exposure and transfer of immunoglobulin G. Maternal immunoglobulin G does not cross the placenta until the 32nd week of gestation. Risk factors for neonatal osteomyelitis include prematurity, ventilator dependence, and central line and umbilical catheter placement.

Diagnosis in the neonate is challenging. The neonate will usually present with nonspecific signs. Early signs and symptoms include poor feeding, temperature instability, and limited movement or discomfort with movement. Swelling, erythema, and localized tenderness are late manifestations. Additionally, 40% of patients with osteomyelitis will have multiple sites of infection. White blood cell count, CRP level, and ESR are not always elevated in the neonate. MRI and bone aspiration can aid in confirming the diagnosis. *S aureus* is the most com-

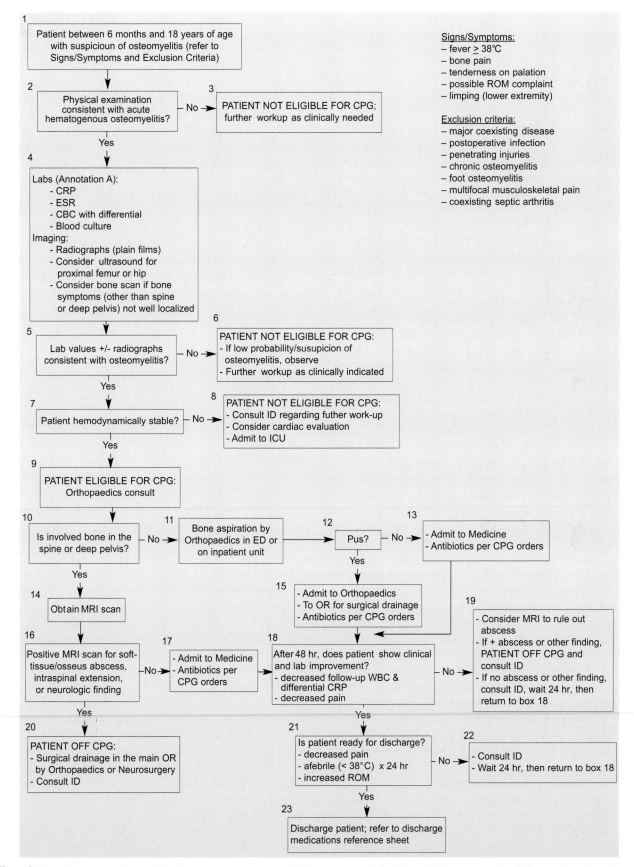

Signs/Symptoms:
– fever ≥ 38°C
– bone pain
– tenderness on palation
– possible ROM complaint
– limping (lower extremity)

Exclusion criteria:
– major coexisting disease
– postoperative infection
– penetrating injuries
– chronic osteomyelitis
– foot osteomyelitis
– multifocal musculoskeletal pain
– coexisting septic arthritis

Figure 4 Clinical practice guidelines (CPG) for the management of acute hematogenous osteomyelitis in children. ROM = range of motion, CBC = complete blood cell count, ID = Infectious Diseases, ICU = intensive care unit, ED = emergency department, WBC = white blood cell count, OR = operating room. *(Copyright © 2002 by Children's Hospital, Boston, MA. Used with permission.)*

mon organism involved in neonatal osteomyelitis, followed by group B β-hemolytic streptococcus, gram-negative organisms, and *Candida albicans*.

Neonates have poor absorption of oral antibiotics. They require a full 4 to 6 weeks of parenteral antibiotics. CRP levels decline quickly in neonates and may be a poor determinate of duration of treatment.

Osteomyelitis in the neonate can be devastating. The shared blood supply of the metaphysis and epiphysis allows infection to cross the physis. This can lead to physeal and epiphyseal damage. Neonates also have substantially thinner cortex and more loosely adherent periosteum, which allow infection to track into the neighboring joints.

Chronic Recurrent Multifocal Osteomyelitis

Chronic recurrent multifocal osteomyelitis is an inflammatory disease of bone. It is characterized by an unpredictable course of exacerbations and spontaneous remissions in multiple sites. In one series, the median number of affected bony sites was four. No causative agent has been found for this illness. This disease affects primarily young girls, with a peak age of onset of 10 years.

The typical features of chronic recurrent multifocal osteomyelitis include local bone pain of gradual onset, multifocal lesions (especially in the long tubular bones, spine, and bones of the foot), inability to culture an infectious agent, and improvement with nonsteroidal anti-inflammatory drugs. Unlike acute hematogenous osteomyelitis, which is characterized by high fevers and leukocytosis, chronic recurrent multifocal osteomyelitis is characterized by a slow onset, low-grade fever, and normal white blood cell count.

Imaging of this condition with radiography demonstrates nonspecific findings such as osteolysis, sclerosis, and new bone formation. These features can mimic osteomyelitis and neoplasms such as Ewing's sarcoma and Langerhans' cell histiocytosis. Multifocal disease can be demonstrated with bone scanning.

The disease course generally runs longer than 6 months with intermittent relapses. Patients with chronic recurrent multifocal osteomyelitis typically show no response to antibiotic therapy. Nonsteroidal anti-inflammatory agents have been used to treat symptoms. Although symptoms can occur into adulthood, most resolve over time. In some patients, a limb-length inequality may result, requiring surgical intervention.

Subacute and Chronic Osteomyelitis

As the infecting organism becomes less virulent and the host resistance increases, subacute osteomyelitis occurs. Subacute osteomyelitis usually passes unnoticed in its early stages. Patients generally respond well to antibiotic treatment. Almost all instances of subacute osteomyelitis are caused by *S aureus*, although streptococcal infections have been reported. Surgery should be re-

served for patients who fail to respond to conservative treatment. All children with suspected subacute osteomyelitis should be ruled out for the presence of a tumor.

In contrast to subacute osteomyelitis, chronic osteomyelitis often requires several surgical procedures and long-term antibiotics. The hallmark of chronic osteomyelitis is bone necrosis. A focal area of necrosis and suppuration may become walled off by granulation tissue forming a Brodie's abscess. Plain radiographs typically reveal extensive bone destruction and new bone formation.

Children with chronic osteomyelitis usually have a history of slow, insidious onset of symptoms such as pain, swelling, and limping. The diagnosis is rarely confirmed by laboratory tests. Histologic confirmation may be required to make the diagnosis.

Antibiotic courses may require 3 to 6 months to be effective. In one series, an average of 3.2 procedures per patient were required. Extensive defects may have to be reconstructed with vascularized bone. Large tibial defects can also be treated by Ilizarov distraction osteogenesis. Recurrence can occur within 2 years in 20% to 30% of patients treated with surgical débridement and antibiotics. If treatment fails, long-term suppressive therapy can be initiated. Hyperbaric oxygen therapy may also play a role in the treatment of chronic osteomyelitis.

Septic Arthritis

True septic arthritis in a child constitutes a surgical emergency. Prompt recognition, diagnosis, and treatment of this entity are essential. Bacterial infection of the joint space results in an inflammatory effusion consisting of up to 90% polymorphonuclear cells. The release of proteolytic enzymes by polymorphonuclear cells and bacteria, in conjunction with increased intra-articular pressure, can result in rapid and irreversible hyaline cartilage degradation in as little as 6 hours in animal studies. If unrecognized or left untreated, this process can result in joint destruction with subsequent severe deformity and devastating lifelong disability. Joint infections can ultimately lead to disseminated infection, systemic bacterial sepsis, multiorgan failure, and death. However, if recognized and treated in a timely fashion with surgical drainage and appropriate antimicrobial therapy, a good outcome with minimal sequelae can be expected. Poor outcomes are most closely associated with a delay in diagnosis. Other factors related to poor outcome include patients younger than 6 months, prematurity, *Staphylococcus* infection, and concomitant osteomyelitis.

Septic arthritis most commonly involves the large joints (hip: 35%; knee: 35%; ankle: 10%; and wrist, elbow, and shoulder: 15% of patients), but it can be seen in small joints as well (2% of patients). The presentation can be only that of a painful, swollen joint and may mimic that of other conditions. The differential diagnosis for septic arthritis includes culture-negative septic arthritis (gonococcal), osteomyelitis, chondrolysis, Lyme disease, viral arthritis, tuberculosis, toxic (or transient) synovitis, poststreptococcal arthritis (acute rheumatic fever), postgastroenteritis arthritis, Reiter syndrome, hepatitis B-associated arthritis, inflammatory bowel disease–associated arthritis, Henoch-Schönlein purpura, hemophilia, sickle cell disease, serum sickness, juvenile arthritis, leukemia, and villonodular synovitis. Reactive arthritis can be seen in association with a bacterial or viral infection and must be differentiated from septic arthritis. Reactive arthritis has been described in association with infection by *Borrelia burgdorferi, Chlamydia, Yersinia, Salmonella, Shigella, Mycoplasma,* and *Campylobacter,* as well as viral infection with hepatitis A and B, human immunodeficiency virus (HIV), mumps, parvovirus B-19, enterovirus, and herpesvirus.

When evaluating the acutely irritable hip, fracture, slipped capital femoral epiphysis, psoas abscess, pyogenic sacroiliitis, and Legg-Calvé-Perthes disease must be ruled out. The differentiation between septic arthritis and transient synovitis is critical and can be difficult based on history and physical examination alone. Transient synovitis is a benign, self-limited, postinfectious, aseptic reactive synovitis that does not require treatment. It frequently occurs in the hip. However, its presentation can be similar to that of septic arthritis, with an acutely irritable hip, inability or refusal to bear weight, fever, limited joint motion, and abnormal serologic markers. Four clinical predictors have been used to assist in the differentiation of these two entities: history of fever greater than 38.5°C, inability to bear weight, ESR greater than 40 mm/h, and white blood cell count greater than 12,000/μL. In one study, the presence of three of four factors was 93.1% predictive of septic arthritis, whereas the presence of all four factors was 99.6% predictive. The predicted probability of septic arthritis using this algorithm has been reported to range from 59% to 99.6%, depending on the study population. These predictors, when used in conjunction with clinical judgment, can be a useful adjunct to the treatment algorithm.

Etiology and Microbiology
Septic arthritis may occur as a result of hematogenous seeding, local spread from a contiguous infection, or primary seeding of a joint secondary to surgery or trauma. In the hip, shoulder, ankle, and elbow (90% of patients), septic arthritis often occurs after metaphyseal osteomyelitis with subperiosteal erosion, abscess formation, and subsequent joint communication (because of the intra-articular location of the metaphyses in these joints). Premature and immunocompromised children are at greater risk. The most commonly identified infecting organisms are *S aureus* (56%), group A streptococci

(22%), *S pneumoniae* (6%), other gram-negative organisms (which may be seen in special hosts or after trauma: *Klebsielleae, Salmonellae, Kingella*), and *Neisseria gonorrhoeae*. Before the advent of an effective vaccine, *H influenzae* B was responsible for up to 40% of instances of septic arthritic, but this incidence has significantly declined because of successful immunization programs. In the neonate, group B β-hemolytic streptococcus and gram-negative bacilli are common infecting agents in addition to *S aureus*. Gram-negative infections are common among intravenous drug abusers. Mycobacteria and fungi must be considered in patients with chronic infections.

Presentation
Children with septic arthritis will often have a history of recent upper respiratory or local soft-tissue infection, as well as a recent course of antibiotics. A high level of suspicion is important when evaluating premature and immunocompromised infants. Septic arthritis is more commonly seen in boys and is most common in children younger than 2 years. Patients may report pain, stiffness, and malaise, but such a history is often impossible to obtain from small children or infants. Fever, a limp, inability or refusal to bear weight, limited and painful range of motion (secondary to capsular stretching), erythema, warmth, tenderness, and swelling are common physical findings. If the hip is involved, the child may report anterior hip, groin, thigh, or knee pain. The child may lie with the hip in external rotation, adduction, and mild flexion to maximize joint volume and decrease capsular stretch. Physical examination of the infant can be challenging and may only demonstrate limited or a lack of active motion in the affected extremity (pseudoparalysis). In general, children with septic arthritis appear more ill than those with osteomyelitis or transient synovitis, with fever, chills, inability to bear weight, an elevated ESR, leukocytosis, reduced hematocrit, and an altered peripheral blood differential.

Laboratory Tests
The currently recommended laboratory workup for septic arthritis includes serum CRP level, ESR, complete blood cell count with differential, blood cultures, throat culture/rapid strep test, and antistreptolysin O titer Lyme disease titers are often added in endemic areas. Blood cultures are positive in 30% to 36% of patients. An infectious organism is identified in 50% to 70% of patients. White blood cell count may be elevated in only 30% to 60% of patients. A left shift is seen in 60% of patients with an elevated white blood cell count. ESR is a more sensitive marker of infection, but it lacks specificity. The ESR is frequently normal when the diagnosis of septic arthritis is established and will frequently rise in the first few days as clinical improvement occurs. The

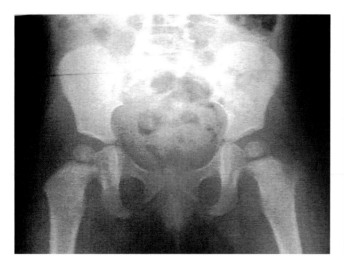

Figure 5 AP pelvis radiograph demonstrating left hip widening from septic arthritis.

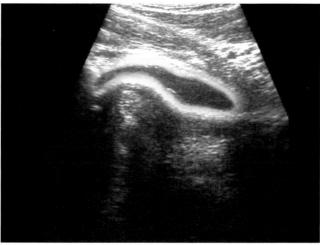

Figure 6 Hip ultrasound demonstrating the presence of effusion.

ESR peaks at day 4 or 5, does not decrease significantly until after approximately day 10, and is of limited utility in monitoring disease resolution. CRP level is probably the most useful marker for monitoring disease progression and response to therapy, and it is a better independent predictor of disease. Adequate treatment results in normalization of CRP level to less than 20 mg/L in 7 days and ESR to less than 25 mm/hr within 3 weeks.

Imaging

Plain radiographs should be obtained for every patient to exclude periarticular bony pathology. Radiographs are usually normal, but they may demonstrate joint space widening, suggesting the presence of an effusion (Figure 5). There may also be evidence of soft-tissue swelling and obliteration of normal fat planes. Joint distention may result in subluxation or even dislocation. Bone destruction can be observed with ongoing infection after 7 to 14 days.

Ultrasound remains the first-line imaging study for the diagnosis of septic arthritis of the hip. Sonography of the hip is an easy, noninvasive technique for detecting joint effusion (Figure 6). If an effusion is present, the fluid should be aspirated under sonographic guidance. The sonographic characteristics of the fluid (clear versus echogenic) do not correlate with the likelihood of infection. Aspiration of other joints can usually be done without imaging guidance. If necessary, guidance in children younger than 8 years is best done with ultrasound because sonography can show cartilaginous structures. In children older than 8 years, fluoroscopy is preferred for guidance of the aspiration. If the patient fails to respond to appropriate antibiotic therapy in 48 hours, MRI should be considered to identify associated osteomyelitis abscess. MRI can demonstrate joint effusion, local abscess, and associated osteomyelitis. CT and bone scanning have a limited role in the diagnosis of septic arthri-

tis. Bone scanning may be useful in locating an infection in the pelvis, hip, ankle, shoulder, foot, and ankle, where the location of the infection can be difficult to identify, or in the neonate with multiple foci of infection.

Aspiration

When clinical, laboratory, and imaging findings suggest septic arthritis, the joint should be aspirated. If no fluid is obtained, arthrography should be performed to confirm intra-articular positioning of the needle. The aspirate should be sent for complete blood cell count with differential, culture (aerobic, anaerobic, and acid-fast bacilli), and Gram stain. A white blood cell count greater than 50,000/µL or a positive Gram stain suggests the presence of septic arthritis and an indication for surgical drainage and initiation of empiric intravenous antibiotic therapy. A white blood cell count of 25,000 to 50,000/µL (with gram-negative stain) suggests the possible presence of septic arthritis, but the probable presence of synovitis. If clinical suspicion remains high, surgical drainage is indicated. A white blood cell count of less than 25,000/µL suggests a reactive arthritis or synovitis, and rheumatology consultation is indicated. Aspirate cultures are positive in 54% to 68% of patients with septic arthritis, and Gram stain is positive in 30% to 50% of patients. Other markers that are suggestive of septic arthritis include a fluid-serum glucose ratio of less than 0.5, increased synovial lactate, and a positive mucin clot test. If gout or pseudogout is suspected in older children, the aspirate should be analyzed for the presence of intracellular crystals.

Treatment

Poor outcome is most closely associated with a delay in diagnosis and subsequent delay in treatment. Once septic arthritis is diagnosed, prompt treatment with adequate surgical drainage and empiric intravenous antimicrobial therapy is essential. Ideally, synovial and blood cultures are obtained before treatment to increase the likelihood of identifying an infecting organism. Open surgical irrigation and débridement to remove the microorganisms, host and bacterial enzymes, and particulate debris is indicated for most patients. However, arthroscopy has been used successfully in the shoulder, elbow, knee, and ankle, but it has not been widely used in the hip. The efficacy of arthroscopic drainage versus open drainage remains unknown. Some authors have reported good results using repeated ultrasound-guided aspirations to treat septic arthritis of the hip joint. Open drainage via an anterolateral or medial approach remains the treatment of choice for septic arthritis of the hip in small children and infants. The posterior approach should be avoided because of concerns about the vascularity of the femoral head.

Empiric intravenous antimicrobial therapy should be initiated as soon as cultures are obtained. Empiric coverage must include an antistaphylococcal agent, either a β-lactamase–resistant penicillin or a first-generation cephalosporin. Cefazolin is recommended for initial empiric therapy because it is effective against *S aureus,* group A streptococcus, and *S pneumoniae*, which should account for nearly all of the infecting organisms in normal hosts with acute hematogenous osteomyelitis. Gram-negative coverage is indicated in the neonate (infecting organisms may also include group B streptococci and gram-negative bacilli) and adolescents (to cover *Gonococcus*). In children who are allergic to penicillin, clindamycin can be used. Ceftriaxone should be considered for coverage of gonococcal arthritis. The antimicrobial regimen is adjusted according to culture speciation; if another organism is identified as the infecting agent, an infectious disease consultation should be sought. Intravenous antibiotics should be continued for 72 hours. If the child shows evidence of clinical improvement (afebrile, decreased localized swelling, decreased/no pain, and increased range of motion) and Lyme disease titers are negative, conversion to oral antibiotics can be considered. The criteria for the use of oral antibiotics include diagnosis within 4 days of the onset of symptoms, no concurrent osteomyelitis, and an ability to tolerate and be rigorously compliant with taking oral antibiotics. Patients treated with cefazolin may be given cephalexin (100 mg/kg/day) divided into four daily doses (maximum dose, 4 g/day), and those treated with ceftriaxone can receive cefixime 8 mg/kg/day every 12 to 24 hours (maximum dose, 400 mg/day) for 21 days. The median duration of intravenous antibiotics is 5 to 15 days, and the total duration of antibiotics has been reported to be 4 to 6 weeks for uncomplicated infections. Physical therapy may be initiated as needed on day 2. Evidence-based clinical practice guidelines for the management of children with septic arthritis are shown in Figure 7.

Other Infections

Diskitis and Vertebral Osteomyelitis

Intervertebral disk infection (diskitis) is uncommon in children. When it does occur in children, it occurs in the lumbar region of those younger than 5 years. This infection begins at the end plates and communicates through vascular channels to the disk space. Younger children are thought to be more susceptible to diskitis because their disks have a rich arterial blood supply that is derived from the vertebral body. In older children, this blood supply is limited.

Children typically present with refusal to walk or a progressive limp. Classically, the younger child will attempt to walk bending forward with the hands on the thighs for support. A low-grade fever may accompany this presentation. This diagnosis may be challenging because of limited physical findings and lack of obvious radiographic abnormalities early in the course of the disease. The hallmark radiographic findings of disk-space narrowing associated with end-plate changes may not be present for 2 to 3 weeks. Increased uptake can be observed using ^{99m}Tc bone scanning. MRI may be useful to assess the disk and two adjacent vertebral bodies for spread of infection. Paravertebral abscesses and spinal cord involvement can also be visualized with MRI.

Most patients with diskitis can be successfully treated with antibiotics. Empiric treatment of *S aureus* is typically initiated. A biopsy is required for atypical patients or when there is a poor response to the antibiotic regimen. Long-term sequelae are rare, but they can include intervertebral fusion, disk-space narrowing, and chronic backache.

Vertebral osteomyelitis typically occurs in older children. They present with back pain in the lumbar, thoracic, or cervical spine. Focal tenderness may be elicited with percussion of the spine. In comparison with children with diskitis, children with vertebral osteomyelitis are more febrile and appear more ill. Osteomyelitis can be detected histologically by obtaining a biopsy specimen of the suspected region. Radiographs may demonstrate rarification of the vertebral body early in the disease process. Bony destruction, usually in the anterior vertebral body, is typically evident in the later stages. Most patients respond well to antibiotics covering *S aureus*. More unusual forms of vertebral osteomyelitis can be caused by *Bartonella henselae* infection (cat-scratch disease).

Human Immunodeficiency Virus Infection

Perinatal transmission is now responsible for a large population of younger children infected with human immunodeficiency virus (HIV). The virus can be transmitted through the intrauterine environment, during delivery, or through breast feeding. Antiretroviral treatment with zidovudine or azidothymidine can significantly de-

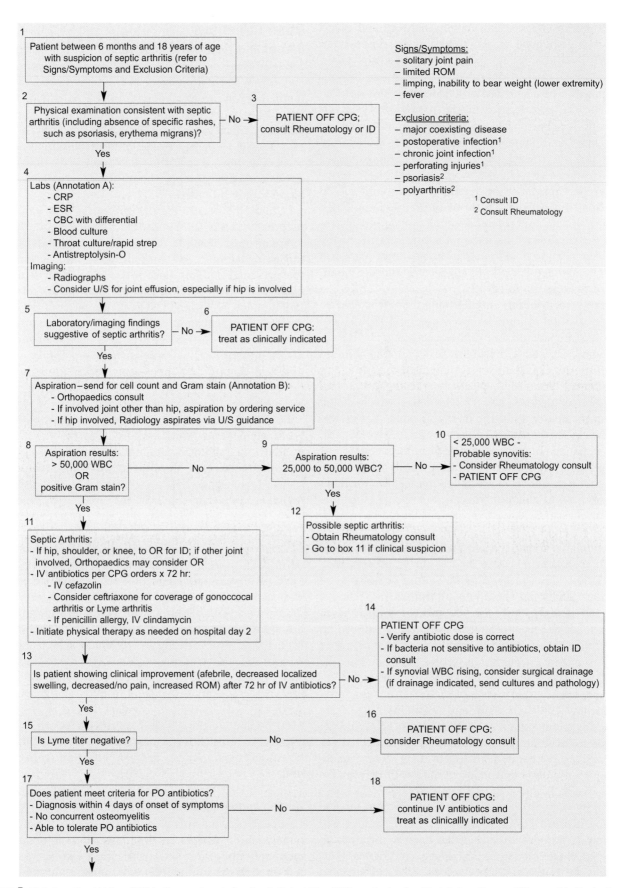

Figure 7 Clinical practice guidelines (CPG) for the management of septic arthritis in children. ROM = range of motion, ID = Infectious Diseases, CBC = complete blood cell count, U/S = ultrasound, OR = operating room, IV = intravenous, PO = oral, WBC = white blood cell count. *(Copyright © 2004 by Children's Hospital, Boston, MA. Used with permission.)*

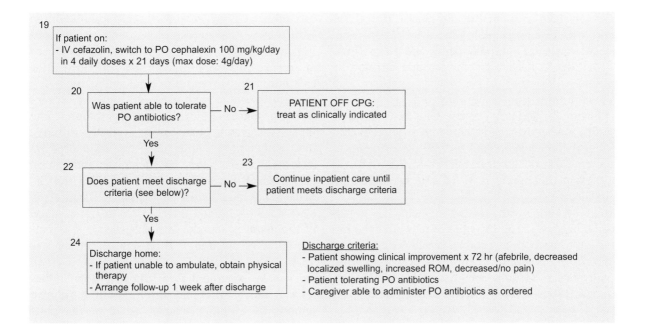

crease the rate of transmission from mother to child.

The virus binds to cells expressing CD4 surface molecules, mainly CD4 lymphocytes. In the immunodeficient state, children are more susceptible to infections such as osteomyelitis and septic arthritis. Central nervous system cells such as microglia, astrocytes, and oligodendrocytes can also be affected. HIV encephalopathy can develop that is either progressive or static. Static encephalopathy can demonstrate many features of cerebral palsy, including muscle imbalance and contractures. In addition, linear growth retardation has been correlated with the level of postnatal HIV viremia. The mechanism is unclear at the present time.

Iliopsoas Abscess

Acute pyogenic abscess of the iliopsoas should be considered in the differential diagnosis for septic arthritis of the hip, osteomyelitis, or appendicitis. Patients with iliopsoas abscesses may present with pain or a mass in the iliac fossa or central abdomen. Pain and flexion deformity of the hip, a limp, and fever may also be present. Unlike other hip infections, passive rotation is usually possible in patients with these abscesses. This diagnosis can be confirmed with ultrasound or CT (Figure 8). Image-guided percutaneous drainage has replaced surgical intervention as treatment for children with iliopsoas abscesses.

Lyme Disease

Lyme disease is a multisystem disease caused by the spirochete *B burgdorferi*. This spirochete is transmitted to humans through the bite of the infected *Ixodes* tick. The disease is most commonly seen in the northeast United States, although it has been reported to occur through-

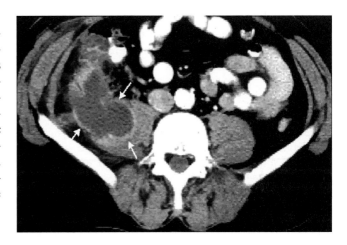

Figure 8 CT scan demonstrating right iliopsoas abscess (arrows).

out the country. This transmission primarily occurs during the months of May through August. Recommendations for avoiding tick bites include wearing long-sleeved shirts tucked into pants and long, light-colored pants tucked into socks or boots. Transmission is thought to occur with tick attachment of more than 24 hours; therefore, removal of the tick may prevent disease.

A characteristic skin lesion, erythema migrans, is present within 3 to 30 days after the tick bite. The erythema migrans lesion is flat, has an erythematous to purplish hue, is warm to the touch, and has a bulls-eye appearance. Many patients are asymptomatic at this stage and only seek medical attention when they experience more disseminated infection. Fever, headache, malaise, arthralgias, and multiple secondary skin lesions may also develop. Untreated Lyme disease can lead to cardiac involvement (atrioventricular block), arthralgias, and neurologic disease (neuropathies). Late manifestations include arthritis, encephalopathy, and polyneuropathies. The knee is the most common joint affected by this arthritis.

Oral antibiotics can successfully treat 90% of infected individuals. The usual course lasts 21 to 28 days. Doxycycline is effective, but it should be avoided in children younger than 8 years and in lactating women; cefuroxime and amoxicillin are effective in these groups. At the present time, there is no vaccine manufactured for Lyme disease.

Further workup with immunoglobulin G anti-*B burgdorferi* antibody requires 4 to 6 weeks after the initial infection to become detectable. Serologic testing can help confirm the diagnosis in the presence of arthritis, neuropathy, or cardiac abnormalities; there is little role for serologic testing early in the course of Lyme disease.

Pyomyositis

Pyomyositis is a primary bacterial infection of skeletal muscle in which the initial clinical features are fever, localized muscle pain and stiffness, swelling, and tenderness. This entity has been described previously in tropical regions. Recent studies, however, indicate that pyomyositis may be more common in temperate climates than previously reported.

Bacterial pyomyositis typically presents in three stages. In the first stage, known as the invasive stage, the patient may have fever, local swelling, mild pain, and minimal tenderness. The muscle itself may have a wooden consistency. These symptoms are frequently ignored by the patient. Because the infection is contained by the overlying fascia, local erythema or heat may be minimal until the infection extends to the subcutaneous tissues. The second stage develops 10 to 21 days later, when the patient experiences distinct muscle tenderness and swelling. This stage, known as the purulent stage, is the most common stage for presentation in temperate climates. The skin is warm but usually not erythematous. The patient is typically febrile. Pus can sometimes be aspirated from the muscle at this point. The last stage of pyomyositis is marked by systemic signs of sepsis and local erythema, extreme tenderness, and fluctuance. The untreated patient may develop metastatic abscesses, shock, and renal failure.

In pyomyositis, laboratory blood testing typically demonstrates a leukocytosis. Eosinophilia is indicative of a parasitic infection. The ESR and CRP level are usually elevated. Muscle destruction can be detected by elevations in serum muscle enzymes. Rhabdomyolysis with myoglobinuria can occur in later stages of the disease.

S aureus is involved in 95% of skeletal muscle infections. Other bacterial species include *Streptococcus pyogenes*, *S pneumoniae*, and gram-negative organisms such as *Escherichia coli*. Adenoviruses, parainfluenza viruses, *H influenzae*, and coxsackievirus have also been isolated in muscle infection. Viral myositis is usually preceded by an upper respiratory infection and primarily affects the calf muscles, preventing normal ambulation. It is frequently associated with markedly elevated serum creatinine phosphokinase without myoglobinuria. The viral illness resolves spontaneously, typically within several days. Other muscle infections may be caused by *Candida* species, toxoplasmosis, trichinosis, and cysticercosis.

Although several imaging modalities can be used, MRI is the modality of choice in the diagnosis of pyomyositis. T1-weighted images demonstrate enlargement of the involved muscle, with an increase in signal intensity in the involved area. High-signal intensity is seen on T2-weighted sequences in the affected muscles. This signal can be separated from the low-signal intensity of normal muscle. MRI may also be useful in ruling out osteomyelitis of the proximal femur or the pelvis, hematoma, soft-tissue tumor, and septic arthritis.

In the early stage of pyogenic disease, antibiotics alone are usually effective. The preferred antibiotic is a penicillinase-resistant penicillin, such as nafcillin or oxacillin. Clindamycin can be used for patients with penicillin allergies. Intravenous antibiotics are initiated and continued until there is evidence of clinical improvement, at which time, oral or parenteral antibiotics are typically administered for 2 to 6 weeks.

Septic arthritis of the hip can be easily mistaken for pyomyositis of the pelvis. In contrast to patients with septic arthritis, patients with pyomyositis have minimal pain with internal and external rotation of the hip.

SAPHO Syndrome

The synovitis, acne, pustulosis, hyperostosis, and osteitis (SAPHO) syndrome is a rare and poorly understood entity that most frequently occurs in Japanese and European children. Dermatologic involvement can be severe, although musculoskeletal symptoms often precede the cutaneous findings and may be the primary symptoms. Patients may report bone and joint pain, which is thought to be related to hyperostosis, aseptic osteomyelitis, or synovitis. In adults, this most commonly presents with osteitis of the sternum, medial clavicle, and anterior portions of the ribs. In children, hyperostosis of the long bones occurs more frequently and may mimic chronic recurrent multifocal osteomyelitis. These patients may report long bone pain and have swelling and tenderness. The clinical findings can often mimic those of bacterial osteomyelitis or septic arthritis. Generalized signs of musculoskeletal inflammation may occur, including arthralgias, synovitis, enthesitis, and tenosynovitis. The etiology and pathophysiology of this condition are unknown. Some studies have suggested a link to infection with the organism *Propionibacterium acnes*, but

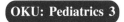

this has yet to be proved. It has also been suggested that the SAPHO syndrome might represent a seronegative spondyloarthropathy. Treatment is generally supportive with analgesics and nonsteroidal anti-inflammatory medications. Antibiotics are ineffective and are not recommended for the SAPHO syndrome.

Sickle Cell Anemia

It is well established that patients with sickle cell anemia are at an increased risk for infections with polysaccharide encapsulated organisms. Osteomyelitis, although uncommon, occurs more frequently in patients with sickle cell anemia than in the general population. This is thought to be because of the presence of bone infarctions, sluggish circulation, and impaired opsonization secondary to hypoasplenia or asplenia. Osteomyelitis is often characteristically seen in the diaphysis of long bones, in addition to the usual metaphyseal location. *Salmonella* infection is the most characteristic of sickle cell disease, but *S aureus* remains the most common infecting organism. It has been reported that 75% of osteoarticular infections (septic arthritis and osteomyelitis) in patients with sickle cell disease can be attributed to *S aureus*, but *Salmonella* is responsible for 60% to 80% of the instances of osteomyelitis.

Osteomyelitis can be difficult to diagnosis in this population and must be differentiated from bone infarctions, which can have a similar clinical and radiographic appearance. Infarction, however, is far more common than infection (50 times higher in some studies). Common physical findings can include fever, swelling, pain, tenderness, warmth, and erythema. White blood cell count and ESR are often elevated in both conditions. Radiographs are often nonspecific, revealing soft-tissue swelling and periosteal reaction. Bone scanning is a sensitive study, but lacks the specificity to differentiate these two entities. Ultrasound can be useful in detecting subperiosteal abscesses. MRI can also be useful in identifying abscesses, but it also lacks specificity. Positive blood cultures and aspiration of purulent material typically confirm the diagnosis of osteomyelitis.

When the diagnosis of osteomyelitis is established, prompt drainage of any abscesses and 6 to 8 weeks of intravenous antibiotics are recommended. Patients typically require a prolonged period of antibiotic therapy secondary to poor bone circulation and an impaired immune status. The usual surgical precautions for sickle cell disease should be undertaken, including exchange transfusion to maintain hemoglobin A levels above 60%, avoidance of tourniquets, and aggressive preoperative hydration.

Tuberculosis

A resurgence of skeletal tuberculosis has occurred in recent years that has been attributed to HIV/acquired immune deficiency syndrome, the emergence of multidrug-resistant strains, increased rates of homelessness, intravenous drug abuse, and reduced emphasis on tuberculosis control programs. Tuberculosis infection can result in osseous or synovial involvement. The causative agents are usually *Mycobacterium tuberculosis*, *M africanum*, or *M bovis*. Extrapulmonary and skeletal tuberculosis are more common among children than adults and characteristically involve the osseous portion of the vertebrae in 50% of patients or the synovium of large joints in 25% of patients. Although less common, solitary osseous lesions and osteomyelitis of the long bones do occur (11% of patients). Clinical presentation may include malaise, pain, fever, night sweats, and weight loss. Spinal involvement can result in significant kyphosis, rigidity, muscle spasm, and focal neurologic deficits. Isolated osseous lesions without pulmonary involvement now more commonly occur (in 50% of patients), and the clinical presentation can be subtle. There are no pathognomonic radiographic characteristics of tuberculosis. These lesions typically involve the metaphyseal regions and can cross the physis of long bones. Radiographs may demonstrate cystic or infiltrative lesions, focal erosions, or spina ventosa (short bone filled with air). Lesions are most commonly radiolucent with marginal sclerosis, round to oval, metaphyseal, and may mimic various benign bone tumors. Other lesions may be more infiltrative and resemble pyogenic osteomyelitis. Lesions are occasionally expansile, resulting in cyst-like, fusiform spina ventosa. Biopsy with histology and culture for acid-fast bacilli is necessary for definitive diagnosis. Wounds should not be left open because sinus tracts that are difficult to close are likely to form. A positive tuberculin purified protein derivative skin test and a chest radiograph demonstrating a Ghon focus is supportive of the diagnosis. The ESR can be normal and the tuberculin purified protein derivative skin test can be negative, but this does not rule out tuberculosis. Treatment is determined by the size and location of the lesion and local demographics of organism drug resistance. Multidrug antitubercular chemotherapeutics are generally required for at least 1 year. A combination of isoniazid, rifampin, pyrazinamide, and ethambutol is most commonly used. Curettage and débridement, usually without bone grafting, is recommended for appendicular lesions. Kyphosis will often improve after adequate medical treatment, but spinal lesions will sometimes require local débridement and stabilization with instrumentation. This most commonly involves the Hong Kong procedure, which involves débridement of the infected bone, decompression of the spinal canal, and correction of the kyphotic deformity using structural grafting. Posterior fusion with instrumentation may be required.

Varicella

Varicella (chicken pox) is usually a self-limiting viral infection. Musculoskeletal manifestations are uncommon. Arthralgia and aseptic arthritis can be seen, but these symptoms generally resolve spontaneously in 72 hours. Soft-tissue infections can be serious and can include necrotizing fasciitis, deep abscess, and toxic shock syndrome, resulting in multiple limb amputations and even death. Secondary bacterial superinfection with resultant septic arthritis or osteomyelitis, although rare, has been described. Fewer than 20 instances of secondary septic arthritis caused by varicella have been reported in the English-language medical literature. The large joints (hip, knee, and ankle) are most commonly involved, but small joint infections have also been reported. The causative agents are most commonly group A β-hemolytic streptococcus and *S aureus*. Superinfection is more common in the immunocompromised patient or those being treated for tumors. Presentation, diagnosis, and treatment are similar to that for septic arthritis and osteomyelitis as outlined previously.

Puncture Wounds

Traumatic wounds to the foot are common in the pediatric population and are often caused by puncture sustained on the plantar surface of the foot after stepping on a sharp object. The classic scenario is that of a child who steps on a rusty nail through a tennis sneaker. These injuries frequently result in soft-tissue or osseous infection. Complications can include pain from a retained foreign body, cellulitis, soft-tissue abscess, metatarsal growth arrest secondary to chronic osteomyelitis, and acute osteomyelitis and intraosseous abscess formation. Obtaining a thorough medical history is essential to evaluate potential sources of infection and to rule out the possibility of a retained foreign body. In the acute setting, plain radiography is indicated to rule out fracture and foreign body retention. Bone scanning or MRI is useful in patients with chronic infection to rule out osteomyelitis and/or abscess. Surgical débridement and intravenous antibiotics are sometimes necessary. *S aureus* is the most common infecting organism. When injury through a sneaker has occurred, *Pseudomonas* infection is most characteristic. Coverage of both of these organisms is recommended. Tetanus immunization status should be determined and prophylaxis instituted when indicated.

Gonococcal Arthritis

Gonococcal arthritis is an infection caused by the organism *N gonorrhoeae*. It is typically characterized by migratory polyarthralgias, rash, and tenosynovitis. In true arthritis, the knee is most commonly involved. Gonococcal infection can occur in sexually active adolescents and sexually abused children and can be transmitted to neonates from their mothers during birth. Diagnosis is confirmed by culture; however, cultures are often negative and must be grown under specific conditions. Gonococcal arthritis is sometimes referred to as culture-negative septic arthritis. Cultures of the blood, synovium, pharynx, genitourinary tract, rectum, and skin lesions should be obtained before initiation of antibiotics. Treatment with penicillin is usually effective, but because resistance has become more common, initial treatment with a third-generation cephalosporin (ceftriaxone) is recommended. Intravenous antibiotic therapy is recommended until clinical improvement occurs, after which oral or intramuscular antibiotics can be administered for a total 7-day course. Unlike other types of septic arthritis, emergent surgical irrigation and débridement is usually not necessary. Open drainage is indicated in the septic hip, but serial aspiration is usually adequate for recurrent effusion in other joints. As a rule, antimicrobial therapy should be initiated and serial aspiration performed as needed. Most patients do well with minimal articular sequelae.

Annotated Bibliography

Osteomyelitis

Duffy CM, Lam PY, Ditchfield M, Allen R, Graham HK: Chronic recurrent multifocal osteomyelitis: Review of orthopaedic complications at maturity. *J Pediatr Orthop* 2002;22:501-505.

Twelve children with chronic recurrent multifocal osteomyelitis were followed for long-term orthopaedic complications. The number of sites affected was 2 to 9 (most commonly the ankle, knee, and clavicle). Five children had leg-length inequalities of at least 1.5 cm. One patient underwent a limb-lengthening procedure.

Gonzalez-Lopez JL, Soleto-Martin FJ, Cubillo-Martin A, et al: Subacute osteomyelitis in children. *J Pediatr Orthop B* 2001;10:101-104.

The authors reviewed 21 instances of subacute osteomyelitis in children. Eleven patients required surgery. Complete healing was achieved in all but one child. Normal growth was seen in all patients. The authors concluded that surgery should be reserved for patients with diagnostic doubts or in those who do not respond favorably to antibiotics.

Hammond PJ, Macnicol MF: Osteomyelitis of the pelvis and proximal femur: Diagnostic difficulties. *J Pediatr Orthop B* 2001;10:113-119.

The authors of this study diagnosed periacetabular infection in 16 children, and radiographs of the pelvis were rarely abnormal within 7 days of the infection. Diagnosis was confirmed with bone scanning and MRI. Only one patient underwent surgery for drainage of an associated septic arthritis. At final follow-up, none of the patients had recurrence or growth asymmetry.

Ibia EO, Imoisili M, Pikis A: Group A beta-hemolytic streptococcal osteomyelitis in children. *Pediatrics* 2003;112(1 Pt 1):e22-26.

In this study, 29 children with group A β-hemolytic *Streptococcus* osteomyelitis were compared with a matched cohort of children with *S pneumoniae* and *S aureus*. Children with group A β-hemolytic *Streptococcus* presented with a marked fever and leukocytosis compared with the other two groups. The authors reported that varicella infection was also associated with group A β-hemolytic *Streptococcus*.

Yeargan SA, Nakasone CK, Shaieb MD, et al: Treatment of chronic osteomyelitis in children resistant to previous therapy. *J Pediatr Orthop* 2004;24:109-122.

In this study, 30 patients with chronic osteomyelitis were reviewed. At an average 2.3-year follow-up, an average of 3.2 procedures per patient was reported. The hospital stay ranged from 2 weeks to 18 months (average, 4.7 months). A good outcome was seen in 80% of patients. Large tibial defects were successfully treated with Ilizarov distraction osteogenesis and tibiofibular synostosis.

Septic Arthritis

Flynn JM, Widmann RF: The limping child: Evaluation and diagnosis. *J Am Acad Orthop Surg* 2001;9:89-98.

The authors review the radiographic, serologic, and clinical evaluation of the limping child.

Givon U, Liberman B, Schindler A, Blankstein A, Ganel A: Treatment of septic arthritis of the hip with repeated ultrasound-guided aspirations. *J Pediatr Orthop* 2004;24: 266-270.

A cohort study of 34 children with septic arthritis of the hip was treated with repeated ultrasound-guided aspirations of the hip joint in lieu of open surgical drainage. Six patients required surgery because of drain dislodgement; 4 of 28 patients treated with aspiration only required open drainage because of failure to improve. The mean number of aspirations was 3.6, and 75% of patients resumed walking within 24 hours. The mean follow-up was 7.4 years, and no complications were reported. The authors recommended serial aspiration as a safe and efficacious option for the treatment of septic arthritis of the hip.

Jung ST, Rowe SM, Moon ES, Song EK, Yoon TR, Seo HY: Significance of laboratory and radiologic findings for differentiating between septic arthritis and transient synovitis of the hip. *J Pediatr Orthop* 2003;23:368-372.

This is a retrospective review of 97 patients with transient synovitis and 27 patients with septic arthritis of the hip. The authors conducted multivariate regression analysis on data obtained from review of medical records, plain radiographs, and clinical findings. Body temperature greater than 37°C, ESR

greater than 20 mm/hr, CRP level greater than 1mg/dL, white blood cell count greater than 11,000/mL, and increased hip joint space of greater than 2 mm were independent multivariate predictors of septic arthritis.

Khachatourians AG, Patzakis MJ, Roidis N, Holtom PD: Laboratory monitoring in pediatric acute osteomyelitis and septic arthritis. *Clin Orthop Relat Res* 2003;409:186-194.

The authors conducted a retrospective review of the medical records of 50 patients who were admitted for acute osteomyelitis, septic arthritis, or both. They reported that the mean number of days to peak and normalization of ESR and CRP levels were twice as long for the surgical group compared with the nonsurgical group.

Kocher MS, Mandiga R, Murphy JM, et al: A clinical practice guideline for treatment of septic arthritis in children: Efficacy in improving process of care and effect on outcome of septic arthritis of the hip. *J Bone Joint Surg Am* 2003;85-A:994-999.

The authors developed guidelines for the treatment of septic arthritis in children and evaluated its efficacy with regard to improving the process of care and its effect on the outcome of septic arthritis of the hip. A historical control group of 30 consecutive children with septic arthritis of the hip treated before the use of the guidelines was compared with a prospective cohort group of 30 consecutive children who were treated with use of the guidelines. The authors reported that the patients treated with use of the guidelines demonstrated less variation in the process of care and improved efficiency of care without a significant difference in outcome.

Kocher MS, Mandiga R, Zurakowski D, Barnewolt C, Kasser JR: Validation of a clinical prediction rule for the differentiation between septic arthritis and transient synovitis of the hip in children. *J Bone Joint Surg Am* 2004;86-A:1629-1635.

The authors reassessed the predictive value of ESR greater than 40 mm/hr, history of fever, inability to ambulate, and white blood cell count greater than 12,000/mL in the differentiation of transient synovitis and septic arthritis of the hip. The area under the receiver operating characteristic curve for the patient population observed in this study was 0.86 compared with 0.96 in the previous study. The authors reported that although their previously published clinical prediction rule was found to have diminished, good diagnostic performance in a new patient population was nonetheless achieved.

Levine MJ, McGuire KJ, McGowan KL, Flynn JM: Assessment of the test characteristics of C-reactive protein for septic arthritis in children. *J Pediatr Orthop* 2003;23: 373-377.

The authors conducted a retrospective review of 133 patients who had synovial fluid aspiration that was sent for culture and Gram stain and had a CRP level determined within

24 hours of presentation. They reported that 39 of the 133 patients had septic arthritis; CRP sensitivity (41% to 90%), specificity (29% to 85%), positive predictive value (34% to 53%), and negative predictive value (78% to 87%) were recorded. The authors concluded that CRP level is a better independent predictor of septic arthritis than ESR, and that CRP level is a better negative predictor of disease than a positive predictor of disease. They also found that if the CRP level was less than 1.0mg/dL, the probability that the patient did not have septic arthritis was 87%.

Luhmann SJ, Jones A, Schootman M, Gordon JE, Schoenecker PL, Luhmann JD: Differentiation between septic arthritis and transient synovitis of the hip in children with clinical prediction algorithms. *J Bone Joint Surg Am* 2004;86-A:956-962.

The authors conducted a retrospective analysis of the predictive value of a clinical algorithm that has been proposed for use in the differentiation of transient synovitis and septic arthritis of the hip using four clinical variables (ESR > 40 mm/hr, white blood cell count >12,000 cells/mm, history of fever, and no weight bearing) in a new patient population that included 163 patients (165 hips). There were 20 instances of true septic arthritis, 27 instances of presumed septic arthritis, and 118 instances of transient synovitis. The authors found the presence of four of the above predictors was only 59% predictive of septic arthritis in contrast to the 99.6% predicted probability in the patient population for which the clinical algorithm was proposed.

Willis AA, Widmann RF, Flynn JM, Green DW, Onel KB: Lyme arthritis presenting as acute septic arthritis in children. *J Pediatr Orthop* 2003;23:114-118.

The authors assessed a series of 10 children who had acute arthritis consistent with septic arthritis and who ultimately were diagnosed with Lyme disease. Seven patients in this series underwent emergent surgical drainage for presumed septic arthritis. The authors suggested evaluation for Lyme disease in all endemic areas and also provide a protocol for the evaluation and management of this disease.

Other Specific Infections

Bickels J, Ben-Sira L, Kessler A, Wientroub S: Primary pyomyositis. *J Bone Joint Surg Am* 2002;84-A:2277-2286.

The authors retrospectively reviewed 676 patients with primary pyomyositis. They reported that pelvis and thigh musculature were the most commonly involved regions and that *S aureus* was the most commonly identified infecting organism (77% of patients). They also reported that the first and second decades of life represented the peak age of presentation.

Rasool MN: Osseous manifestations of tuberculosis in children. *J Pediatr Orthop* 2001;21:749-755.

In this retrospective analysis of 42 children with tuberculous osteomyelitis, 50 osseous lesions were observed. The authors described four types of lesions based on clinical and radiographic appearances: cystic (N = 26), infiltrative (N = 10),

focal erosions (N = 8), and spina ventosa (N = 8). Most lesions were located in the metaphyseal region of long bones. The authors noted that the lesions often radiographically resembled pyogenic and fungal infections as well as benign and malignant tumors. Biopsy was recommended for diagnosis. All patients were treated with curettage and antitubercular chemotherapeutics for 1 year. Most patients had good results at 6-month to 9-year follow-up.

Tay BK, Deckey J, Hu SS: Spinal infections. *J Am Acad Orthop Surg* 2002;10:188-197.

The authors of this article argue that prompt and accurate diagnosis of spinal infections, the cornerstone of treatment, requires a high index of suspicion in at-risk patients and the appropriate evaluation to identify the organism and determine the extent of infection. They also recommended that neurologic function and spinal stability should be carefully evaluated. The goals of therapy should include eradicating the infection, relieving pain, preserving or restoring neurologic function, improving nutrition, and maintaining spinal stability.

Classic Bibliography

Chambers JB, Forsythe DA, Bertrand SL, Iwinski HJ, Steflik DE: Retrospective review of osteoarticular infections in a pediatric sickle cell age group. *J Pediatr Orthop* 2000;20:682-685.

Fernandez M, Carrol CL, Baker CJ: Discitis and vertebral osteomyelitis in children: An 18-year review. *Pediatrics* 2000;105:1299-1304.

Howard AW, Viskontas D, Sabbagh C: Reduction in osteomyelitis and septic arthritis related to Haemophilus influenzae type B vaccination. *J Pediatr Orthop* 1999;19:705-709.

Kocher MS, Zurakowski D, Kasser JR: Differentiating between septic arthritis and transient synovitis of the hip in children: An evidence based clinical prediction algorithm. *J Bone Joint Surg Am* 1999;81:1662-1670.

Jarvis JG, Skipper J: Pseudomonas osteochondritis complicating puncture wounds in children. *J Pediatr Orthop* 1994;14:755-759.

Letts M, Davidson D, Birdi N, Joseph M: The SAPHO syndrome in children: A rare cause of hyperostosis and osteitis. *J Pediatr Orthop* 1999;19:297-300.

Puffinbarger WR, Gruel CR, Herndon WA, Sullivan JA: Osteomyelitis of the calcaneus in children. *J Pediatr Orthop* 1996;16:224-230.

Schreck P, Schreck P, Bradley J, Chambers H: Musculoskeletal complications of varicella. *J Bone Joint Surg Am* 1996;78:1713-1719.

Spiegel DA, Meyer JS, Dormans JP, Flynn JM, Drummond DS: Pyomyositis in children and adolescents: Report of 12 cases and review of the literature. *J Pediatr Orthop* 1999;19:143-150.

Sucato DJ, Schwend RM, Gillespie R: Septic arthritis of the hip in children. *J Am Acad Orthop Surg* 1997;5:249-260.

Wang MN, Chen WM, Lee KS, Chin LS, Lo WH: Tuberculous osteomyelitis in young children. *J Pediatr Orthop* 1999;19:151-155.

Watts HG, Lifeso RM: Tuberculosis of bones and joints. *J Bone Joint Surg Am* 1996;78:288-298.

Chapter 7

Common Musculoskeletal Neoplasms

J. Dominic Femino, MD

Ernest U. Conrad III, MD

Introduction

Although musculoskeletal tumors are uncommon, pediatric orthopaedists commonly perform the initial evaluation for children with musculoskeletal tumors. Patients often present or are referred to pediatric orthopaedists with reports of pain or a mass. Because bone and soft-tissue neoplasms can mimic more common disorders, they present a diagnostic and therapeutic challenge. An index of suspicion for neoplastic disease must always be maintained to make a timely diagnosis and initiate proper management.

Initial Evaluation

History

The medical history for musculoskeletal neoplasms can vary widely with the type of tumor, location, and patient's age. A complete survey of systems, past medical history, and family history is important. The most common symptom for most bone tumors is pain. Pain in a teenager for more than 6 weeks after any injury should be carefully assessed; this assessment should include radiographic imaging. If the radiographs are normal, repeat examinations should be done at 6-week intervals until symptoms resolve. Pain at rest is generally more worrisome than pain with activity and may indicate a greater degree of bone destruction. The most common physical sign is the presence of a bony or soft-tisssue mass. Any child who presents with a mass should be further evaluated for the possibility of a neoplasm. The diagnosis of hematoma may be used for patients who present with a mass, but this diagnosis should be made with caution, a classic traumatic history should be obtained, and follow-up should be vigilant so that a neoplastic process is not overlooked. Typically, a sprain, strain, or even a fracture will resolve or improve significantly over a 6-week observation period. If symptoms are not improved within 6 weeks, further investigation should begin. The age of the patient and duration of the symptoms can also help narrow the differential diagnosis.

Physical Examination

A complete physical examination should be performed, with special attention to sites of possible lymphatic node involvement or lung disease. The musculoskeletal focus should include measurement of the mass if one is present. Attention to the possible depth or superficiality of the mass, along with surrounding or involved neurovascular structures, is important for treatment planning. Limitation of motion, atrophy, the texture of a mass, angular deformity of an extremity, or limb-length discrepancy should be noted. The possibility of multiple site involvement should be evaluated. Tinel's test (percussion of the mass with radiation of pain along the path of the nerve) can be helpful to determine the nerve sheath origin of a tumor.

Diagnostic Imaging

Radiographs are the most important diagnostic imaging modality in the initial evaluation of a bone tumor. A differential diagnosis can be made with careful examination of radiographs for signs that are characteristic of certain tumors. When evaluating the radiographs, answering the following four questions (originally posed by Enneking) will help narrow the differential diagnosis: (1) What is the location of the tumor (epiphyseal, diaphyseal, metaphyseal, surface, cortical, medullary, central, or eccentric)? The age of the patient is also important in answering this question. (2) What is the tumor doing to the bone (expansion, destruction, or bowing)? (3) What is the bone doing in response to the tumor (sclerotic margin, periosteal reaction, onion skinning, or Codman's triangle)? (4) Is there a matrix produced by the tumor (osteoid production, calcifying cartilage, or a ground-glass appearance)?

Answers to these questions should enable orthopaedists to develop a good differential diagnosis based on the radiographs alone. Typically, slow-growing tumors will have well-defined borders, surrounding sclerosis, and mature periosteal reactions because these reactive processes take time to develop. Fast-growing tumors typically will have ill-defined borders and partial peri-

Table 1 | The MSTS Staging System for Benign and Malignant Neoplasms

MSTS Benign Tumor Stage
1 Latent
2 Active
3 Aggressive

MSTS Malignant Tumor Stage
I Low-grade
  A Intracompartmental
  B Extracompartmental
II High-grade
  A Intracompartmental
  B Extracompartmental
III Metastatic disease
  A Intracompartmental
  B Extracompartmental

Table 2 | Definitions of TNM

Primary Tumor (T)	
TX	Primary tumor cannot be assessed
T0	No evidence of primary tumor
T1	Tumor ≤ 8 cm
T2	Tumor > 8 cm
T3	Discontinuous tumors in the primary bone site
Regional Lymph Nodes (N)	
NX	Regional lymph nodes cannot be assessed
N0	No regional lymph node metastasis
N1	Regional lymph node metastasis
Distant Metastasis (M)	
MX	Distant metastasis cannot be assessed
M0	No distant metastasis
M1	Distant metastasis
M1a	Lung
M1b	Other distant sites
Histologic Grade (G)	
GX	Grade cannot be assessed
G1	Well differentiated (low-grade)
G2	Moderately differentiated (low-grade)
G3	Poorly differentiated (high-grade)
G4	Undifferentiated (high-grade)

T = size of the primary tumor, N = spreading into lymphatic nodes, M = spreading into other organs (metastasis)

osteal reactions, such as a Codman's triangle, because the bone has less time to form a mature response to the rapidly growing neoplasm.

MRI is the diagnostic imaging modality of choice for soft-tissue neoplasms. The extent and occasionally tissue type of soft-tissue neoplasms may be distinguished with MRI. CT is most useful in evaluating bone destruction and may be useful in differentiating benign from malignant bone tumors. Axial imaging may be beneficial in diagnosing a lesion that is difficult to detect using plain radiography. Evaluation for metastatic lung disease is most reliably accomplished with chest CT. Bone scintigraphy is useful to determine the activity of the primary tumor and to evaluate polyostotic involvement.

Staging

Staging is the evaluation of the extent and aggressiveness of the neoplasm. The staging systems used by most orthopaedic surgeons were developed by the Musculoskeletal Tumor Society (MSTS) for both benign and malignant neoplasms (Table 1).

In addition to the MSTS staging system, the American Joint Commission on Cancer (AJCC) has updated the TNM staging system for primary bone tumors (TNM is an acronym in which the T category represents the size of the primary tumor, the N category represents spreading into lymphatic nodes, and the M category represents spreading into other organs or metastasis). The TNM staging system includes all primary tumors of bone except lymphomas and myeloma (Table 2). The T category has been redefined as bone tumors that are 8 cm or less in greatest dimension (T1) versus tumors larger than 8 cm (T2). T3 defines a skip lesion within the same bone. The M1 category has been subdivided into M1a (lung metastases only) and M1b (other distant metastases including lymph nodes). Table 3 summarizes the AJCC staging systems for bone and soft-tissue sarcomas. Both the MSTS and AJCC staging systems help determine the prognosis of the patient and guide treatment. Higher-stage tumors generally have a poorer prognosis than lower-stage tumors. In addition, chemotherapy intensification may be used in patients with higher-stage tumors. Surgical planning also may be influenced by the size, location, and stage of the tumor.

Principles of Biopsy

If there is any suspicion of malignancy on the diagnostic imaging evaluation of a tumor, the patient should be referred to an orthopaedic oncologist for additional treatment, including biopsy. Biopsy may be fraught with potential complications that may significantly alter the patient's prognosis or treatment.

Fine-needle aspiration or core needle, incisional, or excisional biopsy all may be adequate, depending on the skill level of the surgeon and pathologist and the size and location of the tumor. Tailoring treatment to the specific clinical scenario and abilities of the pathology department are essential. In general, a well-planned and executed incisional biopsy will yield adequate tissue for

Table 3 | AJCC Staging System for Primary Malignant Bone Tumors

Stage IA	T1	N0	M0	G1,2 low-grade
Stage IB	T2	N0	M0	G1,2 low-grade
Stage IIA	T1	N0	M0	G3,4 high-grade
Stage IIB	T2	N0	M0	G3,4 high-grade
Stage III	T3	N0	M0	Any G
Stage IVA	Any T	N0	M1a	Any G
Stage IVB	Any T	N1	Any M	Any G
	Any T	Any N	M1b	Any G

(Reproduced with permission from AJCC Staging for Primary Malignant Bone Tumors, in The AJCC Cancer Staging Handbook, ed 6. New York, NY, Springer-Verlag, 2002.)

all diagnostic studies and not compromise recovery or future care of the patient.

Avoiding pitfalls is essential when performing a biopsy. The biopsy incision should be along the line of a potential incision for wide resection. This is usually longitudinal in the extremities. If a tourniquet is used, it should be inflated; leg elevation should be used to decrease limb blood volume. Exsanguination should not be done. The contamination of multiple compartments or vital structures should be avoided, which usually means avoiding standard approaches and violating only a single muscle to perform the biopsy. Round or ovoid windows in bone should be used to minimize stress risers. Meticulous hemostasis should also be used to avoid contamination of soft tissues.

Osseous Tumors by Tissue Type
Bone-Producing Tumors
Osteoid Osteoma
Osteoid osteoma is a neoplastic process producing fibrovascular tissue and immature osteoid. By definition, it is less than 1.5 cm in diameter at the nidus and often has dense reactive bone surrounding it. Osteoid osteoma may occur in any bone, but approximately 50% occur in the femur. The clinical characteristics of osteoid osteoma include constant, unremitting pain, which is usually most noticeable at night and is relieved with nonsteroidal anti-inflammatory drugs (NSAIDs) or aspirin. Diagnosis using radiography and CT is recommended. CT axial imaging is most useful to identify the nidus, which may not be apparent on radiographs. Technetium bone scans usually demonstrate a focal, high-intensity signal associated with the lesion. MRI is not particularly useful for identifying this type of tumor because surrounding marrow and soft-tissue edema can be mistaken for Ewing's sarcoma or osteomyelitis. There are three general treatment options for patients with osteoid osteoma: NSAID therapy, surgical resection, and the use of minimally invasive, percutaneous techniques such as radiofrequency ablation (RFA). The first is medical therapy with NSAIDs, which are thought to reduce

prostaglandins produced by the tumor and modulate symptoms of pain. Long-term NSAID therapy is effective in controlling pain, but must be continued until the osteoid osteoma has regressed or burned out, which may take several years; therefore, appropriate liver and kidney function monitoring must be performed in conjunction with NSAID therapy. Surgical resection of the nidus is effective in relieving pain, with reported recurrence rates of 5% to 10%. The entire nidus must be resected to avoid recurrence. The nidus may be localized intraoperatively by a burr-down technique, radiographically, or with tetracycline labeling. Depending on the location and size of resection, bone grafting and/or internal fixation may be required.

Minimally invasive, percutaneous techniques such as RFA have gained popularity in the past 5 years and are becoming the treatments of choice for osteoid osteomas. Under CT guidance, an RFA probe is placed percutaneously into the center of the nidus. High-frequency energy (> 500,000 Hz) is delivered through the probe to the tissue in the nidus. Thermal injury occurs to the tissue in the nidus through resistive heating. The procedure may be performed on an outpatient basis with general or regional anesthetic. Recurrence rates are comparable to those for open surgical resection (5% to 10%), but recovery, cost, and morbidity are significantly decreased. One disadvantage to RFA is that histologic evaluation is difficult because of the small needle sample size. Diagnostic biopsies done in conjunction with RFA are successful only 30% to 50% of the time. Therefore, surgeons should be certain that the clinical symptoms and diagnostic imaging studies are entirely characteristic of osteoid osteoma before performing RFA.

Osteoblastoma
Osteoblastoma is histologically identical to osteoid osteoma, with immature bone production, fibrovascular stroma, and abundant bony reaction. By definition, osteoblastoma is larger than 1.5 cm. It may occur in any bone and accounts for less than 1% of all primary bone tumors. The radiographic appearance of osteoblastoma

may show abundant periosteal reactive bone. Osteoblastoma has a propensity for the axial skeleton, particularly the posterior spinal elements, and bone scanning typically shows increased uptake. Treatment is aimed at relief of pain, usually with aggressive curettage and occasionally with wide resection.

Osteosarcoma

Osteosarcoma is the most common primary malignant bone tumor in children, with a cumulative estimated incidence for ages 5 to 19 years of 29 per 1 million persons. The peak age at diagnosis is 15 years, with 80% of osteosarcomas diagnosed in patients younger than 20 years. A second peak incidence occurs after age 60 years, which is probably related to Paget's osteosarcoma. The most common clinical symptoms are aching pain and the presence of a mass. The most common locations are the distal femur, proximal tibia, and proximal humerus (all areas of rapid bone growth in adolescence). The radiographic appearance of osteosarcoma is variable, but the tumor is usually metaphyseal in origin, with lytic destruction and production of radiodense osteoid. Osteosarcoma typically has an associated soft-tissue mass at presentation. MRI is useful in identifying the extent of tumor and should be used to evaluate patients for skip lesions within the same bone.

Histologically, a malignant spindle-cell stroma produces osteoid. As with the radiographic appearance, the histologic appearance is variable, with osteoblastic, chondroblastic, fibroblastic and giant-cell rich histologic subtypes.

Biopsy and treatment of a suspected osteosarcoma should be performed by an orthopaedic oncologist. Treatment typically includes induction (neoadjuvant) chemotherapy, followed by limb-salvage surgery and then additional chemotherapy. Ninety percent of children in the United States are treated under protocols of the Children's Oncology Group, the surgical goals of which are to achieve a wide margin at the time of resection with normal tissue completely surrounding the tumor. Approximately 90% of patients with osteosarcoma successfully undergo limb-sparing wide resection and reconstruction of their extremities (discussed under the section entitled Limb-Salvage Surgery for Children). Using a combination of multiagent chemotherapy and surgery, the 5-year survival rate is approximately 70%. Patients with metastatic disease at presentation and with less than 90% necrosis of their tumor after induction chemotherapy have a poorer prognosis.

The performance of limb-salvage surgery remains controversial in patients who sustain pathologic fractures either before diagnosis or during induction chemotherapy. A pathologic fracture has been considered an indication for amputation because of soft-tissue contamination with fracture hematoma containing osteosarcoma cells. In a recent multicenter retrospective study conducted by the MSTS, patients who sustained a pathologic fracture had an increased risk of local recurrence and a decreased rate of survival compared with those without pathologic fractures. In these patients with pathologic fractures, however, limb-salvage surgery in carefully selected patients did not appear to adversely affect local recurrence or survival.

The low- and intermediate-grade variants osteosarcoma are rare, representing less than 10% of osteosarcomas. Radiographically, these variants have characteristics that distinguish them from conventional osteosarcoma. Both parosteal osteosarcoma and periosteal osteosarcoma are surface lesions. Parosteal osteosarcoma appears as a stuck-on osteoblastic lesion on the cortex of the bone. Seventy percent are located on the posterior aspect of the distal femur. Axial imaging with MRI or CT is extremely useful to distinguish parosteal osteosarcoma from osteochondroma. Parosteal osteosarcomas are usually low-grade or intermediate-grade lesions, and treatment is surgical wide resection, with chemotherapy usually reserved for the occasional high-grade lesion.

Periosteal osteosarcoma is an intermediate-grade surface osteosarcoma that typically occurs in the diaphyseal region of long bones, particularly the anterior tibia. It occurs under the periosteum and has a significant periosteal reaction. There usually is a significant cartilaginous component. Treatment is with surgical wide resection, with or without chemotherapy.

Telangiectatic osteosarcoma is a medullary lesion that has no significant visible osteoid production on radiographs, making it a challenging diagnosis on biopsy. The appearance is primarily lytic, and evidence of fluid-fluid levels is usually visible on MRI scans; consequently, it may be confused with a benign bone cyst. Histology typically demonstrates malignant spindle cells in the soft-tissue lining, with production of osteoid. Telangiectatic osteosarcoma is usually a high-grade lesion and requires combined chemotherapy and surgical treatment.

Cartilage Tumors

Enchondroma

Enchondromas are benign, intramedullary cartilage tumors. They account for approximately 18% of all bone tumors and are common in adults, but less common in childhood. They are most common in the metaphysis, but may occur in the diaphysis and epiphysis, even in skeletally immature patients. The most common locations are the small tubular bones of the hand (42% of instances), metaphyseal distal femur, and proximal humerus. Enchondromas have a wide age distribution, with approximately 25% occurring in patients younger than 20 years.

Radiographically, enchondromas appear as lytic lesions entirely within the bone. Speckled calcification or "popcorn calcification" of arcs and rings may be visible within the lesion, but calcification may be absent in skeletally immature patients. MRI and CT are helpful in identifying endosteal scalloping or cortical destruction that may be suggestive of chondrosarcoma, which is rare in children.

Most enchondromas are clinically silent and are identified as an incidental finding on radiographs. Enchondromas of the hand frequently present with fracture. Routine fracture immobilization usually is adequate treatment; however, intralesional curettage and grafting is sometimes required.

Ollier's Disease

Ollier's disease is a nonhereditary condition of multiple enchondromatosis. It is usually diagnosed in the first decade of life as a result of parental concerns of bony deformity. Any bone may be involved, but lesions commonly are in the metaphyseal long bones, often unilaterally. Limb-length discrepancy, angular deformity, short stature, and pain are frequent clinical features.

Recent studies have led to the development of a model in which the Indian hedgehog gene and parathyroid hormone-related protein (PTHrP) are involved in a feedback loop controlling chondrocyte differentiation and proliferation in the growth plate. The formation of multiple enchondromas is a result of an increase in PTHrP signaling that leads to a decrease in chondrocyte differentiation in the growth plate.

Radiographically, Ollier's disease appears as multiple enlarged metaphyseal lytic lesions with expansion of bone. Calcification and trabeculation within the lesions are variable. Management is aimed at preventing deformity, equalizing leg lengths, preventing fracture, and reducing pain. Observation is sufficient for most patients with this type of lesion, but some require surgical intervention. Corrective osteotomies and physeal stapling procedures are useful for angular correction. The use of Ilizarov external fixation for treatment of limb-length discrepancy in patients with Ollier's disease was recently reported. Distraction was performed through the enchondromas with resultant conversion of abnormal cartilage into histologically mature bone in the distraction sites.

Patients with Ollier's disease require lifetime monitoring for malignant transformation. The risk of malignant degeneration in patients with Ollier's disease is approximately 25%. In patients with Maffucci's syndrome (multiple enchondromas associated with vascular malformations), some studies report the risk of malignant transformation to be approximately 100%.

Osteochondroma

Solitary osteochondromas are benign bony protuberances with cartilage caps that grow on the surface of a bone. Osteochondromas have been described as the most common bone tumor treated, although the exact incidence is unknown.

The peak incidence for osteochondromas is in the second decade of life, and the most common locations are the metaphyseal regions of the distal femur, proximal tibia, and proximal humerus. Osteochondromas, however, may occur in any site. The lesion can continue to increase in size until the patient is skeletally mature, but the rate of growth is not predictable. Osteochondromas should not continue to grow in adulthood. If enlarging in adulthood, the patient should be evaluated for malignant transformation to chondrosarcoma.

Radiographically, there are two forms of osteochondroma: pedunculated and sessile. Both types have the characteristic feature of communication between the medullary canal of the bone and the base of the osteochondroma. The cortex of the bone also is in continuity with the cortex of the osteochondroma. Although standard radiographs usually are diagnostic of osteochondromas, occasionally axial imaging with MRI or CT is necessary to differentiate osteochondromas from other lesions such as parosteal osteosarcoma. The characteristic medullary continuity between the bone and osteochondroma should be apparent on axial images.

Treatment of osteochondromas is based on symptoms, and most do not require surgical resection. Osteochondromas may cause pain from local compression on muscles and tendons, nerves, or vessels. Overlying bursa formation may become painful. Occasionally, a pedunculated osteochondroma may fracture, causing pain. In addition, osteochondromas may cause angular deformity of the limb in the growing child or limited range of motion. Symptomatic lesions may be excised. The osteochondroma should be removed flush with the underlying cortex. Care should be taken to avoid damage to the physis, which can be in close proximity. Asymptomatic lesions should be assessed annually or biannually in the skeletally immature child to monitor for angular deformity during growth.

The risk of malignant degeneration for solitary osteochondromas is approximately 1% over the lifetime of the patient. Radiographic signs of sarcomatous degeneration include irregularity of the margin, inhomogeneous mineralization, and an associated soft-tissue mass. Young children may have thick (> 1 cm) cartilaginous caps, but a thick and irregularly calcified cartilage cap after skeletal maturity suggests sarcomatous degeneration. Enlargement of the cartilaginous cap at any age is of concern and should be investigated.

Hereditary Multiple Exostoses

Hereditary multiple exostoses (HME) is an autosomal-dominant disorder characterized by the development of multiple osteochondromas. HME has an estimated incidence of at least 1 in 50,000 individuals.

The *EXT* family of genes has been characterized with the presence of inactivating *EXT1* and *EXT2* mutations on chromosomes 8 and 11, respectively, in HME. These genes encode the copolymerase responsible for the biosynthesis of heparan sulfate, which, when altered, appears to lead to the ectopic bone growth characteristic of HME. A variety of mutations occur in these genes that likely account for the difference in severity of phenotypic expression of the disease. *EXT1* mutations have been associated with a more severe clinical form of the disease.

The most common clinical symptoms associated with HME include localized and generalized pain, short stature, limb-length discrepancies, valgus deformities of the knee and ankle, shortening of the ulna with radial bowing and radial head subluxation, limited range of motion, and coxa valga. The rate of malignant transformation in patients with HME is much higher than for those with solitary osteochondromas, with most estimates being approximately 6% and ranging from 0.5% to 25%.

The treatment of pain in patients with HME is similar to the treatment of patients with solitary osteochondromas. Special attention to deformity and growth is required because these problems are common in patients with HME. Patients should be evaluated annually for deformity and limb-length discrepancy until skeletal maturity. Use of hemiepiphysiodeses, epiphysiodeses, or osteotomies may be necessary to maintain lower extremity alignment and equality. Upper extremity Madelung's disease-like deformity is generally well tolerated and causes little functional impairment. There is some support for radial osteotomy and ulnar lengthening, although the functional benefits are not well established.

Chondroblastoma

Chondroblastoma is a rare, benign, cartilage tumor that occurs in the epiphyseal or apophyseal regions of long bones. It can cause significant damage to joints because of the proximity to the articular surface. Chondroblastoma has a peak incidence in the second decade of life and accounts for 1% of all bone tumors and 5% to 10% of cartilage tumors. The proximal tibia, distal femur, and proximal humerus are the most common locations.

The clinical presentation of patients with chondroblastoma typically includes persistent aching pain in and around a joint. There may be a sympathetic joint effusion with limited motion or even tumor extension through the epiphysis into the joint.

Radiographs typically show a well-circumscribed, lytic lesion with a sclerotic border in the epiphysis. Occasionally, cartilage stippling is visible. Chondroblastoma may be difficult to identify on standard radiographs, and MRI is helpful in identifying the extent of the tumor.

Surgical excision is the standard of care for chondroblastoma. Because of the epiphyseal location, the surgical approach may be complicated. Either a transepiphyseal or transmetaphyseal approach may be used with intralesional curettage and grafting. Adjuvant phenol, cauterization, or cryotherapy has been used. Autograft, allograft, synthetic bone graft substitutes, and methylmethacrylate all have been used effectively to fill the defect. Local recurrence is common.

Although chondroblastomas are benign tumors, they can rarely metastasize to the lungs. CT imaging for pulmonary metastases should be performed at the time of diagnosis. Lung nodules should be biopsied to confirm a diagnosis of chondroblastoma. Surgical resection can be performed. Lesions may not always progress, and there is little evidence of effective adjuvant chemotherapy or radiation therapy.

Fibrous Tumors

Fibrous Dysplasia

Fibrous dysplasia is a sporadic skeletal disorder in which normal bone and bone marrow is replaced by benign fibrous tissue. The peak age at diagnosis is the second decade of life. Fibrous dysplasia most commonly occurs in the femur, tibia, ribs, and skull. The natural history is variable. Lesions may remain stable for decades or may progress relentlessly, causing deformation and pathologic fractures. Progression may be more rapid in the immature skeleton.

The cellular etiology of fibrous dysplasia is an activation mutation of the gene encoding Gs-α protein on chromosome 20q13. Activation of Gs-α activates adenylate cyclase, thus generating high levels of cyclic adenosine monophosphate (cAMP). These cAMP-dependent pathways may mediate the phenotypic effects of the mutation in bone.

Radiographs demonstrate a metaphyseal or diaphyseal lesion with a lytic or ground-glass appearance. There may be expansion of the bone. There is usually sharp margination of the lesion. Bowing or pathologic fractures are common. Bone scanning is helpful in defining the extent of polyostotic disease.

Histologic analysis typically demonstrates proliferating fibroblasts with dense collagenous matrix, irregular trabeculae (alphabet soup), and absence of rimming osteoblasts.

Treatment varies depending on the degree of involvement and symptoms. Observation is adequate for asymptomatic patients, which should include a yearly evaluation to monitor deformity. Surgical intervention is indicated for patients with deformity and for fracture management. Surgical options include osteotomies, bone grafting, and internal fixation with rods or plates. Surgical curettage of these lesions has a high recurrence rate after treatment. Bisphosphonate therapy has been proved effective to decrease bone pain, decrease markers of bone turnover, and increase bone density in areas

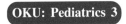

of fibrous dysplasia. Patients with McCune-Albright syndrome (endocrinopathy, fibrous dysplasia, and café-au-lait spots) should be referred to a pediatric endocrinologist for management. Fibrous dysplasia has the potential for malignant transformation in adult patients.

Osteofibrous Dysplasia

Osteofibrous dysplasia is an entity distinct from fibrous dysplasia, and it does not share the Gs-α protein mutation of fibrous dysplasia. Osteofibrous dysplasia typically presents in the first decade of life with a mass or bowing of the anterior tibia. It almost exclusively occurs in the tibia or fibula, although there are sporadic reports of osteofibrous dysplasia occurring at other sites. It is a cortically based, expansile, lytic lesion originating in the anterior diaphyseal cortex. As it enlarges, it may expand into the medullary canal and cause anterior bowing or pathologic fracture of the tibia.

Treatment of children with osteofibrous dysplasia is centered on management of pain and prevention of deformity and fracture. Osteofibrous dysplasia may spontaneously regress or become stagnant in older adolescents or adults. Therefore, nonsurgical management with fracture bracing or casting usually will control pain and prevent fracture in young children. Occasionally, surgical intervention is required if symptoms cannot be controlled nonsurgically. Attempts at aggressive curettage and bone grafting carry a high recurrence rate. Osteotomy and intramedullary rodding with a locked nail in skeletally mature adolescents will correct deformity and help control pain.

It may be difficult to distinguish osteofibrous dysplasia from adamantinoma in some instances, and vigilant radiographic evaluation for progressive cortical destruction is required. If there is suspicion for adamantinoma, multiple biopsies may be necessary to confirm a diagnosis. If adamantinoma is identified, the patient's lesion should be staged and treated with a wide resection.

Nonossifying Fibroma

Nonossifying fibroma, or fibroxanthoma, is a benign fibrous lesion that is often noted incidentally on radiographs. It is probably the most common benign lesion in bone, but the true incidence is unknown. The diagnosis almost always can be made based on the radiographic appearance. The lesion tends to occur in the metaphyseal regions of long bones. It is eccentric and usually cortically based. Smaller lesions may appear as ovoid lucencies within the cortex. Larger lesions may expand into the medullary canal, thin the cortex, and have a bubbly, multiloculated sclerotic border. The lesions are usually solitary, but the incidence of multifocal nonossifying fibroma may be underestimated.

Small or asymptomatic lesions do not require surgical intervention and may be observed with serial radiographs. Lesions that cause pain, pathologic fracture, or

are of significant size (> 3 cm or > 50% of the diameter of the involved bone) should be considered for surgical treatment. Predicting the risk of pathologic fracture in patients with benign skeletal lesions is difficult, but essential to the management and counseling of the patient and family. The risk of pathologic fracture depends on several factors, including the patient's height, weight, activity level, and loading regimen. The use of quantitative CT to measure bending and torsional rigidity has been shown to be more accurate than standard radiographic criteria for predicting pathologic fracture through benign bone lesions in children.

When clinical symptoms or the risk of pathologic fracture necessitate surgery, biopsy followed by intralesional curettage and bone grafting is effective in eradicating the lesion and relieving pain. When a patient presents with a pathologic fracture, the fracture may be treated initially with casting, and curettage and bone grafting may be performed if there is persistent nonossifying fibroma after fracture healing.

Miscellaneous Bone Tumors and Tumor-like Conditions

Ewing's Sarcoma

Ewing's sarcoma is the second most common malignant tumor of bone in children. It occurs in approximately 3 per 1 million Caucasian children per year and is rarer in Asian and African-American children. The peak incidence of Ewing's sarcoma is in the second decade of life, with 80% of patients younger than 20 years. The tumor was first described in 1921 by James Ewing as a diffuse endothelioma of bone. It is a malignant neoplasm of primitive mesenchymal cell origin and is part of the family of small round blue-cell tumors.

The location of Ewing's sarcoma may be in any bone, but it is most common in the diaphyseal and metadiaphyseal regions of long bones. It occurs more commonly than osteosarcoma in central locations such as the pelvis and spine. The lower extremities are more frequently involved than the upper extremities.

Pain and swelling or a mass are the most common presenting symptoms. Approximately 20% of patients present with fever, and orthopaedists must be careful not to confuse this symptom with fever related to osteomyelitis or a soft-tissue abscess. Diagnostic imaging with radiographs and MRI will help make the distinction because patients with Ewing's sarcoma usually have a large surrounding soft-tissue mass or an infection, whereas patients with Langerhans cell histiocytosis will not. Radiographs typically show a permeative, lytic lesion with ill-defined borders. There may be cortical destruction and periosteal reactive bone. The radiographic appearance is variable. MRI is helpful to assess the associated soft-tissue mass, bone marrow, neurovascular structures, and response to chemotherapy.

If Ewing's sarcoma is suspected based on the patient's history, physical examination, and imaging studies, the patient should be referred to an orthopaedic oncologist for treatment. Treatment, after staging and biopsy, begins with induction chemotherapy, usually with a Children's Oncology Group protocol. Most patients will undergo limb-sparing wide resection with reconstruction. Limb-sparing internal hemipelvectomy has become a viable alternative for local control, with reported recurrence rates being better or equal to those treated with local radiation. Ewing's sarcoma is a radiosensitive tumor, and radiation therapy is sometimes used for local control, lung disease, or for positive surgical margins. Adjuvant chemotherapy and/or bone marrow transplant completes the standard treatment. The survival rate at 5 years is 65% to 70% for patients with extremity disease and 40% to 50% for those with central lesions.

Giant Cell Tumor

Giant cell tumor of bone is a benign tumor of fibroblastic mononuclear cells and multinucleated giant cells. It may behave aggressively, causing local bone destruction of the physis and cortex. This is one of the few bone tumors that will cross the physis into the epiphysis. The peak incidence is in the third and fourth decades of life, but occasionally it occurs in adolescents, including those who are skeletally immature. The most common location is around the knee, although it may occur in any bone, including the pelvis.

The radiographs show a purely lytic lesion of the metaphysis and epiphysis, with expansion of bone and thinning of the cortex. There may be expansion into the soft tissues. Radiographs or CT scans of the lungs should be obtained at the onset of treatment to evaluate for lung metastases, which are present in approximately 3% of patients.

Intralesional curettage with a high-speed burr is the standard treatment of giant cell tumor. Adjuvant therapy with phenol or liquid nitrogen may reduce local recurrence. Cementation or bone grafting are both used to fill the defect, with recurrence rates slightly lower using cementation, presumably as a result of marginal cell necrosis from the cement's exothermic reaction during curing. Internal fixation with intramedullary Steinmann pins may increase the strength of the reconstruction. Local recurrence rates are 10% to 25%. Patients with metastatic lung disease should be considered for adjuvant chemotherapy.

Unicameral Bone Cyst

Unicameral bone cysts, also known as solitary or simple bone cysts, are intraosseous, fluid-filled lesions with a membranous lining. They occur most commonly in children in the proximal humerus and proximal femur, but

may occur in almost any bone. Unicameral bone cysts represent 3% of all bone lesions and are extremely rare in adults. They typically are discovered on radiographs after a pathologic fracture, activity-related pain, or as an incidental finding. Radiographs usually are diagnostic, showing a central, metaphyseal, lytic lesion with a well-demarcated border. There may be expansion of the bone and cortical thinning or fracture. A "fallen-leaf" sign is the radiographic appearance of a fractured cortical fragment that has fallen into the cyst. CT can be helpful to evaluate the thickness of the cortex in determining healing or return to activities. MRI may be useful to confirm the presence of fluid within the lytic lesion. Unicameral bone cysts that are less than 1 cm from the growth plate have been defined as active, and those that are more than 1 cm from the growth plate have been defined as inactive; however, it is unclear whether these labels are clinically relevant in predicting fracture potential.

The etiology of unicameral bone cysts remains unknown. The most popular theory involves venous stasis causing increased bone marrow pressure, bone necrosis, fluid collection, and the release of bone resorptive factors. Other hypotheses include metaphyseal trauma, physeal microtrauma, or healing from a preexisting tumor.

The natural history of unicameral bone cysts begins with a lytic lesion adjacent to the physis, and with time the physis grows away from the cyst. Lesional growth and local bone destruction is extremely variable, but as many as 75% of patients present with pathologic fractures. Only 10% to 15% of unicameral bone cysts will resolve after fracture healing, leaving the orthopaedic surgeon with the challenging task of estimating the risk of future fractures. There is no standard method to predict pathologic fractures in patients with unicameral bone cysts, but variables to consider include location of the cyst, size of the cyst, cortical thinning, activity level, and pain. Recently, the use of quantitative CT to calculate bending and torsional rigidity has been proposed to predict pathologic fractures in patients with benign skeletal lesions. If no intervention is performed, there is still a 10% reported risk of physeal arrest from the cyst or from fracture through the cyst. Many believe that unicameral bone cysts will resolve spontaneously because they are relatively common in children and rare in adults; however, no longitudinal radiographic studies have documented the validity of this theory.

Gross findings typically show a membrane or no tissue in an osseous cavity, and serous or hemorrhagic, straw-colored fluid is present. The cyst lining is a thin rim of fibroconnective tissue with occasional giant cells. There is no cytologic atypia.

Unicameral bone cysts have been subjected to a multitude of treatments, with no single technique demonstrating complete efficacy. Unicameral bone cysts are most commonly treated with aspiration and injection techniques developed in the 1970s, which usually involves a two-needle technique and the injection of methylprednisolone. More recently, aspiration and injection with bone marrow or bone marrow combined with demineralized bone matrix has been used. Others report injecting calcium sulfate pellets. Although injection techniques are minimally invasive, they usually require two or more injection procedures with 2 to 3 months between injections to achieve adequate healing. One should confirm the diagnosis during needle aspiration/injection by noting the presence of straw-colored fluid, cystogram to demonstrate a fluid-filled cavity, and/or needle biopsy of the membrane.

Open curettage and bone grafting for unicameral bone cysts also yields good results, with recurrence rates of 12% to 20%, which are equivalent to or slightly better than injection techniques. Although this procedure is more invasive than needle injections, it usually requires only one anesthetic. Adjuvants such as liquid nitrogen and phenol have been used to reduce recurrence rates with open curettage.

Several other techniques have aimed at reducing potential intraosseous pressure from the unicameral bone cyst to cause resolution of the cyst and include placement of cannulated screws, intramedullary rodding, and trepanation.

Although there are a multitude of accepted treatments for unicameral bone cysts, surgeons should keep in mind that the goal of treatment is to return the patient to activities without symptoms or fracture. Immediate complete radiographic resolution of the lesion is not necessary to achieve this goal, and care should be taken to not make the treatment worse than the disease.

Aneurysmal Bone Cyst

Aneurysmal bone cysts are benign, locally aggressive bone tumors. They cause expansile lesions of bone with mixed blood-filled cavities and fibroconnective tissue. Peak incidence is in the second decade of life, but aneurysmal bone cysts have been reported up to the seventh decade of life. Metaphyseal regions of long bones are the most common area of occurrence, but aneurysmal bone cysts may occur in any bone.

Gross examination typically reveals blood-filled lakes with moderate to abundant soft tissue within the bone. Microscopically, the cyst walls show spindled fibroblastic cells with multinucleated giant cells and thin strands of bone. The spaces lack endothelial lining. Cytogenetic aberrations establishing a neoplastic basis of primary aneurysmal bone cysts recently have been identified, most commonly featuring chromosome band 17p13 rearrangements.

Radiographic distinction between aneurysmal bone cysts and unicameral bone cysts may be challenging. An-

eurysmal bone cysts are usually medullary based and may be centric or eccentric. Rarely, they may be subperiosteal. Lysis is always present with no visible matrix, and cortical thinning is almost always present. Aneurysmal bone cysts usually have well-defined margins and may have a multiloculated or soap-bubble appearance. There usually is enlargement of the bone, hence the label aneurysmal. MRI is useful in demonstrating the presence of a double-density fluid level and multiple septations within the lesion.

Aneurysmal bone cysts typically are more aggressive than unicameral bone cysts, causing progressive bone destruction, pain, pathologic fractures, and physeal arrests. Although spontaneous regression of aneurysmal bone cysts has been reported, the usual natural history is progressive local destruction of bone; therefore, surgical intervention, rather than observation, usually is indicated for aneurysmal bone cysts.

Treatment of aneurysmal bone cysts primarily is with open curettage and bone grafting, using allograft, autograft, or any type of bone-graft substitutes; adjuvant liquid nitrogen or phenol is frequently used. A wide range of recurrence rates has been reported using this technique (11% to 70%), but most recurrence rates are in the 20% range. Recently, a large series found no difference in recurrence rates related to age of the patient. Several series of percutaneous treatment of aneurysmal bone cysts using Ethibloc injections (Ethicon/Johnson and Johnson, Norderstedt, Germany) with moderate success have been reported in the European literature.

Langerhans Cell Histiocytosis

Langerhans cell histiocytosis is a clonal proliferation of histiocytic cells, which can affect various organs. There is a spectrum of clinical involvement, ranging from single-bone or single-organ involvement to multisystem disease. Organ system involvement may include bone, bone marrow, lung, liver, pituitary-thalamic axis (characterized by diabetes insipidus), skin, spleen, gastrointestinal tract, and lymph nodes. The spectrum of Langerhans cell histiocytosis encompasses the historical terms eosinophilic granuloma, Hand-Schuller-Christian disease, and Letterer-Siwe disease.

Although Langerhans cell histiocytosis may occur at any age, 50% of patients are children, and the average age of onset is 1.8 years. The incidence in the pediatric population is 5 per 1 million annually, and the adult incidence is unknown.

Painful bone lesions are typical at presentation. A third of patients have a unifocal bone lesion at presentation, and 19% have isolated multifocal bone involvement. Any bone may be affected, but lesions of the spine, skull, ribs, and pelvis are most common. In long bones, the lesions tend to be diaphyseal. Radiographically, Langerhans cell histiocytosis is considered a great mimicker because its appearance is highly variable. Lytic bone destruction and abundant periosteal reaction are common in patients with Langerhans cell histiocytosis and may be confused with the radiographic appearance of malignant bone tumors such as Ewing's sarcoma.

Histologically, the Langerhans cell appears as a histiocytic cell with a coffee-bean–shaped nucleus that has a central cleft. Cell surface expression of CD1a is diagnostic for Langerhans cells, and the cells do not show dysplasia or atypia (features of malignant cells). Langerhans cell histiocytosis lesions contain a mixture of Langerhans cells, macrophages, T cells, eosinophils, and granulocytes.

Baseline evaluation to establish the extent of disease includes a skeletal survey, chest radiograph, complete blood cell count with differential, liver function tests, coagulation studies, and urine osmolality measurement. Radionuclide bone scanning is not as sensitive as radiographic survey in detecting these lesions. Biopsy of a skeletal lesion often is required to establish a definitive diagnosis.

Treatment of Langerhans cell histiocytosis depends on the extent of disease. Children with solitary skeletal lesions may resolve spontaneously over months to years. Surgical intervention with curettage or internal fixation and bone grafting may be necessary to manage skeletal pain, deformity, or pathologic fractures. Intralesional injection of corticosteroids also has been used effectively for treatment of skeletal lesions. Vertebral lesions usually can be managed with bracing until the patient is asymptomatic. Most patients with single skeletal lesions will achieve disease-free survival without progression of disease. Patients with multisystem disease should be treated with multiagent chemotherapy. There are several current treatment protocols, and prognosis is poor in patients with greater organ involvement and in those younger than 2 years.

Other Tumors With Skeletal Lesions

Neuroblastoma and acute lymphoblastic leukemia are childhood malignancies that frequently develop musculoskeletal sequelae. In a report of 648 metastatic neuroblastoma patients being treating in accordance with Children's Oncology Group protocols, 55% were found to have metastases to bone, and 70% were found to have metastases to bone marrow. Surgical biopsy may be useful for diagnosis or staging in patients with neuroblastoma; however, most skeletal lesions will resolve with chemotherapy or radiation therapy, and orthopaedic surgical intervention rarely is indicated.

Musculoskeletal symptoms may accompany acute leukemia in up to 30% of patients at presentation. Osteopenia, bone pain, metaphyseal bands, and osteolytic lesions are the most frequent manifestations. The orthopaedist should be cognizant of the musculoskeletal symptoms of leukemia to assist in the diagnosis and timely initiation of systemic treatment. In addition, osteonecrosis occurs in approximately 15% of patients with leukemia who are treated with high-dose corticosteroids as part of their cancer therapy. Osteonecrosis in young patients with cancer is challenging to treat. If possible, corticosteroids should be reduced or discontinued. Surgical intervention with core decompression, osteotomy, bone grafting, or joint arthroplasty should be considered to relieve pain.

Common Soft-Tissue Tumors

Popliteal Cysts

Popliteal, synovial, or Baker cysts are common occurring masses in the posterior knee of children that can be confused with soft-tissue neoplasms. They are most common in the posteromedial knee in children between the ages of 4 and 8 years. Popliteal cysts are usually asymptomatic and not associated with intra-articular pathology. Because popliteal cysts in children typically will spontaneously resolve and require no treatment, distinguishing a popliteal cyst from a soft-tissue sarcoma or other solid tumor is critical. A history of fluctuating size is consistent with the presence of a popliteal cyst, whereas a soft-tissue sarcoma will not decrease in size and will become progressively larger. Transillumination of the mass or ultrasound can help verify the cystic nature of the lesion. If there is any question on ultrasound, MRI will reliably identify the fluid-filled popliteal cyst versus any soft-tissue tumor.

Once a diagnosis of popliteal cyst is made by examination or diagnostic imaging, serial observation and parental assurance is the treatment of choice. Rarely, a painful cyst will require surgical resection, and recurrence rates are significant.

Hemangioma

Hemangiomas are benign proliferations of blood vessels. They are the most common soft-tissue tumors of infancy and childhood and account for approximately 7% of all benign tumors. The characterization and anatomic distribution of hemangiomas vary widely. Hemangiomas may occur in virtually any anatomic location.

Capillary hemangiomas, capillary-sized proliferations of blood vessels occurring in the skin or subcutaneous tissue in the first few weeks or months after birth, are the most common subtype of hemangioma. They appear as elevated, red or purple masses and may enlarge rapidly, usually achieving their largest size in 6 to 12 months. Most capillary hemangiomas (75% to 90%) spontaneously resolve within several years. When the tumor occurs during the rapid-growth phase, there is a tendency to intervene with treatment; however, because of the natural history of spontaneous regression, treatment is rarely necessary. Management with skilled observation and parental assurance is optimal in most instances.

Cavernous hemangiomas occur less frequently than capillary hemangiomas, but are also most common during childhood. Cavernous hemangiomas differ from capillary hemangiomas in that they are larger, less circumscribed, and have large, dilated, blood-filled vessels. They more frequently involve deep structures, including muscle and synovium.

Many patients with cavernous hemangiomas may have minimal symptoms. Some patients may have symptoms of aching pain that worsen with activity or dependent positioning. They may have compression of neighboring structures, muscle spasm or contracture, or joint destruction (if intra-articular).

Diagnostic imaging studies of cavernous hemangiomas often demonstrate phleboliths on standard radiographs. Radiographs also may show bone or joint erosions from local compression and repeated intra-articular hemorrhage. MRI scans are most valuable in evaluating these tumors and can be virtually diagnostic; the characteristic pattern is a "serpiginous" mixture of high- and low-signal intensity on T1- and T2-weighted images.

Treatment should be individualized based on symptoms. Unlike capillary hemangiomas, cavernous hemangiomas have little tendency to regress. Progression usually is slow and limited. A combination of compression stockings and NSAIDs may benefit some patients. Embolization and sclerotherapy have been reported to have limited success. Surgical resection may be necessary for the most symptomatic patients. A wide surgical margin is preferable, but often not achievable to spare vital functional structures. Recurrence rates are substantial. Radiation therapy should be avoided for hemangiomas because of associated risks, including radiation-induced sarcomas. Interferon-2A and other antiangiogenesis agents have been used for the control of large or life-threatening hemangiomas that cannot be treated surgically.

Rhabdomyosarcoma

Rhabdomyosarcomas are a heterogeneous group of malignancies of mesenchymal cell origin. Although rhabdomyosarcomas may arise from sites of skeletal muscle, this is not always true, suggesting they arise from undifferentiated cells. Rhabdomyosarcoma is the most common soft-tissue sarcoma in children, accounting for approximately 50% of soft-tissue sarcomas of childhood. Two percent of rhabdomyosarcomas may be present at birth, 5% are diagnosed in the first year of life, and more than 50% occur in the first decade of life.

Histologic classification conventionally recognizes several subtypes: embryonal, botryoid, alveolar, and ple-

omorphic rhabdomyosarcomas. The alveolar subtype generally has the poorest prognosis, and also is the most common subtype in the extremities. Rhabdomyosarcoma arises in three predominant anatomic regions: the head and neck, the genitourinary tract and retroperitoneum, and the extremities. Orthopaedic surgeons will typically encounter rhabdomyosarcomas in the extremities, which account for 15% to 20% of all rhabdomyosarcomas.

Treatment of rhabdomyosarcoma has improved dramatically over the past 40 years. Radical surgical resections during the 1960s resulted in significant functional loss and disfigurement, with a survival rate of less than 10%. Using multiagent chemotherapy, radiation therapy, and surgery, the overall 5-year survival rates are now 71%; however, alveolar subtypes have a much poorer prognosis (an overall 5-year survival rate of 38%).

A wide margin of resection of rhabdomyosarcomas is recommended to decrease the risk of local recurrence. If possible, a limb-sparing wide resection can be performed while preserving the functional and cosmetic status of the limb. The size and location of the tumor and the involvement of the major nerves usually dictate the ability to salvage a functional limb. Involved vessels may be bypassed, and functional free muscle flaps may be used for soft-tissue reconstruction. The sacrifice of one major nerve to an extremity may be preferable to an amputation. If an adequate surgical margin cannot be obtained while sparing the limb, then amputation should be performed.

Orthopaedic surgeons should be aware of the risk for regional lymph node metastases in patients with rhabdomyosarcoma, which at 10% to 15% is higher than that for other soft-tissue sarcomas. Sentinel lymph node mapping and biopsy should be considered.

Synovial Sarcoma

Among the nonrhabdomyosarcoma soft-tissue sarcomas, the most common in children is synovial sarcoma, which accounts for approximately 5% to 10% of soft-tissue sarcomas in children and adolescents. Despite the name, the origin of synovial sarcoma from synovial tissues has never been proved. Although synovial sarcoma occurs primarily in the periarticular regions of the extremities, it may occur in any location.

Clinical signs and symptoms may be more prolonged for patients with synovial sarcoma than for those with rhabdomyosarcoma, with many reported instances of masses or pain being present for more than 2 years before treatment. A slow-growing mass is the most common sign of synovial sarcoma, and pain is a frequent symptom.

Radiographs for patients with synovial sarcoma demonstrate calcifications within the soft-tissue mass in approximately 30% of patients. MRI typically shows a heterogeneous, solid soft-tissue tumor that is characteristic of most soft-tissue sarcomas.

The histology associated with synovial sarcoma has a classic biphasic type, monophasic fibrous type, or monophasic epithelial type. Recent molecular genetic findings have shown a balanced reciprocal translocation, t(X;18) (p11.2;q11.2), in more than 90% of synovial sarcomas. Two fusion genes have been identified (*SYT-SSX1* and *SYT-SSX2*), but their clinical difference with regard to metastatic potential is not clear.

Surgical wide resection is the primary treatment of synovial sarcoma. For large tumors around the ankle or foot, this often requires amputation because of soft-tissue and reconstructive limitations. Smaller tumors and those in other locations often are amenable to limb-sparing wide resection. Radiation therapy or brachytherapy may be considered for adjuvant local control in situations with less than optimal surgical margins. The Children's Oncology Group has several ongoing chemotherapy trials for children with synovial sarcoma.

Limb-Salvage Surgery in Children

Oncologic reconstruction in the growing child is complicated by accommodations for continued growth. Many surgical options are available to accommodate for potential limb-length inequality in the growing child, including epiphysiodesis, acute shortening, distraction osteogenesis, amputation, rotationplasty, modular endoprosthetics, and noninvasive expandable endoprosthetics. All of these options should be in the orthopaedic surgeon's armamentarium, and surgical decisions should be made individually by consulting with the patient, family, and medical team to devise the best overall treatment plan.

The overall consideration of salvaging a limb versus amputation involves several factors. The primary oncologic consideration for patients with high-grade sarcomas is to achieve a wide resection margin. If the tumor surrounds major nerves or vital structures to the limb, and achieving a wide margin would render the limb functionless, then amputation is the better choice. In children younger than 5 years, reconstruction with limb equalization becomes extremely difficult. In the upper extremity, limb preservation should be attempted despite compromise of limb length or shoulder function if function of the hand can be preserved. The oncologic margin should not be compromised.

If amputation is chosen, the amputation level should be as distal as possible for both upper and lower limb amputations while still ensuring a wide surgical margin and optimum local control. Consideration should be given to disarticulation when margins and soft-tissue coverage allow. Disarticulation at the knee allows some end bearing and continued growth of the residual limb and also eliminates stump overgrowth, which can occur in up to 50% of transosseous skeletally immature amputees. Painful stump overgrowth often requires revision amputation surgery.

Rotationplasty is an intercalary amputation that converts an above-knee amputation to a functional below-knee amputation. After resection of a distal femoral or proximal tibial tumor and knee joint, the ipsilateral ankle is rotated 180° and reattached to the remaining femur. The rotated ankle then functions as a knee joint with a specialized external prosthesis. Limb-length discrepancy issues also are eliminated by rotationplasty if the rotated ankle and contralateral knee joint are placed at a level that will be equal at skeletal maturity. The rotationplasty prosthesis is adjusted during growth to accommodate limb-length differences. The advantages include a durable reconstruction of native bone that is amenable to athletic and high-impact activities, whereas the disadvantages primarily are cosmetic, and many families in the United States have difficulty accepting the appearance of a rotated limb despite its functionality. Derotation of the limb during growth is not as common in oncology patients when compared with rotationplasty for patients with congenital limb deficiency.

Limb-salvage endoprosthetic designs have advanced in the past 5 years with attempts to accommodate for growth and prosthetic durability. These implants have been successful from a tumor perspective, but high implant revision rates are of concern. Modular endoprostheses can be lengthened in the growing child, but this requires a large open surgery with removal of periprosthetic scar tissue, which has associated risks of infection, neurovascular injury, and extended convalescence and rehabilitation. The Repiphysis prosthesis (Wright Medical Technology, Arlington, TN) accommodates for growth by expanding in a noninvasive manner. The prosthesis contains a compressed spring that is encased within polyethylene. To expand the prosthesis, an electromagnet is placed over the spring, melting the polyethylene, and releasing stored energy in the spring to lengthen the prosthesis. Expansions usually are performed in 7- to 10-mm increments to keep up with the growth of the contralateral limb until skeletal maturity. Early results in 18 patients have shown an average expansion of 38 mm per patient over 2 years. One failure of expansion has been reported as well as several component fractures requiring revision.

Prosthetic stem fixation, whether cemented or cementless, becomes a problem in the child because of aseptic loosening. Activity levels of children and adolescents generally are higher than in adults, placing more stress on prosthetic fixation. Prosthetic loosening may result in multiple revision surgeries over a patient's lifetime. A new device that addresses prosthetic fixation is the Compress System (Biomet, Warsaw, IN). The system uses compliant prestress fixation with a stacked series of

Belleville washers compressed within the prosthesis to achieve immediate rigid fixation without a standard stem. Forces generated by compression stimulate bone hypertrophy and ingrowth at the bone-prosthetic junction. Encouraging early results have been reported for this design, particularly in young patients who put high demands on their prosthesis for many years.

Annotated Bibliography
Initial Evaluation

Greene FL, Page DL, Fleming ID, et al (eds): AJCC Cancer Staging Handbook, in *AJCC Cancer Staging Manual, ed 6.* New York, NY, Springer-Verlag. 2002, pp 213-219.

This handbook contains the full TNM parameters, stage grouping, explanatory text, and features all of the required fields for the AJCC-approved hospital cancer programs.

Osseous Tumors by Tissue Type

Ahmed AR, Tan TS, Unni KK, Collins MS, Wenger DE, Sim FH: Secondary chondrosarcoma in osteochondroma: Report of 107 patients. *Clin Orthop* 2003;411:193-206.

This retrospective study revealed that irregularity of the margin, inhomogeneous mineralization, and an associated soft-tissue mass were radiographic signs of sarcomatous degeneration in patients with solitary osteochondromas.

Bielack SS, Kempf-Bielack B, Delling G, et al: Prognostic factors in high-grade osteosarcoma of the extremities or trunk: An analysis of 1,702 patients treated on neoadjuvant cooperative osteosarcoma study group protocols. *J Clin Oncol* 2002;20:776-790.

The authors present an analysis of data from the European Cooperative Osteosarcoma Study Group. They found that tumor size, site, primary metastasis, response to chemotherapy, and extent of surgery were of independent prognostic value.

DiCaprio MR, Enneking WF: Fibrous dysplasia: Pathophysiology, evaluation and treatment. *J Bone Joint Surg Am* 2005;87:1848-1864.

The authors provide a comprehensive overview of fibrous dysplasia, with emphasis on pathophysiology of the Gs-α activating mutation, clinical decision making, and treatment options.

Ghanem I, Collet LM, Kharrat K, et al: Percutaneous radiofrequency coagulation of osteoid osteoma in children and adolescents. *J Pediatr Orthop B* 2003;12:244-252.

This is the only report of radiofrequency ablation exclusively in children and adolescents. The authors retrospectively reviewed 23 patients and found that 21 patients had relief of pain with one radiofrequency ablation.

Goorin AM, Schwartzentruber DJ, Devidas M, et al: Presurgical chemotherapy compared with immediate surgery and adjuvant chemotherapy for nonmetastatic osteosarcoma: Pediatric Oncology Group study POG-8651. *J Clin Oncol* 2003;21:1574-1580.

The authors of this prospective, randomized clinical trial of 100 patients found no difference in event-free survival for patients having immediate surgery followed by chemotherapy versus surgery at week 10 of the chemotherapy protocol. They also reported no difference in the rate of limb salvage.

Pierz KA, Stieber JR, Kusumi K, Dormans JP: Hereditary multiple exostoses: One center's experience and review of etiology. *Clin Orthop* 2002;401:49-59.

The authors reviewed clinical data on 43 patients with hereditary multiple exostosis. They discuss the clinical spectrum of the disease and provide a good review of the *EXT* family of gene mutations responsible for the disease.

Porter DE, Lonie L, Fraser M, et al: Severity of disease and risk of malignant change in hereditary multiple exostoses. *J Bone Joint Surg Br* 2004;86:1041-1046.

The authors conducted a single-blinded, prospective study of 172 individuals (78 families) with hereditary multiple exostosis. They reported that patients with the *EXT1* mutation had significantly worse phenotypic expression of the disease in three of five parameters. The authors also found a higher association between the *EXT1* mutation and malignant transformation to chondrosarcoma.

Potter BK, Freedman BA, Lehman RA Jr, Shawen SB, Kuklo TR, Murphey MD: Solitary epiphyseal enchondromas. *J Bone Joint Surg Am* 2005;87:1551-1560.

The authors conducted a retrospective review of 33 patients with epiphyseal enchondromas, which is twice the number previously reported in the literature. The radiographic and clinical features of epiphyseal enchondromas are discussed.

Scully SP, Ghert MA, Zurakowski D, Thompson RC, Gebhardt MC: Pathologic fracture in osteosarcoma: Prognostic importance and treatment implications. *J Bone Joint Surg Am* 2002;84-A(1):49-57.

In this retrospective study that was conducted with the cooperation of the MSTS, 52 patients with osteosarcoma and pathologic fractures were compared with 55 patients with osteosarcoma and no fractures. The authors reported that the 5-year estimated survival rates were 55% in the patients with pathologic fractures and 77% in the patients with no fractures ($P = 0.02$). They also reported that performance of a limb-salvage procedure in selected patients with pathologic fractures did not increase the risk of local recurrence or death.

Miscellaneous Bone Tumors and Tumor-like Conditions

Bacci G, Ferrari S, Longhi A, et al: Local and systemic control in Ewing's sarcoma of the femur treated with chemotherapy, and locally by radiotherapy and/or surgery. *J Bone Joint Surg Br* 2003;85:107-114.

The authors from the Rizzoli Institute performed a retrospective review of 91 patients to compare surgery alone, surgery and radiotherapy, and radiotherapy alone in patients with Ewing's sarcoma of the femur. Survival and local recurrence were improved with surgical treatment (with or without radiotherapy) compared with radiotherapy alone.

Dormans JP, Hanna BG, Johnston DR, Khurana JS: Surgical treatment and recurrence rate of aneurysmal bone cysts in children. *Clin Orthop* 2004;421:205-211.

The authors conducted a retrospective study of 45 pediatric patients with aneurysmal bone cysts and compared recurrence rates stratified by age groups. They found no difference in persistence or recurrence rates based on age.

Oliveira AM, Perez-Atayde AR, Dal Cin P, et al: Aneurysmal bone cyst variant translocations upregulate USP6 transcription by promoter swapping with the ZNF9, COL1A1, TRAP150, and OMD genes. *Oncogene* 2005;24(21):3419-3426.

The authors discuss chromosome 17p13 rearrangements in aneurysmal bone cysts and provide characterization of four different aneurysmal bone cyst translocations involving 17p13, each of which is associated with a novel *USP6* fusion oncogene.

Snyder BD, Hauser-Kara DA, Hipp JA, Zurakowski D, Hecht AC, Gebhardt MC: Predicting fracture through benign skeletal lesions with quantitative computed tomography. *J Bone Joint Surg Am* 2006;88:55-70.

Quantitative CT was used in 36 pediatric patients with benign bone lesions to predict the risk of pathologic fracture. A combination of bending and torsional rigidity was used to calculate the risk of fracture with 97% accuracy.

Other Tumors With Skeletal Lesions

Kobayashi D, Satsuma S, Kamegaya M, et al: Musculoskeletal conditions of acute leukemia and malignant lymphoma in children. *J Pediatr Orthop B.* 2005;14(3):156-161.

The authors of this retrospective study evaluated and discuss the orthopaedic radiographic and clinical manifestations of leukemia and lymphoma.

Common Soft-Tissue Tumors

Guillou L, Benhattar J, Bonichon F, et al: Histologic grade, but not SYT-SSX fusion type, is an important prognostic factor in patients with synovial sarcoma: A multicenter, retrospective analysis. *J Clin Oncol* 2004;22: 4040-4050.

In contrast to previous studies, the authors of this study reported that the *SYT-SSX* fusion type was not found to be a prognostic indicator of metastasis or survival.

Okcu MF, Munsell M, Treuner J, et al: Synovial sarcoma of childhood and adolescence: A multicenter, multivariate analysis of outcome. *J Clin Oncol* 2003;21:1602-1611.

The authors of this study identified the prognostic factors related to outcome in 219 patients with synovial sarcoma by using multivariate analysis. They report that clinical group, tumor size, and invasiveness were important prognostic factors.

Punyko JA, Mertens AC, Baker KS, Ness KK, Robison LL, Gurney JG: Long-term survival probabilities for childhood rhabdomyosarcoma: A population-based evaluation. *Cancer* 2005;103:1475-1483.

This is a statistical analysis of data on 848 children with rhabdomyosarcoma; the data were obtained from the Surveillance, Epidemiology, and End Results Program. The authors report that significant variations in 5-year survival rates were found based on patient age and tumor characteristics.

Limb-Salvage Surgery in Children

Kumta SM, Cheng JC, Li CK, Griffith JF, Chow LT, Quintos AD: Scope and limitations of limb-sparing surgery in childhood sarcomas. *J Pediatr Orthop* 2002;22: 244-248.

The authors conducted a retrospective review of 43 pediatric limb-salvage cases and present an algorithm for limb-sparing versus amputation surgery.

Neel MD, Wilkins RM, Rao BN, Kelly CM: Early multicenter experience with a noninvasive expandable prosthesis. *Clin Orthop* 2003;415:72-81.

The authors conducted a retrospective multicenter study of 15 pediatric patients who received 18 noninvasive expandable prostheses. They report that 60 expansions were successful in gaining an average of 8.5 mm per lengthening and that revision rates were high for patients with component fractures.

Classic Bibliography

Allen PW, Enzinger FM: Hemangioma of skeletal muscle: An analysis of 89 cases. *Cancer* 1972;29:8-22.

Bini SA, Johnston JO, Martin DL: Compliant prestress fixation in tumor prostheses: interface retrieval data. *Orthopedics* 2000;23(7):707-711.

Enneking WF (ed): *Limb Salvage in Musculoskeletal Oncology.* New York, NY, Churchill Livingstone, 1987.

Enneking WF, Spanier SS, Goodman MA: A system for the surgical staging of musculoskeletal sarcoma. *Clin Orthop* 1980;153:106-120.

Gitelis S, Wilkins R, Conrad EU III: Benign bone tumors. *Instr Course Lect* 1996;45:425-426.

Mankin HJ, Mankin CJ, Simon MA: The hazards of the biopsy, revisited: Members of the Musculoskeletal Tumor Society. *J Bone Joint Surg Am* 1996;78:656-663.

Rougraff BT, Simon MA, Kneisl JS, Greenberg DB, Mankin HJ: Limb salvage compared with amputation for osteosarcoma of the distal end of the femur: A long-term oncological, functional, and quality-of-life study. *J Bone Joint Surg Am* 1994;76:649-656.

Simon MA, Aschliman MA, Thomas N, Mankin HJ: Limb-salvage treatment versus amputation for osteosar-coma of the distal end of the femur. *J Bone Joint Surg Am* 1986;68:1331-1337.

Widhe B, Widhe T: Initial symptoms and clinical features in osteosarcoma and Ewing sarcoma. *J Bone Joint Surg Am* 2000;82:667-674.

Winkelmann WW: Rotationplasty. *Orthop Clin North Am* 1996;27:503-523.

Section 2

Neuromuscular Disorders and Metabolic Bone Diseases

Section Editor:
William G. Mackenzie, MD

Chapter 8

Cerebral Palsy

Kirk W. Dabney, MD

Freeman Miller, MD

Introduction

Cerebral palsy is a heterogeneous condition characterized by a nonprogressive injury to the immature motor cortex of the brain. The size and location of this lesion determines not only the severity of motor involvement, but also the concomitant involvement of the child's speech, cognition, and sensation. Modern technology has improved the survival rate of children with cerebral palsy; it is now the most prevalent neuromuscular disorder in children.

Classification

Because of its heterogeneity, cerebral palsy is commonly classified physiologically, anatomically, and functionally. The physiologic classification defines the motor characteristics and reflects the location of the brain lesion. There are four types of cerebral palsy: spasticity, dyskinesia, ataxia, and a mixed type, which is a combination of two or more of the first three types.

Spasticity, the most common type of cerebral palsy, occurs when the pyramidal area of the brain is involved. Dyskinesia occurs when the extrapyramidal region of the brain is involved and is characterized by involuntary motor movements. Dyskinesia includes athetosis, rigidity, and dystonia. Ataxia is uncommon and occurs when the cerebellar region of the brain is involved. Ataxia is characterized by a disturbance in balance and a patient's inability to coordinate voluntary movements. The mixed type of cerebral palsy often results in spasticity and dyskinesia.

The anatomic classification describes the number of limbs involved: quadriplegia (all four extremities), diplegia (lower extremity involvement greater than upper extremity involvement), and hemiplegia (arm and leg involvement on one side of the body, usually with greater upper extremity involvement). Other descriptions include variable anatomic involvement, such as triplegia, double hemiplegia, asymmetric diplegia, and triplegia. Unfortunately, overlaps in the anatomic classification of cerebral palsy can result in confusion (for example, severe diplegia may overlap with less severe quadriple-

gia). For this reason, a functional classification, which is descriptive (community ambulator, household ambulator, exercise ambulator, or nonambulator), is often more useful. Additional descriptors further describe function (for example, a community ambulator with an assistive device and ankle-foot orthosis [AFO]). More recently, the Gross Motor Function Classification System, a five-level grading system, has been devised that describes the spectrum of function in children with cerebral palsy (Table 1). Level I is the most advanced gross motor skill and self-mobility level and level V is the most restricted level in self-mobility, even with the use of assistive technology. Distinctions among the levels is based on self-initiated movement, with a particular emphasis on sitting and walking, and functional limitations (the need for assistive mobility devices, wheeled mobility, and to a lesser extent quality of movement). Functional limitations have been established as guidelines for each of the five levels within four specific age categories (birth to 2 years, 2 to 4 years, 4 to 6 years, and 6 to 12 years). Interrater reliability is high using this classification system, and its ability to reliably predict motor function is good. Recently, this classification system has also been shown to correlate strongly with transfer and mobility abilities, sports and physical function, and gait velocity and oxygen consumption data during gait analysis in ambulatory children with cerebral palsy. Classification schemes have also been established for hemiplegia (types 1 through 4) and more recently for diplegia. The classification scheme for diplegia is based on five sagittal gait patterns derived from a combination of kinematic gait data and pattern recognition.

Prevalence and Etiology

The prevalence of cerebral palsy is variable and ranges from 1.5 to 3 per 1,000 live births. The neonate who is premature and weighs less than 1,500 g has a 90 per 1,000 prevalence of cerebral palsy. In addition to premature birth, other risk factors include chorioamnionitis, placental complications, third trimester bleeding, maternal epilepsy, severe toxemia, and low Apgar scores (< 3

Table 1 | Gross Motor Function Classification System

Level	Function	Limitations
I	Walk/run indoors and outdoors without braces or assistive devices	More advanced gross motor skills (speed, balance, and coordination)
II	Walk without assistive devices	Running; walking on uneven surfaces/inclines (outdoors) and in crowds/confined spaces (community)
III	Walk indoors or outdoors on a level surface with an assistive mobility device; good upper extremity function	Require self-propelled wheelchair or transport for long distance or uneven terrain
IV	May at best walk short distance with a walker; need trunk support for upper extremity function	Require transport or power mobility outdoors and in the community
V	Some children achieve power mobility with extensive adaptations	Self-mobility is severely limited even with the use of assistive technology; poor trunk and upper extremity function

at 10 minutes after birth). Multiple etiologies can cause insult to the immature brain and include cerebral anoxia, intraventricular hemorrhage, infection (bacterial and viral), maternal drug and alcohol use, various other teratogens, and numerous genetic syndromes. Mental retardation is seen in 60% to 65% of children with severe cerebral palsy (quadriplegia). Seizure disorders may occur in up to 30% of children with cerebral palsy. Swallowing difficulties, gastroesophageal reflux, and associated aspiration pneumonias are more common in children with more severe motor involvement. Children with more severe cerebral palsy, therefore, often require the involvement of multiple medical specialists, including the orthopaedic surgeon.

Goal Setting and the Orthopaedic Surgeon

From the orthopaedic surgeon's vantage point, it is helpful to divide goal setting into four main age groups. From ages 0 to 3 years, physical therapy is a main focus. The therapist is therefore often the primary care provider and goal setter for patients in this age group. From ages 4 to 6 years, therapy remains important; however, this is also the ideal age for orthopaedic intervention in children with the appropriate indications. In patients in this age group, functional issues become apparent, and orthopaedic surgery is least disruptive to the child's education. During age 7 to 18 years, the educational and psychological needs of the patient should be the primary focus. Orthopaedic surgery is still important in many children in this age group, but disruptions in the child's education should be minimized. After age 18 years, integrating the patient into the work force, addressing independence and residential issues, and considering future relationships/marriage are issues of primary concern.

Initially, the primary concern of parents of children with cerebral palsy is usually whether their child will walk. Ambulatory potential depends on several factors, including balance and coordination, overall muscle strength, various biomechanical factors such as skeletal deformity and muscle tendon length, and supplying the energy demands necessary to walk. Several prognostic indicators for future ambulation have been cited as important; the persistence of two or more primitive reflexes after the age of 12 months is considered a poor prognostic indicator for future ambulation. If children are not sitting independently by the age of 5 years and not walking by the age of 8 years, they are also unlikely to be independent ambulators. Although ambulation is a primary concern, the functional priorities of the adult with cerebral palsy in order of importance are typically communication, activities of daily living, and mobility. Walking is inclusive, but not exclusive within mobility. The physician should always be mindful that the family and health care team have limited time, resources, and energies to devote to all of these priorities during a single period. From the orthopaedist's perspective, it is helpful to devise long-term goals based on the level of motor involvement and the age of the child.

Ambulatory Patients

A normal gait pattern is typically established when children are approximately 3½ years of age. Normal gait requires a normal control system (motor cortex) and energy source, properly aligned and functioning skeletal levers, and adequate motors. Damage to the central control system in children with cerebral palsy causes a loss of selective muscle control, a dependence on primitive reflex patterns, abnormal muscle tone, a relative imbalance between muscle agonists and antagonists, and a deficiency of normal equilibrium reactions. All of these conditions cause the pathologic gait patterns seen in children with cerebral palsy. Gait patterns can be qualified as a loss of one or more of the following prerequisites necessary for a normal gait: an unstable stance limb, insufficient foot clearance during the swing phase of gait, inappropriate prepositioning of the foot at the end of swing phase of gait, an inadequate step length, and overall inadequate energy conservation throughout the gait cycle. The astute orthopaedist must distinguish

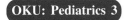

between primary abnormalities (muscle spasticity, loss of balance, and loss of selective muscle control), secondary abnormalities (fixed muscle/tendon contractures and bony deformities), and tertiary abnormalities (compensatory or coping responses). The goals of the orthopaedic surgeon are to reestablish as many of the normal gait prerequisites as possible, improve abnormal muscle tone and difficulties with motor control, and optimize energy expenditure. This requires a detailed clinical examination to assess strength, muscle tone, selective motor control, balance and equilibrium, the presence of dynamic versus fixed muscle contractures, and the presence of any bone deformities (femoral and tibial torsional deformities and foot deformities). It is imperative to minimize the number of surgical events by performing multilevel procedures as needed. This results in less psychological trauma to the child, less burden to the family, easier rehabilitation, less interruption in the child's education, and fewer hospital admissions. Computerized three-dimensional gait analysis is recommended in children with complex gait patterns to assist with decision making.

Gait Analysis

Routine physical examination cannot always characterize the complex nature of the many abnormal gait patterns that occur in children with cerebral palsy. Computerized three-dimensional gait analysis is an extremely useful tool that provides the clinician with a more descriptive and quantitative means of analyzing the abnormal gait patterns that occur in these children. It should consist of (1) a detailed physical examination measuring tone, strength of individual muscles, range of motion of each joint, muscle contractures, and motor function (using, for example, the Gross Motor Function Measure, (2) temporal and spatial data, (3) videotaped observational analysis, (4) kinematic data, (5) kinetic data, (6) dynamic electromyography, and (7) pedobarography to measure foot pressure and energy consumption data.

Recently, a classification scheme based on physical examination and three-dimensional gait analysis was described for spastic diplegia that characterized five common sagittal gait patterns based on a cross-sectional study of 187 children with spastic diplegia. Children with pattern I (true equinus) have ankle equinus and the knee and hip extend fully. The pelvis is in normal position or tilted anteriorly. In children with pattern II (jump gait), the ankle is in equinus; however, the hip and knee do not reach full extension. The pelvis is in normal position or tilted anteriorly. Children with pattern III (apparent equinus) have normal ankle range of motion; however, the knee and hip are excessively flexed. The pelvis is in normal position or tilted anteriorly. Children appear to be in equinus because of excessive hip knee and flexion contracture. Children with pattern IV (crouch gait) have excessive hip and knee flexion, but there is excessive dorsiflexion at the ankle. The pelvis is in normal position or tilted posteriorly. Children with pattern V have an asymmetric gait pattern with each of their lower limb patterns belonging to different groups. In this study, 34 children were followed longitudinally for a period of 1 year. The classification demonstrated both intrarater and interrater reliability.

Although controversy still exists regarding surgical intervention for children with cerebral palsy, most ambulatory children with cerebral palsy who are being considered for surgical intervention should also undergo full three-dimensional gait analysis because preliminary data have shown its value in guiding and altering surgical decision making.

Hip

Hip subluxation and dislocation is uncommon in ambulatory patients with cerebral palsy. More commonly, ambulatory patients with cerebral palsy have difficulty with a scissoring gait because of adductor muscle spasticity. Inadequate foot clearance occurs during the swing phase of gait because one extremity gets caught on the opposite extremity. Treatment includes surgical lengthening of the adductor longus and gracilis muscles.

Hip flexor or iliopsoas tightness causes the patient to walk with a flexed hip posture, often with an increase in lordosis. Gait analysis typically shows decreased hip extension in the sagittal plane and increased anterior pelvic tilt, often with a double-bump pattern during stance (Figure 1). Weakness of hip extensors and ankle plantar flexors is often concomitant with hamstring tightness, making it difficult to discern the ideal treatment. When an obvious hip flexion contracture exists, an intramuscular iliopsoas lengthening is the treatment of choice. This procedure may be done over the brim of the pelvis or through the groin if accompanied by adductor tenotomy.

Increased femoral anteversion resulting in a toe-in gait pattern is also commonly encountered in children with cerebral palsy and is thought to produce lever arm dysfunction; bone malrotation can lead to less effective hip flexor and extensor muscle function. The normal infant is born with increased femoral anteversion of approximately 40° to 45°, which decreases to approximately 15° in the normal adult. Persistence of this infantile anteversion is common in many children with cerebral palsy. In one study of 147 patients with cerebral palsy, femoral anteversion was similar to that in healthy children at an early age. As age increased, however, anteversion improved in healthy children, but it did not change in those with cerebral palsy. Assessment of femoral anteversion can be difficult. The use of CT has been described for the assessment of femoral anteversion in patients with cerebral palsy; however, its value is contro-

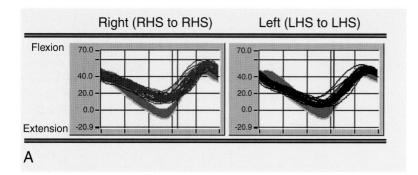

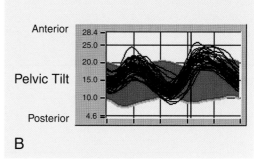

Figure 1 Kinematic findings characteristic of hip flexion (iliopsoas) contracture. **A,** Sagittal plane kinematics of the hip show decreased hip extension compared with normal (gray) in stance. **B,** Sagittal plane pelvic kinematics show data from a patient with a typical double-bump pattern (black) during stance compared with normal range (gray). RHS = right hip stance, LHS = left hip stance.

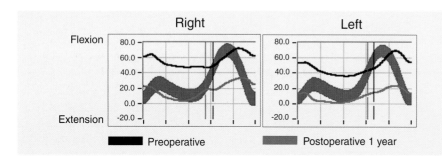

Figure 2 Kinematic findings on gait analysis characteristic of hamstring tightness show increased knee flexion at initial contact and decreased knee extension at terminal swing. This child from whom these data were derived has rectus femoris spasticity. Postoperative kinematics after hamstring lengthening shows a shift in the entire pattern down, correcting excessive knee flexion in stance but not providing the correction to restore the necessary peak knee flexion in swing. This child may benefit from a rectus femoris transfer.

versial. One recent study using model femurs showed accurate assessment of anteversion to be highly dependent on optimum positioning within the CT scanner. Measurement using three-dimensional CT techniques showed a statistically significant increase in accuracy over two-dimensional CT when positioning was optimum. Preoperatively, assessment of femoral alignment in the transverse plane by gait analysis gives an accurate, real-time assessment of femoral alignment, but it may be dependent on marker placement.

Rotational osteotomies of the proximal or distal femur have each been shown to have comparable results in the correction of rotational alignment. In children with hemiplegia, correction of femoral anteversion may also assist in correcting transverse plane pelvic rotational alignment.

Knee
Hamstring tightness is a frequent contributor to a crouched gait in children with cerebral palsy. Patients typically have an increase in popliteal angle on physical examination. Kinematic evaluation on gait analysis shows increased knee flexion at initial foot contact in the stance phase of gait and decreased knee extension in the terminal swing phase of gait (Figure 2). Increased knee flexion may persist through midstance if the gastrocnemius muscle is too weak. Medial hamstring lengthening is performed initially. If severe crouch is present, lateral hamstring lengthening is also performed.

A stiff-knee gait pattern is common in this patient population and is typically characterized by toe dragging during the swing phase of gait and frequent tripping. There are several causes of a stiff-knee gait in children with cerebral palsy, including poor hip flexion, poor hip strength, and an overactive rectus femoris muscle. On physical examination, increased rectus femoris muscle tone is common, but it is not always observed in patients with a positive Duncan-Ely test. This pattern is caused by abnormal activity of the rectus femoris muscle during the swing phase of gait, which can be identified with the use of dynamic electromyography (Figure 3). Children with a stiff-knee gait pattern also have decreased and/or delayed peak flexion during the swing phase of gait on sagittal knee kinematics causing inadequate foot clearance. A transfer of the rectus femoris to one of the knee flexors is the recommended treatment to improve knee flexion during the swing phase of gait when abnormal rectus femoris swing phase activity is present. Recently, three-dimensional computerized modeling created from MRI scans obtained after rectus transfer suggests that the beneficial effects of the procedure result from reducing the effect of the rectus femoris muscle as a knee extensor rather than converting it to a knee flexor.

Anterior knee pain is common in preadolescents or adolescents with cerebral palsy. Patients are frequently crouched secondary to hamstring spasticity and may also have increased rectus femoris spasticity. Patellae alta is usually identified on routine radiographs.

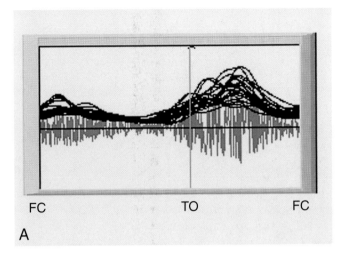

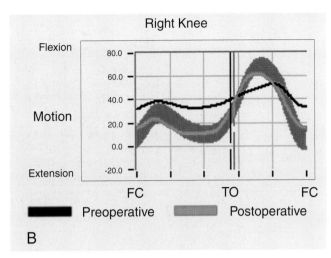

Figure 3 **A,** Typical electromyographic findings with a stiff-knee gait resulting from abnormal swing phase activity of the rectus femoris muscle. The rectus femoris muscle should be relatively inactive during swing phase. FC = foot contact. **B,** Preoperative (black) sagittal plane knee kinematics typically shows both delayed and decreased swing phase peak knee flexion. After rectus femoris transfer and hamstring lengthening (dark gray), the sagittal plane kinematics are within a normal range (light gray). Peak knee flexion (60° to 70°) should occur at approximately one third of the way into swing phase. FC = foot contact.

Occasionally, a stress fracture of the inferior pole of the patellae is found in this patient population, which is typically exhibited as tenderness over the distal patellae. Conservative treatment usually involves hamstring stretching exercises. Hamstring lengthening for contractures may help if pain is not relieved. Excision of the inferior pole patellar fragment may be required for patients with patellar pole fractures who continue to experience pain. Uncommonly, children with spasticity and anterior knee pain will have subluxation or dislocation of the patellae. Treatment consists of lengthening the spastic hamstring muscle and soft-tissue realignment of the patellae. In skeletally mature children, medial transfer of the tibial tubercle may be performed.

Foot and Ankle

Full function of the foot and ankle are important for children to have stable limbs while standing and proper prepositioning of the foot before initial contact during gait. The most common foot and ankle deformities in children with cerebral palsy include equinus, equinovarus, planovalgus deformities, and torsional deformities of the tibia. Many children with spastic diplegia also develop a compensatory external tibial torsion to femoral anteversion. Deformities of the great and lesser toes may also be present. Restoration of normal sagittal ankle kinematics and kinetics is critical to successful treatment of these patients because the ankle is the primary source of power during normal walking (Figure 4, *A*). Lever-arm dysfunction is a common denominator in children with cerebral palsy and can negatively impact ankle power, making the correction of rotational alignment critical (Figure 4, *B*).

Equinus deformity is a result of spasticity of the gastrocnemius-soleus muscle complex. Clinically, two

patterns typically occur: a toe-walking gait pattern, which usually occurs in younger children, and a back-knee gait pattern, which occurs more commonly in older children. Younger children without a fixed contracture can usually be treated with an AFO. Another option is the use of a botulinum toxin injection into the gastrocnemius muscle to control dynamic spasticity. In children with more fixed contractures and when the use of an AFO is not effective, a gastrocnemius recession or Achilles tendon lengthening can be performed. The need for the latter is usually ascertained with the patient under anesthesia by testing ankle dorsiflexion with the knee in both extension and flexion. Equinus with the knee extended but dorsiflexion above neutral ankle position with the knee flexed indicates primarily gastrocnemius tightness, in which instance a recession can be performed without lengthening the soleus. Inability to dorsiflex the ankle above neutral with the knee flexed usually indicates the need for Achilles tendon lengthening. A gastrocnemius recession has been shown to result in better push-off power, and over-lengthening is less common than with Achilles tendon lengthening. Kinematics and kinetics are usually improved, however, after both procedures. Overlengthening of the gastrocnemius-soleus muscle complex can result in an increase in knee crouch and poor push-off power; therefore, this should be avoided. Equinus may recur as children continue to grow.

Equinovarus deformity is most frequently caused by spasticity of the tibialis posterior muscle and the gastrocnemius-soleus muscle complex. Spasticity of the tibialis anterior muscle may also contribute to the deformity. Equinovarus deformity occurs more commonly in children with spastic hemiplegic involvement. Clinically, the child toe-walks with increased foot pressure on the outer border of the foot, causing an unstable limb during

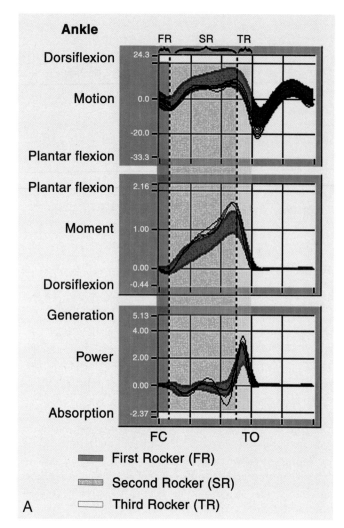

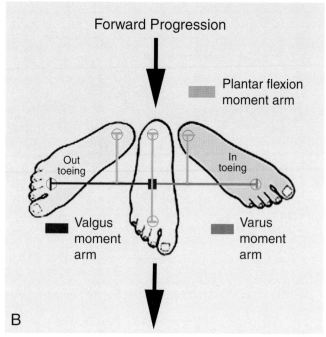

Figure 4 **A,** Normal ankle kinematics and kinetics of three ankle rockers. For the first ankle rocker, the foot plantar flexes from foot contact (FC) to foot flat and is controlled by eccentric contracture of the tibialis anterior. For the second ankle rocker, the foot dorsiflexes relative to the ankle during midstance and is controlled by eccentric contracture of the gastrocnemius-soleus complex. For the third ankle rocker, the foot plantar flexes during toe-off and is controlled by concentric contracture of the gastrocnemius-soleus complex. Note the sharp positive moment and power generated by the third rocker. **B,** The plantar flexion moment arm is determined by the cosine of the angle of rotation; therefore, greater than 30° of rotation rapidly decreases the moment arm length, decreasing the moment (force × moment arm length) and power (moment × angular acceleration). *(Reproduced with permission from Miller F: Gait, in Dabney K, Alexander M (eds): Cerebral Palsy. New York, NY, Springer, 2005, p 294 and p 317.)*

stance. In addition, the child is unable to adequately preposition the equinovarus foot before foot contact. Pedobarographs show increased lateral forefoot pressures in these patients. As with equinus deformity, younger children are usually adequately treated using an AFO. Botulinum toxin injection into the involved muscle groups may also be helpful if the deformity is dynamic. As the child grows, the deforming muscle typically becomes more fixed, in which instance lengthening of the gastrocnemius-soleus muscle complex and intramuscular lengthening or split transfer of the tibialis posterior tendon to the peroneus brevis can produce good long-term results. The split portion of the tibialis posterior tendon can be attached to the peroneus brevis proximal or distal to the lateral malleolus with equally good results. Tibialis posterior tendon surgery in children younger than 8 years, especially those with diplegia, can result in overcorrection into planovalgus as patients approach adolescence. The determination to perform a split tibialis posterior versus a split tibialis anterior tendon transfer is best based on both physical examination and gait analysis.

Dynamic electromyography should be used to monitor both the gastrocnemius and tibialis anterior muscles with surface electrodes and the tibialis posterior muscle with fine wire electrodes. If the tibialis posterior muscle does not have a fixed contracture and electromyography shows constant activity with varus throughout stance, a split tibialis posterior transfer is indicated. If varus is present during swing phase and the tibialis anterior shows constant activity or throughout most of stance, a split transfer of the tibialis anterior tendon is indicated. If both the tibialis anterior and tibialis posterior tendons show constant activity, either split transfer of both tendons or a myofascial lengthening of the tibialis posterior plus a split transfer of the tibialis anterior tendon should be considered. Older children with rigid equinovarus may not achieve correction without osteotomies in addition to soft-tissue balancing. Occasionally, a painful severe arthritic foot deformity may be treated with subtalar or triple arthrodesis.

Planovalgus deformity is common in children with spastic diplegia and quadriplegia. This deformity results from a combination of factors, including spasticity of the gastrocnemius-soleus muscle complex and peroneal muscles as well as tibialis posterior weakness. These children typically walk with increased foot pressure on the medial side of the foot, especially over the talar head. Pain may occur over this area, and a hallux valgus deformity may develop. These children typically have an unstable limb during stance, and the lever arm of the foot during the push-off phase of gait is significantly decreased, resulting in a marked decrease in push-off moment and power in the terminal stance phase of gait (Figure 5).

Standing AP and lateral radiographs of the foot and ankle should be obtained for this patient population. Valgus deformity of the ankle joint may be part of the deformity along with hindfoot valgus and forefoot abduction. Weight-bearing radiographs will also help identify the presence of hindfoot equinus. Mild planovalgus feet in younger patients can be treated with a supramalleolar orthosis, whereas moderate deformities may be better treated with an AFO. In younger children, a calcaneal lengthening elongates the lateral column of the foot and can correct both forefoot abduction and hindfoot valgus in those with mild to moderate deformities. Compensatory midfoot supination may become more apparent after calcaneal lengthening and is treated with plantar flexion osteotomy of the medial cuneiform or first metatarsal; peroneus brevis lengthening is often performed concomitantly. Lengthening of the peroneus longus should be avoided because this can lead to further first ray dorsiflexion. In older children with more severe deformities, a subtalar joint fusion with or without a midfoot arthrodesis can provide good long-term results. If hindfoot equinus is present, the gastrocnemius-soleus muscle complex should be lengthened as well.

Torsional deformities of the tibia are also common in children with cerebral palsy and result in lever-arm dysfunction, which in turn causes a decrease in ankle push-off power. Derotational osteotomy of the tibia (supramalleolar) is a common and effective treatment and often does not require a concomitant fibular osteotomy.

Great toe deformities are common in children with cerebral palsy. Hallux valgus (bunion) deformity usually occurs with planovalgus foot deformity (Figure 6). Untreated hallux valgus usually worsens with time in children with cerebral palsy. Mild to moderate hallux valgus can be treated with an AFO with an extended toe plate. A hallux strap can be added to the AFO that helps hold the great toe in a more neutral position. Surgical correction of moderate to severe planovalgus foot deformity may stop the progression of mild hallux valgus deformity. Metatarsophalangeal joint fusion is the most reliable surgical procedure used to correct moderate to severe bunions in children with cerebral palsy, especially for those who are marginal ambulators or nonambulators. In children who are good ambulators, soft-tissue balancing procedures and metatarsal osteotomy may be an option, but this procedure has a higher recurrence

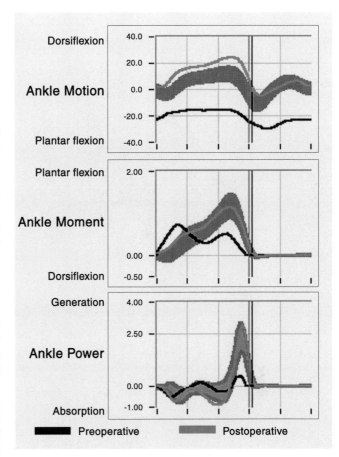

Figure 5 Preoperative (dark gray) sagittal kinematics and kinetics of the ankle in a patient with equinus and planovalgus foot deformity showing a decrease in the moment and power. Postoperative (light gray) kinetics shows marked improvement in both moment and power.

rate than metatarsophalangeal joint fusion. In addition, a significant number of children with cerebral palsy and bunions also have valgus interphalangeus, which requires osteotomy of the proximal phalanx.

Nonambulatory Patients

The major goals of treating nonambulatory children with cerebral palsy are to prevent hip subluxation/dislocation, maintain a comfortable sitting position, and assist with custodial care and hygiene. Some children with severe cerebral palsy are predisposed to fractures of the long bones because of osteoporosis and/or osteomalacia. It is critical in the treatment of children with quadriplegia that parental and/or caretaker goals are well aligned with the treating orthopaedist's goals because treatment is directed toward enhancing the quality of life rather than bringing about functional changes that are not likely to occur.

Hip

One area in which the orthopaedist can have a positive impact on nonambulatory children with spastic cerebral

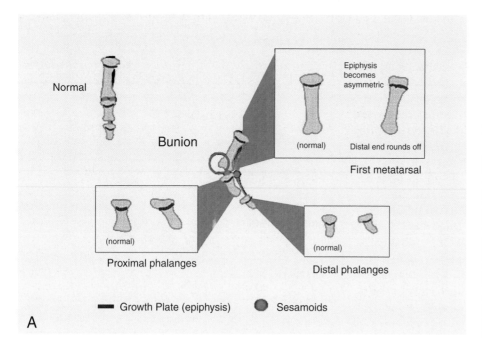

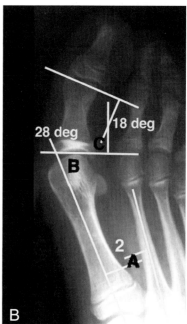

Figure 6 **A,** Planovalgus foot deformity in the child with spastic cerebral palsy causes increased laterally directed pressure to the medial side proximal phalanx causing hallux valgus. The first metatarsal is forced into varus through the medial cuneiform-first metatarsal joint. If the foot is in equinus, weight bearing shifts distally deforming the proximal phalanx and sometimes the distal phalanx (hallux interphalangeus). **B,** Radiograph of a spastic bunion deformity shows first metatarsal varus (A) and hallux valgus (B) and valgus (C) of the proximal phalanx. *(Reproduced with permission from Miller F: Knee, leg, and foot, in Dabney K, Alexander M (eds): Cerebral Palsy. New York, NY, Springer, 2005, pp 779-780.)*

palsy is to prevent spastic hip subluxation/dislocation. Most spastic hip subluxations/dislocations occur posterosuperiorly, the primary cause of which is spasticity of the adductor muscles, with spasticity of the iliopsoas and hamstrings being a contributory cause. These muscles develop increased contracture with growth. Secondary pathology can occur over time and include femoral neck valgus, persistence of infantile femoral anteversion, and acetabular dysplasia. The natural history of the disease involves a progression from mild subluxation to complete dislocation and eventually severe arthritic changes. According to reports in the orthopaedic literature, 50% to 75% of dislocated hips eventually become painful in this patient population.

Physical examination is the most important tool for screening and monitoring patients with spasticity who are at risk for hip subluxation and dislocation. This involves measurement of hip abduction with the patient's hips and knees fully extended. Early detection and treatment in one population-based study showed a significant decrease in dislocation compared with children who did not participate in a monitoring program. Monitoring is typically performed every 6 to 12 months until at least 8 years of age. If abduction is less than 45°, the monitoring process should include a supine AP radiograph of the pelvis and hips with each lower extremity in a neutral position. Reimer's migration percentage is measured as a percentage of the width of the femoral head that is lateral to Perkin's line (Figure 7). Treatment

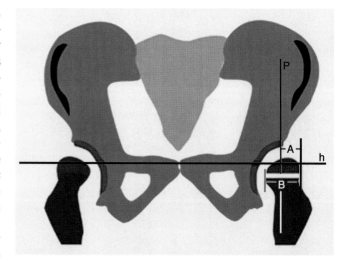

Figure 7 Schematic representation showing how Reimer's migration percentage is measured from an AP radiograph. Hilgenreiner's (h) and Perkin's (P) lines are drawn. Distance A (the distance from P to the lateral border of the femoral epiphysis) is divided by distance B (the width of the femoral epiphysis) and multiplied by 100 to calculate Reimer's migration percentage (A/B × 100). *(Reproduced with permission from Miller F: Hip, in Dabney K, Alexander M (eds): Cerebral Palsy. New York, NY, Springer, 2005, p 532.)*

is based on the age of the child, the amount of hip abduction, and the migration percentage. Treatment can be divided into prevention, reconstruction, and palliation. Preventive treatment consists of soft-tissue release of the adductor longus and proximal gracilis. The adductor brevis is partially or completely released if necessary until 45° of hip abduction is obtained. The iliopsoas is completely released in nonambulatory patients, and an intramuscular tendon release of the psoas is performed in children with some ambulatory potential. In children younger than 8 years, soft-tissue release is indicated when the migration percentage is between 25% and 60% and hip abduction is less than 30°. Long-term follow-up using this treatment protocol shows good to excellent results in 70% of patients.

Reconstruction involves the correction of secondary deformities (femoral neck valgus, femoral anteversion, and acetabular dysplasia) and muscle lengthening. Treatment guidelines for hip reconstruction include a migration index greater than 60% in children 8 years of age or younger, and a migration index greater than 40% in children older than 8 years. Femoral anteversion and femoral neck valgus are corrected with proximal femoral varus derotational osteotomy. The goal of reconstruction of the acetabulum should be correction of the posterior and lateral dysplasia. Ideally, symmetric motion and limb length should be restored after reconstruction. Both femoral and acetabular reconstruction is best performed before there is excessive femoral head deformity. Two studies have reported 95% success rates with femoral varus derotational osteotomy and pelvic osteotomy (San Diego osteotomy and peri-ileal osteotomy). Recently, incomplete peri-ileal osteotomy has also been described in patients with closed triradiate cartilage; poor results included pain and redislocation.

Palliative treatment is reserved for patients with painful hips who do not respond favorably to hip reconstruction and those with painful hips with severe degenerative arthritis. Several procedures have been recommended for these patients, including resection arthroplasty, interposition arthroplasty, total hip arthroplasty, valgus osteotomy, and hip fusion. The goal of each of these procedures is pain relief and to help the patient achieve a good sitting position.

Spine

Spinal deformity is common in children with cerebral palsy. Scoliosis is the most prevalent spinal deformity; however, kyphosis and hyperlordosis may also occur. The incidence of scoliosis is highest in nonambulatory patients, with a reported prevalence of up to 74%. Progression of scoliosis is common, and the rate of progression can be 2° to 4° per month among adolescents with cerebral palsy. Progression also occurs after skeletal maturity and in patients with spinal curves greater than 40°. Spinal curves in the 60° to 90° range affect sitting, arm position, and head control. Further progression may prevent patients from sitting in an upright position. Conservative treatment with chair modifications and bracing may temporarily help with sitting, but do not stop spinal curve progression. Bracing is commonly

helpful in younger children with flexible scoliosis to temporarily maintain upright sitting posture. Eventually, however, as the spinal curve progresses, the parent or caregiver must decide whether definitive treatment with spinal fusion and instrumentation should be undertaken.

Indications for instrumentation and spinal fusion are not precise, but they are based on symptoms (pain) and other quality of life considerations, such as sitting alignment and sitting tolerance. Spinal fusions are often done for patients with spinal curves greater than 50°. Anterior diskectomies are done for those with rigid deformities, such as spinal curves approaching 90° on sitting radiographs or greater than 40° on supine traction radiographs. Techniques of spinal deformity correction for neuromuscular curves typically include segmental fixation using wires, hooks, or screws. Pelvic fixation utilizing the Galveston technique, a unit rod, or iliac screws is commonly used to treat concomitant pelvic obliquity. Anterior diskectomy and spine osteotomies are done for patients with more rigid deformities such as severe scoliosis approaching 100° or in those whose traction radiographs show spinal curves greater than 70°. Similarly, sagittal plane deformities that are rigid, such as those that occur with severe kyphosis or lordosis, may necessitate anterior release and/or osteotomy.

Once orthopaedists and parents agree to proceed with surgery, preoperative workup should be done to assess the child's overall medical and nutritional status, both of which should be optimized before surgery. Posterior spinal fusion is the preferred approach. Multiple methods of instrumentation have been described; however, segmental instrumentation with sublaminar wires and cantilever correction of pelvic obliquity with the Galveston technique should still be considered the gold standard for scoliosis correction in this patient population. Dual rods with cross-links or a unit rod has the advantage of preventing rod rotation or shift. Unless the child has good standing balance and is a good ambulator, the fusion levels typically extend from the first or second thoracic vertebrae down to include the pelvis (to correct pelvic obliquity). Ambulatory potential, which is usually limited in this patient population, does not seem to be affected with fusion to the pelvis as long as sagittal balance is normalized. In children who have undergone previous dorsal rhizotomy, pedicle screws may be necessary if the posterior elements are missing.

Instrumentation should produce a scoliosis correction between 70% and 80% of the preoperative curve magnitude and an 80% to 90% correction of pelvic obliquity. The head should be well centered over the center of the sacrum, and sagittal alignment should normalize thoracic kyphosis and lumbar lordosis. Complications are common and include excessive intraoperative bleeding, neurologic complications, atelectasis, pneumonia, prolonged postoperative ileus, pancreatitis, and wound infection. Mechanical or technical complications can also occur and include rod or wire prominence, pseudarthrosis, rod penetration through the pelvis, and curve progression after fusion because of the crankshaft phenomenon. In one study, postoperative complications were highly correlated with the magnitude of the child's spinal curve, preoperative pulmonary status, and the more severe the degree of neurologic involvement. Despite complications, one survey of 190 parents and caregivers assessing outcomes in children with cerebral palsy after undergoing posterior spinal fusion found that 95.8% of parents and 84.3% of caregivers would recommend spinal surgery again. Positive responses included improved appearance, overall function, quality of life, and ease of care. Overall life expectancy of children with cerebral palsy after undergoing posterior spinal fusion is also critically important. A survival analysis showed that the presence of severe preoperative thoracic hyperkyphosis and the number of postoperative days in the intensive care unit correlated with decreased life expectancy.

Although hyperkyphosis or hyperlordosis are less common in this patient population than scoliosis, both can nonetheless cause difficulty with seating if severe. Hyperlordosis may result in pain. Little is known about the etiology and natural history of these sagittal plane spinal deformities. Hamstring contracture may be associated with excessive thoracolumbar kyphosis. Hip flexion contracture may be associated with hyperlordosis. Multiple level laminectomies after dorsal rhizotomy may also result in hyperlordosis. Orthotic devices may be helpful in treating flexible mild to moderate kyphosis. In symptomatic children with severe hyperlordosis or hyperkyphosis greater than 70°, surgical correction can be considered. Posterior fusion alone with instrumentation can be done in patients with a more flexible deformity, whereas anterior release and/or osteotomies are used in those with rigid deformity. As with scoliosis, unit rod instrumentation or cross-linked dual rods with segmental fixation provides effective correction. A recent study of 24 children with cerebral palsy and sagittal plane spinal deformity reported successful treatment with unit rod instrumentation and improved sitting position and pain.

Bone Density and Fractures

Low bone mineral density and increased risk of fracture can occur in nonambulatory children with cerebral palsy. Fractures can be a costly problem in this group of patients. In one study, bone mineral density was studied in 139 patients with spastic cerebral palsy. Bone mineral density was measured using dual-energy x-ray absorptiometry (DEXA) and averaged 1 standard deviation below age-matched normal control subjects. Low bone mineral density correlated most highly with ambulatory

status; nutritional status was the second most significant factor. Other less significant factors included the type of cerebral palsy, duration of immobilization, and calcium intake. Other studies have reported that the use of anticonvulsants correlates with low bone mineral density. Low impact-type fractures are most commonly seen in metaphyseal bone, especially the proximal tibia and distal femur. Short-term splinting with a well-padded bulky dressing is recommended to prevent extended periods of immobilization and further disuse osteoporosis.

Children with more than one fracture episode should undergo workup for metabolic bone disease; baseline serum calcium, phosphorus, and alkaline phosphatase levels should be assessed and a bone density measurement should be done using DEXA. Bone density measurement at the distal femur has been recommended by some to be more reliable than spine or proximal femoral measurements because of the frequent presence of hardware after spinal fusion and hip osteotomy in children with cerebral palsy. In a recent study, treatment with intravenous pamidronate improved bone mineral density and stopped fracture occurrences. In children with a history of three or more fractures and low bone mineral density with Z scores measured by DEXA to be less than 2 standard deviations, treatment with intravenous pamidronate should be considered (Figure 8). Treatment is given every 3 months over a 1-year period. A recent randomized-controlled trial of standing programs showed increased standing time to improve bone mineral density in nonambulatory children with cerebral palsy.

Upper Extremity

The upper extremity is commonly involved in patients with quadriplegic or hemiplegic cerebral palsy. In infancy, the hand is commonly fisted, with the thumb in the palm, the wrist palmar flexed, the forearm pronated, and the elbow in a flexed position. Occupational therapy is typically initiated to encourage the child to use the arm; two-handed play activities with toys are particularly encouraged. Splinting of the involved extremity is sometimes disadvantageous because covering the hand only discourages use. Recently, constraint-induced movement therapy in patients with hemiplegia has been used with short-term success by casting the uninvolved extremity to encourage use of the involved arm. Botulinum toxin injection has been shown to be helpful in younger children with dynamic deformities. When children with cerebral palsy are between the ages of 6 and 9 years, fixed contractures typically begin to develop, and surgical intervention can be considered. Functional improvement in patients with hemiplegia is most successful in those with spastic cerebral palsy who have voluntary grasp and release, proprioception, and sensibility. Appropriate intelligence quotient and surgery

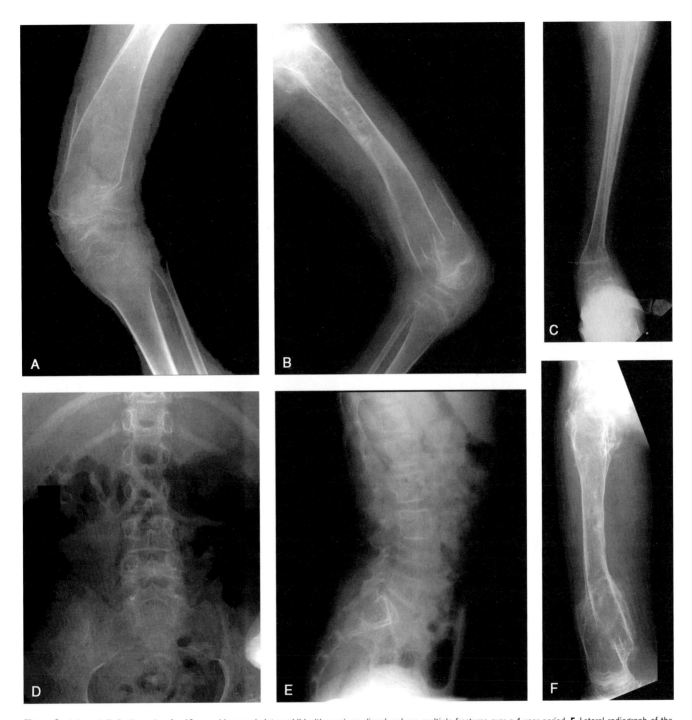

Figure 8 **A** through **E,** Radiographs of a 12-year-old nonambulatory child with a seizure disorder shows multiple fractures over a 1-year period. **F,** Lateral radiograph of the femur after a course of intravenous pamidronate shows healing and increased bone density; the child did not experience any subsequent fractures.

done between the ages of 8 and 12 years are factors associated with more favorable functional outcomes. Improvement of the extremity's function as a helper hand is a realistic outcome. For children in whom functional gains are not expected, cosmesis may be an important consideration in surgically correcting the extremity. In children with quadriplegia, functional gains and cosmesis are rarely indicated; however, improved hygiene and ease of care are primary considerations. Surgery aims to

correct all deformities in one stage and may include the correction of wrist drop, pronation contracture, thumb adduction contracture, and elbow flexion contracture.

Other Treatments
Physical Therapy
Physical therapy has long been the primary mode of nonsurgical treatment for children with cerebral palsy.

Critical periods for physical therapy include early intervention from birth to age 3 years and postoperative rehabilitation. School therapy also aims to optimize the child's function as it relates to education. Controversy exists as to the effectiveness of physical therapy on long-term functional outcome in children with cerebral palsy. One study showed no difference between traditional physical therapy and more intensive physical therapy. In addition to stretching spastic muscles, strength training has been shown to be important in improving function in children with cerebral palsy.

Alternative forms of therapies have been described. Electrical stimulation to selected muscle groups, aquatic therapy, hippotherapy (horseback riding therapy), and hyperbaric oxygen therapy are all current forms of alternative therapy. A blinded, randomized-controlled trial with blinding failed to show benefits on motor function from hyperbaric oxygen treatments.

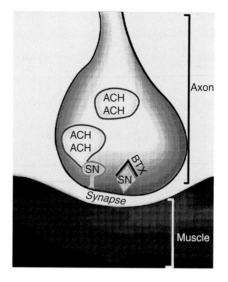

Figure 9 Mechanism of action for botulinum toxin. Synaptosomal vesicles bind to synaptic protein (SN) and release acetylcholine (ACH). Botulinum toxin (BTX) permanently attaches to SN and prevents binding to synaptosomal vesicles. (*Reproduced with permission from Miller F: Neurologic control of the musculoskeletal system, in Dabney K, Alexander M (eds): Cerebral Palsy. New York, NY, Springer, 2005, p 120.*)

Oral Medications

Oral baclofen is a gamma-aminobutyric acid (GABA) analog, an inhalational neurotransmitter, and binds to GABA receptors in the spinal cord after crossing the blood-brain barrier. Diazepam also blocks GABA. Both drugs reduce muscle tone; however, they cause sedation and are associated with tolerance and withdrawal reactions if abruptly discontinued. Both baclofen and Valium are frequently used to manage hypertonia in children with cerebral palsy. Valium is helpful in the immediate postoperative control of spasticity.

Botulinum Toxin

Botulinum toxin, a neurotoxin extracted from *Clostridium botulinum*, affects the neuromuscular junction by irreversibly binding to synaptic proteins to prevent the release of acetylcholine (Figure 9). Both botulinum toxin type A and type B are commercially available. The US Food and Drug Administration has approved botulinum toxin for use in patients with strabismus, blepharospasm, and cervical dystonia. However, botulinum toxin has been used extensively to control spasticity in children with cerebral palsy. Botulinum toxin is injected directly into the spastic muscle at its neuromotor junction rich zone, resulting in 3 to 6 months of denervation, after which time the neuromuscular junction reestablishes conduction, presumably via new axon terminals sprouting. Pediatric dosages are better outlined for botulinum toxin type A than type B. A botulinum toxin type A dosage of 1 to 2 U/kg for most small target muscles, 3 to 6 U/kg for most large target muscles, and limited to a total of 10 to 20 U/kg (maximum dose, 400 U) typically allows clinicians to treat local spasticity in two to three muscle groups per session. Some children develop tolerance after repeat injections. Botulinum toxin should be used to treat dynamic spasticity only. A recent study showed that the combination of botulinum toxin type A with serial casting was not advantageous in improving fixed equinus contractures in children with cerebral palsy.

Intrathecal Baclofen

Baclofen given intrathecally has an advantage over oral baclofen in that it bypasses the blood-brain barrier. For this reason, smaller dosages are given intrathecally with a much lower risk of systemic adverse effects. A battery-powered pump is implanted subcutaneously in the abdomens of larger children or beneath the rectus abdominis fascia in those with little subcutaneous fat (Figure 10, *A*). A flexible catheter is tunneled subcutaneously around the lateral trunk from the pump to the intrathecal space. The tip of the catheter is usually placed at the midthoracic level (Figure 10, *B*); more recently, it has been described with higher placement in the cervical spine to provide better upper extremity control of spasticity. The dosage is adjusted based on clinical signs and symptoms using computerized telemetry, and the pump reservoir is filled by injection through the overlying skin. Intrathecal baclofen is usually indicated in nonambulatory children with cerebral palsy who have generalized moderate to severe spasticity (Ashworth scale score ≥ 3), symptoms of pain, and/or difficulty with positioning or dressing. Complications include cerebral spinal fluid leakage, infection, mechanical problems with the catheter (breakage, kinking, and disconnection) leading to acute baclofen withdrawal (causing rebound spasticity, hallucinations, and possible seizures), wound dehiscence, and baclofen overdose. Recent preliminary reports show a possible increased development of scoliosis after intrathecal baclofen. A recent caregiver survey indicates favorable quality of life benefits for patients who received intrathecal baclofen. The use of intrathecal baclofen in ambulatory children with cerebral palsy and severe spasticity is still under investigation.

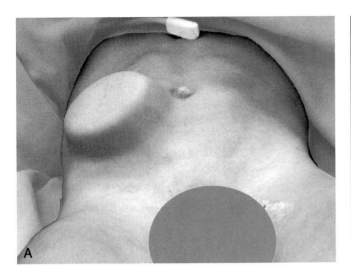

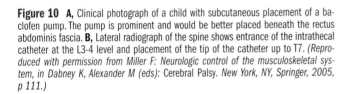

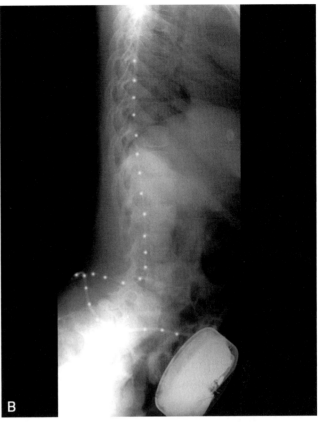

Figure 10 A, Clinical photograph of a child with subcutaneous placement of a baclofen pump. The pump is prominent and would be better placed beneath the rectus abdominis fascia. **B,** Lateral radiograph of the spine shows entrance of the intrathecal catheter at the L3-4 level and placement of the tip of the catheter up to T7. *(Reproduced with permission from Miller F: Neurologic control of the musculoskeletal system, in Dabney K, Alexander M (eds): Cerebral Palsy. New York, NY, Springer, 2005, p 111.)*

Selective Dorsal Rhizotomy

Selective dorsal rhizotomy (SDR) reduces spasticity by selectively cutting dorsal nerve rootlets between L1 and S1, which prevents sensory feedback through afferent sensory nerves from the muscle spindles. Limiting the percentage of dorsal rootlets cut is important in preventing loss of motor strength and control. The ideal patient for SDR is a diplegic child with significant spasticity who is between 3 and 8 years old and is believed to be a good ambulator, has good motor strength and trunk balance, can cooperate with an intensive postoperative physical therapy program, and has good intelligence and motivation. A reduction in spasticity was observed in children with cerebral palsy who were treated with SDR and physical therapy when compared with those who received physical therapy alone in a meta-analysis of three randomized-controlled trials. However, functional outcomes were minimal. Other investigators have shown that 24% to 51% of children who have undergone SDR will still need orthopaedic procedures. Complications include decreased sensation, bowel and bladder dysfunction, hip subluxation/dislocation, scoliosis, kyphosis, lordosis, and spondylolisthesis. A multidisciplinary team is often needed to evaluate children before undergoing SDR and receiving intrathecal baclofen. This multidisciplinary team may include an orthopaedist, neurosurgeon, physiatrist, developmental pediatrician, and physical therapist.

Outcome Measures

Although central nervous system injury does not typically progress in children with cerebral palsy, progression of physical and functional impairments is common with growth. Outcome measures provide an objective tool to measure changes that occur with growth and treatment. In the past, physical examinations and radiographs have been used to measure these changes. More objective measurement using three-dimensional instrumented gait analysis has not only been shown to positively affect treatment decisions, but also to document changes after treatment. Over the past several years, this has also included energy consumption data. The Gross Motor Function Measure, which is used to assess gross motor function in children with cerebral palsy, includes five dimensions: lying and rolling, sitting, crawling and kneeling, standing, and walking, running, and jumping. The Pediatric Outcomes Data Collection Instrument (PODCI) was developed as a pediatric tool to measure the patient's and/or parent's perception of function as well as participation in community activities. The domains of the PODCI include upper extremity function, transfer and mobility, sports and physical function, comfort, expectations for treatment, happiness, and satisfaction. Over the past 5 years, several investigators have found statistical correlation between many of these outcome measures as well as used them to document changes after treatment. Recently, a multicenter study correlated the relationship between different levels of severity of ambulatory children with cerebral palsy as measured by the Gross Motor Function Classification System with several other pediatric outcome tools (the Gross Motor Function Measure, PODCI, temporospatial gait parameters, and oxygen cost).

Summary

Cerebral palsy is a static yet heterogeneous condition with multiple etiologies. Because of its heterogeneity, goal setting aimed at the individual child involved is imperative. In addition to a detailed physical examination, newer classification schemes aim to characterize motor function as well as predict future function of the child. Treatment of nonambulatory patients should focus on improving sitting position, dressing and hygiene, and occasionally function. In particular, the prevention and treatment of hip dislocation and treatment of spinal deformity are important in the totally involved child. In ambulatory patients, physical examination, classification of motor function, and three-dimensional gait analysis assist with outlining treatment. Treatment may include a number of modalities (some in combination), including physical therapy, bracing, medication to control spasticity, Botox injection, intrathecal baclofen, and orthopaedic procedures. Although several randomized trials suggest the beneficial effects of several treatments (Botox, SDR, and constraint therapy), there are no completed clinical trials to help choose the best treatment available for children with cerebral palsy. A number of outcome measures have been described and provide objective measures to document changes in function with growth and treatment. As more long-term randomized data are gathered that correlate various treatment methods with outcome measures, the objectives and satisfaction from different treatment modalities will become better understood.

Annotated Bibliography

General

Miller F (ed): *Cerebral Palsy*. New York, NY, Springer Science and Business Media, Inc, 2005.

This is a comprehensive text on all aspects of cerebral palsy.

Classification

Rodda JM, Graham HK, Carson L, Galea, Wolfe R: Sagittal gait patterns in spastic diplegia. *J Bone Joint Surg Br* 2004;86:251-258.

This cross-sectional study of 187 children with cerebral palsy was conducted to develop a classification of sagittal gait patterns in patients with spastic diplegic cerebral palsy based on pattern recognition and kinematic data. A longitudinal study of 34 children followed for greater than 1 year demonstrated the reliability of this classification system.

Ambulatory Patients

Aminian A, Vankoski SJ, Dias L, Novak RA: Spastic hemiplegic cerebral palsy and the femoral derotation osteotomy: Effect at the pelvis and hip in the transverse plane during gait. *J Pediatr Orthop* 2003;23:314-320.

In this study, nine patients with spastic hemiplegia underwent femoral derotational osteotomy. The authors reported that both femoral rotation and pelvic transverse plane rotation improved postoperatively.

Asakawa DS, Blemker SS, Rab GT, Bagley A, Delp SL: Three-dimensional muscle tendon geometry after rectus femoris tendon transfer. *J Bone Joint Surg Am* 2004;86-A:348-354.

In this study, a three-dimensional computer model was created from the MRI scans of five patients who underwent rectus femoris transfers. Results suggested that a rectus femoris transfer is beneficial by reducing the effects of the muscle as a knee extensor rather than converting the muscle to a knee flexor.

Bell KJ, Ounpuu S, DeLuca PA, Romness MJ: Natural progression of gait in children with cerebral palsy. *J Pediatr Orthop* 2002;22:677-682.

In this study, 28 children were assessed with two gait analyses spaced over an average of 4.4 years. The authors reported that overall gait function decreased longitudinally with time.

Davids JR, Marshall AD, Blocker ER, Frick SL, Blackhurst DW, Skewes E: Femoral anteversion in children with cerebral palsy: Assessment with two and three-dimensional computed tomography scans. *J Bone Joint Surg Am* 2003;85-A:481-488.

Because optimal alignment of the femur within the CT scanner is required for accurate measurement of anteversion, the authors of this study compared two- and three-dimension CT scans and reported that three-dimensional scanning was more accurate.

Kay RM, Rethlefsen SA, Hale JM, Skaggs DL, Tolo VT: Comparison of proximal and distal femoral osteotomy in children with cerebral palsy. *J Pediatr Orthop* 2003;23: 150-154.

The authors of this study found comparable results when derotational osteotomies were performed proximally (intertrochanteric) and distally (distal femur). They also reported that static and dynamic measures of femoral rotation improved in both groups with no difference in the complication rates.

Kay RM, Rethlefsen SA, Kelly JP, Wren TA: Predictive value of the Duncan-Ely test in distal rectus femoris transfer. *J Pediatr Orthop* 2004;24:59-62.

In this retrospective review, 94 patients undergoing rectus femoris transfer underwent preoperative and postoperative gait analysis. Results indicated that a positive preoperative

Duncan-Ely test may be a positive predictor of good outcome after rectus femoris outcome.

Murray-Weir M, Root L, Peterson M, et al: Proximal femoral varus rotation osteotomy in cerebral palsy: A prospective gait study. *J Pediatr Orthop* 2003;3:321-329.

In this study, 37 patients were prospectively studied with preoperative and 1-year postoperative gait analyses after undergoing proximal femoral varus rotation osteotomy of the femur. The authors reported that the procedure resulted in objective improvement in gait parameters.

Ryan DD, Rethlefsen SA, Skaggs DL, Kay RM: Results of tibial rotational osteotomy without concomitant fibular osteotomy in children with cerebral palsy. *J Pediatr Orthop* 2005;25:84-88.

This review of 72 distal tibial osteotomies without concomitant fibular osteotomy showed that this procedure is effective and safe for correcting tibial torsion in patients with cerebral palsy.

Schwartz MH, Viehweger E, Stout J, Novacheck TF, Gage JR: Comprehensive treatment of ambulatory children with cerebral palsy: An outcome assessment. *J Pediatr Orthop* 2004;24:45-53.

This retrospective study was conducted to evaluate the outcome of treatment in 135 ambulatory children with cerebral palsy who underwent surgical treatment guided by gait analysis. The authors reported that a majority of subjects (79%) improved on a predominance of outcome measures.

Nonambulatory Patients

Hagglund G, Anderson S, Duppe H, Lauge-Pederson H, Nordnark E, Westbomj L: Prevention of dislocation of the hip in children with cerebral palsy: The first ten years of a population-based prevention programme. *J Bone Joint Surg Br* 2005;87:95-101.

The authors of this study reported that a population-based prevention program of early detection and intervention of hip dislocation in children with cerebral palsy was shown to be highly effective when compared with a control group.

Henderson RC, Lark RK, Kecskemethy HH, Miller F, Harcke HT, Bachrach SJ: Bisphosphonates to treat osteopenia in children with quadriplegic cerebral palsy: A randomized, placebo-controlled clinical trial. *J Pediatr* 2002;141:644-651.

The authors of this double-blind, placebo-controlled clinical trial found pamidronate to be safe and effective in the treatment of osteopenia in children with quadriplegic cerebral palsy. They reported that bone mineral density increased by 89% in the treatment group compared with only 9% in the control group.

Lipton GE, Letonoff EJ, Dabney KW, Miller F, McCarthy HC: Correction of sagittal plane spinal deformities

with unit rod instrumentation in children with cerebral palsy. *J Bone Joint Surg Am* 2003;85-A:2349-2357.

In this study, 24 patients with sagittal plane spinal deformity (hyperkyphosis and hyperlordosis) underwent successful treatment with spinal fusion and unit rod instrumentation. The primary indications for treatment were loss of sitting ability or balance and back pain.

Presedo A, Oh CW, Dabney KW, Miller F: Soft-tissue releases to treat spastic hip subluxation in children with cerebral palsy. *J Bone Joint Surg Am* 2005;87:832-841.

In this study, 65 children with spastic hip subluxation were subjected to a treatment protocol based on age, hip abduction, and hip migration index. At mean 10.8-year follow-up, open adductor tenotomy and iliopsoas recession was found to be effective in 67% of children. The authors reported that hip migration index at 1 year postoperatively was a predictor of final outcome.

Taub E, Ramey SL, DeLuca S, Echols K: Efficacy of constraint-induced movement therapy for children with cerebral palsy with asymmetric motor impairment. *Pediatrics* 2004;113:305-312.

This randomized controlled clinical trial showed that children with constraint-induced therapy (consisting of bivalved casting of the less effected arm and intensive therapy of the more effected arm) acquired significantly more gains in motor skills compared with children treated with conventional therapy.

Terjesen T, Lie GD, Hyldmo AA, Knaus A: Adductor tenotomy in spastic cerebral palsy: A long-term follow-up study of 78 patients. *Acta Orthop* 2005;76:128-137.

In this study, adductor tenotomy was performed in 78 children with cerebral palsy. After an average 10-year follow-up, the authors reported favorable outcomes in two-thirds of patients and that outcomes were best when the migration percentage was less than 50%.

Tsirikos AI, Chang WN, Dabney KW, Miller F: Comparison of parents' and caregivers' satisfaction after spinal fusion in children with cerebral palsy. *J Pediatr Orthop* 2004;24:54-58.

In this study, a questionnaire was used to assess functional improvement after spinal fusion in children with cerebral palsy. Of the 190 parents who completed the questionnaire, most parents (95.8%) and caregivers (84.3%) reported that they would again recommend spine surgery.

Tsirikos AI, Chang WN, Shah SA, Dabney KW, Miller F: Preserving ambulatory potential in pediatric patients with cerebral palsy who undergo spinal fusion using unit rod instrumentation. *Spine* 2003;28:480-483.

The authors of this study reported that ambulatory function was preserved in 24 patients who underwent spinal fusion extending to the pelvis with unit rod instrumentation.

Tsirikos AI, Chang WN, Dabney KW, Miller F, Glutting J: Life expectancy in pediatric patients with cerebral palsy and neuromuscular scoliosis who underwent spinal fusion. *Dev Med Child Neurol* 2003;45:677-682.

Kaplan-Meier survival analysis was performed in 288 patients with severe cerebral palsy who underwent spinal fusion. The authors reported that the number of days in the intensive care unit and the presence of preoperative thoracic hyperkyphosis were statistically significant in predicting decreased life expectancy after spinal fusion in children with cerebral palsy.

Other Treatments

Gooch JL, Oberg WA, Grams B, Ward LA, Walker ML: Care provider assessment of intrathecal baclofen in children. *Dev Med Child Neurol* 2004;46:548-552.

A caregiver survey was given to care providers of 80 children who were managed with intrathecal baclofen. The authors reported that 95% of care providers would agree to having the procedure performed again.

Johnson MB, Goldstein L, Thomas SS, Piatt J, Aiona M, Sussman M: Spinal deformity after SDR in ambulatory patients with cerebral palsy. *J Pediatr Orthop* 2004;24: 529-536.

The authors of this study reported that spinal deformity developed in 30 of 34 patients after SDR and included lumbar hyperlordosis, scoliosis, and spondylolisthesis. No difference, however, was reported to have occurred when comparing patients who underwent laminectomy and those who underwent laminoplasty.

Kay RM, Rethlefsen SA, Fem-Buneo A, Wren TA, Skaggs DL: Botulinum toxin as an adjunct to serial casting treatment in children with cerebral palsy. *J Bone Joint Surg Am* 2004;86-A:2377-2384.

This prospective, randomized trial compared children with cerebral palsy with ankle equinus contractures who were treated using serial casting alone or serial casting plus botulinum toxin type A. The authors reported that patients who underwent serial casting alone had a later recurrence of contracture.

McLaughlin J, Bjornson K, Temkin N, et al: Selective dorsal rhizotomy: Meta-analysis of three randomized controlled trials. *Dev Med Child Neurol* 2002;44:17-25.

The authors of this meta-analysis found that SDR was shown to be efficacious in reducing spasticity.

Oeffinger DJ, Tylkowski CM, Rayens MK, et al: Gross Motor Function Classification System and outcome tools for assessing ambulatory cerebral palsy: A multi-center study. *Dev Med Child Neurol* 2004;46:311-319.

The gross motor function classification system was assessed in a range of severities of ambulatory children with cerebral palsy and compared with several pediatric outcome tools. The authors reported that the gross motor function clas-

sification system correlated with other tools, thereby establishing justification of its use.

Classic Bibliography

Bleck EE: Locomotor prognosis in cerebral palsy. *Dev Med Child Neurol* 1975;17:18-25.

Bobroff ED, Chambers HG, Sartoris DJ, Wyatt MP, Sutherland DH: Femoral anteversion and neck-shaft angle in children with cerebral palsy. *Clin Orthop Relat Res* 1999;364:194-204.

Chad KE, Bailey DA, McKay HA, Zello GA, Snyder RE: The effect of a weight-bearing physical activity program on bone mineral content and estimated volumetric density in children with spastic cerebral palsy. *J Pediatr* 1999;135:115-117.

Damiano DL, Abel MF: Functional outcomes of strength training in spastic cerebral palsy. *Arch Phys Med Rehabil* 1998;79:119-125.

DeLuca PA, Davis RB, Ounpuu S, Rose S, Sirkin R: Alterations in surgical decision making in patients with cerebral palsy based on three-dimensional gait analysis. *J Pediatr Orthop* 1997;17:608-614.

Dias RC, Miller F, Dabney K, Lipton G, Temple T: Surgical correction of spinal deformity using a unit rod in children with cerebral palsy. *J Pediatr Orthop* 1996;16: 734-740.

Gage JR (ed): *The Treatment of Gait Problems in Cerebral Palsy*. London, England. MacKeith Press, 2004.

Henderson RC, Lin PP, Greene WB: Bone-mineral density in children and adolescents who have spastic cerebral palsy. *J Bone Joint Surg Am* 1995;77:1671-1681.

Jenter M, Lipton GE, Miller F: Operative treatment for hallux valgus in children with cerebral palsy. *Foot Ankle Int* 1998;19:830-835.

Koman LA, Mooney JF III, Smith BP, Walker F, Leon JM: Botulinum toxin type A neuromuscular blockade in the treatment of lower extremity spasticity in cerebral palsy: A randomized, double-blind, placebo-controlled trial: Botox study group. *J Pediatr Orthop* 2000;20:108-115.

Miller F, Dias RC, Dabney KW, Lipton GE, Triana M: Soft-tissue release for spastic hip subluxation in cerebral palsy. *J Pediatr Orthop* 1997;17:571-584.

Miller F, Girardi H, Lipton G, Ponzio R, Klaumann M, Dabney KW: Reconstruction of the dysplastic hip with peri-ileal pelvic and femoral osteotomy followed by immediate mobilization. *J Pediatr Orthop* 1997;5:592-602.

Mosca VS: Calcaneal lengthening for valgus deformity of the hindfoot: Results in children who had severe, symptomatic flatfoot and skewfoot. *J Bone Joint Surg Am* 1995;77:500-512.

Mubarak SJ, Valencis FG, Wenger DR: One-stage correction of the spastic dislocated hip: Use of pericapsular acetabuloplasty to improve coverage. *J Bone Joint Surg Am* 1992;74:1347-1357.

Ounpuu S, Muik E, Davis RB III, Gage JR, DeLuca PA: Rectus femoris surgery in children with cerebral palsy: Part I: The effect of rectus femoris transfer location on knee motion. *J Pediatr Orthop* 1993;13:325-330.

Ounpuu S, Muik E, Davis RB III, Gage JR, DeLuca PA: Rectus femoris surgery in children with cerebral palsy: Part II: A comparison between the effect of transfer and release of the of the distal rectus femoris on knee motion. *J Pediatr Orthop* 1993;13:331-335.

Reimers J: The stability of the hip in children: A radiological study of the results of muscle surgery in cerebral palsy. *Acta Orthop Scand Suppl* 1980;184:1-100.

Rose SA, DeLuca PA, Davis RB III, Ounpuu S, Gage JR: Kinematic and kinetic evaluation of the ankle after lengthening of the gastrocnemius fascia in children with cerebral palsy. *J Pediatr Orthop* 1993;13:727-732.

Silver RL, Rang M, Chan J, de la Garza J: Adductor release in nonambulant children with cerebral palsy. *J Pediatr Orthop* 1985;5:672-677.

Chapter 9

Myelomeningocele

Jeffrey D. Thomson, MD

Introduction

Myelomeningocele (also called meningomyelocele) is one entity in a spectrum of congenital malformations of the spinal column and spinal cord known as spina bifida of which there are two broad divisions: spina bifida occulta and spinal bifida cystica. Spina bifida occulta is a typically benign defect of the posterior vertebral elements of the fourth and fifth lumbar vertebrae and first sacral vertebrae. Approximately 10% to 15% of the population may have spina bifida occulta. Although it is usually not associated with any abnormalities, spina bifida occulta rarely can be associated with symptomatic lower spinal cord malformations, such as lipomeningocele and tethered cord, with possible progressive neurologic symptoms. Spina bifida cystica can be differentiated into meningocele, myelomeningocele, myelocele, and lipomeningocele. Meningocele is defined as a cyst of the meninges through a defect in the posterior vertebral elements; however, the underlying spinal cord and nerve roots are not involved in the cyst. Myelomeningocele occurs when the spinal cord and/or the spinal nerve roots protrude outside the spinal canal through a defect in the posterior arch along with the meninges. Myelocele, which is also known as rachischisis or myeloschisis, is the most severe form of spinal bifida cystica in which the neural plate is exposed with no overlying tissue cover. Lumbosacral lipoma is a descriptive term that includes lipomeningocele, intraspinal lipoma, and lipoma of the filum terminale. Lumbosacral lipomas typically consist of skin-covered subcutaneous lipomas that are connected to intraspinal lipomas and most often occur in the lumbosacral spine. They can be associated with spinal cord tethering and neurologic symptoms as well as diastematomyelia.

Myelomeningocele, which represents about 90% of all instances of spina bifida cystica, is thought to occur in approximately 1 in 20,000 live births. Maternal serum α-fetoprotein level and ultrasound are commonly used for prenatal screening. Positive findings from either of these two diagnostic modalities can be followed with amniocentesis, detailed sonography, or both. Cesarean section, which is the preferred method of delivery for neonates with spina bifida cystica, is thought to avoid trauma to the myelomeningocele sac; it is also done after intrauterine closure of spina bifida because the forces of labor may produce a dehiscence.

Four risk factors have been strongly associated with spina bifida: a history of previously affected pregnancy with the same partner, inadequate maternal intake of folic acid, pregestational maternal diabetes, and in utero exposure to valproic acid or carbamazepine.

Folic acid dietary supplementation has been shown to reduce the incidence of neural tube defects. One study reported a 72% reduction in neural tube defects at birth in a high-prevalence area of Northern China. As a result, women without a family history of neural tube defects who anticipate a pregnancy are advised to take 0.4 to 0.8 mg of folic acid daily. Women with a positive history (first-degree relative with a neural tube defect or a prior pregnancy affected by neural tube defect) should take 4 mg of folic acid per day at least 1 month before conception.

To date, intrauterine repair of myelomeningocele has not been associated with improvement in lower extremity neurologic function. However, an unexpected positive result has been seen in the reduction of the anatomic Chiari type 2 malformation and a potential decrease in the need for a cerebral spinal fluid shunt. Currently, a multicenter prospective randomized trial is underway to determine the benefits of intrauterine repair.

Closure of the myelomeningocele is usually done within 48 hours of birth; if signs of hydrocephalus are apparent, a shunt is usually placed when the lesion is closed. The rate of survival is about 87%, and approximately 78% of all individuals with spina bifida survive to the age of 17 years. Persons with spina bifida continue to have significant orthopaedic, neurosurgical, and urologic problems. It has been well established that the level of neurologic deficit is the main determent of disability.

A dedicated multidisciplinary team of physicians should be involved in the care of children with myelomeningocele. Ideally, the team should consist of an orthopaedic surgeon, a neurosurgeon, a urologist, a physiatrist or pediatrician who can coordinate and oversee over all medical care, and a dedicated nurse to act as liaison with the patient, family, and medical care providers.

The role of the orthopaedic surgeon is to make the patient as orthopaedically functional as possible, which entails maximizing function and minimizing deformity. The role of nursing is especially important as traditional multidisciplinary spina bifida clinics close. The patient with spina bifida also requires regular occupational and physical therapy visits and yearly manual muscle tests. Ongoing wheelchair assessments and regular orthotic modifications require the presence of dedicated specialists.

Perhaps the most challenging issue for patients with spina bifida is the transition from childhood and adolescence into adulthood. Teenagers with spina bifida especially have problems finding peer groups, which can result in social isolation. As adults, this patient population can also have tremendous difficulty finding suitable employment.

Neurosurgical Issues and Tethered Cord

Clinical signs of tethered cord occur in approximately 15% of patients with spina bifida. The clinical signs include changes in urologic function, development of spasticity in the lower extremities, leg weakness, foot deformity, scoliosis, back pain, increased lumbar lordosis, and sensory changes. It is important to be aware that almost all children with myelomeningocele show tethering of the spinal cord on MRI scans, but they may not have clinical manifestations. If clinical reasons to suspect a tethered cord exist, the patient should be evaluated using MRI; it is also important to rule out shunt malfunction. Urodynamics can be useful as they can show signs of tethered cord before there are orthopaedic manifestations. Neurosurgical detethering has been shown to be of benefit in patients presenting with tethered cord syndrome. Detethering generally stabilizes neurologic status and prevents further deterioration. Some patients have recovery of lost motor function, whereas a small percentage of patients may lose some function. Alternatively, patients with tethered cord syndrome can undergo end organ surgery, which may include symptomatic treatment of their orthopaedic and urologic conditions. However, it has been shown that 90% of patients treated thus required additional orthopaedic or urologic procedures because of further symptoms of tethered cord. Tethered cord can cause scoliosis, and curves less than 40° may benefit from detethering. Conversely, another study showed that patients with curves greater than 40° did not have any decrease in their curves after tethered cord release.

One study reported that 20% of children with myelomeningocele had sleep-disordered breathing, with a higher prevalence occurring in patients who were nonambulatory, patients with abnormal pulmonary test results, and patients with severe Chiari malformation. Sleep-disordered breathing and sudden unexplained death during sleep were associated with up to 22% of deaths in patients with myelomeningocele. Overnight polysomnography is the gold standard for diagnosis in this patient population. Although treatments are variable and depend on the diagnosis, they may include pharmacologic management, pulmonary measures, otolaryngological procedures, and neurosurgical procedures. Periodic neurosurgical follow-up of children with myelomeningocele who have cerebral spinal fluid shunts is vital.

Upper Extremity Dysfunction

Impaired upper extremity function commonly occurs in children with myelomeningocele and can be caused by hydrocephalus and/or shunt problems. A syrinx in the cervical spine can be another cause and can present as asymmetric hand strength. Periodic monitoring of grip strength by an occupational therapist is an excellent screening modality. Ongoing assessments and therapy are useful to maximize function and to identify new problems that can be the first manifestation of neurologic changes.

Spine Deformities

A high incidence of scoliosis and kyphosis occurs in children with spina bifida (approximately 60%). Most spinal curves are paralytic, but a 15% incidence of congenital spinal deformity has been reported as well.

The definition of scoliosis should be a curve greater than 20°. Many children with spina bifida can sit in an asymmetric pattern and provide the false impression of a curve. Although most curves manifest in children younger than 10 years, some curves can develop as late as age 15 years. The last intact laminar arch has been found useful to determine the incidence of scoliosis. If the last intact laminar arch is in the thoracic level, then the incidence of scoliosis is approximately 90%. In patients with a last intact laminar arch below L4, the incidence of scoliosis is approximately 10%. Curves less than 20° should be observed. Curves ranging from 20° to approximately 40° can be braced to provide better sitting balance for the patient; however, this treatment has not been shown to be effective in preventing curve progression. Furthermore, patients are susceptible to skin breakdown with the use of braces. Tethered cord should be evaluated in patients with progressive scoliosis between 20° and 40°. Other sources for curve progression include shunt problems and syringomyelia, which can be evaluated using CT and MRI, respectively.

Curves greater than 50° can affect sitting balance because of pelvic obliquity and lead to pressure sores. Severe scoliosis can lead to restrictive pulmonary disease, which can be improved with surgical treatment consisting of combined anterior and posterior spinal fusion. However, in selected patients, anterior fusion alone or posterior spinal fusion with instrumentation can be safely performed. This is especially true with the increasing use of pedicle screw fixation. In general, many factors need to be considered when performing scoliosis surgery on children with spina bifida, including the age of the child, location of curve, level of paralysis, and ambulatory status. Longer fusions are usually safer; if there is more than 10° of pelvic obliquity in a nonambulatory child, the instrumentation should be extended to the pelvis. In an ambulatory child with less than 10° of pelvic obliquity, stopping instrumentation short of the pelvis can be considered. There is a potential for Charcot joint development at the L5/S1 junction, but this has not been well documented.

When performing anterior and posterior spinal fusion, the anterior release is usually performed first. Anterior instrumentation is controversial and with the advent of posterior pedicle screws may not be necessary. The anterior release and fusion is especially necessary when the posterior elements in the lumbar spine are deficient, as typically occurs in the thoracic level in children with spina bifida. Anterior fusion and instrumentation alone can be performed in patients with a thoracolumbar curve less than 75°, a compensatory proximal curve less than 40°, no significant kyphosis in the primary curve, and no evidence of a syrinx. Posterior instrumentation and fusion alone can be performed in patients who have most of the posterior elements intact and if the dysraphic part of the lumbar spine can be fixed with pedicle screws. Complications have been reported to occur in 10% to 30% of patients and include loss of neurologic function, decrease in independence, potential loss of the ability to self-catheterize, loss or diminishment of transfer skills and mobility, infection, pseudarthrosis, and skin breakdown. Despite the recommendation for surgical treatment of patients with severe scoliosis, few high-quality outcome studies have been conducted to help determine whether these procedures have a significant effect on duration and quality of life.

Kyphosis occurs in approximately 8% to 15% of all children with spina bifida and can be an especially challenging problem to manage. Untreated, the kyphosis can lead to loss of truncal height and decreased respiratory capability secondary to increase of abdominal pressure into the chest. The kyphosis can also lead to skin breakdown. Bracing is extremely difficult, and the kyphosis tends to progress relentlessly.

Kyphectomy can be performed in newborn patients at the time of sac closure. In young children presenting with significant kyphosis, limited vertebral body resec-

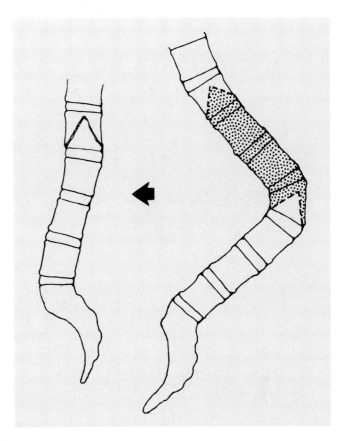

Figure 1 The rigid S-shaped kyphosis is corrected by excising the vertebrae between the apex of the kyphosis and the lordosis and fusing the apical vertebrae. *(Reproduced with permission from Lindseth RE: Myelomeningocele, in Morrissy RT (ed): Lovell and Winters' Pediatric Orthopaedics, ed 3. Philadelphia, PA, JB Lippincott, 1990, p 522.)*

tion and wire fixation has been described. Bringing the erector spinae muscles posterior to the spinal column is considered an essential step that will help counteract the flexion deformity. Substantial correction of the kyphosis can be achieved, but some recurrence of the curve can be expected, although many patients do not need further surgery.

Another option in the treatment of children with significant kyphosis is to perform a resection of the kyphotic segment (excision or subtraction osteotomy), fuse the resected segment, stabilize with posterior instrumentation, and use the Luque trolley technique in the thoracic spine to allow longitudinal spinal growth. This involves performing extraperiosteal exposure in the thoracic spine with use of sublaminar wires or cables attaching the rods to the spine but not performing a fusion. The goal is to allow the thoracic spine to grow along the Luque rods; results of this procedure, however, have been unpredictable.

Kyphectomy, which involves resection of vertebrae just cephalad to the apex of the kyphosis combined with instrumentation, has been the classic approach (Figure 1). This technique is used in patients with stiff, rigid deformities. Conversely, subtraction (decancellization) of

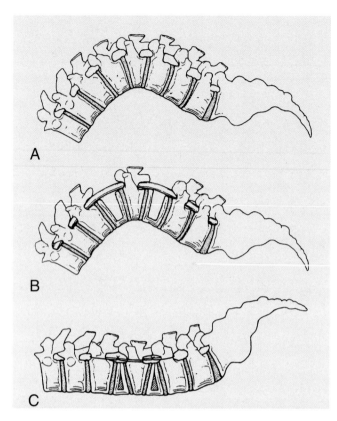

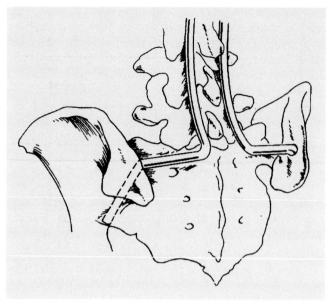

Figure 3 Diagram shows the Galveston method of fixing the pelvic limb of the rod to the posterior column of the ilium. Because the construct extends through two planes, this provides triangulation, which is a biomechanically important feature contributing to stability. *(Reproduced from Banta JV, Drummond DS, Ferguson RL: The treatment of neuromuscular scoliosis.* Instr Course Lect 1999;48:551-562.)

Figure 2 A, The C-shaped kyphosis before removal of the ossific nucleus from its vertebrae. **B,** The spinous process, lamina, pedicle, and ossific nucleus have been removed from the vertebrae above and below the apical vertebrae. The growth plate, disk, and anterior cortex are left intact. **C,** The deformity is reduced by pushing the apical vertebrae forward and tension-band wiring around the pedicles. *(Reproduced from Lindseth RE: Spine deformity in myelomeningocele.* Instr Course Lect 1991;40: 273-279.)

the vertebrae about the apex has been shown to be useful and result in fewer complications than the classic resection method. Decancellization vertebrectomy involves removing a wedge of bone from each vertebra about the apex (Figure 2). The pseudarthrosis rate is much lower than resection kyphectomy when using this procedure, and the neural placode can be preserved by mobilization and provide extra posterior coverage. Annulotomy can also be performed, which involves incising the disk fibers over the apex of the deformity to gain further correction.

Instrumentation extending from the upper thoracic level to the sacrum is required for successful treatment of kyphosis; fixation to the pelvis is required. The Galveston technique (Figure 3), the Fackler technique (Figure 4), and the S-rod fixation technique (Figures 5 and 6) have proved useful.

Complications in kyphectomy surgery are similar to those in scoliosis surgery. Special precautions need to be taken if the thecal sac over the kyphosis is resected to prevent acute hydrocephalus. Overlengthening of the spinal column can result in stretching of the great vessels, but preservation of the anterior longitudinal liga-

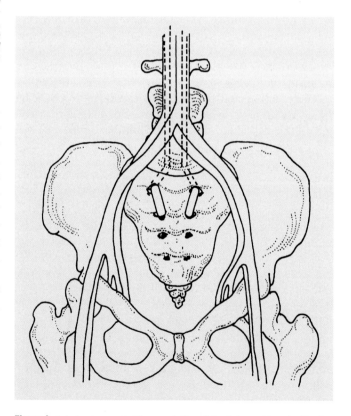

Figure 4 Anterior placement of Luque rods through the first sacral foramina. The first sacral foramina are medial to the internal iliac vessels. *(Reproduced with permission from Warner WC Jr, Fackler CD: Comparison of two instrumentation techniques in treatment of lumbar kyphosis in myelodysplasia.* J Pediatr Orthop 1993;13(6):704-708.)

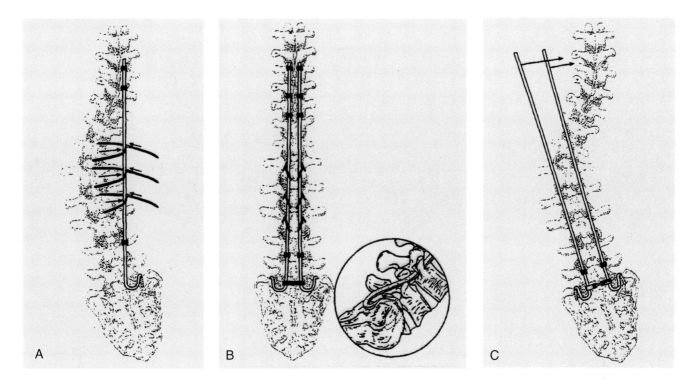

Figure 5 **A** through **C,** Diagrams of S-rod usage for scoliosis. The S-rod can be used as part of a system that corrects with distraction/translation or with cantilever forces. The distraction/translation system uses hooks or a combination of hooks and screws for distraction across the concavity of a scoliotic curve with sublaminar wires or cables for translation of the apical segments. *(Reproduced with permission from McCarthy R: S-rod fixation, in McCarthy R (ed):* Spinal Instrumentation Techniques: Scoliosis. Pelvic Fixation. *Rosemont, IL, Scoliosis Research Society, 1998, pp 1-8.)*

ment should prevent this catastrophic complication. Intraoperative monitoring of pedal pulse oximetry or lower extremity blood pressure can be done to monitor lower extremity blood flow during kyphosis correction.

Bracing and Gait Analysis

In children with thoracic and upper lumbar level spina bifida, extensive bracing with parapodiums, reciprocating gait orthoses (RGOs), or hip-knee-ankle-foot orthoses (HKAFOs) is required for the child to be upright. It is unknown whether such children are better off in a standing and ambulation program for which they may require significant physical therapy, expensive orthotic devices, and possibly surgery versus using a wheelchair exclusively. With braces, most children with myelomeningocele at the lower thoracic/upper lumbar neurosegmental level can walk, but by approximately 10 to 12 years of age, most choose a wheelchair as a more energy-efficient means of mobility. It is generally believed that children should be allowed to participate in a walking/standing program, but allowed to stop participating if so inclined. Patients and parents may enjoy the upright experience and the satisfaction of achieving upright mobility, but they may also experience significant disappointment when the child inevitably stops walking. Criteria for successful use of an RGO include lower thoracic/lumbar level lesion, parental cooperation,

access to a treatment center, symmetric motor function and upper-limb strength, no obesity, no mental retardation, minimal scoliosis, and no significant lower limb contractures. One report proposed a trial use of an RGO and recommended prescription of an RGO only when the child can take more than 10 strides on repeated occasions.

Although standing programs have been promoted as being beneficial for children with myelomeningocele, a recent study found no difference between patients with high-level myelomeningocele who used a parapodium and those who use a wheelchair. The same study also reported no difference between patients in terms of renal health, number of fractures, obesity, participation in sports, incontinence, activities of daily living, or orthopaedic procedures. Sacral pressure sores were more common in children using wheelchairs, whereas skin sores were more common in the parapodium group.

HKAFOs appear to be more energy efficient than RGOs for patients with high-level myelomeningocele. Although most children with high-level myelomeningocele will eventually stop walking, it has been shown that children walking with HKAFOs into adolescence had a faster velocity and lower oxygen expenditure than children who discontinued use of HKAFOs. A reasonable protocol for upright ambulation in a patient with upper level paralysis (L3 and higher) may start with RGOs, with children switching to HKAFOs when upper ex-

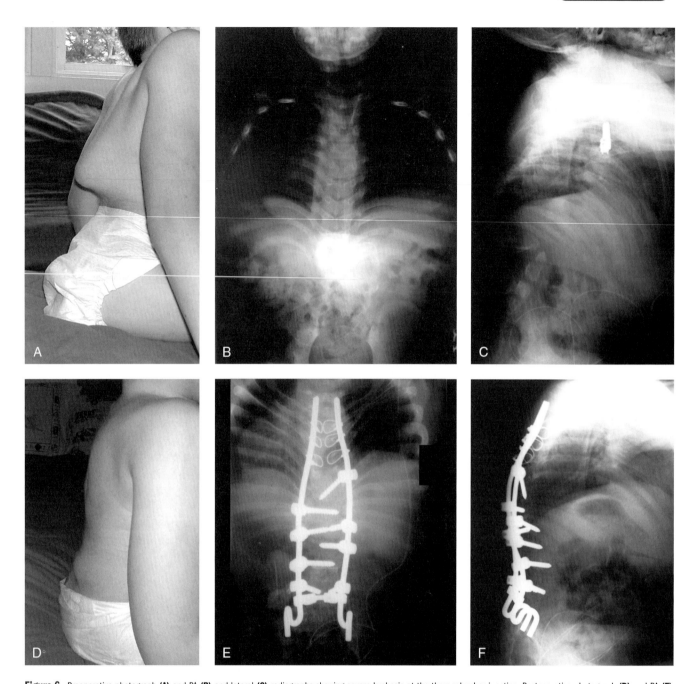

Figure 6 Preoperative photograph **(A)** and PA **(B)** and lateral **(C)** radiographs showing severe kyphosis at the thoracolumbar junction. Postoperative photograph **(D)** and PA **(E)** and lateral **(F)** radiographs of the same patient after undergoing S-rod fixation instrumentation using lumbar and thoracic pedicle screws with thoracic sublaminar cable.

tremity strength improves and walking speed is of importance. The child may opt to switch to wheelchair mobility when speed and a more energy-efficient method of community mobility are important. However, a recent meta-analysis found little benefit to walking with a parapodium, HKAFO, or RGO in patients with upper level paralysis.

In children with low-level myelomeningocele (L4, L5, S1), the literature supports the use of an ankle-foot orthosis (AFO). This brace improves the velocity of walking, decreases time spent in the double-limb phase

of gait, and decreases excessive ankle dorsiflexion. The AFO, however, prevents the ankle and subtalar joint from absorbing forces, which are then transmitted to the knee. Increased transverse plane knee rotation has been documented in patients with low-level myelomeningocele who walk with an AFO compared with those who walk without an AFO, which raises concerns about the development of osteoarthritis. Crutches can improve the kinematics of the knee and reduce transverse plane rotation, which potentially reduces the risk of knee instability and osteoarthritis. This may be especially beneficial to patients with weak hip abductors in whom excessive knee valgus force has been documented. Some patients with excessive external tibial torsion may benefit from tibial derotational osteotomy, but weakness of the hip abductor muscle is much more determinant of knee valgus then external tibial torsion.

In patients with knee valgus, knee-ankle-foot orthoses (KAFOs) are an option to minimize or prevent knee valgus forces. To date, however, no study has demonstrated that KAFOs can prevent detrimental knee valgus forces or that KAFOs provide significant benefits for the knee. In sagittal plane analysis, few if any differences between AFOs and KAFOs have been shown.

In patients with L3/L4 myelomeningocele who ambulate using AFOs and crutches, the swing-through gait is more energy efficient than reciprocal walking; as a result, the swing-through gait should not be discouraged because it appears to allow children to function best with their peers.

Not all patients with low-level myelomeningocele will walk. Balance disturbances, spasticity in the knee and hip joints, and increased number of shunt revisions can adversely affect a child's ability to achieve ambulation. Neurologic deterioration, knee and hip contractures, low back pain, lack of motivation, and serious major medical events have also been found to adversely effect walking ability.

Treatment

The orthopaedic management of patients with myelomeningocele consists of preventing or correcting the deformity while maximizing mobility and independence consistent with the patient's functional neurosegmental level. All treatment is based on the patient's functional neurosegmental level, a stable neurologic state, and knowledge of the natural history of spina bifida.

The functional motor level of a patient is of prime importance in determining prognosis, treatment, and outcome. Several different systems have been developed to classify the neurologic level of involvement in patients with myelomeningocele. Unfortunately, no consistent correlation among the numerous systems exists. It is imperative to use the same classification system when assessing and discussing patients. The International Myelodysplasia Study Group has proposed a straightforward and easy-to-use system (Table 1).

Periodic manual muscle testing is important. If done by the same examiner, results are generally reliable, but not until the child is approximately 5 to 6 years of age. Also up to 60% of children with myelomeningocele may have an upper motor neuron lesion that can present as spasticity. Patients can also have gaps in their neurosegmental levels that can make classification difficult. All of these factors make manual muscle testing challenging. Gait analysis, conversely, provides an objective and reproducible kinetic, kinematic, and video record of the patient's function.

Thoracic to Upper Lumbar (L1/L2)

The main treatment goals for children with thoracic/upper lumbar level (L1/L2) myelomeningocele are to maintain spinal balance, a level pelvis, and mobile hips, knees, and plantigrade feet. Approximately 70% to 90% of patients with myelomeningocele at this level will develop scoliosis and require spinal fusion. Because of deficient posterior elements, most of these patients will require anterior and posterior spinal fusion with fusion to the pelvis. Patients with myelomeningocele at this level also frequently have significant kyphosis that can be treated with formal kyphectomy or wedge resection osteotomies and instrumentation.

In children with thoracic and/or upper lumbar level spina bifida, reconstructive procedures to correct hip dysplasia or dislocation are usually not indicated because the status of the hip has no influence on the ability to walk. It is controversial whether these children should be placed into an exclusive wheelchair program or encouraged to walk. Hip surgery in patients with thoracic and upper lumbar level spina bifida is indicated for those with flexion contractures greater than 25° to 30° that interfere with bracing. The sartorius, rectus femoris, iliopsoas, and tensor facia lata can be released through an anterior approach. The anterior hip capsule can also be released if it is tight. It is vital to maintain the hips in an extended position for the first 2 weeks after surgery. Adduction contractures can be relieved via simple myotomy of the adductor longus and the adductor brevis if necessary.

Knee flexion contractures are common in patients with thoracic and/or upper lumbar level spinal bifida. Contractures greater than 20° to 25° may impair bracing, and surgery may be indicated. The posterior knee capsule is often tight, and posterior capsulotomy may be required if hamstring lengthening is not effective; however, neurovascular structures may still limit full extension. Posterior capsulotomy can be done through a single midline posterior incision or two separate incisions (one posteromedial and one posterolateral). Extension osteotomy of the distal femur can be performed, but rapid recurrence of deformity is common if this is done at a young age.

In patients with thoracic and/or upper lumbar level spina bifida, a supple flexible flail foot should be the ultimate goal of treatment. Simple tenotomies of tight or spastic tendons should be performed to achieve a plantigrade foot.

Although almost any foot deformity can occur at any given neurosegmental level, equinus foot deformity is common in patients with thoracic and/or upper lumbar level spina bifida, and prevention of deformity with

Table 1	International Myelodysplasia Study Group Criteria for Assigning Neurosegmental Levels
Neurosegmental Level	**Criteria**
T10 or above	Determine based on sensory level and/or palpation of abdominals
T11*	
T12	Some pelvic control in sitting or when supine, which may originate in the abdominals or back; hip hiking may be noted
L1	Weak iliopsoas (grade 2)
L1-2*	
L2	Iliopsoas, sartorius, adductors all grade 3 or higher
L3	Meet criteria for L2 and quadriceps are grade 3 or higher†
L3-4	
L4	Meet criteria for L3 and have medial hamstrings grade 3 or higher and anterior tibialis grade 3 or higher (may also have weak peroneus tertius)
L4-5*	
L5	Meet criteria for L4 and have lateral hamstrings grade 3 or higher plus one of the following:
	Gluteus medius grade 2 or higher
	Peroneus tertius grade 4 or higher
	Posterior tibialis grade 3 or higher
L5-S1*	
S1	Meet criteria for L5 plus two of the following:
	Gastrocnemius-soleus complex grade 2 or higher
	Gluteus medius grade 3 or higher
	Gluteus maximus grade 2 or higher (puckering of buttocks)
S1-2*	
S2	Meet criteria for S1 and gastrocnemius-soleus muscle complex grade 3 or higher and gluteus medius and maximus grade 4 or higher
S2-3	All muscles in lower extremities of normal strength, though may be grade 4 in one or two muscle groups; also includes normal-looking infants to be bowel and bladder trained
No loss	Meets criteria for S2-3 and has no bowel/bladder loss
L1-3	Weak hip flexors, adductors, and weak quadriceps (weak innervation through L3)
L2-4	Strong hip flexors, but weak knee flexion and extension

* Assign to this level when the child exceeds the criteria for the preceding level but does not meet the criteria for next lower level

† "Meet criteria for" indicates that the strength of the muscles listed in the preceding levels should be increasing

(Reproduced from Wright JG: Neurosegmental level and functional status, in Sarwark JF, Lubicky JP (eds): Caring for the child with spina bifida. Rosemont, IL, American Academy of Orthopaedic Surgeons, 2001, p 71.)

an AFO is always the best initial treatment. If the deformity is mild, a simple tenotomy can be performed followed by a short leg cast, but some recommend an open tenotomy with a 2-cm excision of tendon to prevent recurrence. For patients with more severe deformity, open capsulotomy with tendon excision through a longitudinal incision may be needed.

Clubfoot can also occur in children with thoracic and/or upper lumbar level myelomeningocele and can be treated with stretching and casting, although this is usually not successful. Radical posteromedial and lateral release with tendon excision via the Cincinnati incision is the treatment of choice. Postoperative position is held with prolonged casting for 3 to 4 months, after which an AFO brace is used.

Talectomy is a salvage procedure for nonambulatory children for whom treatment fails or clubfoot deformity recurs. The lateral column may be shortened by either calcaneal shortening osteotomy or calcaneal cuboid fusion to correct foot deformity. In general, foot arthrodesis surgery is contraindicated in patients with spina bifida, but limited arthrodesis of the calcaneocuboid joint in conjunction with talectomy can be beneficial in nonambulatory patients to create a plantigrade foot (Figure 7).

Vertical talus can be seen in patients with thoracic and/or upper lumbar level myelomeningocele and is best treated surgically through a dorsal approach to release the tight anterior structures. Transferring the anterior tibialis into the neck of the talus has been reported to help prevent recurrence. The posterior structures can

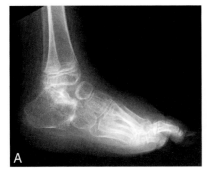

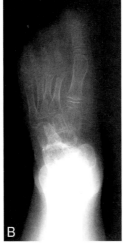

Figure 7 Postoperative lateral **(A)** and AP **(B)** foot radiographs after talectomy and calcaneocuboid fusion.

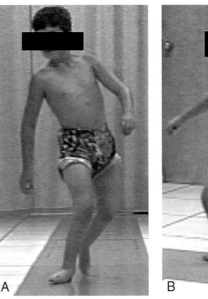

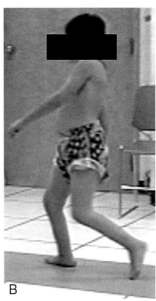

Figure 8 **A** and **B**, Photographs of a patient with weak abductor muscles exhibiting valgus knee position. *(Reproduced with permission from Iunpuer S: Gait analysis in orthopaedics, in Fitzgerald AR, Kaufer H, Malkani AL (eds): Orthopaedics. Philadelphia, PA, Mosby, 2002, p 103.)*

be released by percutaneous tenotomy or open tenotomy if so desired. A Kirschner wire is driven antegrade into the navicular, cuneiform, and first metatarsal and then retrograde into the talus while the joint is held in a reduced position. The Kirschner wire can be removed 8 weeks later. Three to 4 months of postoperative casting is recommended to prevent recurrence.

Midlumbar Level (L3/L4)

Patients with midlumbar level (L3/L4) myelomeningocele have good quadriceps function but poor hamstring function. These patients can be household walkers or limited community walkers using HKAFOs, KAFOs, or AFOs and crutches. Only 1 in 5 patients with myelomeningocele at this level will have normal and reduced hips. Dysplasia and dislocation occur frequently in this patient population; when this occurs, release of hip contractures that interfere with ambulation or bracing are indicated. It has not been demonstrated that patients with midlumbar level myelomeningocele have better ambulatory potential with located versus dislocated hips. In general, if both hips are dislocated they are probably best left untreated. Although a unilateral dislocation may warrant surgical treatment, this is controversial because recurrent dislocation is so common. The recent trend is to treat the contracture if it interferes with bracing or walking but not reduce the hip.

Patients with midlumbar level myelomeningocele do not have a functional hip abductor and therefore are at risk for developing valgus knees because of the significant lateral sway when walking while using AFOs. The use of crutches with AFOs or KAFOs is recommended to protect the knees. These patients can have significant knee valgus secondary to their weak hip abductor muscles and associated lateral trunk shift during ambulation (Figure 8). The knee valgus can be compounded by external tibial torsion and femoral anteversion. Distal tibial derotational osteotomy may be indicated for these

patients, but it does not necessarily eliminate the valgus at the knee joint. These patients may benefit from KAFOs after surgery, and the use of crutches is another method for reducing knee valgus.

In patients with midlumbar level myelomeningocele, knee flexion contractures greater than 20° typically result in increased energy use because of a crouched gait. Hamstring release or lengthening and posterior capsulotomy with release of the origin of the gastrocnemius is therefore indicated. A long leg cast is used for approximately 3 weeks; subsequent splinting to maintain correction may be of benefit, but high-quality outcome studies of this treatment approach are lacking.

Foot deformity is best treated with tenotomy to achieve a flail but supple foot that fits into a brace. Calcaneal foot deformity occurs in this patient population because of the unopposed action of the anterior tibialis. Simple tenotomy is recommended because transfer of the anterior tibialis through the interosseus membrane to the calcaneus has not been reported to have resulted in antigravity plantar flexion strength. Patients still require the use of AFOs. The transfer of the distal Achilles tendon into the distal fibula also has not been shown to result in greater longitudinal growth of the distal fibula. Equinovarus can be treated with simple tenotomy of the posterior tibialis and other involved tendons; if there is still residual hindfoot varus, a lateral closing wedge calcaneal osteotomy or a lateral displacement horizontal calcaneal osteotomy can be performed. Residual forefoot adduction can be treated with an opening wedge osteotomy of the cuneiform and closing wedge osteotomy of the cuboid bone.

Equinovalgus foot deformity can be treated with soft-tissue releases of the peroneus brevis and longus and calcaneal lengthening. With calcaneovalgus foot deformity, the peroneus tertius may be involved and need release. The lesser toe extensors can also be potential deforming forces that may require tenotomy. The distal tibial plafond may be in valgus position and must be evaluated. If patients are younger than 8 years, a valgus tibial plafond can be treated with a temporary distal medial tibial hemiepiphyseodesis using a screw or a staple. An osteotomy is required if the growth plate is closed.

Low Lumbar Level (L5)

Patients with low lumbar level (L5) myelomeningocele have strong quadriceps and knee flexor function; more importantly, they have grade 2 or greater hip abductor strength (International Myelodysplasia Study Group criteria). Hip abduction and extensor strength is an important determinant in walking because it stabilizes the trunk and pelvis during gait and reduces knee valgus. Patients with grade 2 hip abductor strength may not have sufficient strength to avoid demonstrating the Trendelenburg sign (gluteal fold that drops while standing on one foot, signifying muscular weakness of the opposite weight-bearing hip), but they compensate by shifting the trunk over the stance phase limb. Patients with grade 3 or greater hip abductor strength will have less, if any, trunk sway as they walk. In general, most patients with L5 involvement can walk with an AFO, and the incidence of hip problems in this patient population is low, as is the incidence of scoliosis. Foot and ankle deformities frequently occur in this patient population, with calcaneal deformity being the most common type because of poor or absent gastrocnemius-soleus function. A release of the anterior tibialis is as effective as transfer in eliminating calcaneal deformity. Significant ankle valgus at the level of the tibial plafond can occur and can be addressed as discussed previously in the Midlumbar Level (L3/L4) section.

High Sacral Level

Patients with high sacral level myelomeningocele usually become community walkers using AFOs. The incidence of scoliosis in this group is less than 5%; if detected in this patient population, the possibility of a tethered cord must be considered. Hip instability (especially if unilateral) should be treated with tendon releases, muscle transfers, and bony surgery as needed to achieve concentric hip reduction and concentric coverage. Preoperative three-dimensional CT is recommended. The Sharrard iliopsoas transfer does not provide active extension or hip abduction power because it results in an out of phase muscle that, when transferred, results in the loss of hip flexion strength. The external oblique muscle is small and does not have the cross-section of the hip abductor; therefore, it cannot provide the same muscle power when transferred.

Foot abnormalities are seen in approximately 50% of patients with high sacral level myelomeningocele; these patients may have equinus, cavus, or valgus deformities. These patients in particular are at high risk for skin breakdown over the feet because they are ambulatory yet have deficient sensation on the plantar surface of the feet. Cavovarus deformity can be treated with radical plantar fascia release if the varus is supple. If the varus is rigid, then dorsiflexion osteotomy of the first metatarsal and/or lateral closing wedge osteotomy of the calcaneus should also be performed. Soft-tissue imbalance must be corrected at the same time. Patients with a tethered spinal cord can present with foot deformity, especially if there is any spasticity. Neurosurgical consultation should be obtained for any new onset of foot deformity in this patient population.

Summary

The management of patients with myelomeningocele remains a significant challenge. Clinicians must be diligent in assessing patients for tethered cord. Most patients who undergo detethering show improvement, but some patients will have a decline in function and some patients will experience retethering. Improvement in spinal deformity correction has resulted from the use of pedicle screws and better pelvic fixation techniques. Substraction osteotomy rather than excisional osteotomy for the treatment of kyphosis has decreased the number of complications. In general, most surgeons advocate not reducing a hip dislocation except for rare instances of unilateral dislocation in patients with a low-level lesion. Hip flexion contractures and knee flexion contractures should be treated to facilitate bracing. There has been a significant amount of research in spinal bifida utilizing gait analysis techniques, which has helped improve the understanding of energy consumption and the effect of braces. Furthermore, gait analysis has shown the limited value of reducing hip dislocations in patients with spina bifida. The role of in utero closure of myelomeningocele defects is being studied and may result in the placement of fewer shunts and hopefully preservation of more neurosegmental levels.

Annotated Bibliography

Neurosurgical Issues and Tethered Cord

Phuong LK, Schoeberl KA, Raffel C: Natural history of tethered cord in patients with myelomeningocele. *Neurosurgery* 2002;50:989-995.

In this study, 45 patients with myelomeningocele who developed symptoms of tethered cord did not undergo detethering. Treatment focused on end-organ surgery, treating bladder spasticity, or orthopaedic foot deformity. Forty of 45 myelomeningocele patients (88.9%) who underwent bladder augmentation or contracture release subsequently required additional surgical procedures because of complications of tethered cord.

Schoenmakers MA, Gooskens RH, Gulmans VA, et al: Long-term outcome of neurosurgical untethering in neurosegmental motor and ambulation levels. *Dev Med Child Neurol* 2003;45:551-555.

In this study, 16 patients with myelomeningocele underwent neurosurgical untethering. Four years after the procedure, 3 patients had deterioration of motor level, 10 were unchanged, and 3 seemed improved.

Upper Extremity Dysfunction/Spine Deformities

Adzick NS, Walsh DS: Myelomeningocele: Prenatal diagnosis, pathophysiology and management. *Semin Pediatr Surg* 2003;12:168-174.

The authors discuss advances in prenatal care and intrauterine myelomeningocele sac closure.

Crawford AH, Strub WM, Lewis R, et al: Neonatal kyphectomy in the patient with myelomeningocele. *Spine* 2003;28:260-266.

In this study, 11 patients underwent neonatal kyphectomy at the time of myelomeningocele closure. Wound closure was successful in all patients; initial correction averaged 77°, but average loss of correction at follow-up was 55°. Only one patient required repeat kyphectomy and spinal fusion. The authors reported that eventual recurrence of deformity was common, but such deformities were longer and more rounded and may therefore be easier to surgically address if required.

Nieto A, Mazon A, Pamies R, et al: Efficacy of latex avoidance for primary prevention of latex sensitization in children with spina bifida. *J Pediatr* 2002;140:370-372.

The authors of this study reported that the prevalence of latex sensitization fell from 27% to 5% in children with spina bifida who were treated in a latex-free environment from birth.

Nolden MT, Sarwark JF, Vora A, Grayhack JJ: A kyphectomy technique with reduced perioperative morbidity for myelomeningocele kyphosis. *Spine* 2002;27: 1807-1813.

The authors of this study reported that decancellation subtraction vertebrectomies with preservation of the thecal sac was highly effective in achieving and maintaining correction of kyphosis without the need for excision of vertebral bodies.

Sarwark JF, Lubicky JP (eds): *Caring for the Child With Spina Bifida*. Rosemont, IL, American Academy of Orthopaedic Surgeons, 2001.

This compilation of a symposium held in April 2000 provides an outstanding summary of the state of the art regarding spina bifida.

Bracing and Gait Analysis

Bare A, Vankoski SJ, Dias L, Danduran M, Boas S: Independent ambulators with high sacral meningocele: The relationship between walking kinematics and energy consumption. *Dev Med Child Neurol* 2001;43:16-21.

The authors of this study reported that hip abductor strength (possibly more than other muscle groups) plays an important role in its predictive value for mobility and in the energy cost of walking.

Bartonek A, Saraste H: Factors influencing ambulation in myelomeningocele: A cross-sectional study. *Dev Med Child Neurol* 2001;43:253-260.

The authors of this study found that balance disturbances, the occurrence of spasticity in knee and hip joints, and an increasing number of shunt revisions were detrimental to expected ambulatory level.

Gabrieli AP, Vankoski SJ, Dias LS, et al: Gait analysis in low lumbar myelomeningocele patients with unilateral hip dislocation or subluxation. *J Pediatr Orthop* 2003;23: 330-336.

The authors of this study concluded that no attempt to should be made to reduce unilateral hip dislocation or subluxation in children with low lumbar level spina bifida. They also recommended that if asymmetric gait exists, then treatment should focus on the contracture.

Mazur JM, Kyle S: Efficacy of bracing the lower limbs and ambulation training in children with myelomeningocele. *Dev Med Child Neurol* 2004;46:352-356.

The authors conducted a meta-analysis to examine the efficacy of bracing and ambulation training in children with myelomeningocele and found little benefit to walking with a parapodium, HKAFO, or RGO for children with high-level paralysis. In patients with low-level paralysis, the literature supports the use of an AFO.

Thomas SS, Buckon CE, Melchionni J, Magnusson M, Aiona MD: Longitudinal assessment of oxygen cost and velocity in children with myelomeningocele: Comparison of the hip-knee-ankle-foot orthosis and the reciprocating gait orthosis. *J Pediatr Orthop* 2001;21:798-803.

In this study, 23 children with myelomeningocele were evaluated to determine whether differences in oxygen consumption, cost, and velocity exist in children who walk with HKAFOs versus those who use RGOs. The authors found that children using HKAFOs had similar oxygen cost compared with that for children using RGOs; children using HKAFOs were found to have achieved a faster velocity than those using RGOs; and children using HKAFOs into adolescence had a faster velocity and lower oxygen cost than children who discontinued use. No significant differences were identified in velocity or oxygen cost when comparing children who continued using RGOs and those who discontinued use of RGOs.

Classic Bibliography

Banta JV: Combined anterior and posterior fusion for spinal deformity in myelomeningocele. *Spine* 1990;15: 946-952.

Beaty JH, Canale ST: Orthopaedic aspects of myelomeningocele. *J Bone Joint Surg Am* 1990;72:626-630.

Burke SW, Weiner LS, Maynard MJ: Neuropathic foot ulcers in myelodysplasia. *Orthop Trans* 1991;15:102.

Dias LS: Surgical management of knee contractures in myelomeningocele. *J Pediatr Orthop* 1982;2:127-131.

Fraser RK, Hoffman EB, Sparks LT, Buccimazza SS: The unstable hip and mid-lumbar myelomeningocele. *J Bone Joint Surg Br* 1992;74:143-146.

Kirk VG, Morielli A, Brouillette RT: Sleep-disordered breathing in patients with myelomeningocele: The missed diagnosis. *Dev Med Child Neurol* 1999;41:40-43.

Lintner SA, Lindseth RE: Kyphotic deformity in patients who have a myelomeningocele: Operative treatment and long-term follow-up. *J Bone Joint Surg Am* 1994;76:1301-1307.

Mazur JM, Shurtleff D, Menelaus M, Colliver J: Orthopaedic management of high-level spina bifida: Early walking compared with early use of wheelchair. *J Bone Joint Surg Am* 1989;71:56-61.

Menelaus MB: Talectomy for equinovarus deformity in arthrogryposis and spina bifida. *J Bone Joint Surg Br* 1971;53(3):468-473.

Pierz K, Banta J, Thomson J: Gahm, Hartford J: The effect of tethered cord release on scoliosis in myelomeningocele. *J Pediatr Orthop* 2000;20:362-365.

Rodrigues RC, Dias LS: Calcaneus deformity in spina bifida: Results of anterolateral release. *J Pediatr Orthop* 1992;12:461-464.

Selber P, Dias L: Sacral-level myelomeningocele: Long-term outcome in adults. *J Pediatr Orthop* 1998;18:423-427.

Sponseller PD, Young AT, Sarwark JF, Lim R: Anterior only fusion for scoliosis in patients with myelomeningocele. *Clin Orthop Relat Res* 1999;364:117-124.

Swank M, Dias L: Myelomeningocele: A review of the orthopaedic aspects of 206 patients treated from birth with no selection criteria. *Dev Med Child Neurol* 1992; 34:1047-1052.

Tosi LL, Slater JE, Shaer C, Mostello LA: Latex allergy in spina bifida patients: Prevalence and surgical implications. *J Pediatr Orthop* 1993;13:709-712.

Williams JJ, Graham GP, Dunne KB, Menelaus MB: Late knee problems in myelomeningocele. *J Pediatr Orthop* 1993;13:701-703.

Chapter 10

Progressive Neuromuscular Diseases

Michael D. Sussman, MD

Introduction

The motor unit consists of the anterior horn cell in the spinal cord, the peripheral nerve that emanates from this cell, the neuromuscular junction, and the muscle. The group of diseases that affect the motor unit have many common characteristics. For physicians treating this patient population, it is important to be aware of the characteristics these diseases have in common and to have specific information regarding the most prevalent neuromuscular diseases likely to be seen by orthopaedists.

Motor Unit Diseases

There are three primary characteristics of most motor unit diseases: they are genetically based, progressive, and weakness is the major manifestation.

Most diseases of the motor unit are heritable (autosomal dominant, autosomal recessive, or X-linked). In addition, there are some dominant conditions wherein the length of repeating nucleotide triplets increases from generation to generation, thereby increasing the severity of the disease. The identification of the genetic basis of these diseases has allowed for specific molecular diagnoses to be made. Conditions that were once thought to be homogeneous or relatively homogeneous, such as Charcot-Marie-Tooth disease type I, have now been shown to have multiple subtypes, each because of a different gene mutation (genotype), but with a similar disease pattern (phenotype). Invasive studies such as nerve conduction velocity studies, electromyography, and muscle biopsies may be avoided because of the specificity of these gene tests. In addition, identifying the gene has allowed investigators to develop many potentially productive approaches for therapy. Some of these may involve direct manipulation of the gene, but others may involve attempts to influence the gene product (the protein that is produced by that gene). In addition, animal models have been developed by production of transgenic animals that then become carriers of the gene and can be used for research.

Some of motor unit diseases manifest at birth, such as spinal muscular atrophy type I and congenital myotonic dystrophy. Some manifest during the first decade of life, such as Duchenne muscular dystrophy and spinal muscular atrophy types II and III. Others manifest later in a variable fashion, such as Charcot-Marie-Tooth disease and Becker muscular dystrophy.

All motor unit diseases result in progressively increasing weakness, although there are a few of these conditions that are relatively static. The weakness is generally not homogeneous. In most conditions, weakness tends to progress from a proximal to a distal fashion, with proximal weakness much more severe than distal weakness. Myotonic dystrophy and hereditary sensory motor neuropathies, however, are exceptions in that the weakness is predominantly distal. In addition, weakness can affect specific muscle groups, such as the peroneal muscles in the leg and intrinsic muscles in the upper extremity in patients with Charcot-Marie-Tooth disease and the facial and periscapular muscles in patients with fascioscapulohumeral dystrophy.

Functional Deficits and Secondary Musculoskeletal Problems Associated With Weakness

Hip Dislocation

When weakness becomes profound before age 10 years and walking ability is lost before this time, patients are prone to hip dislocation. In patients who never walk or lose this ability by age 5 years, dislocation of one or both hips is almost universal, such as those with spinal muscular atrophy I and II. Hip dysplasia can also be seen in patients with Charcot-Marie-Tooth disease, but the explanation for this is unclear because these patients are fully ambulatory. Hip dysplasia may occur in patients with Duchenne muscular dystrophy, but it is rarely symptomatic. With dislocations resulting from flaccid muscle weakness in nonambulatory patients, pain is not typically a prominent complaint, and decreased range of motion is not a clinical problem. This is in contrast to the spastic dislocations in patients with cerebral palsy, which are often stiff and painful.

Scoliosis

Scoliosis is caused by a loss of muscular support of the vertebral column with subsequent development of postural curvature, which becomes progressive and results in structural scoliosis. Therefore, scoliosis is most likely to develop in patients who lose the ability to stand and become full-time sitters before the onset of puberty. When the ability to stand is lost after skeletal maturity, the risk of development of scoliosis is minimal.

Respiratory Muscle Weakness

As generalized weakness progresses, the muscles of respiration will also be affected, including the intercostal muscles and the diaphragm. Patients will develop chronic respiratory insufficiency and have problems clearing secretions. Respiratory insufficiency (chronic or acute or secondary to acute respiratory infection) is most frequently the cause of death. Respiratory function can be supported by assisted bilevel positive pressure ventilation at night. Providing this type of ventilatory support reduces muscle fatigue, provides better daytime function, and may prolong life. In some patients, life can be prolonged for years and even decades with full-time assisted ventilation. A position statement recently published by the American Thoracic Society provides guidelines for pulmonary management for patients with Duchenne muscular dystrophy.

Cardiac Dysfunction

In some muscle diseases such as Duchenne muscular dystrophy and Becker muscular dystrophy, associated cardiomyopathy can occur, which can be aggravated by pulmonary insufficiency. Treatment with corticosteroids as well as with angiotensin-converting enzyme inhibitors and beta blockers have been shown to decrease cardiac dysfunction in patients with Duchenne muscular dystrophy. In addition, some neuromuscular degenerative conditions such as Emery-Dreifuss dystrophy, myotonic dystrophy, and Friedreich's ataxia are associated with conduction abnormalities that can lead to fatal ventricular arrhythmia.

Gastrointestinal Abnormalities

Some muscle diseases, such as Duchenne muscular dystrophy, are associated with gastric hypomotility and hypomotility of the bowel because of smooth muscle dysfunction. This can lead to acute gastric dilatation and contribute to problems of chronic constipation.

Contractures

Contractures regularly occur in patients who become nonambulatory as muscle weakness worsens. Some patients with conditions such as Duchenne muscular dystrophy and Emery-Dreifuss dystrophy seem to be particularly prone to rapid development of contractures as weakness progresses because there is a fibrosing compo-

Table 1	Common Characteristics of Contractures in Patients With Motor Unit Diseases	
Flexion contractures	Most contractures of the extremity are flexion contractures (plantar flexion at the ankle, flexion at the knees and hips, and elbows); this may be because the flexors tend to remain stronger than the extensors or there may be some positional contribution in that when sitting, the hips and knees tend to remain in flexion for prolonged periods
Neck extension contractures	The cervical spine tends to go into extension and relatively severe neck extension contractures can develop
Foot deformity	As weakness progresses, foot deformity can occur in a consistent pattern for each specific condition
Equinovarus	Occurs in patients with Duchenne muscular dystrophy, Becker muscular dystrophy, and spinal muscular atrophy
Cavovarus	Patients with Charcot-Marie-Tooth disease develop a characteristic cavovarus deformity with dynamic hyperextension of toes, contracture of the plantar fascia, and elevation of the longitudinal arch in association with dorsiflexion at the ankle joint (these patients are not in equinus)
Pure equinus	Patients with congenital myotonic dystrophy develop equinus

nent of the disease, whereas other patients have smaller degrees of contracture. Therefore, there are biologic mechanisms that lead to contracture in patients with muscle weakness that segregate independently of those issues that cause the weakness. The recently discovered molecule titin may play a significant role in contracture development. Contractures in patients with motor unit diseases have several common characteristics (Table 1).

Diagnosis

Because manual muscle testing is difficult to perform in children, a functional examination must be used to assess for weakness. In children, motor milestones are critical, and any child who walks later than 18 months should be examined for an underlying problem. Assessment of the walking child must include a careful visual assessment of gait. Particular attention should be given to identifying signs of side-to-side sway of the trunk while walking (Trendelenburg gait) and anterior pelvic tilt associated with excessive lumbar lordosis. If the walking is reasonably normal, children can be assessed for the presence of other abnormalities by asking them to run and go up and down stairs. In addition, children can be asked to sit down and rise from the floor to assess whether they use Gowers' maneuver or a modification thereof, which is indicative of quadriceps and gluteus maximus weakness. Although Gowers' maneuver is seen in all boys with Duchenne muscular dystrophy, it is also associated with other conditions in which patients have proximal muscular weakness. To assess upper extremity and shoulder girdle weakness, children can be asked to get down on all fours, at which time the examiner picks up their legs and asks them to use a wheelbarrow race type of function (walking on the hands with the legs held by the examiner). Another test is the Meryon's sign, which is elicited when children are lifted up under the arms, are not able to support themselves, and slip through the examiner's hands.

Muscular Dystrophy

Duchenne muscular dystrophy is the most common motor unit disease in children. The incidence is 1 in 3,500 male children, and it is inherited in an X-linked fashion; therefore, Duchenne muscular dystrophy affects boys, although by quirks of genetic sorting, girls are rarely affected. One third of the instances of Duchenne muscular dystrophy are the result of new mutations that are thought to occur during spermatogenesis on the paternal side of the mother and manifest in male offspring.

Natural History

Duchenne muscular dystrophy, unlike many conditions treated by pediatric orthopaedists, has a very predictable clinical course. When seen soon after birth, boys affected with Duchenne muscular dystrophy have a fairly normal neuromuscular examination, but by the age of 1 year they will demonstrate some difficulty in keeping themselves extended when held prone in the horizontal position. Another useful test is to have the patients lie supine with their shoulders at the edge of the examination table. The neck flexors manifest weakness early in the disease and affected patients will be unable to support their heads. Unless there is a family history, patients are not usually diagnosed until the age of 3 to 6 years. The typical chief complaint is abnormal gait. Affected boys walk late (> 18 months) and always have a wide base, abductor lurch, increased lumbar lordosis, and never run or walk on stairs normally. Walking begins to markedly deteriorate between the ages of 6 and 8 years. By age 12 years, most patients with Duchenne muscular dystrophy are no longer able to walk. At this point, when they become full-time wheelchair users, scoliosis develops in 90% of patients. Once the scoliosis begins, it always relentlessly progresses, resulting in severe spine deformity that limits the ability to sit and causes a great deal of discomfort during the teenage years. Death usually occurs toward the end of the second decade of life because of chronic respiratory decompensation or acute decompensation following a respiratory infection.

Pathophysiology

The pathophysiology of Duchenne muscular dystrophy is an absence of the muscle protein dystrophin. This is a long, rigid molecule that constitutes only a small portion (< 0.01%) of total muscle protein, but it is critically important for the physical as well as metabolic stability of the myofiber membrane. Dystrophin is linked to a series of extracellular dystrophin associated proteins, including dystroglycans, sarcoglycans, merosin, and laminin, which link the myofibers to the extracellular matrix. Dystrophin is completely absent in patients with Duchenne muscular dystrophy and is present in reduced quantities of a smaller molecular weight in patients with a milder form of the disease, Becker muscular dystrophy. Duchenne muscular dystrophy and Becker muscular dystrophy are classified as dystrophinopathies.

The dystrophin protein abnormality is the result of an abnormality in the gene for dystrophin, which is found on the X chromosome. In two thirds of affected patients, there is a deletion of a segment of the dystrophin gene. In patients with Duchenne muscular dystrophy, this deletion occurs within a triplet reading frame (frame-shifting mutation); therefore, when the gene is spliced back together, the reading frame is disrupted and no protein is produced. In 20% to 25% of patients, instead of a deletion, there is a stop codon, which is a point mutation that causes cessation of transcription of the mRNA. In addition, point mutations can occur, resulting in altered splicing. In some patients (< 5%), a duplication of the gene occurs. In all of these situations, no dystrophin is produced.

In Becker muscular dystrophy, the deletion is between the reading frames, usually in a noncoding region; therefore, when the gene is spliced back together, there is a normal reading frame, and thus a truncated dystrophin is produced. There may also be point mutations (single nucleotide substitution) that cause skipping of an exon, with resultant synthesis of truncated dystrophin. Improved understanding of these genetic mutations has allowed for more precise diagnosis of patients with Duchenne muscular dystrophy and Becker muscular dystrophy and has led investigators to a number of novel potential therapies.

The consequence of the absence of dystrophin is increased fragility of the myofiber membrane, which results in several problems. Cellular contents, including proteases, leak into the extracellular space, causing an inflammatory response and resulting in fibrosis. This fibrosis may be as important, if not more so, as the loss of muscle fibers to the muscle dysfunction and development of contractures. Because of the leakage of proteases, the metabolic pathways that support muscle cell metabolism are disrupted; therefore, muscles cannot function efficiently. Evidence in experimental systems has also revealed that eccentric muscle activity may be particularly damaging and lead to much more rapid progression of the disease.

Laboratory Diagnosis

When the diagnosis of Duchenne muscular dystrophy or Becker muscular dystrophy is suspected, the first test to be done is to determine the creatine kinase level in the blood. In normal patients, the creatine kinase level is less than 300 U/L, whereas in dystrophinopathies this level may be greater than 10,000 U/L.

If the creatine kinase level is elevated, then blood should be sent for genetic testing for Duchenne muscular dystrophy and Becker muscular dystrophy. Standard clinically available techniques yield positive results in approximately two thirds of patients; however, more recently available techniques that fully sequence the gene provide an absolute diagnosis of dystrophinopathy in 95% of patients.

In the small percentage of patients who have negative results on genetic testing, a muscle biopsy and Western blot test for dystrophin can provide an absolute diagnosis. Those patients who have Duchenne muscular dystrophy will show total absence of dystrophin on the Western blot test, whereas those who have Becker muscular dystrophy will demonstrate a reduced quantity of a truncated dystrophin. Biopsy is now rarely indicated for the diagnosis of Duchenne muscular dystrophy because of the increased precision of DNA testing. Biopsy, however, is the only way to definitively distinguish Duchenne muscular dystrophy from Becker muscular dystrophy.

Medical Treatment

The biggest advance in the treatment of Duchenne muscular dystrophy has been the use of corticosteroid therapy. Although several early studies indicated that corticosteroid therapy may be of benefit in this patient population, the results reported were relatively short term, with the longest follow-up being 3.25 years. In these studies, the cumulative muscle strength score showed dramatic differences when compared with cumulative muscle strength scores of the natural history when patients were maintained on prednisone at 0.75 mg/kg/d. Smaller doses and alternate day doses were not as effective, and larger doses had no greater degree of effectiveness.

The role of corticosteroid therapy, however, has been further clarified. One study offered deflazacort; a corticosteroid derived from prednisolone, to a group of 78 patients who were carefully followed by objective measures. In this study, 40 self-selected patients received daily deflazacort at 0.9 mg/kg/day with a minimum of

4 years of treatment; 48 patients whose families chose no treatment served as control subjects. Patients were assessed at 4- to 6-month intervals. Significant and dramatic differences in walking, pulmonary function, scoliosis, cardiac function were reported between the two groups. The authors reported that no control subjects were walking at 12 years, whereas one third of the patients in the treatment group were still walking at 18 years. When pulmonary function was assessed, forced vital capacity was found to be the same in both groups at age 10 years; however, by age 15 years the forced vital capacity of the control subjects was reduced to 44%, whereas the treated patients were at 85%. At age 18 years, the forced vital capacity was 33% in the control subjects and 73% in the treated patients. Eight years after the study was initiated, approximately 70% of the control subjects had scoliosis greater than 20°, whereas only 20% of the treated patients had a comparable degree of scoliosis. Although data have not been reported, anecdotal evidence indicates that once patients receive corticosteroid therapy, they do not show significant scoliosis progression, even when they develop minor degrees of scoliosis. Cardiac function, which was assessed using echocardiography, was significantly better in the treated patients than the control subjects.

Significant adverse effects are associated with the use of corticosteroids. Reduction in height was noted in the deflazacort study; patients in the treatment group were reported to be 20 to 25 cm shorter at skeletal maturity than the control subjects. Patients receiving corticosteroid therapy may also develop cushingoid facies and may gain a significant amount of weight; however, weight gain is much less with deflazacort than prednisone. Cataracts were identified in one third of the patients in the treatment group of the deflazacort study, but none were symptomatic enough to require treatment. No difference in fracture rate was reported when comparing patients in the treatment group and control subjects. Behavioral issues associated with corticosteroid therapy may be a significant problem and lead many families to discontinuation.

The current consensus is that the optimum age for instituting treatment is 5 to 7 years, although some recommend initiating corticosteroid therapy earlier. The long-term effects of weight gain and other developmental effects must be considered and balanced against the protective effect of corticosteroids on the muscle. Deflazacort is not approved for use in the United States; therefore, unless patients choose to acquire the drug independently from overseas pharmacies, they should receive prednisone at 0.75 mg/kg/day and be carefully monitored for adverse effects. A recently published practice parameter supported by the American Academy of Neurology recommends the use of corticosteroid therapy in patients with Duchenne muscular dystrophy.

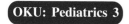
The proposed mechanisms of action of corticosteroids involves stabilization of the myofiber membrane, reduction of the inflammatory response associated with the leaky myofiber membrane (thereby reducing fibrosis), enhancement of muscle regeneration, and upregulation of the gene for calcineurin, which in turn increases the synthesis of utrophin (a functional substitute for dystrophin).

Another promising treatment is use of gentamicin or an experimental drug, PTC124, to reverse the effects of some specific pathologic stop codons (particularly the UGA stop codon). PTC124 is currently in phase II clinical trials. Another approach involves the use of an antisense oligoribonucleotide to block the area surrounding a frame-shifting deletion or pathologic point mutation, resulting in a premature stop codon to allow synthesis of a truncated dystrophin and thereby convert a Duchenne muscular dystrophy phenotype with no dystrophin to a milder Becker muscular dystrophy form with a truncated but partially functional dystrophin.

The ultimate treatment of Duchenne muscular dystrophy and Becker muscular dystrophy will repair the gene defect or involve insertion of a normal dystrophin gene into the genome to allow synthesis of dystrophin in affected patients. Although there are significant technical problems in achieving this goal there is a great deal of research currently being conducted in this area.

Rehabilitation and Orthopaedic Treatment

Because of the muscle weakness and development of contracture, patients with Duchenne muscular dystrophy lose function over time. Adaptive equipment, particularly power wheelchairs, are essential to maintain function as boys with Duchenne muscular dystrophy become progressively weaker. Many of these patients are in school physical therapy programs that emphasize stretching exercises. Stretching, although widely applied to this patient population, has never been proven to be effective and can cause discomfort. Nighttime ankle-foot orthotic devices are used to prevent equinus contracture. However, providing patients with positional alternatives such as standing frames may be beneficial psychologically and physically to these patients. It is important to maintain an activity level that can be tolerated without inducing fatigue; however, eccentric activity should be avoided because there are experimental data in animal models that indicate that this type of activity is damaging to dystrophin-deficient muscles.

Prophylactic surgery in patients with Duchenne muscular dystrophy or Becker muscular dystrophy who are 5 to 7 years of age is practiced, particularly in Europe, and includes release of the flexors at the hip, iliotibial band, knee, and ankle. However, data supporting this approach do not show dramatic differences in prolonga-

tion of walking. Some patients may develop early contractures and still have enough strength to stand and walk; in this patient group, contracture release with immediate resumption of standing and walking may prolong function, but this occurs infrequently. Foot surgery, including posterior tendon transfer and Achilles tendon lengthening, may prolong walking in some patients, but once patients cease walking, the presence of foot deformity does not affect long-term comfort or function. The recurrence of contractures following release is extremely common in this patient population.

The main role of orthopaedic surgery in the treatment of patients with Duchenne muscular dystrophy has been to address scoliosis. This treatment paradigm was established in the 1980s, when it was noted that nonsurgical methods did not prevent progression of scoliosis, and as scoliosis progressed in the early teen years, there was concomitant reduction of pulmonary function. Therefore, if surgery is delayed in these patients, pulmonary function would be reduced to a level that would make surgery dangerous. Because all spinal curves progress once they reach 20°, the principle has been established that early spinal instrumentation and fusion should be done once curve onset is noted and while the curves are still small. Surgery should extend from the upper thoracic spine to L5 or to the pelvis and sacrum in patients with established pelvic obliquity.

The use of corticosteroids has dramatically altered the natural history of scoliosis. The likelihood of developing a spinal curve is greatly reduced in patients receiving adequate corticosteroid treatment, and there is strong anecdotal evidence suggesting that when small spinal curves develop in these patients, they do not progress in the same relentless fashion as in the untreated patients; therefore, it may be appropriate to follow these patients through skeletal maturity and only surgically intervene when curves exceed 40°. However, data on this topic are not yet available.

As respiratory function declines in patients in their late teens, chronic respiratory insufficiency develops. With use of bilevel positive pressure ventilation at night, function, comfort, and life span may be increased. In addition, some patients may choose tracheostomy with long-term ventilation that may prolong their life span by many decades, although they will require total care. The ultimate life span of patients receiving corticosteroid therapy is not known, but it is likely that corticosteroid treatment will extend the expected life span by a significant number of years and maintain them during this time at a comfortable functional level.

Limb Girdle Muscular Dystrophy

Limb girdle muscular dystrophy is not a single muscle disease, but a large group of muscle diseases that are all characterized by progressive deterioration of muscle function and a dystrophic appearance of muscle biopsy specimens. Most are autosomal recessive, although there are rare autosomal dominant types. Because limb girdle muscular dystrophy includes a multitude of different diseases, the onset, clinical course, and findings are quite variable. The creatine kinase level in patients with limb girdle muscular dystrophy may be mildly to greatly elevated. Muscle biopsy will show histologic evidence of dystrophic changes with normal dystrophin, but precise diagnosis can be made by analysis of immunohistochemical staining of muscle specimens.

Recent studies have shown that half of the patients with limb girdle muscular dystrophy have genetically defined abnormalities. Most of the abnormalities are relatively equally distributed among defects in dysferlin, calpin-3, sarcoglycan, and alphadystroglycan, all of which are sarcolemmal proteins. As experience is gained with more precise genetic diagnosis, clinical characteristics of the individual types of limb girdle dystrophy will be better defined.

The prevalence of limb girdle muscular dystrophy has not been clearly established and estimates range from 1:14,500 to 1:123,000; thus, the incidence is much less than that of Duchenne muscular dystrophy, Becker muscular dystrophy, and many of the other entities previously discussed. The onset of weakness may be in childhood, but is generally in adolescence or adulthood; therefore, patients with limb girdle muscular dystrophy tend to make up a small percentage of those seen in pediatric neuromuscular clinics. In making the diagnosis, other causes of progressive weakness must be ruled out, including Duchenne muscular dystrophy, Becker muscular dystrophy, facioscapulohumeral muscular dystrophy, Emery-Dreifuss muscular dystrophy, and others. If limb girdle muscular dystrophy is suspected, patients should first be tested for abnormalities in the dystrophin gene, which can be done with a blood test as outlined previously. If the results of the blood test are normal, then a muscle biopsy should be done and processed by immunohistochemical techniques to define abnormalities in specific muscle proteins known to be associated with limb girdle muscular dystrophy. In addition, molecular genetic studies can be done on blood samples. Treatment is based on specific deformities that may occur. Scoliosis is uncommon in this population because patients usually present after skeletal maturity.

Myotonic Dystrophy

Myotonic dystrophy is the most prevalent neuromuscular disease in adults and affects 13 per 100,000 live births. It is inherited in a dominant form, but the severity is variable. Pediatric orthopaedists will most likely treat patients with congenital myotonic dystrophy. These children will be severely hypotonic at birth and may require full-time assisted ventilation for weeks to months

before they become strong enough to be weaned from the ventilator. Seventy-five percent of patients with this form of myotonic dystrophy will survive. Those who do survive will become progressively stronger with time, although they will be severely delayed in both motor and cognitive development. Most patients with myotonic dystrophy are able to walk by age 5 years, and essentially all will be independent walkers. Equinus contracture in this patient population is common, and many patients are unable to walk until this is surgically corrected. Scoliosis or kyphosis may occur (it is infrequent but not rare).

In the mild form of myotonic dystrophy, children may present with developmental delay and possibly toe walking, which can be confused with idiopathic toe walking. They will have distal weakness and motor as well as cognitive delay. The mildest form of myotonic dystrophy may typically have mild symptoms, and many affected adults may not realize that they have myotonic dystrophy until they have a child who manifests a more severe form of the disease, at which time the parent is also diagnosed.

A thorough history and careful physical examination will show evidence of distal weakness in addition to myotonia, and many affected adults will relate an inability to remove jar lids from screw top jars. In the teenage years, myotonia may develop, wherein when patients perform a maximal muscle contraction (such as tightly gripping an object), the muscle maintains this contraction even when the patient tries to relax. Patients with Steinert's disease (myotonia congenita) also exhibit myotonia, but they do not have progressive weakness or any of the other characteristics of myotonic dystrophy. All patients with myotonic dystrophy have a characteristic drooping face, particularly those who are more severely affected. The appearance is so characteristic of the disease that patients tend to resemble one another more than other family members. Adults, even those with a mild form of disease, may also have cardiomyopathy and cardiac conduction abnormalities that can cause spontaneous ventricular arrhythmias and lead to sudden death. Therefore, careful monitoring of cardiac function in adults is essential. A significant number of patients develop cataracts because of the effect of the trinucleotide repeat on an adjacent gene to the one responsible for myotonic dystrophy.

Myotonic dystrophy is caused by an expanded CTG nucleotide repeat in a noncoding region on chromosome 9 adjacent to the myotin protein kinase gene, resulting in deficient synthesis of the myotin protein kinase protein, which is important for RNA metabolism. The severity of the disease is proportional to the number of trinucleotide repeats (Table 2).

A phenomenon known as amplification, in which during oogenesis the number of these trinucleotide repeat units increases, resulting in a mother with only mild

Table 2 | The Severity of Myotonic Dystrophy as Determined by the Number of Trinucleotide Repeats

No. of Trinucleotide Repeats	Disease Severity
3 to 37	Normal
28 to 50	Premutation
50 to 150	Mild
> 150	Severe
> 500	Congenital myotonic dystrophy

Table 3 | Characteristics of the Two Major Forms of Charcot-Marie-Tooth Disease

Charcot-Marie-Tooth disease type I	Demyelinating peripheral neuropathy 60% to 80% of all patients with Charcot-Marie-Tooth disease Decreased nerve conduction velocity on electrodiagnostic studies
Charcot-Marie-Tooth disease type II	Axonal neuropathy 20% to 40% of all patients with Charcot-Marie-Tooth disease Normal or mildly decreased nerve conduction velocity Decreased amplitude of muscle action potential

and unapparent disease with less than 100 trinucleotide repeats who may have a child with severe congenital myotonic dystrophy with over 1,000 repeating subunits. The affected mother frequently does not realize that she has the disease until she has a child with myotonic dystrophy. This same type of amplification does not occur during spermatogenesis; therefore, only the children of affected mothers tend to present with severe congenital myotonic dystrophy.

Diagnosis

In the past, electromyography, which provided the typical and diagnostic "dive bomber" response, was used to diagnose patients with myotonic dystrophy. Currently, however, it is less traumatic to the child and more precise to obtain DNA studies that will provide an absolute diagnosis along with the number of CTG repeats. Once the diagnosis is established in the child, parents should be tested so that appropriate genetic counseling can be done.

Treatment

The survivors of congenital myotonic dystrophy, although profoundly hypotonic at birth, become progressively stronger with time. Equinus contracture, when present, will impair standing balance; once equinus is surgically corrected, patients will begin to stand and walk. Patients eventually become independent ambulators, usually by age 5 years. If surgery for any reason is necessary, it should be noted that these patients are typically quite sensitive to anesthetic gases as well as local anesthesia used in epidural pain control and opiates. Scoliosis and kyphosis, although not common in patients with myotonic dystrophy, may occur with increased frequency in this patient population, and those affected should be monitored for spinal alignment during growth. In the second and third decades of life, patients should be monitored for cardiac conduction abnormalities.

Dermatomyositis

Juvenile dermatomyositis, which may cause severe disability in childhood, is one of the few degenerative diseases of the motor unit that is not genetically based. It appears to be an autoimmune disease that presents with

acute onset of weakness in childhood after normal early development, along with a facial rash. Patients will have markedly elevated creatine kinase levels in the range of 5,000 to 10,000 U/L, which is comparable to the levels found in patients with Duchenne muscular dystrophy. Patients with dermatomyositis will also have a high erythrocyte sedimentation rate. Additionally, patients will have a characteristic electromyogram, and muscle biopsy will show normal dystrophin, but characteristic inflammatory changes will be apparent. Some of these patients will have spontaneous recovery, and for those who do not, corticosteroid treatment may be effective. If corticosteroid treatment is not effective, other therapies include chloroquine, methotrexate, cyclosporine, cyclophosphamide, and intravenous immunoglobulin. Patients may have persistent disease, which can be extremely disabling; these patients will develop profound weakness, ultimately require mechanical ventilation in spite of treatment, and for some the disease can be fatal.

Charcot-Marie-Tooth Disease

Charcot-Marie-Tooth disease, a group of diseases that affect the peripheral nerve, is moderately common, with an incidence of 1 in 2,500 individuals. All forms of the disease manifest as distal weakness primarily in the foot and ankle; somewhat later in life the hand may be affected as well. The classic description of Charcot-Marie-Tooth disease is peroneal muscle weakness resulting in cavovarus deformity. There are two major forms of the disease (type I and type II), the characteristics of which are listed in Table 3.

Natural History

Patients with Charcot-Marie-Tooth disease type I usually present toward the end of the first decade of life with progressive cavovarus deformities of the feet associated with dorsiflexion of the toes during the swing phase of gait and contracture of the plantar fascia. Muscle testing typically demonstrates weakness of the peroneal musculature, with relative preservation of the anterior and posterior tibialis and toe dorsiflexor muscles. Radiographic studies of patients with Charcot-Marie-Tooth disease have demonstrated that most patients have dorsiflexion of the hindfoot with concomitant forefoot equinus, which results in a true cavus foot. Because the hindfoot is in dorsiflexion, Achilles tendon lengthening should be avoided unless true equinus is radiographically confirmed on lateral weight-bearing radiographs (a situation that is rarely encountered). If left untreated, these patients will go on to develop severe and disabling cavovarus deformities. In Charcot-Marie-Tooth disease type II, patients may exhibit cavovarus, but more frequently have a more balanced weakness throughout the foot, resulting in relatively normal appearance of the foot; a drop foot, however, is usually present because of marked dorsiflexor weakness.

Pathophysiology

There are over 30 genes that now have been described in association with the different forms of hereditary motor sensory neuropathy. With Charcot-Marie-Tooth disease type I, 70% of patients show a duplication of the peripheral myelin protein (PMP) gene on chromosome 22. This duplication causes an overproduction of the gene product, PMP-22, which results in demyelination of the nerves with resulting neural dysfunction. The second most prevalent type of Charcot-Marie-Tooth disease type I is the X-linked form associated with a deficiency in the connexin gene, which is responsible for 15% to 20% of all instances of Charcot-Marie-Tooth type I disease and 90% of X-linked forms.

Medical Treatment

There are no clinically proven treatments for Charcot-Marie-Tooth disease, but there are some promising new treatment approaches being studied. The first of these involves administration of ascorbic acid (vitamin C). In a mouse model, a clinical, physiologic, and histologic improvement was demonstrated after administration of the equivalent of 4 g of ascorbic acid once per week. Another study has shown efficacy in an experimental animal model after administration of an antagonist of progesterone.

Orthopaedic/Rehabilitation Treatment

The major disability in children with Charcot-Marie-Tooth disease is foot deformity. In patients with Charcot-Marie-Tooth disease type IA, a progressive foot deformity occurs that is consistent in its clinical presentation, but somewhat variable in the age of onset. A progressive varus deformity of the heel typically occurs in association with plantar flexion of the first metatarsal, elevation of the longitudinal arch, and tightness

of the plantar fascia. In patients with early onset deformity, plantar fasciotomy may help to reverse this deformity, albeit temporarily. As the disease progresses, so does foot deformity. When the deformity becomes more severe but before it becomes rigid, multiple tendon transfers to help rebalance the foot will maintain foot balance as the muscles undergo further deterioration. The latter treatment consists of transfer of the extensor hallucis longus to the first metatarsal neck (Jones transfer), accompanied by fusion of the interphalangeal joint of the great toe to prevent excessive interphalangeal toe flexion. In skeletally immature patients, instead of interphalangeal fusion, the stump of the extensor hallucis longus should be side-to-side tenodesed to the extensor digitorum brevis. Transfer of the extensor digitorum longus tendons as a group to the lateral cuneiform (Hibbs transfer), transfer of the anterior tibial tendon to the lateral cuneiform, and transfer of the posterior tibial tendon through the interosseous membrane to the lateral cuneiform should also be performed in the typical patient. If the first metatarsal is in fixed plantar flexion, a dorsal closing wedge osteotomy of the first metatarsal may need to be added. Some surgeons also add a Dwyer lateral closing wedge or sliding type calcaneal osteotomy for correction of varus heel.

The Coleman block test is often used to differentiate a rigid from a supple hindfoot deformity. Triple arthrodesis should be avoided if possible, although in some patients with persistent progression and severe rigid deformity, this may be the only means to obtain a plantigrade foot.

Spinal Muscular Atrophy

Spinal muscular atrophy is the most common genetic disease resulting in death during childhood. It affects 1 out of 10,000 live births, and the carrier frequency is 1 of 50 individuals. The condition is inherited in an autosomal recessive manner; therefore, both parents must be carriers, in which instance each child has a 1 in 4 chance of being affected. There is much variability in the severity of the disease, which correlates with the age of onset. However, if there is more than one child in a family, the degree of involvement is similar in all affected children. The major manifestation of spinal muscular atrophy is weakness, which is typically more profound proximally than distally and becomes progressively worse with time.

Classification

Spinal muscular atrophy is divided into three subtypes (type I [Werdnig-Hoffman Disease], type II, and type III), the onset and expected functional levels and life expectancy of which are listed in Table 4. In type I and II spinal muscular atrophy, the cause of death is typically respiratory failure; longer lifespan is possible with assisted ventilation.

Table 4 | Disease Onset, Functional Level, and Life Expectancy of Patients With Spinal Muscular Atrophy

Subtype	Onset (Months)	Highest Level of Function	Life Expectancy (Years)
Type I (Werdnig-Hoffman disease)	0 to 6	Sits with support	< 2
Type II	6 to 18	Sits unassisted	15 +
Type III	> 18	Independent walking	15 to normal

Natural History

The primary characteristic of spinal muscular atrophy is progressive muscle weakness, which is caused by progressive loss of alpha-motor neurons in the anterior horn of the spinal cord. Fasciculations, which are caused by spontaneous firing of the damaged anterior horn cells, can be observed on electromyography as spontaneous motor potentials and are characteristic of spinal muscular atrophy. Because only a thin membrane covers the tongue, fasciculations are easily observed; they can also be observed in the hand and fingers as a fine tremor at rest. Patients with severe spinal muscular atrophy become progressively weaker and ultimately die as a result of respiratory failure.

Spinal Muscular Atrophy Type I

Although some patients with spinal muscular atrophy type I (Werdnig-Hoffman disease) present at birth with severe weakness, others are normal at birth and begin to manifest weakness during the first few months of life. In patients with spinal muscular atrophy type I, progression is rapid and death typically occurs as a result of respiratory failure by age 2 years. If patients receive artificial ventilation via tracheostomy, survival may be longer, and patients will manifest profound weakness as well as all of the complications of spinal muscular atrophy, including hip dislocation, scoliosis, and joint contracture.

Spinal Muscular Atrophy Types II and III

Spinal muscular atrophy types II and III represent a spectrum of the disease; the arbitrarily set dividing point between type II and type III is the ability to stand independently. Although it is not clear that muscles actually become weaker, function clearly diminishes with time; therefore, patients acquire skills more slowly than normal individuals, never achieve many motor milestones, and lose skills that they have acquired earlier in childhood. Problems secondary to the weakness include hip dislocation, scoliosis, and joint contractures. Treatment of deformities is designed to improve the quality of life. Spine fusions are done to preserve sitting mobility. Contractures are released if they interfere with hygiene or care.

Pathophysiology

Spinal muscular atrophy is caused by a deficiency of the survival motor neuron (SMN) protein, which is reduced by 5% to 95% in patients with spinal muscular atrophy. The severity of the disease is directly related to the amount of reduction in levels of the circulating SMN protein. This protein is involved in messenger and ribosomal RNA transcription and processing; however, it is not known why the defect manifests only in anterior horn cells. Deficiency of the SMN protein leads to progressive loss of anterior horn cells and thereby progressive weakness.

The reason for the deficiency in the SMN protein is an abnormality in the *SMN* genes, which are located on chromosome 5. There are two alleles of *SMN-I* in a telomeric position on chromosome 5, and several copies of a similar (but not identical) gene (*SMN-II*) in a centromeric location on the same chromosome. This *SMN-II* gene produces a functional but shorter and less functional SMN protein because one exon is not transcribed as a result of a single nucleotide difference between the *SMN-I* and *SMN-II* genes. Affected patients with all types of spinal muscular atrophy will have functional loss of both copies of the *SMN-I* gene. However, the disease severity is determined by the number of functional copies of *SMN-II* that are present. Therefore, patients with spinal muscular atrophy type I have function of only one *SMN-II* gene that produces low levels of SMN protein, whereas patients with milder disease may have multiple copies of the *SMN-II* gene that produce higher levels of the protein. Complete absence of SMN protein is lethal, whereas loss of the *SMN-II* copy alone does not result in disease.

This *SMN-I* gene abnormality is detectable in blood DNA analysis in 95% of patients with all forms of spinal muscular atrophy. A positive test result is absolutely diagnostic, and a negative test result indicates a greater than 5% chance that the patient may have classical spinal muscular atrophy. Muscle biopsy is rarely indicated in this population. The carrier state cannot be detected by routine clinical analysis at present, but this is available as a research tool.

Treatment

No effective medical treatment is currently available for patients with spinal muscular atrophy. Clinical trials of riluzole have shown some response to treatment, but results have not been dramatic.

There are a variety of genetically based research studies for treatment of spinal muscular atrophy. One approach targets the single nucleotide difference on *SMN-II*, which causes skipping of an exon and results in a functional but less stable SMN protein. Investigators are using antisense oligoribonucleotides to block this site and allow synthesis of a full-length SMN protein.

As in other conditions resulting in muscle weakness, the general principles for provision of adaptive equipment are important for patients with spinal muscular atrophy. Patients with spinal muscular atrophy type II and advanced forms of spinal muscular atrophy type III will require powered mobility and should be supplied with this as early as age 2 years if they are not walking.

Although all patients with spinal muscular atrophy type I or II and many of those with spinal muscular atrophy type III will develop a dislocation of one or both hips, no treatment (either prophylactic or salvage) is indicated. The hip dislocation is rarely symptomatic and does not seem to impair function. If pain does occur, patients should be counseled that in all likelihood the pain will resolve within 6 months to 1 year; therefore, surgical intervention should be delayed. In the rare patient with persistent hip pain, proximal femoral resection or proximal femoral valgus osteotomy may provide resolution of symptoms. Attempt at reduction is not warranted.

Scoliosis is a significant problem for patients with spinal muscular atrophy. In patients with more severe spinal muscular atrophy type II, the onset of scoliosis may occur by the second or third year of life and progression may be rapid. Although there are limited studies of bracing for patients with spinal muscular atrophy, treatment with a thoracolumbar sacral orthosis improves sitting stability and may slow curve progression to allow for greater spinal growth until spinal surgery is ultimately performed. Because respiration is supported to a large extent by diaphragmatic motion in these patients, a large abdominal hole should be placed in the orthotic device to allow for abdominal expansion with breathing. For younger patients, the soft Boston thoracolumbosacral orthosis will provide sufficient support, but in older patients, more rigid materials will be required. When curves progress past 50° to 60°, spinal fusion and stabilization is indicated, even though this will reduce spinal growth in these young children. Because of their relative small size and reduced growth potential, there is a limited amount of anterior spinal growth, and it is not clear whether the risks of anterior fusion to prevent crankshaft deformity are worth the potential benefits in these patients who are full-time sitters. Unlike Duchenne muscular dystrophy, in which the spine becomes quite rigid because of the muscular fibrosis, in these patients the spine remains relatively flexible, and a significant amount of correction may be obtained, even in patients with more severe curves, with posterior surgery alone. Newer techniques of instrumentation, such as the vertical, expandable prosthetic titanium rib system that has been advocated for patients with thoracic insufficiency, may prove efficacious for young patients with spinal muscular atrophy type II with curves greater than 50°.

Patients with spinal muscular atrophy will develop hip and knee flexion contractures as well as equinovarus contracture at the foot. Foot deformity may occur while patients still have relatively good preservation of strength of the extremity. In these instances, correction of the foot deformity by tenotomy of posterior tibial, flexor digitorum longus, and flexor hallucis longus tendons may allow for prolongation of standing and walking and should be performed. Once knee and hip contractures reach 30° to 40°, release of the hamstrings typically has not yielded significant enough improvement to warrant intervention. However, in patients with lesser degrees of contracture, hamstring release may be indicated if patients seem to have enough strength to continue to walk. This is only infrequently indicated and should only be done in patients who have a strong motivation to walk.

Role of the Muscular Dystrophy Association

Patients with most motor unit diseases fall under the umbrella of the Muscular Dystrophy Association (MDA), which supports clinics throughout the United States. The MDA provides excellent informational brochures, patient support groups, and supports a 1-week summer camp, which is the highlight of the year for many patients with these conditions. In addition, the MDA supports a tremendous amount of basic and clinical research, and many of the advances in the understanding and treatment of diseases of the motor unit has come from MDA-funded studies.

Summary

This group of diseases presents a multitude of diagnostic and therapeutic challenges to the pediatric orthopaedist. Although the orthopaedic issues are significant and orthopaedic interventions may provide great functional benefits, these constitute only a small portion of the medical issues presented by this patient population. The care of patients with progressive neuromuscular diseases requires a team approach and should include a geneticist, a neurologist, physical and occupational therapists, a social worker for psychological support, and a coordinator to tie all the services together. Consultants need to be available in cardiology, pulmonology, and other medical areas. Most patients with these conditions will be followed in an MDA-sponsored clinic, and many of these clinics can benefit from the addition of a knowledgeable pediatric orthopaedist.

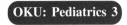

Annotated Bibliography
Motor Unit Diseases

Gene Reviews Web site. Available at: http://www.genetests.org. Accessed March 2, 2006.

This Web site posts review articles on specific neuromuscular diseases and is updated every 2 years.

Neuromuscular Disease Center. Washington University Neuromuscular Web site. Available at: http://www.neuro.wustl.edu/neuromuscular/. Accessed January 6, 2006.

This is a continuously updated, comprehensive reference source in outline form on the Web for all neuromuscular diseases.

Muscular Dystrophy

Alman B, Raza S, Biggar W: Steroid treatment and the development of scoliosis in males with Duchenne muscular dystrophy. *J Bone Joint Surg Am* 2004;86-A:519-524.

The authors of this study documented a marked reduction in the incidence of scoliosis in boys with Duchenne muscular dystrophy who were being treated with corticosteroids.

Biggar W, Gingras M, Fehlings D, Harris F, Steele C: Deflazacort treatment of Duchenne muscular dystrophy. *J Pediatr* 2001;138:45-50.

This article describes the significant benefits of using deflazacort in the treatment of patients with Duchenne muscular dystrophy.

Biggar W, Klamut H, Demacio P, Stevens D, Ray P: Duchenne muscular dystrophy: Current knowledge, treatment, and future prospects. *Clin Orthop Relat Res* 2002;401:88-106.

The authors provide a review of the pathophysiology of Duchenne muscular dystrophy and the Becker form of muscular dystrophy.

Cripe LH: Cardiovascular health supervision for individuals affected by Duchenne or Becker muscular dystrophy. *Pediatrics* 2005;116:1569-1573.

The authors, in association with the section on cardiology and cardiac surgery of the American Academy of Pediatrics, provide recommendations for cardiovascular assessment and treatment of patients with Duchenne muscular dystrophy or Becker muscular dystrophy.

Finder J, Birnkrant D, Carl J, et al: Respiratory care of the patient with Duchenne muscular dystrophy: ATS consensus statement. *Am J Respir Crit Care Med* 2004;170:456-465.

The authors describe the practice parameters for all phases of respiratory care for patients with Duchenne muscular dystrophy.

Flanigan K, von Niederhausern A, Dunn D, Alder J, Mendell J, Weiss R: Rapid direct sequence analysis of the dystrophin gene. *Am J Hum Genet* 2003;72:931-939.

The authors discuss the technique and results of using rapid direct sequence analysis to assess genetic defects in patients with Duchenne muscular dystrophy. They report that laboratories using this approach can diagnose 95% of patients using DNA analysis.

Gaine WJ, Lim J, Stephenson W, Galasko CS: Progression of scoliosis after spinal fusion in Duchenne's muscular dystrophy. *J Bone Joint Surg Br* 2004;86:550-555.

The authors report on the long-term follow-up of 85 patients with Duchenne muscular dystrophy who underwent spinal fusion. At a mean 49-month follow-up, they found that fusion to L5, S1, or the ilium provided similar initial curve correction and maintenance of stability, whereas fusion to L4 or above provided less optimal outcomes. One perioperative death occurred, and there were three wound infections and two symptomatic pseudarthroses.

Lu QL, Rabinowitz A, Chen YC, et al: Systemic delivery of antisense oligoribonucleotide restores dystrophin expression in body-wide skeletal muscles. *Proc Natl Acad Sci USA* 2005;102:198-203.

The authors of this article discuss a novel and promising molecular treatment of patients with Duchenne muscular dystrophy. They systemically injected a specific modified oligoribonucleotide into mdx mice with a point mutation and found generalized expression of dystrophin in skeletal but not cardiac muscle.

Moxley R, Ashwal S, Pandya S, et al: Practice parameter: Corticosteroid treatment of Duchenne dystrophy. Report of the quality standards subcommittee of the American Academy of Neurology and the Practice Committee on the Child Neurology Society. *Neurology* 2005;64:13-20.

The authors of this article provide a review of the published literature on the corticosteroid treatment of Duchenne muscular dystrophy and provide medication treatment recommendations.

Sussman M: Duchenne muscular dystrophy. *J Am Acad Orthop Surg* 2002;10:138-151.

This is a general review of Duchenne muscular dystrophy, including a discussion of pathophysiology, natural history, and treatment.

Limb Girdle Muscular Dystrophy

Gordon E, Pegoraro E, Hoffman E: Limb girdle muscular dystrophy overview, in Gene Reviews. (Revised February 2006). Available at: http://www.genetests.org. Accessed March 2, 2006.

The authors provide an overview of this complex series of diseases with documentation of the specific molecular defects responsible for many of the subtypes of limb girdle muscular dystrophy.

Myotonic Dystrophy

Campbell C, Sherlock R, Jacob P, Blayney M: Congenital myotonic dystrophy: Assisted ventilation duration and outcome. *Pediatrics* 2004;113:811-816.

The authors reviewed the outcomes of patients with congenital myotonic dystrophy who received assisted ventilation and found that those requiring more than 30 days of assisted ventilation had a 25% mortality rate in the first year, whereas no child in the shorter-term assisted ventilation group died. The mortality rate after 1 year was similarly low, but patients in the shorter-term assisted ventilation group had better motion, language, and activities of daily life scores at all ages.

Logigian E, Moxley R IV, Blood C, et al: Leukocyte CTG repeat length correlates with severity of myotonia in myotonic dystrophy type I. *Neurology* 2004;62:1081-1089.

This is a study of the molecular pathophysiology of myotonic dystrophy.

Dermatomyositis

Sallum A, Kiss M, Sachetti S, et al: Juvenile dermatomyositis: Clinical, laboratorial, histological, therapeutical and evolutive parameters of 35 patients. *Arq Neuropsiquiatr* 2002;60:889-899.

This is a retrospective analysis of 35 patients who were followed for a mean of 3 years and 10 months. All patients met clinical criteria for juvenile dermatomyositis and underwent a muscle biopsy to confirm the diagnosis.

Charcot-Marie-Tooth Disease

Passage E, Norreel J, Noack-Fraissignes P, et al: Ascorbic acid treatment corrects the phenotype of a mouse model of Charcot-Marie-Tooth disease. *Nat Med* 2004; 10:396-401.

The authors of this study reported evidence of response to a novel treatment of Charcot-Marie-Tooth disease using a transgene mouse model.

Saifi G, Szigeti K, Snipes G, Garcia C, Lupski J: Molecular mechanisms, diagnosis, and rational approaches to management of and therapy for Charcot-Marie-Tooth Disease and related peripheral neuropathies. *J Investig Med* 2003;51:261-283.

This is a comprehensive review of the diagnosis and pathophysiology of Charcot-Marie-Tooth disease. (The senior author originally described the duplication of PMP 22 in

Charcot-Marie-Tooth IA.) The authors present a coherent stepwise approach to diagnosis and a clear diagnostic classification.

Sereda M, Meyer zu Horste G, Suter U, Uzma N, Nave KA: Therapeutic administration of progesterone antagonist in a model of Charcot-Marie-Tooth disease (CMT-IA). *Nat Med* 2003;9:1533-1537.

The authors of this study reported evidence of response to a novel treatment of Charcot-Marie-Tooth disease in a transgene mouse model.

Spinal Muscular Atrophy

Iannaccone S, Smith S, Simard L: Spinal muscular atrophy. *Curr Neurol Sci Rep* 2004;4:74-80.

The authors present a review of the natural history and current management of spinal muscular atrophy and discuss medications used in current clinical trials.

Jablonka S, Sendtner M: Molecular and cellular basis of spinal muscular atrophy. *Amyotroph Lateral Scler Other Motor Neuron Disord* 2003;4:144-149.

This is a discussion of the function of the SMN protein.

Prior T, Russman B: Spinal muscular atrophy, in *Gene Reviews*. Available at: http://www.genetests.org.

The authors present a thorough review of clinical issues and pathophysiology of spinal muscular atrophy, which is updated every 2 years.

Wirth B: Spinal muscular atrophy: State of the art and therapeutic perspectives. *Amyotroph Lateral Scler Other Motor Neuron Disord* 2002;3:87-95.

The authors discuss the genetic defect and gene-based therapeutic possibilities for patients with spinal muscular atrophy.

Role of the Muscular Dystrophy Association

Muscular Dystrophy Association Web site. Available at: http://www.mdausa.org/. Accessed January 12, 2006.

Classic Bibliography

Fenichel G, Florence JM, Pestronk A, et al: Long-term benefit from prednisone therapy in Duchenne muscular dystrophy. *Neurology* 1991;41:1874-1877.

Hoffman E, Fischbeck KH, Brown RH, et al: Characterization of dystrophin in muscle-biopsy specimens from patients with Duchenne's or Becker's muscular dystrophy. *N Engl J Med* 1988;318:1363-1368.

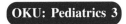

Read L, Galasko CS: Delay in diagnosing Duchenne muscular dystrophy in orthopaedic clinics. *J Bone Joint Surg Br* 1986;68:481-482.

Russman B, Buncher C, White M, Samaha F, Iannaccone S, Group DS: Function changes in spinal muscular atrophy II and III. *Neurology* 1996;47:973-976.

Sussman M: Advantage of early spinal stabilization and fusion in patients with Duchenne muscular dystrophy. *J Pediatr Orthop* 1984;4:532-537.

Wilkins KE, Gibson DA: The patterns of spinal deformity in Duchenne muscular dystrophy. *J Bone Joint Surg Am* 1976;58:24-32.

Chapter 11

Arthrogrypotic Syndromes and Osteochondrodysplasias

François Fassier, MD, FRCSC

Reggie C. Hamdy, MD, MSc, FRCSC

Arthrogrypotic Syndromes

The word *arthrogryposis* is derived from the Greek roots *arthro* (joint) and *gryposis* (curved). Arthrogryposis is not a diagnosis but rather a term used by clinicians to describe multiple contractures present at birth. There are over 150 different syndromes associated with congenital contractures, the most common being arthrogryposis multiplex congenita (amyoplasia affecting all four limbs).

Etiology

The main cause of arthrogryposis is diminished fetal movement, resulting from either fetal or maternal abnormalities. The decreased fetal movement ultimately leads to development of multiple joint contractures. There are numerous causes of diminished fetal movement, including neuropathic abnormalities, muscle abnormalities, abnormalities of connective tissue, space limitations of the fetus, intrauterine vascular compromise, and maternal diseases. Prenatal diagnosis may be possible by using repeated ultrasound studies to evaluate fetal movements and characteristic fetal positions. The incidence of arthrogryposis (as a whole) is approximately 1 per 3,000 live births, and the incidence of amyoplasia is approximately 1 in 10,000 live births.

Classification

Arthrogryposis multiplex congenita can be classified into three broad categories according to the presence or absence of associated visceral and central nervous anomalies. Group 1 disorders affect only the limbs (amyoplasia). Group 2 disorders affect the limbs with involvement of other parts of the body. Group 3 disorders affect the limbs with associated central nervous system involvement.

Group 1 disorders are usually seen by orthopaedic surgeons, and the most common disorder of this group is amyoplasia (which literally means no muscle growth). Distal arthrogryposis type 1 is a specific type of congenital contractures involving the distal joints only and is inherited as an autosomal dominant trait. Affected children show a typical positioning of the hands, medially overlapping fingers, clenched fists, ulnar deviation of the fingers, and camptodactyly. Distal arthrogryposis type 1 is associated with foot contractures. Other more proximal joints may be involved to a milder degree. Children with distal arthrogryposis type 1 typically respond well to physical therapy.

Group 2 disorders include multiple pterygium syndromes, some forms of skeletal dysplasia such as diastrophic dysplasia, and Larsen's syndrome.

Group 3 disorders include numerous syndromes with involvement of the central nervous system; patients with group 3 disorders can have associated congenital contractures.

Genetic Aspects

Arthrogryposis is a component of numerous genetic syndromes. About half of the conditions associated with arthrogryposis have an underlying genetic abnormality.

Workup

Any infant or child with multiple contractures should have a thorough family history obtained, physical examination, and additional studies if necessary. It should be determined during the physical examination whether the arthrogryposis involves only the limbs or also other parts of the body, specifically the neurologic and muscular systems. It is also important to determine which parts of the limbs are involved, and to what extent. The range of motion of each joint should be carefully recorded. Radiographs of the spine, hips, and feet should be obtained.

It is essential to determine whether this condition is genetic or nongenetic, not only for management, but also for counseling the parents on the risks that may be associated with future pregnancies. Genetic investigations should include assessment of blood cells and skin fibroblasts because in some patients mosaicism may exist (when chromosomal studies on blood cells are normal, but an abnormality is detected in the skin fibroblasts). The most common form of arthrogryposis,

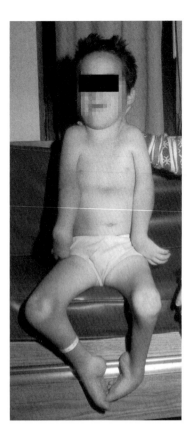

Figure 1 Photograph of a 5-year-old child with arthrogryposis shows typical upper and lower limb deformities.

amyoplasia, is not a hereditary condition, and no specific etiology can be determined. Nerve conduction velocity studies and electromyography may be indicated.

Prognosis

Most patients with arthrogryposis do not have intellectual impairment or sensory deficits. The functional long-term prognosis is usually good for most of these patients, unlike patients with other neuromuscular conditions. The contractures are usually most severe at birth and then gradually improve. The overall good prognosis should be clearly explained to the parents.

Clinical Picture

A child with arthrogryposis typically presents with the shoulders internally rotated and adducted, the elbows extended, the forearms pronated, and the wrist and fingers flexed (Figure 1). This clinical presentation is often described as a policeman's hand or a waiter's tip hand. In the lower limbs, the foot is most commonly affected (approximately 90% of patients), followed by knee deformities (approximately 70% of patients), and then hip deformities (approximately 40% of patients). Loss of skin creases is typically detectable across the joints, and dimpling can be noted at the sites of the joints. The muscles are severely atrophied. All children with arthrogryposis have a normal intelligence quotient and normal sensation.

General Management

Children with arthrogryposis multiplex congenita should be managed in a multidisciplinary clinic. The overall goal in the management of these children is to improve function and ambulation while allowing the child to develop as normally as possible. If possible, multiple surgeries should be combined so that hospitalizations can be minimized.

Lower Limb Deformities

Initial treatment of clubfoot deformity consists of repeated weekly casting. Conservative treatment, however, is unlikely to be successful in this patient population; therefore, radical posteromedial release is usually necessary at approximately 1 year of age followed by prolonged splinting to prevent or minimize recurrence of deformities. Talectomy should be reserved for patients with severe or recurrent deformities. The goal of talectomy is to obtain a painless, plantigrade foot; however, because talectomy only addresses the hindfoot deformity, additional surgery may be required for correction of forefoot deformities. Talectomy should be used with caution because long-term complications are commonly associated with this procedure and include pain, tibiocalcaneal arthritis, and recurrence of deformity. Gradual correction using a circular external fixator is another option for the correction of complex foot deformities.

The treatment of vertical talus usually requires surgical intervention. Early casting may help in stretching the tissues, but it is unlikely to correct the deformity. A radical single-stage release is usually performed when patients are approximately 1 year of age. A high recurrence rate has been reported with this procedure. If it is impossible to reduce the talus, then a talectomy may be performed. Care should be taken to carefully position the os calcis underneath the tibia (Figure 2).

Flexion contractures are the most common knee deformities in children with arthrogryposis multiplex congenita. The goal in the management of knee flexion deformities is to facilitate ambulation, sitting, and standing. Initial treatment in the neonate and infant consists of stretching and bracing. Mild deformities of up to 20° are compatible with an excellent function and do not need any specific treatment other than physiotherapy and night bracing. More severe deformities of the knee can be managed with posterior soft-tissue release, femoral shortening, supracondylar extension osteotomy, or a combination of these three procedures. Supracondylar extension osteotomy has been reported to have a high rate of recurrence in this patient population (Figure 3). Gradual correction with an Ilizarov circular fixator is another option for patients with severe deformities (Figure 4). Prolonged postoperative bracing is typically necessary to prevent or minimize recurrence.

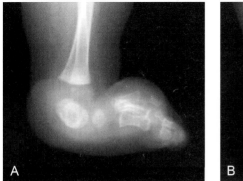
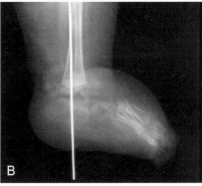
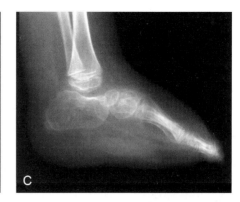

Figure 2 **A,** Radiograph showing vertical talus in a 2-year-old child with arthrogryposis. **B,** Radiograph obtained after talectomy was performed shows good position of the calcaneus underneath the tibia. **C,** Radiograph obtained 4 years postoperatively.

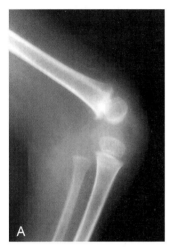
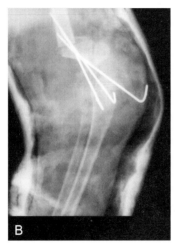
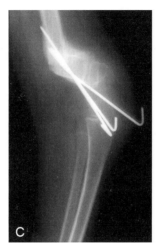
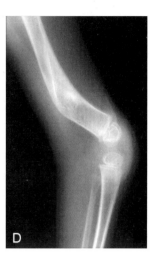

Figure 3 **A,** Preoperative radiograph shows a severe knee flexion deformity in a 5-year-old child with arthrogryposis. **B,** Postoperative radiograph after supracondylar osteotomy was performed. **C,** Radiograph obtained 2 months postoperatively. **D,** Radiograph obtained 1 year postoperatively shows remodelling.

Knee extension contractures are much less common than flexion contractures. Initial treatment consists of stretching the quadriceps and repeated castings. If this fails to correct the hyperextension or subluxation of the knee, then quadricepsplasty is recommended.

Hip deformity occurs in 50% to 80% of patients with arthrogryposis multiplex congenita and includes dislocations, subluxations, and contractures. There is consensus in the literature for the need to reduce a unilateral hip dislocation to prevent pelvic obliquity and scoliosis. Closed reduction, however, always fails to reduce a hip dislocation. Most orthopaedists will perform an open reduction via an anterior Smith-Petersen approach, although a medial approach has been reported to yield good results (Figure 5).

The management of patients with bilateral hip dislocation remains controversial. Although many orthopaedists do not perform open reduction to avoid increasing stiffness and the development of osteonecrosis of the femoral head, others recommend open reduction for this patient population. The typical hip deformity in pa-

tients with arthrogryposis is flexion, abduction, and external rotation. The treatment of a hip flexion contracture becomes necessary if it exceeds 30° to 40° because a hip flexion contracture this severe may interfere with walking or bracing. Soft-tissue release is recommended (iliopsoas release). A femoral extension osteotomy may be performed for patients with more severe and complex deformities. Patients with abduction contractures may be treated with iliotibial band release with or without a varus femoral osteotomy. Femoral derotation osteotomy is recommended for patients with external rotation contractures.

Upper Limb Deformities

Upper limb deformities in patients with arthrogryposis multiplex congenita typically include adduction and internal rotation of the shoulder, extension of the elbow, flexion and ulnar deviation of the wrist, and stiff fingers with thumb in palm deformity. The goal in the management of patients with upper limb deformities is to maximize functional independence by positioning the limbs

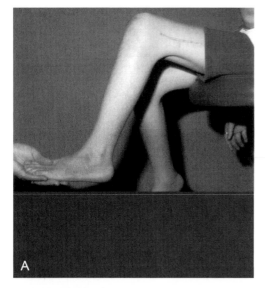
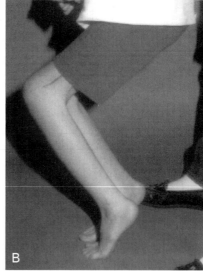
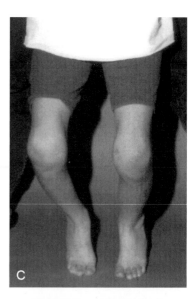
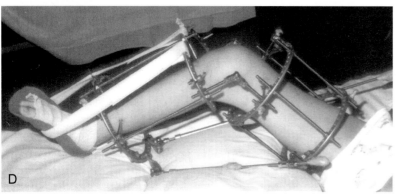
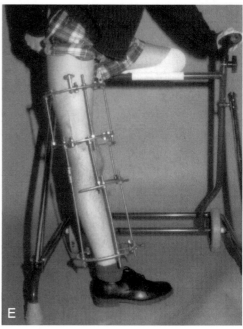

Figure 4 **A,** Photograph shows a severe knee flexion deformity in a 10-year-old patient with arthrogryposis (who previously had soft-tissue releases). **B** and **C,** Photographs show that the patient had difficulty standing with this degree of knee flexion contracture. **D,** Photograph shows gradual correction with a circular external fixator. **E,** Photograph shows full correction has been obtained.

for optimal use. It was long believed that the best position of the upper limbs should be one limb in full extension and one in flexion; however, because the absence of a strong unilateral grasp renders the use of bimanual function necessary, preservation of the bimanual use pattern of the upper limbs has been recently recommended. Ideally, the limbs should be positioned at tabletop level to facilitate self-care, self-feeding, and computer use.

Shoulder adduction and external rotation contractures can be corrected with a derotation osteotomy of the proximal humerus. Before proceeding with correction of a fixed elbow extension contracture, a good passive range of motion of the elbow should be first obtained by a posterior elbow release and tricepsplasty.

With regard to the wrist, the typical deformity in patients with arthrogryposis multiplex congenita is flexion and ulnar deviation. Proximal row carpectomy, shortening dorsal radial wedge resection osteotomy, and wrist arthrodesis at skeletal maturity have been recommended for the correction of this deformity. One report described resection of a biplanar wedge of midcarpus to treat this deformity.

The thumb-in-palm deformity is very disabling and can be addressed using a comprehensive thenar release. The fingers may be very rigid in patients with arthrogryposis multiplex congenita; therefore, most studies recommend using continuous passive stretching, casts, and orthotic devices to treat this patient population. Surgical release may result in additional stiffness. High-quality

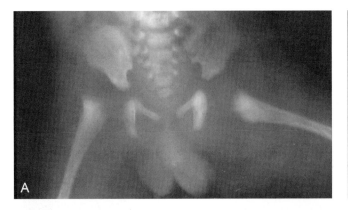

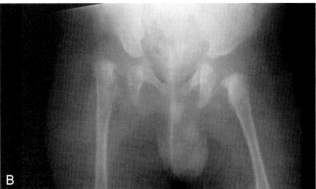

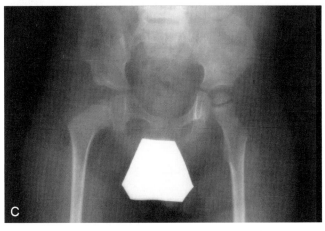

Figure 5 A, Radiograph shows a unilateral hip dislocation in a neonate with arthrogryposis. The contralateral hip shows an abduction contracture. **B,** Radiograph shows failed closed reduction of the right hip and the abduction contracture of the contralateral hip has been successfully treated with physiotherapy. **C,** Postoperative radiograph obtained after open reduction.

outcome studies are not available to assess the effectiveness of these procedures in this heterogeneous group of patients.

Scoliosis
The incidence of scoliosis in patients with arthrogryposis multiplex congenita ranges from 2.5% to 69.6%. No single spinal curve is typical in these patients, but congenital, paralytic, and idiopathic types of scoliosis have been reported. Treatment recommendations tend to follow those for the spinal curve type as outlined in chapter 28.

Larsen's Syndrome
Larsen's syndrome is a genetic disorder that is classified within group 2 disorders. It is inherited either as autosomal dominant or recessive form. Although the symptoms of Larsen's syndrome may be confused with those of arthrogryposis at birth, patients with Larsen's syndrome are easily differentiated by facial appearance (flattening of the face, prominent forehead, depressed nasal bridge, and widely spaced eyes). Patients with Larsen's syndrome also typically have ligamentous hyperlaxity, multiple joint dislocations (hips, knees, shoulder, and elbows), hand deformities with long cylindrical fingers, feet deformities in the form of equinovarus and equinovalgus, and a high incidence of spine anomalies

(specifically cervical kyphosis) caused by hypoplasia of vertebral bodies. Congenital cardiac and respiratory anomalies may also be present in this patient population, but intelligence is normal. Nonsurgical management of congenital knee dislocation is usually unsuccessful. Surgical intervention (including lengthening the quadriceps) is typically required. The treatment of bilateral hip dislocations is controversial. Equinovarus deformities are treated with posteromedial release. Because of the potential morbidity of cervical kyphosis, early posterior cervical fusion is recommended.

Popliteal Pterygium Syndrome
Popliteal pterygium syndrome is a rare disorder that affects 1 in every 300,000 live births. It is inherited as autosomal dominant with a wide pattern of expression. It is part of a group of disorders encompassing multiple pterygia. The key features include genitourinary, craniofacial, and extremity malformations in association with popliteal webs that vary greatly in severity. The edge of the pterygium consists of a dense fibrotic band that extends from the ischium to the os calcis. The foot of a patient with popliteal pterygium syndrome is typically held in fixed equinus and the knee in flexion. The sciatic nerve is usually shortened and lies deep to the dense fibrotic band, posterior to its normal position. The fixed knee and ankle deformities associated with popliteal

Table 1	Superti-Furga Classification of Osteochondrodysplasias	
Type	**Characteristics**	
G2.1	Defects in extracellular structural proteins	
G2.2	Defects in metabolic pathway	
G2.3	Defects in folding and degradation of macromolecules	
G2.4	Defects in hormones and signal transduction mechanisms	
G2.5	Defects in nuclear protein and transcription factors	
G2.6	Defects in oncogenes and tumor suppressor genes	
G2.7	Defects in RNA and DNA processing and metabolism	

Table 2	Alman Classification of Osteochondrodysplasias	
Type	**Characteristics**
I	Structural (bone, cartilage, ligaments, and tendon)
II	Tumor and cell regulatory (cell growth)
III	Developmental (organ patterning)
IV	Protein processing (enzymes)
V	Important in nerve and muscle function
VI	Large chromosomal abnormalities

Table 3	Kornak Classification of Osteochondrodysplasias	
Type	**Characteristics**
1	Disorders of skeletal patterning
2	Disorders of early differentiation
3	Disorders of growth
4	Disorders of skeletal homeostasis

pterygium syndrome render ambulation difficult. Conservative treatment in the form of physiotherapy, traction, and casting is usually unsuccessful. Careful preoperative planning using MRI for preoperative assessment is vital to delineate the exact anatomic position of the sciatic nerve. When the popliteal webbing is mild, multiple skin Z-plasties, excision of the dense fibrotic band, hamstring lengthening, posterior capsulotomy, and Achilles tendon lengthening are recommended. When the deformity is severe, femoral shortening and extension osteotomy with soft-tissue release may be an option. Another option has been reported to give good results in patients with severe deformities is gradual correction using a circular fixator, excision of the dense fibrotic band, and multiple Z-plasties of the skin.

Osteochondrodysplasias

The osteochondrodysplasias (derived from the Greek root *plassein* [to form]) is a heterogeneous group of disorders that affect the development of different components of the skeleton (cartilage and bone) in their size, shape, and organization, often resulting in disproportionate short stature. Nonskeletal manifestations may also be present in patients with osteochondrodysplasia. More than 250 different types of osteochondrodysplasia have been described, ranging from the lethal forms occurring at birth to mild forms with bony anomalies that are typically detected later in life. Most types of osteochondrodysplasia are caused by genetic abnormalities, and recent advances in molecular genetics have elucidated the underlying genetic defects associated with many of these disorders. Individual dysplasias are rare, with the overall incidence being 2 to 5 per 10,000 live births. Although the prenatal diagnosis of osteochondrodysplasia using ultrasound has been reported to be correct in approximately one third of patients, the ability to predict prognosis and lethality with ultrasound has been

shown to be accurate in 90% of patients. Amniocentesis and chorionic villi sampling may identify the genetic defect in some patients.

Classification

The classification of this large, clinically diverse group of disorders constitutes a major challenge. The first classification, the Paris Nomenclature of Constitutional Disorders of Bone, was completed in 1972 and largely based on clinical and radiographic findings. The classification has evolved over the years to include the dysostosis group of skeletal dysplasias as well as the latest data on the underlying molecular genetic defects of various dysplasias. Most recently, other classifications have been reported that specifically address the molecular aspects, embryology, and pathogenesis of these disorders, including the Superti-Furga (Table 1), Alman (Table 2), and Kornak (Table 3) classifications.

Workup

Clinical, radiographic, morphologic, and laboratory assessments are required in the evaluation of children with skeletal dysplasia. Obtaining a careful history is essential, specifically one that includes family history and age of onset of growth retardation (because some dysplasias are not recognized at birth). Physical examination should include anthropometric measurements, including height, weight, head circumference, arm span, upper/lower segment ratio, and growth curves. If the child has a disproportionately short stature, it should be determined whether this is a short-limb or a short-trunk dwarfism; additionally, it should also be determined which segment of the limb is affected: rhizomelic (proximal), mesomelic (middle), or acromelic (distal). General examination is important to detect other nonskeletal anomalies, specifically facial dysmorphism.

Radiographic evaluation includes AP and lateral views of the skull, spine, chest (to assess the ribs), AP of the pelvis, AP of all tubular bones (which can be limited to one side if no asymmetry is suspected), radiographic assessment of bone age (left hand), and lateral radiograph of the knee (to assess the patella). Radiographic assessment is important to determine not only which bones are affected, but also which parts of the bone are involved in the disease process: the epiphysis, growth plate, metaphysis, or diaphysis. Morphologic examination (bone biopsy) may be indicated if other surgical procedures are performed. Laboratory tests include biochemical studies (for example, in patients with mucopolysaccharidosis) and molecular genetic testing. Superimposed inflammatory conditions in skeletal dysplasias are not rare and can be managed by medical treatment.

Achondroplasia

Achondroplasia is the most common skeletal dysplasia and is caused by a mutation of the fibroblast growth factor receptor 3 (*FGFR3*) gene. It is autosomal dominant (although 90% of instances are the result of new mutations), and it affects primarily enchondral bone formation (intramembranous bone formation is normal in this patient population). As a result, the trunk length is normal, and the limbs are short (rhizomelic shortening). The face has typical features (frontal bossing, midface hypoplasia), and short and broad trident hands are also characteristic of patients with achondroplasia. The spine and lower extremities are most commonly affected. Neurologic complications such as apnea, hypotonia, and hydrocephalus may be caused by stenosis of the foramen magnum and result in a risk of sudden death during the first 2 years of life. CT and MRI can help assess the foramen magnum and ventricular size, particularly when direct signs (head perimeter enlargement) or indirect signs (general fatigue or irritability) of hydrocephalus are present. Thoracolumbar kyphosis is common in patients with achondroplasia and usually resolves with independent ambulation. Thoracolumbar kyphosis may require bracing if it persists beyond the age of 3 years. If the kyphosis (particularly that caused by a wedge-shaped vertebra) progresses despite bracing, then anterior and posterior arthrodesis is recommended (Figure 6). Careful attention is required when instrumenting the spine because spinal stenosis often occurs in this patient population. Thoracolumbar sacral decompression may be indicated later in life in symptomatic patients. Lumbar hyperlordosis is common in patients with achondroplasia; lumbar lordosis (particularly the sacral tilt) may be improved by femoral lengthening.

Genu varum and internal tibial torsion commonly occur in patients with achondroplasia, usually as a result of a tibial bow with a relatively longer fibula. Bracing is of little value in the management of this condition, and surgical correction is indicated in symptomatic patients (Figure 7). Any associated collateral ligament hyperlaxity should be taken into consideration during surgical procedures because it may lead to intraoperative errors during realignment procedures. Because the varus may occur in the distal femur, proximal or distal tibia, and through the knee joint, osteotomies may need to be done at multiple levels. The value of using epiphysiodesis or shortening of the fibula to prevent these deformities has yet to be demonstrated.

The treatment of the short stature remains a challenge. Exogenous growth hormone has little impact on final height. Bone lengthening in children with achondroplasia is controversial and not recommended by most centers in North America, despite the fact that many patients are satisfied with the results of these lengthening procedures. The height achieved using lengthening procedures remains below that of an average adult, and dysmorphic features are still present. Numerous complications may also be encountered during these extensive and lengthy procedures. Preoperative psychological assessment is recommended for patients with achondroplasia before undergoing bone lengthening. If the lower limbs are lengthened, then lengthening of the humeri is necessary to restore body proportions and improve function.

Hypochondroplasia

Hypochondroplasia is caused by a different mutation of *FGFR3*, resulting in milder clinical symptoms. Facial abnormalities and tibial bowing are less pronounced in children with hypochondroplasia than in children with achondroplasia.

Pseudoachondroplasia

Pseudoachondroplasia is caused by a mutation of the cartilage oligomeric matrix protein gene on chromosome 19. Patients with this type of dwarfism typically present with severe hyperlaxity and epiphyseal involvement. The epiphyseal involvement results in premature osteoarthrosis. The face of a patient with pseudoachondroplasia is normal, and growth retardation is not apparent before 2 years of age (fingers are small and hyperflexible). The shortening is typically rhizomelic, and the lower extremities may exhibit valgus, varus, or windswept deformities. Surgical correction of these deformities is indicated for patients with progressive deformities or those who are symptomatic, but recurrence is common. Platyspondyly is a constant feature in this patient population, but no spinal stenosis occurs in children with pseudoachondroplasia as in children with achondroplasia. Atlantoaxial instability is not uncommon.

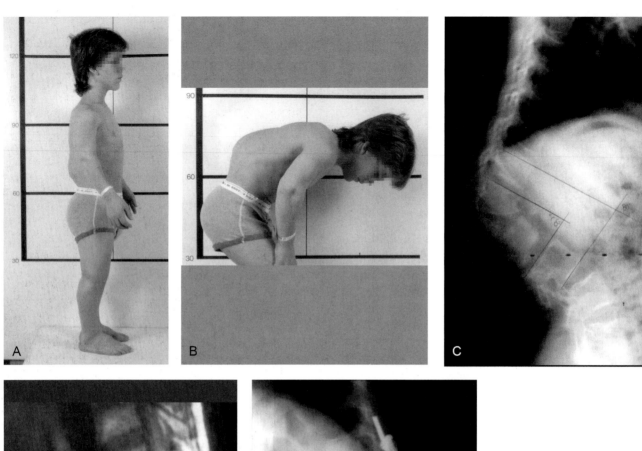

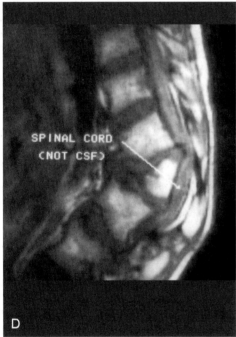

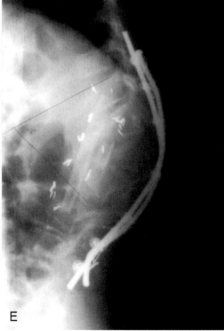

Figure 6 **A** and **B,** Photographs of a 13-year-old patient with achondroplasia show thoracolumbar kyphosis. **C,** Radiograph of the same patient shows the wedge vertebra and severe kyphosis. **D,** MRI scan of the same patient. CSF = cerebrospinal fluid. **E,** Postoperative radiograph shows that the patient underwent a two-stage procedure (anterior fusion with a fibular strut graft and a posterior fusion).

Spondyloepiphyseal Dysplasias

Spondyloepiphyseal dysplasias are characterized by disproportionate short trunk dwarfism and are caused by a mutation in the gene coding for type II collagen. The severity of spondyloepiphyseal dysplasia varies from a lethal form (achondrogenesis type II) to a mild form (spondyloepiphyseal dysplasia tarda) diagnosed late in childhood or in young adults. Kniest dysplasia and Stickler's syndrome are also type II collagenopathies.

Patients with these disorders also have platyspondyly and delayed ossification of the epiphyses. Spondyloepiphyseal dysplasia congenita is challenging to treat orthopaedically because of the presence of upper cervical instability, scoliosis, severe hip involvement, and genu valgum. The cervical instability is often caused by ligamentous laxity and a hypoplastic odontoid and may lead to myelopathy if left untreated. Surgical stabilization (C1-C2 fusion and/or decompression) is indicated in such patients (Figure 8).

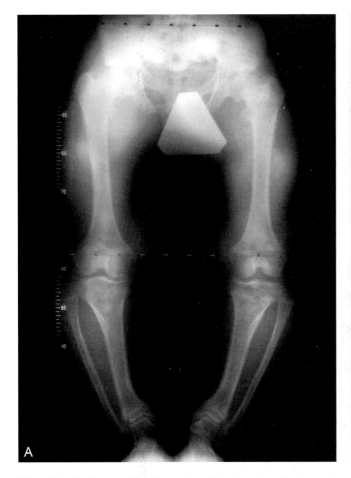
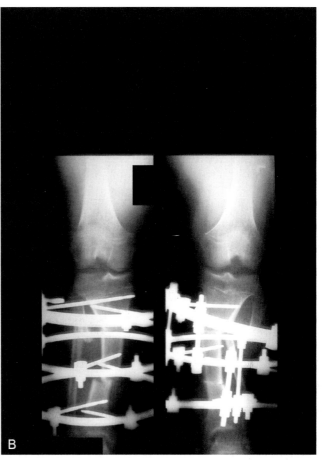

Figure 7 **A,** AP radiograph of the pelvis and lower limbs of a patient with achondroplasia shows severe deformities of the tibia and fibula, including proximal and distal varus of the tibia and overgrowth of the fibula. **B,** Postoperative radiograph shows that correction was achieved using an Ilizarov frame and a double tibial osteotomy.

Hip involvement includes marked coxa vara, hip flexion contracture, and delayed ossification of proximal femoral epiphyses. These deformities may require surgical treatment (femoral and/or pelvic osteotomies). Nevertheless, no long-term study data support the value of these treatments in preventing or reducing the rate of degenerative joint disease. Patients may require total hip arthroplasties as early as the second decade of life. Technical difficulties are to be expected when performing total hip arthroplasty, particularly with the large size of the implants required. Extraskeletal manifestations include ophthalmologic involvement, which requires regular ophthalmologic evaluations.

Multiple Epiphyseal Dysplasias

Multiple epiphyseal dysplasias are characterized by mild dwarfism (near normal vertebrae). Patients with multiple epiphyseal dysplasia typically present with early osteoarthrosis resulting from abnormal endochondral ossification of the epiphyses. The defect is caused by a mutation in the gene coding for the cartilage oligomeric matrix protein (the same gene as for pseudoachondroplasia, but a different mutation occurs, causing a differ-

ent phenotype) or a mutation in a gene coding for collagen type IX. The weight-bearing joints (particularly the hip) are the most severely affected joints. The irregular aspect of the proximal femoral epiphyses is similar to that observed in patients with Legg-Calvé-Perthes disease. However, in patients with multiple epiphyseal dysplasia, the radiographic changes affect both hips in a symmetric fashion; furthermore, other epiphyses are involved. Osteonecrosis and osteochondritis dissecans of the proximal femoral epiphysis can complicate the evolution of this disease. Surgical procedures aiming at containment of the femoral head have not yet proved to be effective in reducing the incidence of osteoarthrosis in this patient population. Ultimately, most patients affected with this autosomal dominant condition will need total hip arthroplasties. Lower extremity angular deformities can occur in children with multiple epiphyseal dysplasia and may require realignment procedures (stapling and/or osteotomies).

Metaphyseal Chondrodysplasias

Metaphyseal chondrodysplasias comprise a group of disorders characterized by abnormal development of the

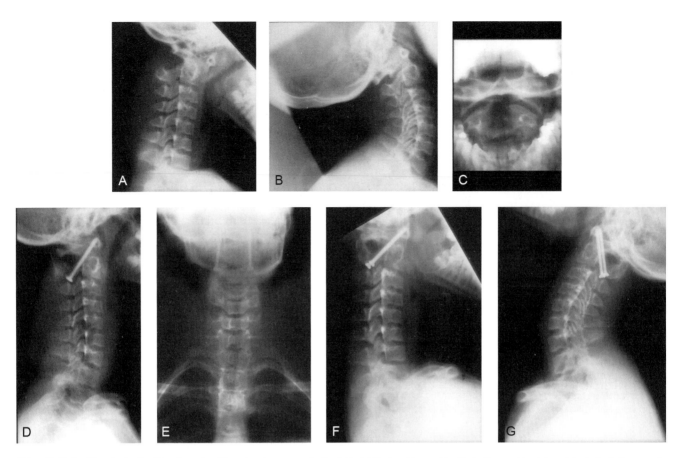

Figure 8 Flexion **(A)** and extension **(B)** radiographs of the spine show severe atlantoaxial instability in a 14-year-old patient with spondyloepiphyseal dysplasia. **C,** Open mouth radiograph shows absence of the odontoid process. **D,** Postoperative lateral radiograph shows C1-C2 fusion was performed. **E,** Postoperative AP radiograph shows the position of the two screws. Postoperative lateral flexion **(F)** and extension **(G)** radiographs show no instability.

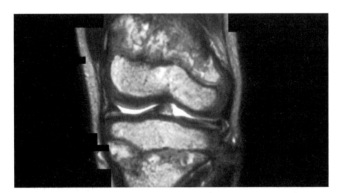

Figure 9 MRI scan of the knee in a patient with Shwachman-Diamond syndrome shows severe metaphyseal involvement.

metaphysis of the tubular bones that lead to deformities of the lower extremities while the epiphyses remain normal (Figure 9). Several types of metaphyseal chondrodysplasias have been described, the most common being the Schmidt type and the McKusick type (cartilage-hair hypoplasias). The Schmidt type is caused by a mutation affecting the collagen X gene. Although the gene defect in the McKusick type has been identified, the exact pathogenesis of this syndrome is still not known. Pa-

tients with each type of metaphyseal chondrodysplasia present with bow legs and a mildly short stature. The hips are affected in patients with the Schmidt type (coxa vara), but not in those with the McKusick type. The McKusick type is associated with blond or light hair and systemic problems (immunologic and malabsorption). The McKusick type has been reported to occur frequently in the Amish population. Both types must be differentiated from rickets. Lower-limb deformities may be corrected with femoral and/or tibial osteotomies; stapling can also be considered. Rare types of metaphyseal chondrodysplasias may be associated with hypercalcemia (for example, the Jansen type, which is caused by a mutation of the parathyroid hormone-related protein receptor gene or Shwachman-Diamond syndrome, which results in pancreatic exocrine insufficiency).

Diastrophic Dysplasia

Diastrophic dysplasia is a severe short stature syndrome caused by a mutation in the *DTDST* gene that affects a sulfate transporter, resulting in undersulfation of proteoglycans in cartilage matrix and subsequent loss of its hydraulic properties. The incidence of diastrophic dysplasia is high in Finland. Affected individuals have dis-

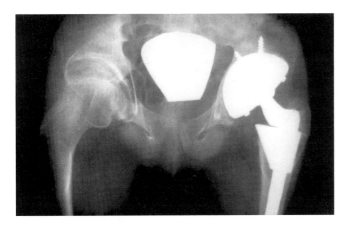

Figure 10 AP radiograph of the pelvis and hips of a child with diastrophic dwarfism shows total hip replacement has been performed.

tinctive hand (hitchhiker thumb) and ear (cauliflower ear) anomalies. The orthopaedic manifestations of this rare syndrome are often multiple and severe, specifically in the spine, hips, and feet. Spine deformities commonly occur before the age of 5 years and include cervical kyphosis and thoracolumbar scoliosis. Cervical kyphosis may lead to neurologic symptoms. In patients with progressive kyphosis that does not resolve during childhood, surgical stabilization may be required.

Bilateral clubfoot deformity is common in this patient population and often difficult to correct, even with extensive surgical procedures (including talectomy). Joint contractures are common (90% of patients), progressive, and resistant to soft-tissue or bone surgery. The hip joints are specifically affected in patients with diastrophic dysplasia (Figure 10). The short-term benefits of correcting flexion contractures in these patients must be weighed against the long-term wheelchair requirements for many affected with this disorder. Open reduction of bilateral hip dislocation remains controversial, and its long-term effect in decreasing the incidence of degenerative arthritis in this patient population has yet to be demonstrated. Although total hip arthroplasties may be technically easier to perform on a reduced hip, from a prognostic standpoint, the primary pathology exists in the cartilage; as a result, early degenerative arthritis of weight-bearing joints (knees and hips) is expected in patients with diastrophic dysplasia regardless of surgical treatment. There is a high incidence of mortality in early childhood in patients with diastrophic dysplasia (as a result of tracheomalacia), but thereafter life expectancy is usually normal.

Multiple Hereditary Exostosis

Multiple hereditary exostosis is caused by a mutation in one of the three *EXT* genes that code for development of chondrocytes in the growth plate (through the Indian hedgehog pathway). It is also called multiple osteocarti-

laginous exostoses or osteochondromatosis. Multiple hereditary exostosis results from chondrocytes growing in the wrong direction. Although the exostoses may affect any part of the endochondral skeleton, the long bones are predominantly involved. The number and size of exostoses vary among patients, and they may cause several orthopaedic problems during or after growth. Only symptomatic lesions need to be resected. Indications for excision include lesions that mechanically interfere with joint mobility or with tendon movements, suspicion of malignant transformation (development of pain or rapidly growing tumors), pressure on nerves or vessels, and extremely large lesions. The anatomic localization of these lesions is important because some complications are specific to the site affected. For example, a proximal fibular exostosis may compress the common popliteal nerve, and an exostosis growing between two bones may lead to progressive dislocation (of the radial head) or diastasis (of the ankle joint), which could be prevented by early recognition and treatment.

Growth is often affected in patients with multiple hereditary exostosis, resulting in angular deformities or limb-length discrepancies. Asymmetric growth in the forearm results in ulnar shortening, with progressive radial bow affecting pronation-supination and radial head dislocation. After growth, osteochondromas stop enlarging, and any symptoms such as onset of pain and increase in size should raise the suspicion of malignant transformation, in which instance the osteochondroma should be removed. It has been reported that the development of chondrosarcoma occurs in less than 1% of lesions. A recent study showed that patients with *EXT 1* mutations seem to have a higher frequency of malignant transformation. Surgical excision of osteochondromas must follow the principles of en bloc resection, including resection of the cartilaginous cap to avoid recurrence. Special care must be taken to avoid damaging the nearby growth plate.

Angular deformities and limb-length discrepancies may occur and require osteotomies and/or epiphysiodesis. The treatment of forearm deformities includes observation in patients with good function and lengthening of the ulna in symptomatic patients (with osteotomy of the radius if necessary). The dislocated radial head can be treated by excision once skeletal maturity is achieved. Epiphysiodesis of the medial malleolus has been recently proposed to correct the ankle valgus in symptomatic patients older than 6 years with a valgus deformity greater than 8°.

Enchondromatosis (Ollier's Disease)

Enchondromatosis (Ollier's disease) is caused by a mutation in parathyroid hormone receptors; this causes the differentiation of chondrocytes in the growth plate to be altered, and as a result, portions of the growth plate are

Table 4 | Other Osteochondrodysplasias Requiring Orthopaedic Intervention

Type of Osteochondrodysplasia	Cause	Characteristics	Orthopaedic Issue
Cleidocranial dysplasia or dysostosis	Mutation of the *CBFA1* gene (which regulates osteoblasts differentiation)	Absent or hypoplastic clavicles Lack of development of pubic bones	Coxa vara (osteotomies)
Nail-patella syndrome	Mutation in the *LMX1B* gene (which regulates gene expression in skeletal and renal development)	Absent or hypoplastic patellae Nail dysplasia Radial head dislocations Iliac horns on radiographs Nephropathy	Knee contractures (soft-tissue and bony procedures) Extensor mechanism realignment
Chondroectodermal dysplasia (Ellis-van Creveld syndrome)	Mutation localized on the 4p16 chromosome, but gene product unknown	Polydactyly Nail and dental anomalies Heart disease	Severe genu valgum (hypoplastic lateral tibial plateau) Realignment osteotomies Medial proximal tibial stapling
Trichorhinophalangeal dysplasia	Mutation in the *TRPS1* gene, but gene product unknown	Facial dysmorphism Clinodactyly	Osteonecrosis of femoral epiphyses (Legg-Calvé-Perthes disease)
Dysplasia epiphysealis hemimelia (Trevor's disease or tarsomegaly)	Unknown	Unilateral involvement of knee and foot with progressive intra-articular deformities	Limb-length discrepancies Genu valgum Foot deformities (equinovalgus) Intra-articular surgery necessary
Leri-Weill dyschondrosteosis	Mutation in the gene *SHOX*, product unknown	Short stature Madelung deformities Limited elbow motion	Osteotomy of radius and realignment of wrist may be necessary (recurrence of deformity during growth) Ligament resection has recently been described

left behind and continue to grow on their own. This disorder is characterized by multiple enchondromas in the metaphyseal region (specifically the metacarpals) that are often asymmetric and sometimes unilateral. The cartilaginous lesions can lead to altered growth, bony deformities, and pathologic fractures. As a result of the altered growth, limb-length discrepancies and angular deformities are frequent and more severe in patients with enchondromatosis than in those with osteochondromatosis.

The forearm deformities that occur in patients with enchondromatosis are quite similar to those in patients with osteochondromatosis, with shortening of the ulna. Bone lengthening may be indicated in patients with ulnar shortening, and the resulting new bone that is being formed at the distraction zone is good despite the bony pathology present. If the multiple osteochondromas are associated with hemangiomas, then this condition is called Maffucci's syndrome. Malignant transformation of enchondromas (into low-grade chondrosarcomas) occurs more frequently in patients with Maffucci's syndrome than in those with enchondromatosis.

Mucopolysaccharidoses

Mucopolysaccharidoses comprise a group of disorders caused by a defect in various enzymes that degrade glycosaminoglycan in the lysosomes. The products of in-complete degradation accumulate in different organs. Many types of mucopolysaccharidoses have been described, and most of them are autosomal recessive, except Hunter type (which is X-linked recessive).

Clinical findings present in patients with any type of mucopolysaccharidoses include visceromegaly, corneal clouding, cardiac disease, and deafness. From an orthopaedic perspective, these patients usually have short stature, their epiphyses are affected (particularly the proximal femoral epiphysis), and most important of all, they have spine involvement with cervical instability. Hurler's syndrome (mucopolysaccharidosis 1-H) is the most common and most severe type of mucopolysaccharidosis, with life expectancy usually not exceeding the second decade of life. Bone marrow transplantation performed early (established brain and skeletal damage are not reversible) has been reported to modify the life expectancy of children with Hurler's syndrome; however, this will not stop the progression of the musculoskeletal disease.

Patients with Hunter's syndrome (mucopolysaccharidosis II) have a normal life expectancy, and their orthopaedic management does not differ from those with Morquio's syndrome (mucopolysaccharidosis IV). Mental deterioration in patients with Hunter's syndrome is progressive. Patients with Morquio's syndrome have a normal intellect, cervical instability, and spinal and limb deformities. The presence of a hypoplastic odontoid leads to cervical instability. C1-C2 fusion is often indicated in this patient population before the age of 10 years. In addition to this instability, intraspinal compression may be related to thickening of extradural soft tissues. Regularly performed dynamic MRI is recommended, particularly in patients with nonspecific symptoms such as fatigue and decreased endurance. Although thoracolumbar kyphosis is common in patients with Morquio's syndrome, it can remain stable, and observation is advocated. Anterior and posterior arthrodeses are indicated when progression and/or neurologic compromise is demonstrated. A relative spinal stenosis caused by thick ligaments should be considered during intraspinal instrumentation with hooks. Genu valgum is common in these patients, and surgical correction by osteotomies and/or epiphysiodesis is indicated if it is greater than 25° to 30°. A high recurrence rate during growth is to be expected. The hips are particularly involved in patients with Morquio's syndrome, with involvement of the acetabulum (severe dysplasia) and proximal femoral epiphysis. Acetabular procedures to increase femoral head coverage and correct the acetabular dysplasia (Shelf procedures) seem to provide good short-term results.

The possible treatment of mucopolysaccharidoses with enzyme therapy raises hopes for the future. The treatment, which was initially used to treat patients with Gaucher's disease type I, has now been extended to patients with mucopolysaccharidosis I. No study data, however, are available yet on the long-term results of this medical treatment. Other osteochondrodysplasias requiring orthopaedic intervention are listed in Table 4.

Annotated Bibliography

Arthrogrypotic Syndromes

Asif S, Umer M, Beg R, Umar M: Operative treatment of bilateral hip dislocation in children with arthrogryposis multiplex congenital. *J Orthop Surg (Hong Kong)* 2004;12:4-9.

The authors of this study reported that eight hips in four patients had open reduction with good results. Follow-up averaged 4 years. Mean age at surgery was 23 months. The authors recommended open reduction in patients with bilateral hip dislocation at an early age to obtain good results.

Bernstein RM: Arthrogryposis and amyoplasia. *J Am Acad Orthop Surg* 2002;10:417-424.

The author provides a concise overview of the orthopaedic management of patients with arthrogryposis and amyoplasia.

Goldfarb CA, Burke MS, Strecker WB, Manske PR: The Steindler flexorplasty for the arthrogrypotic elbow. *J Hand Surg [Am]* 2004;29:462-469.

In this study, 17 elbows in 10 patients (average age, 7 years) were treated with Steindler flexorplasty. At an average follow-up of 5 years, the authors reported excellent functional outcome. They recommend use of this procedure to increase active elbow function and increase patient independence.

Parikh SN, Crawford AH, Do TT, Roy D: Popliteal pterygium syndrome: Implications for orthopaedic management. *J Pediatr Orthop B* 2004;13:197-201.

The authors of this study reviewed eight patients who underwent orthopaedic management for popliteal pterygium syndrome. They recommended using soft-tissue procedures for the treatment of patients with mild deformities, whereas femoral extension and shortening osteotomies with soft-tissue release were recommended for those with severe deformities. The authors also emphasized the importance of preoperative MRI to locate the sciatic nerve.

Smith DW, Drennan JC: Arthrogryposis wrist deformities: Results of infantile serial casting. *J Pediatr Orthop* 2002;22:44-47.

In this study, 17 patients were reviewed at an average follow-up of 6 years. The authors recommended early casting of infants with wrist deformities and found that casting is effective in treating patients with distal arthrogryposis, with good response noted after the first casting and no recurrences reported.

Yau PW, Chow W, Li YH, Leong JC: Twenty-year follow-up of hip problems in arthrogryposis multiplex congenital. *J Pediatr Orthop* 2002;22:359-363.

In this study, 38 hip problems (dislocations, subluxations, and contractures) in 19 patients were assessed at an average follow-up of 20 years. The authors found that closed reduction always failed in reducing the hips. Although hips that were reduced using open surgery were stiffer, the long-term results were comparable with other forms of treatment.

Osteochondrodysplasias

Ain MC, Shirley ED: Spinal fusion for kyphosis in achondroplasia. *J Pediatr Orthop* 2004;24:541-545.

In this study, four patients with achondroplasia (age range, 4 to 8 years) with progressive thoracolumbar kyphosis underwent two-stage surgery (anterior spinal fusion and instrumentation and posterior spinal fusion, followed by a second [additional] posterior fusion). The authors reported that all four patients achieved solid fusion, and no neurologic complications were reported.

Alman BA: A classification for genetic disorders of interest to orthopaedists. *Clin Orthop Relat Res* 2002;401: 17-26.

The author proposed a broad classification system of genetic disorders of interest to the orthopaedists in five categories based on the function of the causative gene. A sixth group was noted to represent patients with large chromosomal abnormalities. These categories include muscular and neurologically inherited diseases.

Grabowski GA, Hopkin RJ: Enzyme therapy for lysosomal storage disease: Principles, practice, and prospects. *Annu Rev Genomics Hum Genet* 2003;4:403-436.

The authors of this article reviewed the concept and application of enzyme therapy in the treatment of patients with Gaucher's disease, Fabry's disease, and mucopolysaccharidosis I.

Hall C: International nosology and classification of constitutional disorders of bone (2001). *Am J Med Genet* 2002;113:65-77.

This article is an update of the International Classification of Constitutional Disorders of Bone. In this evolving classification, 33 groups of osteochondrodysplasias and 3 groups of localized dysostoses are now listed.

Helenius I, Remes V, Tallroth K, Peltonen J, Poussa M, Paavilainen T: Total hip arthroplasty in diastrophic dysplasia. *J Bone Joint Surg Am* 2003;85-A:441-447.

The authors reviewed 41 total hip arthroplasties in 24 patients with diastrophic dysplasia at an average follow-up of 7.8 years (minimum follow-up, 5 years). They reported that the rate of complications and revisions for this group of patients was 24% and 12%, respectively. The mean Harris hip score increased from 44 points (range, 25 to 66 points) before surgery to 70 points (range, 37 to 89 points) at the time of final follow-up ($P < 0.001$). The technical difficulties of performing this procedure in the patient population are discussed.

Kornak U, Mundlos S: Genetic disorders of the skeleton: A developmental approach. *Am J Hum Genet* 2003; 73:447-474.

In this article, the authors presented a classification based on a combination of molecular pathology and embryology. Their classification system emphasizes how the gene defect affects the development (patterning, differentiation, and growth) or the homeostasis of the skeleton.

Muenzer J, Fisher A: Advances in the treatment of mucopolysaccharidosis type I. *N Engl J Med* 2004;350:1932-1934.

The authors of this article summarized the knowledge in the treatment of mucopolysaccharidosis I. Bone marrow transplantation, which has been used since 1981, is the treatment of choice for treating patients with Hurler's syndrome who are younger than 2 years and have minimal or no neurologic impairment. Bone marrow transplantation was reported to have no effect on skeletal manifestations of the disease.

Parilla BV, Leeth EA, Kambich MP, Chilis P, MacGregor SN: Antenatal detection of skeletal dysplasias. *J Ultrasound Med* 2003;22:255-258.

Over an 8-year period, 37 instances of skeletal dysplasias were antenatally diagnosed. Follow-up was completed in 31 patients. The authors reported that antenatal diagnosis was correct in 65% of patients, with two false-positive diagnoses. The ability to predict lethality was 100%, with no false-positive diagnosis.

Park H-W, Kim H-S, Hahn S-B, et al: Correction of lumbosacral hyperlordosis in achondroplasia. *Clin Orthop Relat Res* 2003;414:242-249.

In this study, the sacral inclination angle and the sacrohorizontal angle were compared before and after lower extremity lengthening in 10 children with achondroplasia. Femoral lengthening resulted in improvement of the sacral tilt compared with tibial lengthening. The lumbar lordosis angle remained unchanged.

Porter DE, Lonie L, Fraser M, et al: Severity of disease and risk of malignant change in hereditary multiple exostoses: A genotype-phenotype study. *J Bone Joint Surg Br* 2004;86:1041-1046.

The authors conducted a prospective genotype-phenotype study using molecular screening and clinical assessment in 172 patients with hereditary multiple exostoses. They reported that only one sarcoma developed in an *EXT2* mutation carrier compared with seven sarcomas in *EXT1* mutation carriers.

Weisstein JS, Delgado E, Steinbach LS, Hart K, Packman S: Musculoskeletal manifestations of hurler syndrome: Long-term follow-up after bone marrow transplantation. *J Pediatr Orthop* 2004;24:97-101.

The authors reported on the orthopaedic outcomes in seven patients who underwent bone marrow transplant (mean follow-up, 7.6 years). They found that bone marrow transplant does not appear to alter the natural history of the musculoskeletal disorders in patients with Hurler's syndrome.

Classic Bibliography

Abel MF, Blanco JS, Damiano DL, Skinner S, Ballock RT: Neuromuscular conditions, in *Orthopaedic Knowledge Update 7*. Rosemont, IL, American Academy of Orthopaedic Surgeons, 2002, pp 219-234.

Aldegheri R, Dall'Oca C: Limb lengthening in short stature patients. *J Pediatr Orthop B* 2001;10:238-247.

Canepa G, Maroteaux P: *Syndrome Dysmorphiques et Maladies Constitutionnelles du Squelette*. Padoue, Italy, Riccin, 1999.

Choi IH, Yang MS, Chung CY, Cho TJ, Sohn YJ: The treatment of recurrent arthrogrypotic clubfoot in children by the Ilizarov method: A preliminary report. *J Bone Joint Surg Br* 2001;83:731-737.

Goldberg MJ: *The Dysmorphic Child: An Orthopedic Perspective*. New York, NY, Raven Press, 1987.

Staheli LT, Hall JG, Jaffe KM, Paholke DO: *Arthrogryposis: A Text Atlas*. New York, NY, Cambridge University Press, 1998.

Brunner R, Hefti F, Tgetgel JD: Arthrogrypotic joint contracture at the knee and the foot: Correction with a circular frame. *J Pediatr Orthop B* 1997;6:192-197.

DelBello DA, Watts HG: Distal femoral extension osteotomy for knee flexion contracture in patient with arthrogryposis. *J Pediatr Orthop* 1996;16:122-126.

Ezaki M: Treatment of the upper limb in the child with arthrogryposis. *Hand Clin* 2000;16:703-711.

Hall JG: Arthrogryposis multiplex congenita: Etiology, genetics, classification, diagnostic approach, and general aspects. *J Pediatr Orthop B* 1997;6:159-166.

Kopits SE: Orthopedic complications of dwarfism. *Clin Orthop Relat Res* 1976;114:153-179.

Laville JM, Lakermance P, Limouzi F: Larsen's syndrome: Review of the literature and analysis of thirty-eight cases. *J Pediatr Orthop* 1994;14:63-73.

Legaspi J, Li YH, Chow W, Leong JC: Talectomy in patients with recurrent deformity in clubfoot: A long-term follow-up study. *J Bone Joint Surg Br* 2001;83:384-387.

Niki H, Staheli LT, Mosca VS: Management of clubfoot deformity in amyoplasia. *J Pediatr Orthop* 1997;17:803-807.

Oppenheim WL, Larson KR, McNabb MBB, Smith CF, Setoguchi Y: Popliteal pterygium syndrome: An orthopaedic perspective. *J Pediatr Orthop* 1990;10:58-64.

Stevens PM, Belle RM: screw epiphysiodesis for ankle valgus. *J Pediatr Orthop* 1997;17:9-12.

Superti-Furga A, Bonafé L, Rimoin DL: Molecular-pathogenetic classification of genetic disorders of the skeleton. *Am J Med Genet* 2001;106:282-293.

Szoke G, Staheli LT, Jaffe K, Hall JG: Medial-approach open reduction of hip dislocation in amyoplasia-type arthrogryposis. *J Pediatr Orthop* 1996;16:127-130.

Yingsakmongkol W, Kumar SJ: Scoliosis in arthrogryposis multiplex congenital: Results after nonsurgical and surgical treatment. *J Pediatr Orthop* 2000;20:656-661.

Chapter 12

Osteogenesis Imperfecta and Metabolic Bone Disease

Arabella I. Leet, MD

Introduction

Normal longitudinal growth occurs at the growth plate, or physis, where a single layer of germinal cells at the base of the growth plate generate columns of cartilaginous cells organized into zones. Cells are maturing at the growth plate, and at the end of maturation produce mineralized matrix. Hormones, both systemic and local, regulate the degree of maturation of these cells: growth hormones and androgens increase growth, whereas estrogens and thyroid hormone act to diminish growth and close the physis at the end of puberty (Table 1).

As growth occurs, the skeleton is in a continuous balance of formation and resorption of bone. For example, as growth occurs in the diaphysis, there must be apposition of bone at the outer cortex while there is resorption of bone at the inner cortex. In addition, the metaphysis continuously becomes the new diaphysis; therefore, the outer edges of the distal metaphysis form a region of high resorption that is balanced by the bone formation at the physis at the opposite end of the metaphysis. In patients with osteopetrosis, the osteoclasts are not able to resorb bone; thus, the metaphysis remains wide, forming the classic "flask" characteristic of the disorder. Osteoblast and osteoclast activity are governed by systemic hormones (parathyroid hormone and calcitonin) as well as local hormones (interleukin-1, transforming growth factor β, and tumor necrosis factor). In children, constitutional delay in growth is produced by systemic hormones such as growth hormone, thyroxine, or sex hormones, which cause a proportionate growth failure equally affecting growth throughout the skeleton. Disproportionate growth failure (as can be seen in patients with Marfan syndrome or rickets) occurs with interference of bone metabolism, resulting in changes in the levels of phosphate, calcium, or calcitriol. This chapter explores some of the major metabolic disorders of the skeleton that affect children.

Rickets and Osteomalacia

Rickets and osteomalacia are caused by decreased levels of calcium or phosphate, leading to abnormal mineralization of the skeleton. Rickets occurs in growing children, and both the cartilage of the physes and the bones are involved. Osteomalacia, by definition, occurs in skeletally mature individuals, and the effect of abnormal mineralization is seen only in bone.

During calcium and phosphate homeostasis neither element is freely soluble in the body, and at critical solubility, precipitation of salts occurs. To avoid ectopic ossification, serum and urine levels of calcium and phosphate are carefully regulated in the body. Calcium transport into the cell is increased by parathyroid hormone and 1,25 dihydroxyvitamin D_3 and decreased by elevations in the serum phosphate concentration. In the past, phosphate regulation was thought to be largely under the control of parathyroid hormone, resulting in the renal tubule system either excreting or resorbing phosphate. In this traditional model of calcium and phosphate homeostasis, bone was always acted upon by other agents; however, the identification of a new hormone, fibroblast growth factor-23 (FGF-23), has changed this classic paradigm of phosphate regulation.

FGF-23 has been recently identified as the protein that is mutated (and in this altered form resistant to degradation) in autosomal dominant hypophosphatemic rickets, and overproduced in mesenchymal soft-tissue tumors that result in oncogenic osteomalacia, otherwise known as tumor-induced osteomalacia. Patients with these tumors have low serum phosphate levels, phosphaturia, low levels of 1,25 dihydroxyvitamin D_3, and osteomalacia severe enough to cause fractures. Removal of the tumor results in the normalization of the skeleton. FGF-23 appears to be produced, under physiologic conditions, in human osteoblast-like cells. Transgenic mice that overexpress FGF-23 have demonstrated hypophosphatemia, increased urinary phosphate levels, and decreased levels of serum 1,25 dihydroxyvitamin D_3.

Commercial assays are now available to measure levels of serum FGF-23 in humans. High levels of serum FGF-23 have also been demonstrated in more than half of all patients with X-linked hypophosphatemic rickets and all patients with fibrous dysplasia of bone who have renal phosphate wasting and hypophosphatemia.

Table 1 | Summary of Bone-Hormone Interactions

Disease	Gene Location	Defect	Diagnostic Modalities or Laboratory Test Results	Radiographs	Phenotype
X-linked rickets	*PHEX*	Decreased FGF-23	Decreased phosphate Increased alkaline phosphatase	Widening and cupping of the physes	Small stature Bowing
Renal osteo-dystrophy	Varied	Increased PTH Dysfunction of eCaSR	Increased or normal PTH Decreased 1,25 vitamin D Increased phosphate (end stage)	Widening physes, SCFE Bowing Calcification of vessels in soft tissues	Short stature + bowing deformity
Osteogenesis imperfecta	Multiple mutations in *COL1A1* *COL1A2*	Abnormal pro-collagen Abnormal differentiation of stromal cells	Fibroblast analysis for defective collagen from a skin biopsy	Wormian bones Multiple fractures	Short stature Deformity Blue sclera Dentogenesis imperfecta Hyperlaxity of joints
Fibrous dysplasia	*GNAS1* causing activating mutation of the GS-α1 protein	Bone marrow stromal cells cannot differentiate to form osteoblasts and remain in a fibrous state of arrested development	Rule out endocrinopathies: precocious puberty phosphate wasting (arrive) IGF-1 Increased TSH Increased control Increased FGF-23	"Ground glass" appearance Lytic or sclerotic lesions of bone	Variable depending on disease burden Deformity Scoliosis Short stature
Osteopetrosis	*CLCN7* *TC1RG1*	Chloride channel defect or H+ adenosinetriphos-phatase proton pump defect	Decreased Ca +2 Secondary increased PTH Increased BB-CK	Dense bone Loss of marrow cavity "Rugger jersey" spine	Short stature Anemia Recurrent fractures Frontal bossing Splenomegaly
Marfan syndrome	*FBN1* or TGF-βR2	Fibrillin mutation or TGF-βR2	None	Scoliosis Spondylolysis Spondylolisthesis Protrusio acetabuli	Ligamentous laxity Arachnodactyly Pectus excavatum Scoliosis Disproportionate skeleton Superior lens dislocation

TGF-βR2 = transforming growth factor beta receptor 2, eCaSR = extracellular calcium receptor, BB-CK = brain isoenzyme of creatine kinase, SCFE = slipped capital femoral epiphysis, TSH = thyroid-stimulating hormone

FGF-23 may interact with a phosphate-regulating gene with homologies to endopeptidases on the X chromosome (*PHEX*), mutations of which are responsible for X-linked hypophosphatemic rickets. The relationship between *PHEX* and FGF-23 has yet to be elucidated, and it is unclear whether, and if so how, FGF-23 and *PHEX* interact.

The recent discovery of FGF-23 as a hormone produced by bone and as a major regulator of phosphate metabolism makes bone now an active participant as an endocrine organ in the regulation of phosphorus and vitamin D. Continued studies of the role that FGF-23 plays in rickets resulting from genetic disorders are ongoing.

Clinical Picture

Rickets and osteomalacia are diagnosed microscopically with evidence of widening of the osteoid seam, the layer of unmineralized bone that forms around mineralized bone in the outer cortex and inner trabeculae. In the growing child with rickets, the defective mineralization affects the physis with loss of columnization in the maturation zone and a gain in height of this zone compared with normal mineralization; the zones of provisional calcification and primary spongiosa demonstrate lack of mineralization. Macroscopically, a child with rickets may have radiographic evidence of widening of the metaphyses and the appearance of flaring or cupping at the physis.

Other effects of rickets on children include growth retardation, lethargy, bowing of the limbs, and prominence of the osteochondral junction of the ribs (the pathognomonic rachitic rosary). Children may present to the emergency department with seizures, tetany, or fractures; a recent increase in breastfeeding has been associated with an increase in the prevalence of vitamin D–deficient rickets.

Treatment

Any patient with clinical rickets requires an endocrinologic workup to assess etiology. Medical treatment with calcium, active vitamin D, calcitonin, or phosphorus can be used to replace specific deficiencies. Medical treatment can result in more normal-appearing radiographs in as little as 2 to 3 weeks and can significantly improve bowing deformities in the limbs. Bowing deformities that do not resolve with medical management can be treated with surgical realignment techniques (hemiepiphysiodesis and osteotomy).

Renal Osteodystrophy

Renal osteodystrophy occurs in the presence of end-stage kidney disease. Renal disease that causes phosphate wasting secondary to tubulopathies with acidosis occurs most commonly in children. Aluminum toxicity can also cause renal osteodystrophy by directly inhibiting parathyroid hormone (PTH). Renal osteodystrophy can occur as both a high and low bone turnover state. High bone turnover is associated with increased PTH levels, whereas more normal PTH levels accompany low bone turnover (adynamic osteodystrophy).

Pathophysiology

Children with end-stage renal disease have decreased synthesis of calcitriol (1,25 dihydroxyvitamin D) in the kidneys; thus, serum levels of calcitriol are also diminished, causing a decrease in the absorption of calcium across the gastrointestinal tract. With decreased calcitriol levels comes an accompanying decrease in the vitamin D receptor in the parathyroid gland, causing secondary hyperparathyroidism. The fact that PTH levels are elevated but calcium levels stay the same indicates that there is an accompanying dysfunction of the extracellular calcium receptor in the parathyroid gland. With continued renal disease, there is phosphate retention, which also contributes to increased levels of PTH and a high bone turnover state. The parathyroid gland may begin to hypertrophy in response to loss of the local negative feedback inhibition that normally accompanies PTH production, and this etiology of increased PTH is known as tertiary hyperparathyroidism.

Children with renal osteodystrophy also have other endocrinopathies, including abnormal gonadotropin production, causing delay of menarche and a reduction in the length of puberty. The growth hormone–insulin-like growth factor 1 (IGF-1) axis is disturbed, resulting in anomalies in the production and cyclical release of growth hormone and inability for growth hormone and IGF-1 to act on the target organs, including the growth plate, with resultant decrease in overall stature.

Clinical Picture

Renal osteodystrophy is associated with many skeletal manifestations, including slipped capital femoral epiphysis, bowing of the extremities (similar in appearance to rickets), osteonecrosis, spontaneous tendon ruptures, and fractures. The etiology of skeletal disease is thought to be not only related to growth plate disturbances, but also resulting from the direct effect of calcium, phosphorus, PTH, and vitamin D–modulating osteoblastic activity and consequently bone formation. In addition, patients with renal osteodystrophy have failure of linear growth accompanied by delay in skeletal maturation and epiphyseal closure. Increased stature is not seen with kidney transplantation, but it can be improved with administration of growth hormone. Children can develop myopathies that can be progressive and cause gait disturbance. In addition, calcifications in the blood vessels can be noted in plain radiographs that include the soft tissues.

Clinical Treatment

Treatment of renal osteodystrophy includes assessment of hyperparathyroidism and 25 hydroxy vitamin D and administration of active vitamin D metabolites accompanied with dietary control of phosphate or calcium-free phosphate binding agents. Clinical trials are underway using calcimimetics, drugs that activate the extracellular calcium sensing receptor; however, the effect that these agents will have on bone is unclear.

Orthopaedic management consists of in situ pinning for slipped capital femoral epiphysis and management of other deformities as the patient's overall health allows.

Osteogenesis Imperfecta

The treatment of osteogenesis imperfecta has undergone recent changes in both medical and surgical options. Trials are being conducted to test different drug treatments; a newly designed rod aimed at eliminating some of the complications associated with the use of former telescopic rods is now approved by the US Food and Drug Administration (FDA).

Genetics

Osteogenesis imperfecta can occur from various mutations in the genes *COL1A1* and *COL1A2* that code for type 1 collagen. The phenotype is incredibly broad and has been traditionally classified using the Sillence classification into four main phenotypes, ranging from neonatal demise to a nearly normal individual phenotype with a history of multiple fractures. Type 1 collagen has a complicated three-dimensional structure, with three polypeptide chains winding into a triple helix. The phenotype is determined by which of the chains carries the mutation, by the resulting amino acid substitution, and by the position in the helix that is occupied by the substituted amino acid. Thus, in osteogenesis imperfecta, the number or extent of the genetic mutations does not correlate well with the severity of the disease (phenotype). For example, if a point mutation causes a premature stop codon, the transcription fragments can be removed through a process called nonsense mediated decay. Individuals with these types of mutations will have normal type 1 collagen produced, but at a much lower rate than normal, leading to defective collagen strength and function. By this process many different mutations can result in a similar phenotype.

Pathophysiology

In osteogenesis imperfecta, the mesenchymal stromal cells with mutations have an arrested development and produce abnormal osteoblasts that, in turn, produce an abnormal bone matrix. Thus, the extracellular matrix in patients with osteogenesis imperfecta shows decreased levels of osteonectin, chondroitin sulfate, heparan sulfate, and bone cell proteoglycans, such as biglycan and d*Eco*RIn, when compared with the bone extracellular matrix of age-matched control subjects. Histologic examination of bone from patients with osteogenesis imperfecta demonstrates a decreased number of trabeculae and a decreased cortical thickness. More osteoblasts and osteoclasts than normal are seen microscopically, and mineralization of bone is also deranged so that bone is more dense (but also more brittle) than normal bone.

Clinical Picture

There is a broad spectrum of phenotypes of osteogenesis imperfecta, including patients with fragile bones and short stature, skeletal deformity, blue sclera, dentogenesis imperfecta, and triangular facies. Other clinical signs include hyperlaxity of joints and skin, hearing impairment, and wormian bones in the skull. Although blue sclera is thought to be pathognomonic for osteogenesis imperfecta, many healthy infants can have muddy or dark sclera.

To further confirm the diagnosis of osteogenesis imperfecta, a skin biopsy can be performed to obtain cultures of fibroblasts from which the structure and amount of collagen can be analyzed. Genomic DNA can be obtained from blood, and the *COL1A1* and *COL1A2* regions can be screened for evidence of a genetic mutation, although this type of testing is often performed under certain research protocols and may not be available clinically. Diagnostic testing is accurate in approximately 90% of patients; however, negative test results do not allow exclusion of the diagnosis of osteogenesis imperfecta, which remains a clinical diagnosis with new phenotypes being continually discovered and described.

The differential diagnosis of osteogenesis imperfecta includes child abuse and osteomalacia. Child abuse must be assessed by the history and whether the events around the injury predict the injury. Abnormal serum calcium and vitamin D levels are found in patients with osteomalacia, but not in those with osteogenesis imperfecta.

Specific orthopaedic concerns in patients with osteogenesis imperfecta are bowing deformities of the upper and lower extremities, coxa vara, pes planovalgus, and other stigmata of ligamentous laxity. In addition, the spine typically shows kyphosis and scoliosis in many patients who have structural deformity of the vertebral bodies. The presence of biconcave vertebral bodies is predictive of scoliosis when six or more are present before puberty.

Fractures of the olecranon are rare in normal children, but are relatively common in children with osteogenesis imperfecta. Often these fractures require surgical intervention and can occur bilaterally. A child presenting with an avulsion of the olecranon apophysis should be evaluated for osteogenesis imperfecta.

Treatment

The treatment of osteogenesis imperfecta includes surgical and nonsurgical management; treatment protocols vary, and some controversies in medical management have yet to be resolved. The aggressiveness of the treatment plan correlates with the severity of the phenotype.

Medical management includes off-label use of oral or intravenous bisphosphonates and growth hormone. Clinical trials are ongoing to determine the dosage and frequency of drug administration as well as the efficacy. Bisphosphonates given intravenously to children with the more severe forms of type 3 and 4 osteogenesis imperfecta have resulted in a decrease in the number of fractures and an improvement in height in reports of a small series of treated children (Figure 1). Bisphosphonates inhibit osteoclast function, thus increasing bone mass by favoring bone formation and inhibiting resorption. Although bone density is improved, controversy continues as to whether bisphosphonates can make bone more brittle or in extreme instances cause an osteopetrotic state with loss of the marrow cavity. Because a dosing regimen for children has not been established, differences in the amount of total bisphosphonate given and interactions between the drug and many phenotypes both may be responsible for differences in treatment results.

Another area of concern about bisphosphonates is the timing of the drug administration around fractures or osteotomy, when osteoclast inhibition might affect healing. A study that compared healing in patients with osteogenesis imperfecta after bisphosphonates showed delayed healing after osteotomy but not after fractures.

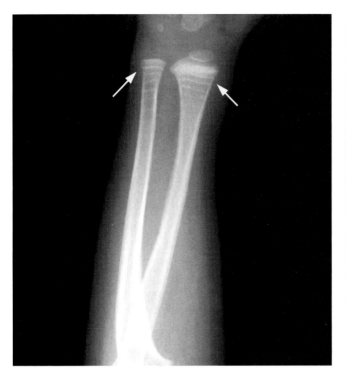

Figure 1 Radiograph of the forearm of a child who has received pamidronate for treatment of osteogenesis imperfecta. The arrows point to the areas of increased bone density resulting from drug treatment. As with rings on a tree, the pamidronate lines can be counted to determine the number of doses administered.

Growth hormone appears to help in the treatment of specific phenotypes of osteogenesis imperfecta, and patients treated with growth hormone and responding with an increase in linear growth also have been shown to have a decrease in the number of fractures. Treatment with growth hormone and bisphosphonates may have a synergistic effect, and more studies will help define the role of growth hormone treatment in children with osteogenesis imperfecta.

Orthopaedic management focuses on preventing fractures, assisting with fracture care, and treating associated scoliosis and limb deformity. Lower extremity bracing with lightweight plastic splints may help prevent fractures when children are learning to ambulate. Having splints available to stabilize bones that fracture frequently can help parents avoid repeated emergency department visits; most parents eventually acquire expertise in determining whether their child has sustained a fracture.

Orthopaedic surgical treatment of long bone deformity (primarily bowing) has shifted from the traditional shish-kabob technique (including extensile exposures with multiple osteotomies along the length of the bone) to a more limited approach, with fewer biplanar osteotomies at the specific level(s) of deformity.

Stabilization of the long bones in a growing child has been challenging, and telescopic rods, such as the Bailey-Dubow rod, are more technically difficult to in-

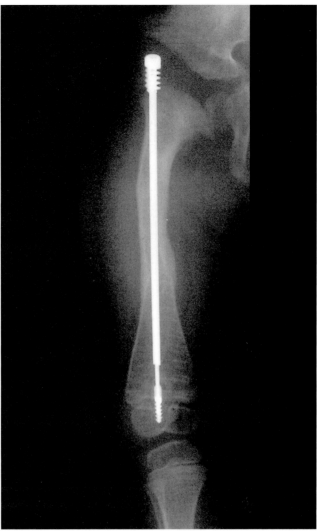

Figure 2 Radiograph of a femur treated with a Fassier-Duval telescoping rod. The rod is made up of two rods; one smaller solid rod fits inside a larger cylinder. The rods lock proximally and distally into the epiphysis.

sert and have increased complication rates compared with static rods, such as Enders and Rush rods. However, static rods do not allow for bone growth and necessitate an increased number of surgical interventions to replace rods with longer versions. The FDA has recently approved a new telescopic intramedullary device, the Fassier-Duval rod, designed specifically for the treatment of osteogenesis imperfecta (Figure 2). The Fassier-Duval rod consists of a proximal cylindrical rod that slides over a distal solid rod, with the ends of both rods held in the epiphysis via a screw system incorporated into the rod. Although initial short-term results from the team that designed this rod are promising, long-term evaluation of the rod at other independent centers and studies comparing the Fassier-Duval rod with other previously popular intramedullary devices, such as the Bailey-Dubow rod, will be necessary to determine the effectiveness of the new rod design.

Treatment of the spine includes assessing patients for basilar invagination. Although radiographic evidence of basilar invagination can be present in up to one fourth of patients, most remain asymptomatic. Patients with severe basilar invagination can present with cranial nerve signs, long tract signs, or respiratory compromise. Treatment for symptomatic patients includes posterior spinal fusion alone or with anterior decompression of C1, the dens, and the clivus.

Progressive scoliosis and kyphosis do not generally respond to brace management. Posterior spinal fusions need to be performed for curve stabilization, although the likelihood of pull-out of the hooks or screws is high in patients with poor bone quality. Thus, fusion to stop curve progression is a more easily attainable surgical goal than curve correction.

Fibrous Dysplasia

Fibrous dysplasia can occur as a single lesion in bone or as multiple lesions, depending on when the genetic mutation occurs during embryologic development. The McCune-Albright syndrome describes the triad that results from the mutation appearing early in embryogenesis, and affects the endoderm, mesoderm, and ectoderm, resulting in bone lesions, endocrinopathy (including precocious puberty), and café-au-lait lesions. The bone lesions in fibrous dysplasia are notorious for dissolving all types of bone graft–allograft or autograft, and skeletal fixation into soft lesions is often tenuous.

Genetics/Pathophysiology

Fibrous dysplasia is caused by an activating mutation of the Gs-α1 protein, which, in bone marrow stromal cells, stops differentiation of these pluripotent cells, preventing them from becoming mature osteoblasts. The proliferating but undifferentiated cells fill the marrow space around spicules of poorly mineralized bone, creating the "Chinese characters" that are the microscopic hallmark of fibrous dysplasia. Because the somatic mutation is lethal, the cells with the mutation are unable to divide. Therefore, clinical improvement can be seen as the ratio of normal to mutated cells increases in the lesions. Radiographically, this change in cell ratio can be observed in lesions; in young children, these lesions have a "ground glass" appearance; in older patients they are more sclerotic appearing.

Clinical Treatment

Fibrous dysplasia often presents with a fracture through a bone lesion. Radiographically, lytic lesions may have a "ground glass" appearance; however, a biopsy is often necessary to confirm the diagnosis. Lesions can occur in any bone, and patients can have varying amounts of disease burden ranging from single lesions (monostotic fibrous dysplasia) to many lesions (polyostotic fibrous dysplasia). Stabilization of lesions can be complex because bone graft is absorbed quickly in the lesions, and metal can cut through the soft bone; thus, screws should be placed in normal bone whenever possible to gain purchase. Intramedullary fixation, if possible, is ideal.

In patients with polyostotic fibrous dysplasia, endocrinopathies should be diagnosed, particularly phosphaturia mediated by FGF-23 produced from the mutated mesenchymal cells in the bone lesions. The presence of untreated endocrinopathies may make fractures occur more frequently and at an earlier age than in patients without endocrinopathies.

The hip is a common location for lesions that can create deformities, such as coxa vara, femoral bowing, or both. The classic shepherd's crook deformity can result in decreased function. Additionally, new bone pain can occur in patients with stress fractures of the femoral neck or a pending fracture through a lesion (Figure 3).

Spinal involvement and scoliosis are common in patients with polyostotic fibrous dysplasia, with the level of the curve corresponding to the presence of a lesion at the same site. The diagnosis of spinal deformity can be difficult to make in patients with severe involvement, including those with deformity of the ribs, pelvis, and lower extremities. The diagnosis of scoliosis should be considered; if scoliosis is present, careful follow-up for signs of progression is warranted. Although the number of reported instances of posterior spinal fusion in patients with polyostotic fibrous dysplasia is small, the results appear to be good at stabilizing the spine and preventing progression.

Medical treatment of patients with fibrous dysplasia with bisphosphonates is controversial, and whether bisphosphonates can reduce bone pain (a common report of patients with fibrous dysplasia) or decrease the fracture rate is not yet known.

Osteopetrosis

With the ability to remove genes or amplify gene products in knockout mice or transgenic mice, many phenotypes of osteopetrosis have been developed in mice. Although this has helped in understanding the function of the osteoclast and the many interactions this cell has with osteoblasts and the bone microenvironment, only three gene defects causing osteopetrosis have been identified in humans so far.

Genetics

In humans, three known mutations, all resulting in failure to acidify and thus resorb bone, can occur. These mutations are in the A3 subunit of the osteoclast-specific H$^+$-adenosine triphosphatase (ATPase) proton pump, in the chloride channel that is coupled to the H$^+$ATPase proton pump, or in carbonic anhydrase II. All three gene defects can occur in the autosomal reces-

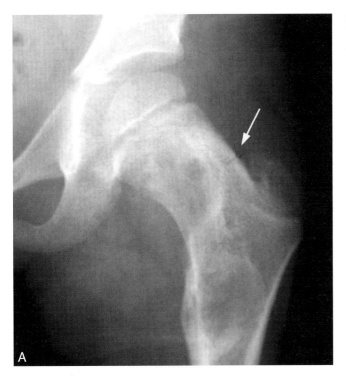
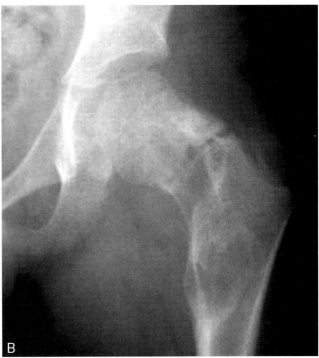

Figure 3 **A,** Radiograph shows a faint tension side femoral stress fracture in the lateral cortex (*arrow*) in this patient with polyostotic fibrous dysplasia and phosphate wasting. **B,** Radiograph of the same patient shows progression to a minimally displaced fracture of the femoral neck, which required surgical intervention.

sive forms of osteopetrosis, whereas only the chloride channel defect (in the *CLCN7* gene) is found in the autosomal dominant form of osteopetrosis. The most common genetic defect (approximately 60% of known instances) occurs in the H$^+$-ATPase proton pump defect (the *TCIRG1* gene).

Pathophysiology

Bone homeostasis occurs when bone formation and bone resorption occur in a balanced state. Bone formation is under the direction of the osteoblast, whereas bone resorption occurs as a function of osteoclast activity. Osteoblasts are derived from mesenchymal stem cells, whereas osteoclasts differentiate from cells of the macrophage-monocyte lines; however, the two cells function in concert via cell signaling. Patients with osteopetrosis currently appear to have identifiable defective osteoclast function. However, many animal models of osteopetrosis exist, often in the form of knockout mouse models in which a gene has been removed. Curiously, only some of the mouse models respond to bone marrow transplantation, creating speculation that some noncellular mechanisms can cause osteopetrosis, with the abnormality arising from the bone microenvironment. Defects in genes controlling osteoblast function have also been identified in mice with the osteopetrotic phenotype, but not yet in humans; these mice have also been successfully treated using bone marrow transplantation. Speculation exists as to whether the clinical fail-

ure of bone marrow transplantation that may occur in some patients represents a noncellular genetic defect that has yet to be found.

Clinical Picture

Osteopetrosis is characterized by dense but brittle bone. There are three main clinical classifications: infantile, intermediate, and autosomal dominant. Radiographically, there is dense bone with loss of the marrow cavity. Without the function of osteoclasts, bone does not remodel with growth; thus, the shape of the long bones can be abnormal. Various morphologic changes to the osteoclast have been reported, including an increase in cell volume, a decrease in cell number, an increase in the number of nuclei, and abnormalities in the ruffled border or clear zone. In patients with osteopetrosis, histologic examination of a bone sample typically demonstrates bone trabeculae interwoven with hyaline cartilage within the medullary cavity. Because the marrow cavity is no longer available for hematopoiesis, hepatosplenomegaly can occur. Children also may present with anemia, thrombocytopenia, and infection. Diagnosis can be made by detection of the brain isoenzyme of creatine kinase in patients with the disease.

Treatment

Allogenic bone marrow transplantation can cure osteopetrosis, and in most patients reverse the phenotype. However, the clinical outcome of bone marrow transplantation can be variable. Failures of bone marrow transplantation may occur when the osteoclasts and osteoblasts are normal, and the pathology is in the bone microenvironment.

Marfan Syndrome

Patients with Marfan syndrome may experience lethal aortic ruptures that can perhaps be obviated with betablockers or corrected surgically. To be treated, the diagnosis of Marfan syndrome must first be established.

Genetics

Marfan syndrome occurs in less than 0.01% of the population and is caused by a mutation in fibrillin (chromosome 15) or possibly in the gene for the transforming growth factor beta receptor 2. Marfan syndrome follows an autosomal dominant inheritance pattern.

Clinical Picture

Patients with Marfan syndrome have skeletal, cardiac, and ocular involvement. Skeletal manifestations include arachnodactyly, pectus excavatum, scoliosis, and protrusio acetabuli. The skeleton is disproportionate, with the upper body to lower body ratio decreased to less than 0.85 (the normal ratio is 0.93). Ligamentous laxity is associated with pes planovalgus and subluxation of the joints (patella and shoulder). Cardiac disease can include aortic dilatation, aortic aneurysm, and mitral valve prolapse. Patients often require treatment with betablockers and other medications to control bone pressure and minimize damage to the aorta. Ocular findings include superior lens dislocations.

Treatment

Spinal fusion should be considered only after a cardiac workup is done. Preoperative CT and MRI are useful for assessment of bone topography and dural ectasia, respectively. Infantile scoliosis should not be treated in children younger than 4 years because this subpopulation is at high risk for cardiac demise. Aggressive correction of large curves tends to cause later decompensation of the spine.

In many patients with Marfan syndrome, the cervical spine is involved; basilar invagination, focal kyphosis, and increased atlantoaxial translation should be ruled out in these patients. In patients with any pathology of the cervical spine, contact sports that involve load to the cervical spine should be avoided. Additional restrictions on sports activities must be made in consideration of aortic dilatation (sports with intense and rapid acceleration and deceleration should be avoided because increased stroke volume and blood pressure over time can increase the rate of aortic dilatation). In addition, isometric exercises (for example, free weights and body

building) should be avoided because the stress of such activities can further weaken the aortic wall.

Approximately 30% of patients with Marfan syndrome develop protrusio acetabuli. Dual-energy x-ray absorptiometry scans of the bone mineral content are similar in patients both with and without protrusio acetabuli. Most patients with protrusio acetabuli are asymptomatic and maintain pain-free and full range of motion of the hips. Although closure of the triradiate cartilage by epiphysiodesis has been suggested as treatment of protrusio acetabuli in patients with Marfan syndrome, there are still no data to suggest any benefit from early surgical intervention.

Surgical treatment of joint subluxation often requires arthrodesis because soft-tissue reconstruction cannot prevent the recurrence of laxity. Physical therapy aimed at strengthening muscle may help stabilize joints, but it must be done in deference to the exercise restrictions necessary in this patient population.

Glucocorticoid Treatment in Children

Glucocorticoids are used for the treatment of many diseases in children, including rheumatoid arthritis, systemic lupus erythematosus, inflammatory bowel disease, glucocorticoid-sensitive nephrotic syndrome, cystic fibrosis, juvenile dermatomyositis, organ transplantation, and as a part of some chemotherapy regimens. The adverse effects of corticosteroid therapy include an inhibitory effect on the growth plate that can cause growth retardation, weight gain that can lead to obesity, and the suppression of bone formation that can potentially lead to osteoporosis. In adults, glucocorticoid therapy (in doses equivalent to 5 mg or more of prednisone) administered for 6 months or longer has been shown to increase the number of fractures in the spine by a factor of five and to double the number of expected fractures at other locations. Controversy continues about whether glucocorticoids increase the fracture rate and decrease bone density in children. Another important difference between children and adults is that children have not yet reached their peak bone mass. Also unclear is the effect of glucocorticoid therapy on the ability of young patients to maximize bone mass by early in the second decade of life or whether corticosteroid therapy contributes to an increase in life-long fractures.

Osteonecrosis is perhaps the most devastating consequence of glucocorticoid treatment. Occurring in the major weight-bearing joints, osteonecrosis results from a transient loss of blood supply to the bone followed by microfracture, subchondral fracture, bone revascularization, and joint collapse. MRI can be used to diagnose osteonecrosis at the earliest stages. How glucocorticoids cause osteonecrosis remains unknown. Surgical treatment can include core decompression, joint stabilization, or replacement procedures. Medical treatment with bisphosphonates or hyperbaric oxygen remains experimental and controversial. Thus, treatment should be individually tailored to the patient based on the degree and location of joint involvement.

The literature both refutes and supports a deleterious effect of glucocorticoids on immature bone. Two factors make demonstrating an effect of glucocorticoids on the bone density of children difficult. First, technical problems exist in determining bone density in children, whose growing bone changes in geometry, which makes comparisons, even with age-matched control subjects, a difficult endeavor. Second, many of the diseases treated with glucocorticoids have an underlining inflammatory component, which may also cause bone resorption independent from the administration of drugs.

Pathophysiology

Glucocorticoids act directly on bone to inhibit bone formation by decreasing the number and function of osteoblasts. In addition, glucocorticoids can act on other target organs, for example, the gut where glucocorticoids decrease the ability of the intestines to absorb vitamin D and calcium. Glucocorticoids increase the excretion of calcium in the urine, thus triggering an increase in parathyroid hormone in response to a lower serum calcium level.

Confounding the effects of glucocorticoids is the release of cytokines as a response to an inflammatory condition that necessitates glucocorticoid treatment. Cytokines are known to cause bone resorption; therefore, differentiating the effect of drugs from the effect of the disease can be challenging.

Clinical Picture

In a recent study, 60 children treated intermittently with glucocorticoids for nephrotic syndrome were compared with a control population. Patients treated with corticosteroids had an increase in body mass index from both weight gain and growth retardation. When adjusted for age, sex, race, and maturity (Tanner stage), the bone mineral content measured by dual-energy x-ray absorptiometry scanning was the same for the spine and the whole body compared with a matched control population. When adjusted for body mass index in addition to the other factors, only the spine in the treatment population demonstrated any difference in bone density. Because bone responds to load, the fact that the treated children had a higher body mass index may explain why the expected effect of glucocorticoid therapy of reducing bone density was not demonstrated.

This study contradicted the findings of an earlier study of 20,000 children given glucocorticoids who demonstrated an increase in fracture risk compared with a matched control group. Although more research needs to be performed to determine the effects of steroids on bone, clinicians should make sure children are receiving adequate vitamin D and calcium in their diets and prescribe supplementation for any child with risk factors for decreased bone density.

Annotated Bibliography
Rickets and Osteomalacia
Bloom E, Klein EJ, Shushan D, Feldman KW: Variable presentations of rickets in children in the emergency department. *Pediatr Emerg Care* 2004;20:126-130.

Three patients with rickets who presented in the emergency department are described, as are the current treatment recommendations for treating rickets.

Jonsson KB, Zahradnik R, Larsson T, et al: Fibroblast growth factor 23 in oncogenic osteomalacia and X-linked hypophosphatemia. *N Engl J Med* 2003;348:1656-1663.

Overproduction of FGF-23 from sarcoma leading to phosphate wasting is described, as is the role FGF-23 plays in X-linked hypophosphatemic rickets.

Mirams M, Robinson BG, Mason RS, Nelson AE: Bone as a source of FGF-23: Regulation by phosphate? *Bone* 2004;35:1192-1199.

Data are presented linking FGF-23 production and phosphate metabolism to bone tissue.

Renal Osteodystrophy
Hernandez JD, Wasserling K, Salusky IB: Role of parathyroid hormone and therapy with active vitamin D sterols in renal osteodystrophy. *Semin Dial* 2005;18:290-295.

The authors discuss updated treatment strategies for patients with renal osteodystrophy, including new vitamin D analogs.

Osteogenesis Imperfecta
Marini JC: Do bisphosphonates make children's bones better or brittle? *N Engl J Med* 2003;349:423-426.

The author recommends cautious use of bisphosphonates because the adverse effects of the drug, proper dosing regime in children, and therapeutic benefits have yet to be determined.

Munns CF, Rauch F, Zeitlin L, Fassier F, Glorieux FH: Delayed osteotomy but not fracture healing in pediatric osteogenesis imperfecta patients receiving pamidronate. *J Bone Miner Res* 2004;19:1779-1786.

Patients who were treated with bisphosphonates were compared with those not receiving drug treatment for speed of healing after fracture and osteotomy.

Zionts LE, Moon CN: Olecranon apophysis fractures in children with osteogenesis imperfecta revisited. *J Pediatr Orthop* 2002;22:745-750.

The authors report that olecranon fractures are rare in children with normal bone density but occur frequently in children with osteogenesis imperfecta.

Fibrous Dysplasia

Leet AI, Magur E, Lee J, Wientroub S, Robey PG, Collins MT: Fibrous dysplasia in the spine: Prevalence of spine lesions and association with scoliosis. *J Bone Joint Surg Am* 2004;86-A:531-537.

The authors of this article reported that lesions of fibrous dysplasia commonly occurred in the spine in patients with polyostotic fibrous dysplasia and correlated with the presence of scoliosis at the same level of the spine.

Osteopetrosis

Tolar J, Teitelbaum SL, Orchard PJ: Osteopetrosis. *N Engl J Med* 2004;351:2839-2849.

Osteoclastic function and genetic mutation are described, as is the osteopetrotic phenotype.

Marfan Syndrome

Jones KB, Erkula G, Sponseller PD, et al: Spine deformity correction in Marfan syndrome. *Spine* 2002;27:2003-2012.

The authors of this article reported that aggressive correction of the spine can lead to decompensation, whereas complications such as infections and dural tears are common in patients with Marfan syndrome.

Glucocorticoid Treatment in Children

Bachrach LK: Bare-bones fact: Children are not small adults. *N Engl J Med* 2004;351(9):924-926.

The author of this article analyzes studies assessing the effect of glucocorticoids on the bones of children and describes the potential negative effects of this drug on the growing skeleton.

Leonard MB, Feldman HI, Shults J, Zemel BS, Foster BJ, Stallings VA: Long-term, high-dose glucocorticoids and bone mineral content in childhood glucocorticoid-sensitive nephrotic syndrome. *N Engl J Med* 2004;351:868-875.

The effect of glucocorticoids on bone density was analyzed in children with nephrotic syndrome. The authors found that intermittent high-dose glucocorticoids did not cause a decrease in bone mineral content when compared with matched control subjects.

Classic Bibliography

Albright F, Butler AM, Hampton AO, et al: Syndrome characterized by osteitis fibrosa disseminate, areas of pigmentation and endocrine dysfunction, with precocious puberty in females: Report of five cases. *N Engl J Med* 1937;216:727-746.

Bianco P, Rimminucci M, Majolagbe A, et al: Mutations of the GNAS1 gene, stromal cell dysfunction, and osteomalacic changes in non-McCune-Albright fibrous dysplasia of bone. *J Bone Miner Res* 2000;15:120-128.

Do T, Giampietro PF, Burke SW, et al: The incidence of protrusion acetabuli in Marfan's syndrome and its relationship to bone mineral density. *J Pediatr Orthop* 2000;20:718-721.

Hobbs WR, Sponseller PD, Weiss AP, Pyeritz RE: The cervical spine in Marfan syndrome. *Spine* 1997;22(9):938-939.

Ishikawa S, Kumar SJ, Takahashi HE, Homma M: Vertebral body shape as a predictor of spinal deformity in osteogenesis imperfecta. *J Bone Joint Surg Am* 1996;78:212-219.

Lazner F, Gowen M, Pavasovic D, Kola I: Osteopetrosis and osteoporosis: Two sides of the same coin. *Hum Mol Genet* 1999;8:1839-1846.

Mankin HJ: Rickets, osteomalacia and renal osteodystrophy: An update. *Orthop Clin North Am* 1990;21:81-96.

Section 3

Lower Extremity Conditions

Section Editor:
Mark J. Romness, MD

Chapter 13

Slipped Capital Femoral Epiphysis and Legg-Calvé-Perthes Disease

Brian G. Smith, MD

Kristan A. Pierz, MD

Janet L. Zahradnik, MD

Slipped Capital Femoral Epiphysis

Slipped capital femoral epiphysis (SCFE) is the most common hip disorder in adolescents. It is by definition a displacement of the femoral head on the neck of the femur, and it occurs most commonly in children from age 10 to 15 years. Specifically, there is a displacement of the femoral head inferiorly and posteriorly or, more accurately, there is translation and migration of the femoral neck anteriorly and superiorly. It is generally believed that the femoral head remains in position and the neck translates on the epiphysis in patients with SCFE. When SCFE occurs in an acute setting, this injury is analogous to a Salter type I fracture of the proximal femoral physis.

Etiology

SCFE typically occurs through the hypertrophic physeal zone. Increases in circulating hormones during puberty (including testosterone) are known to cause elongation of the hypertrophic zone. Mechanical forces may cause physiologic stress within the physis, especially in patients who are particularly at risk for SCFE, such as obese boys with femoral retroversion. The result is a biomechanical failure of the physis that may occur gradually over time, causing the translation of the femoral neck on the head. This is the etiology in most patients with SCFE, the so-called idiopathic type of this disorder.

An atypical type of SCFE occurs in patients with endocrine disorders such as renal osteodystrophy. Additional causes of SCFE include other endocrine disorders such as hypothyroidism or hyperthyroidism. Patients who have undergone radiation therapy or receive growth hormone therapy are also predisposed to SCFE.

SCFE is known to be more common in boys than in girls (a ratio of 2:1), more common in African Americans than Caucasians, and more common in obese patients. Recent studies of the seasonal variation of SCFE have implicated dysfunction or disorders of vitamin D metabolism as a possible factor for predisposing patients to SCFE. One recent study found a seasonal variation in SCFE in the northern United States, with this incidence being more prominent in Caucasians than African Americans. Another recent study found an increase in incidence of SCFE in males in the autumn. Heavier patients are known to have decreased levels of vitamin D, and African-American children tend to be heavier in adolescence than Caucasian children in the United States. Because an association between vitamin D deficiency and SCFE has been demonstrated, it is possible that a disorder in vitamin D synthesis may be involved in SCFE. Decreased vitamin D from absence of sun exposure in the northern United States during the winter may cause a relative vitamin D deficiency, thus potentially increasing the incidence of SCFE.

Incidence

The incidence of SCFE in various reports in the literature varies from less than 1 per 100,000 persons to 61 per 100,000 persons. Boys are at increased risk for SCFE as are African Americans; it has been estimated that cumulative risk for African-American boys may be as high as 1 in 400. Increased body mass index (BMI) has been identified as a possible predictive factor in patients who are predisposed to SCFE. In a recent study, girls age 14 years with SCFE had a BMI of 22.6 versus a normal value of 19.6 and boys age 14 years with SCFE had a BMI of 25.4 versus a normal value of 18.7.

The risk of patients with a single SCFE having a contralateral slip is also quite high and has been the source of recent discussions on prophylactic fixation in patients with SCFE. The incidence of bilateral SCFE has ranged from approximately 10% to 15% in some studies to as high as 40% to 60%. Whereas one in five patients who present with SCFE actually has bilateral SCFE, more than 90% of patients who develop late SCFE on the contralateral side are asymptomatic. It has been calculated that a patient with a single slip is 2,335 times more likely to have a contralateral SCFE than a patient without a slip is to have a SCFE.

Presentation

The classic patient presenting with SCFE is an obese African-American male with left-sided groin pain typically for a duration of weeks to months. The age of presentation is typically between 12 to 16 years for boys (average age, 15.5 years) and 10 to 14 years for girls (average age, 11.5 years). The presentation of SCFE in patients outside of these age ranges should alert physicians to a potential endocrinopathy. Many patients attribute the pain to a pulled groin muscle and often relate a history of mild trauma. Delay in diagnosis of SCFE was recently evaluated at a medical center in a review of nearly 200 patients. The length of delay of diagnosis was correlated with the severity of SCFE. Factors that were associated with an increased delay in diagnosis of SCFE included reports of distal thigh or knee pain, Medicaid coverage, and stable slips.

Historically, SCFE has been classified based on the duration of symptoms. Symptoms of groin, thigh, or leg pain for greater than 3 weeks resulted in a diagnosis of a chronic SCFE. Pain of less than 3 weeks duration was classified as acute SCFE; duration of 3 weeks or longer is considered chronic. Approximately 85% of patients have chronic SCFE at presentation.

More recently, a classification of SCFE based on stability has become more commonly used. By definition, stable SCFE is diagnosed in a patient who is able to walk or bear weight on the leg. Patients may present with an acute, unstable hip or a chronic slip can become acutely unstable such that patients are not able to walk or bear weight on the affected leg. On physical examination, patients with acute unstable SCFE will often not allow any range of motion of the hip. The extremity is usually shortened, abducted, and externally rotated. Patients with chronic SCFE will allow range-of-motion testing and often have good range of motion, with the most common finding being a decrease in internal rotation and some lower extremity shortening.

Patients with acute, unstable SCFE will often present with significant or severe pain, will be unable to bear weight on the affected limb, and will have radiographic evidence of what is essentially a Salter type I fracture through the proximal femoral physis. At the time of surgery, gross instability of the femoral head relative to the neck is often noted on fluoroscopic examination. Unstable SCFE has a much higher incidence of complications, including osteonecrosis and chondrolysis. In a recent study, patients with unstable SCFE comprised approximately 15% of 196 patients who were evaluated for delay in diagnosis. A delayed diagnosis (median delay, 8 weeks) was found to significantly increase the risk of chronic stable SCFE becoming acutely unstable. These findings underscore the need for early diagnosis in patients with this disorder.

Diagnostic Imaging

The standard diagnosis of SCFE is made using an AP pelvis radiograph that includes the hips and a frog lateral radiograph of the hips. Diagnosis is usually straightforward on the radiographs of patients with stable, chronic SCFE. Patients with unstable or acute SCFE may need a true lateral radiograph obtained in the operating room so the patient can be immobilized. CT and MRI play a relatively small role in the initial diagnosis of SCFE. Bone scanning and MRI can be used in the diagnosis of patients with acute, unstable SCFE to assess the femoral head vascularity and viability or to diagnose a "pre-slip" (an inflamed hip that is destined to experience slip).

Radiographs are also used to classify SCFE. The severity of SCFE can be graded based on the percentage of epiphyseal displacement with respect to metaphyseal width of the femoral neck as observed on AP or lateral radiographs. Slippage of 0 to 25% is classified as mild, 26% to 50% is moderate, and greater than 50% is severe. Lateral radiographs can also be used to calculate an angle between a line drawn perpendicular to the base of the epiphysis and a line drawn along the femoral shaft. This head-shaft angle, or slip angle, is classified as grade I (mild) if it is less than 30°, grade II (moderate) if it is between 30° and 50°, and grade III (severe) if it is greater than 50°.

Treatment

The current standard treatment for SCFE is in situ cannulated screw fixation done on an urgent basis. The goal of treatment is to arrest further progression of the slip and to gain closure of the capital femoral physis. Past studies have documented a high complication rate with multiple techniques. One recent study reported a complication rate of 5% with a single cannulated screw technique, which is comparable to findings reported elsewhere in the literature. Patients with SCFE who undergo in situ screw fixation can subsequently be managed with ambulation on crutches and partial weight bearing for 4 to 6 weeks. The recommended best position for single screw placement is the center of the femoral head as identified on both AP and lateral radiographs. Further slippage prior to physeal closure has been reported when less than five threads enter the epiphysis on the frog lateral radiograph. Other reported options for managing patients with SCFE include bone peg epiphysiodesis and cast immobilization, neither of which is currently recommended.

The management of patients with unstable SCFE presents additional challenges. Of greatest concern is the risk of osteonecrosis in patients with an acute unstable slip, the reported incidence of which varies from 3% to 47% of patients. A recent retrospective study at a children's medical center found that of 212 patients

(299 hips) treated primarily with screw fixation, 4 of 27 patients with unstable SCFE developed osteonecrosis, whereas this did not occur in any patients with stable SCFE. In another study, five patients with unstable SCFE were studied with super-selective angiography, and three patients showed no evidence of filling of the superior retinacular artery before reduction of acute SCFE, suggesting the likely etiology of osteonecrosis is a compromise of the blood supply resulting from disruption of the superior retinacular vessels.

Management of patients with unstable SCFE can include in situ cannulated screw fixation, often with two screws. A second screw has been reported in some studies to help enhance stability and maximize rotational control. Other options include primary osteotomy and/or gentle manipulative reduction. One recent study reported that extremely gentle manipulative reduction was not associated with an increased risk of osteonecrosis overall in patients with unstable SCFE, and preoperative traction was not shown to be of any significant benefit. Spontaneous or serendipitous reduction or controlled reduction under fluoroscopic guidance has not been associated with an increased rate of osteonecrosis in patients with unstable SCFE, but excessive internal rotation or forceful maneuvers of reduction are not recommended in these patients.

Prophylactic Pinning of the Contralateral Hip

Prophylactic in situ screw fixation of the contralateral hip has been recommended in patients with chronic SCFE. Recently, it has been argued that the risk of osteonecrosis and chondrolysis from prophylactic in situ screw fixation of the contralateral hip is virtually negligible when using in situ cannulated screw fixation with improved imaging technology and radiolucent tables. In this study, because the percentage of patients with contralateral SCFE ranges anywhere from 20% to 40% (and possibly as high as 60% to 80% in some subsets of patients with endocrine disorders), "decision analysis" was used to assess the risk of prophylactic pinning of the contralateral hip. Prophylactic pinning was found to be beneficial in long-term outcomes based on the rates of sequential slip and the late diagnosis of contralateral slip when compared with the complications associated with prophylactic pinning (Figure 1). A more recent study indicated that the incidence of the contralateral hip slippage would have to be 27% or greater for patients to realize the benefits of prophylactic in situ pinning. Currently, prophylactic contralateral hip fixation is recommended for patients with established metabolic or endocrine disorders and for children with SCFE who are younger than 10 years.

Anatomic parameters have been evaluated to predict which patients are at risk for developing a contralateral SCFE. An increased posterior sloping angle

(> 12°) of the capital femoral physis with respect to the diaphysis on the axial radiograph has been associated with an increased risk of contralateral SCFE.

Further evaluation of the skeletal maturity of patients with SCFE has been advocated to help determine who may be at risk for contralateral slip. A study of the skeletal maturity of patients with SCFE indicated that once the triradiate cartilage was closed, the risk of a contralateral slip was 4%, whereas once Risser stage 1 was achieved, the risk of a contralateral slip was virtually zero.

Complications

Chondrolysis is a complication of SCFE that has often been linked to persistent penetration of a screw in the hip joint after in situ screw fixation. Transient penetration of the joint has not been associated with chondrolysis. Some patients with SCFE are known to have chondrolysis at the time of presentation (Figure 2). It is thought that chondrolysis may be associated with an autoimmune reaction within the joint space. Immune complexes have been identified in the synovial fluid of such patients. Treatment consists of exercises focused at regaining range of motion, decreased weight bearing, and rest, sometimes supplemented or followed with capsulotomy and continuous passive motion exercises. Persistent or severe chondrolysis has a guarded long-term prognosis.

Progression of SCFE after in situ fixation with a screw has also been noted. In the absence of known endocrinopathy, treatment of progressive SCFE despite fixation would be activity restrictions or possibly the addition of a second screw.

The most common and troublesome long-term complication associated with SCFE is osteonecrosis. The incidence of osteonecrosis in patients with unstable SCFE has been reported to be as high as 50%, and a recent study reported a 15% incidence. The authors of this latter study recommended urgent treatment, including gentle closed reduction either by positioning on the bed or some traction with the patient under anesthesia on the fracture table with gentle internal rotation. If this is not successful, the authors recommended open reduction. A percutaneous capsulotomy was also recommended to decrease intra-articular hemarthrosis for patients with unstable SCFE. In a recent series using this protocol, in situ cannulated screw fixation was performed, and only 2 of 16 patients with acute unstable SCFE developed osteonecrosis.

Another large retrospective review of 240 patients showed no associated osteonecrosis in 204 patients with chronic or stable SCFE, regardless of SCFE grade and treatment. Osteonecrosis occurred in 21 patients with unstable SCFE, and the risk was correlated with severity or grade as well as with multiple pin fixation rather

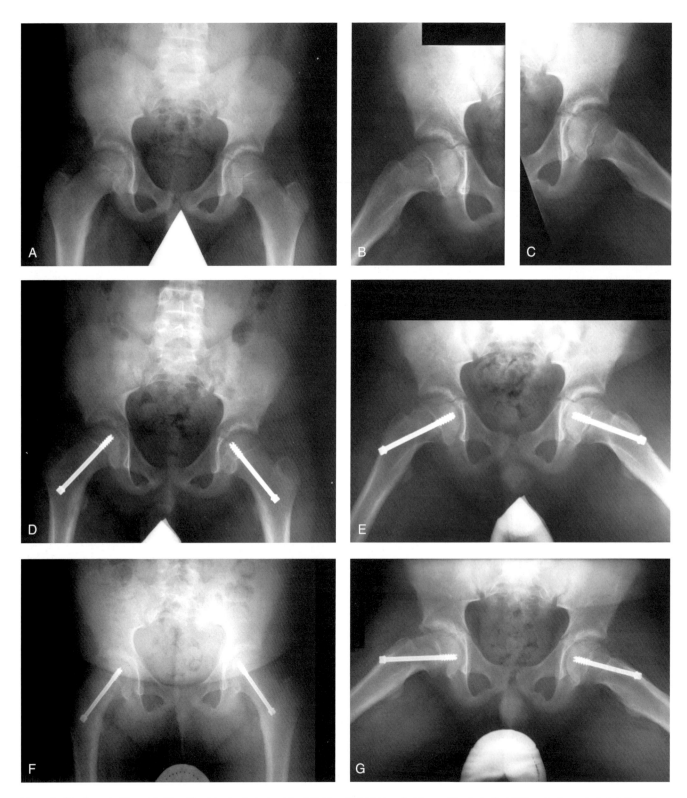

Figure 1 AP radiograph of the pelvis **(A)** and frog lateral radiographs of the right **(B)** and left **(C)** hips of a 10-year-old patient with right hip pain show a grade 1 stable SCFE on the right and no definitive slip on the left. Because of the age of the patient and the presence of open triradiate cartilage, in situ cannulated screw fixation of both hips was performed. AP **(D)** and frog lateral **(E)** radiographs of the pelvis obtained approximately 3 days postoperatively. Weight-bearing AP **(F)** and frog lateral **(G)** radiographs of the pelvis obtained 14 months postoperatively show closure of the proximal femoral physis bilaterally. The weight-bearing AP radiograph demonstrated no significant limb-length inequality.

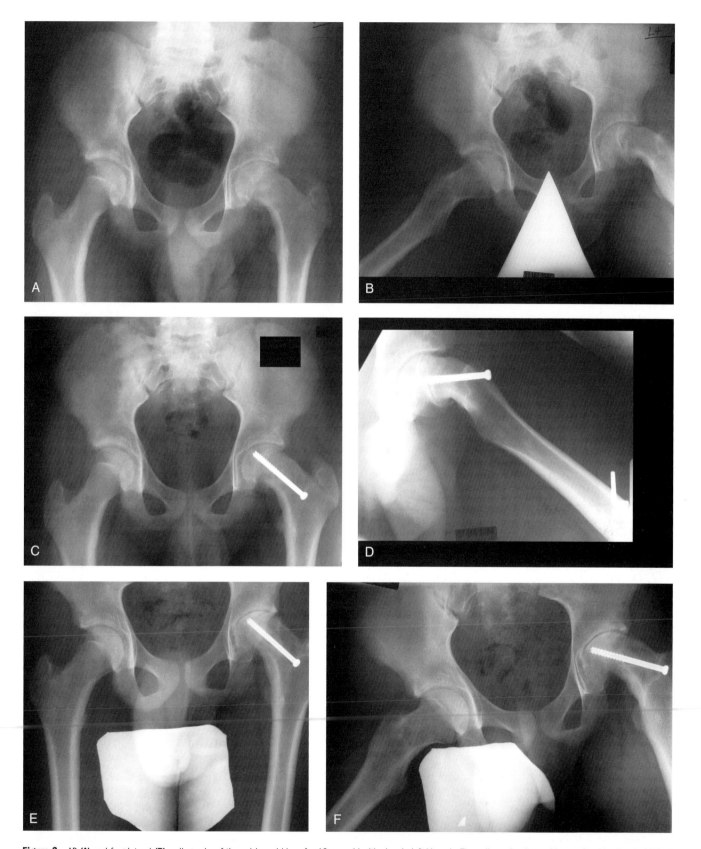

Figure 2   AP **(A)** and frog lateral **(B)** radiographs of the pelvis and hips of a 12-year-old with chronic left hip pain. The radiographs show evidence of stable chronic SCFE of undetermined age. Joint-space narrowing that is already indicative of early chondrolysis is also evident. AP **(C)** and frog lateral **(D)** radiographs obtained approximately 3 weeks after the patient underwent in situ cannulated screw fixation of the SCFE. AP **(E)** and frog lateral **(F)** radiographs of the pelvis obtained approximately 1 year postoperatively show advanced chondrolysis.

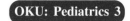

than a single in situ cannulated screw. In this particular series, complete or partial reduction of the unstable slip increased the likelihood of osteonecrosis. The authors, therefore, recommended pinning in situ without reduction with a single cannulated screw for patients with stable or unstable SCFE.

Another study identified anterior physeal separation as a significant risk factor for osteonecrosis in patients with unstable SCFE. Physeal separation is best viewed radiographically on a frog lateral radiograph as separation between the metaphysis and epiphysis that is acute and well demarcated. In a study of 110 hips, seven of eight patients with radiographic evidence of anterior physeal separation developed osteonecrosis.

Treatment of osteonecrosis may involve prolonged restriction of weight bearing depending on whether the involvement of the femoral head is partial or complete. Hip arthrodesis or arthroplasty may be required as symptoms and radiographic findings warrant.

Legg-Calvé-Perthes Disease

Legg-Calvé-Perthes disease is osteonecrosis of the capital femoral epiphysis in children. Treating patients with Legg-Calvé-Perthes disease remains a challenge to orthopaedists in terms of its etiology and management, and continues to be a significant source of disability in children.

Etiology

Although the precise cause of Legg-Calvé-Perthes disease is unknown and traditional etiologies of Legg-Calvé-Perthes disease include trauma and inflammation, recent research suggests an association with disorders of the clotting system, specifically thrombophilia, as a possible mechanism. Protein C, protein S, and antithrombin III are key components of the coagulation cascade, deficiencies of which may cause thrombosis.

The proposed sequence for osteonecrosis in the capital femoral epiphysis is venous stasis or thrombosis causing increased intraosseous pressure in the femoral head, decreased arterial flow, and ischemia, which results in osteocyte death and osteonecrosis.

Recent reports include support for and against thrombophilia as a cause of Legg-Calvé-Perthes disease. A review of 50 consecutive patients with Legg-Calvé-Perthes disease did not identify abnormalities in plasma concentrations of protein C, protein S, or antithrombin III in patients with Legg-Calvé-Perthes disease at a rate or incidence that was higher than what would be expected for the general population.

However, a similar study compared 72 patients with Legg-Calvé-Perthes disease with 197 healthy control subjects and found that the factor-V Leiden mutation and anticardiolipin antibodies were more common at a level of statistical significance in patients with Legg-

Calvé-Perthes disease, suggesting a possible causal relationship.

Systemic Factors

Because children with Legg-Calvé-Perthes disease have been identified as having developmental delays in stature and maturity, a systemic theory for the etiology of Legg-Calvé-Perthes disease has also been proposed. Delay in the development of the ossific nucleus on the unaffected side has recently been identified in patients with Legg-Calvé-Perthes disease, suggesting skeletal dysplasia may have some causal significance. A review of five sets of male twins documented that the lower birth weight twin was the one who developed Legg-Calvé-Perthes disease. This finding argues against a completely genetic cause, but indicates that small stature or environmental factors may predispose to Legg-Calvé-Perthes disease.

Clinical Presentation

The child presenting with Legg-Calvé-Perthes disease is typically a boy with a limp for weeks to months. A history of recent or remote viral illness may be obtained, and persistent inflammation or lingering toxic synovitis has been indicated as a possible risk factor. The onset may be insidious, and pain is often present and localized distally in the thigh or knee. The disorder is more common in boys 4 to 8 years of age, with most studies reporting a boy to girl ratio of 2 or 3:1. Decreased hip range of motion, particularly in abduction and internal rotation, a hip flexion contracture, and slight shortening of the leg are common physical examination findings, especially as the process evolves through the fragmentation and reossification phases and femoral head collapse occurs.

Differential Diagnosis

Bilateral Legg-Calvé-Perthes disease occurs in 8% to 24% of patients and may occur simultaneously or with one hip preceding the other. Blood tests to rule out hypothyroidism should be performed. Other diagnostic considerations include either multiple or spondyloepiphyseal dysplasia and pseudoachondroplasia. One study of more than 600 patients with Legg-Calvé-Perthes disease at a large children's medical center reported a 13% incidence of bilaterality along with the finding that the second side had milder involvement.

Imaging Studies

The diagnosis of Legg-Calvé-Perthes disease is made using plain radiography, which denotes changes in the capital femoral epiphysis that include smaller size, the crescent sign of a subchondral fracture, and flattening of the epiphysis (Figure 3). Bone scanning has been proposed to identify the stage and classification of Legg-Calvé-

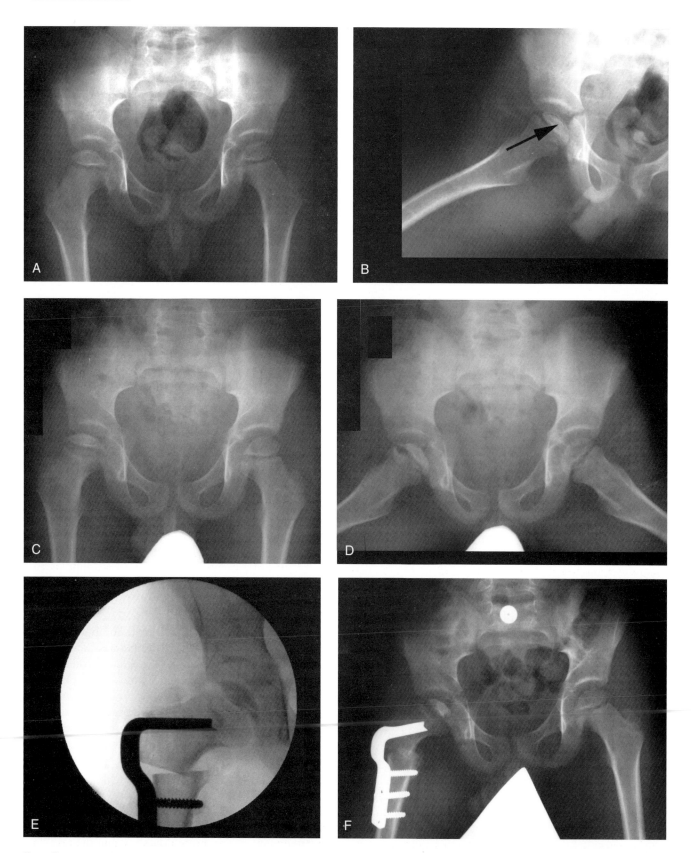

Figure 3   AP **(A)** and frog lateral **(B)** radiographs of the pelvis and right hip of a 5-year-old patient who presented with a limp and thigh pain for several weeks show some sclerosis of the capital femoral epiphysis and some widening of the medial clear space in a smaller epiphysis on the AP view. A classic crescent sign (*arrow*) is visible on the frog lateral view. AP **(C)** and frog lateral **(D)** radiographs of the pelvis 5.5 months after diagnosis show continued sclerosis, some slight lateral uncovering of the epiphysis, and a Herring lateral pillar group C classification. On the frog lateral radiograph, cystic changes in the metaphysis are evident. **E,** Intraoperative radiograph shows excellent coverage of the epiphysis after the patient underwent a varus osteotomy. **F,** AP radiograph obtained approximately 5 weeks postoperatively shows healing of the patient's varus osteotomy of the right hip.

American Academy of Orthopaedic Surgeons

Table 1 | Legg-Calvé-Perthes Disease Classification Systems

Classification System Group or Class				
Herring	Salter	Catterall	Phase/Stage	Treatment Options
A	1	I	Avascular/synovitis	Range-of-motion exercises Casting (Petrie)
		II	Fragmentation/resorption	Abduction orthosis Crutches
B		III	Reossification/regeneration	Varus osteotomy Salter osteotomy
	2			
C		IV	Remodelling/residual	Distraction arthroplasty Contralateral epiphysiodesis Valgus osteotomy/Cheilectomy Shelf procedure

Perthes disease to better determine prognosis and treatment options.

MRI can provide information regarding extent of involvement, vascular status, and sphericity of the femoral head in all planes. In one recent study, deformity of the femoral head and epiphyseal collapse were found to be most significant in the sagittal plane, but better maintenance of sphericity occurred in this plane, reflecting physiologic molding from flexion and extension of the hip.

Arthrography is a useful means of assessing coverage and containment of the femoral head. Epiphyseal extrusion was documented in a recent study to be optimally determined by arthrography, thereby more accurately predicting outcome and guiding appropriate intervention.

Classification

An accurate, reliable, and reproducible classification system is particularly important in a disorder as variable as Legg-Calvé-Perthes disease, especially if it permits early intervention and appropriate treatment that optimizes outcome. The phases and stages for the various classification systems are listed in Table 1. A multicenter study of 345 patients with Legg-Calvé-Perthes disease reviewed the Herring lateral pillar classification scheme, which was modified to include a B/C border group (patients midway between group B and C). In the B/C border group, the lateral border of the femoral head epiphysis is narrow (2 to 3 mm wide) and has greater than 50% loss of height relative to the central pillar. The Herring lateral pillar classification was found to have good to excellent interobserver and intraobserver reliability for Legg-Calvé-Perthes disease.

One difficulty with the Herring lateral pillar classification is the timing of the assessment for the lateral pillar grade. Although the initial study classified the radiographs during the first 6 months of the fragmentation stage, the follow-up study of 275 patients with Legg-Calvé-Perthes disease found that 75% of patients were upgraded from group A to group B and 30% of group B patients were raised to group C, such that only 4% of hips remained classified as group A. The authors found that femoral head deformity was maximal at 7 months after presentation and that 96% of patients had a Herring lateral pillar classification of B or C, suggesting this is essentially a two-grade system.

When the Salter, Catterall, and Herring classifications were compared, the Salter classification and the Herring classification were shown to be more reliable than the Catterall classification. A subchondral fracture, which is required in the Salter classification, was present in only 30% of patients in the study, limiting its usefulness. The Catterall classification was more reliable when combined into two classes, I-II and III-IV. Recently, the Herring lateral pillar classification has been used to predict outcome and to plan treatment for patients with Legg-Calvé-Perthes disease. All of the classification systems demonstrate that the greater collapse or involvement of the lateral femoral head, the poorer the prognosis. Lateral femoral head collapse is more commonly associated with subluxation or extrusion as well as hinge abduction and an aspherical final femoral head shape.

Prognostic Factors

Factors influencing outcome in patients with Legg-Calvé-Perthes disease include range of motion of the hip, the age of onset of the disorder, and the extent of femoral head involvement, position of the femoral head, or containment of the femoral head within the acetabulum.

One study reported on the long-term follow-up of 32 patients (average age, 20 years) and determined that the Herring lateral pillar classification alone was not predictive of outcome based on the Stulberg scoring system, but when related to age (either younger than or older than 9 years), prognostic significance was present. Herring lateral pillar classification group C patients younger than 6 years still had favorable outcomes. Patients presenting with Legg-Calvé-Perthes disease at age 9 years or later tended to have the worst outcomes regardless of classification, which highlights the importance of the remodeling time of the femoral head in patients with this disorder.

Various radiographic findings are predictive of outcome, including the head-at-risk signs noted by Catterall, which include lateral epiphyseal calcification, a horizontal physis, Gage sign (a small osteoporotic segment forming a translucent V on the lateral side of the femoral head epiphysis), and femoral head subluxation. Metaphyseal cysts or changes in the physis resulting in abnormal growth of the femoral head or neck, shortening of the extremity, and greater trochanteric overgrowth may all adversely affect the final outcome. Signs of the femoral head at risk signify that the hip is becoming adducted, the femoral head is subluxating or extruding, and ultimately that an aspherical deformity of the femoral head will result. One study found that epiphyseal extrusion measured on a weight-bearing AP pelvis radiograph or by arthrogram was a more reliable and accurate means of determining coverage of the femoral head in patients with Legg-Calve-Perthes disease.

Clinical Course

Evolution of Legg-Calvé-Perthes disease occurs over months and years, starting with the early synovitis or avascular stage when the child will manifest a limp or stiffness of the hip with little if any pain. During this avascular phase, the subchondral fracture initiates reactive synovitis, causing decreased rotation and limiting joint mobility. Muscle spasm, especially of the adductors, with continued weight bearing on the mechanically compromised femoral head causes further subchondral collapse and contributes to increasing femoral head deformity, flattening, and subluxation. The vascular regeneration via creeping substitution reossifies the femoral head, often resulting in radiographic evidence of femoral head hypertrophy, which may impair containment.

Stulberg described femoral head sphericity based on radiographic evidence of femoral head congruency with the acetabulum at skeletal maturity. Patients with Stulberg class I and class II femoral head sphericity have spherical congruency and a good long-term prognosis, whereas those with Stulberg class V (aspherical incongruity) typically have early degenerative arthritis. Containment and coverage of the femoral head can be inadequately assessed on plain radiographs when the ossified cartilaginous femoral epiphysis appears lateralized yet still covered by the unossified labrum. Arthrog-

raphy and MRI are more valuable in assessing containment than plain radiography and are indicated in some patients.

Nonsurgical Treatment

Containment methods include both nonsurgical and surgical options. The initial and primary component of treatment is preservation of range of motion of the hip. Strategies to maintain range of motion include protected weight bearing with crutches or a walker with a physical therapy program and rest. Another primary goal of treatment of Legg-Calvé-Perthes disease is to maintain coverage and containment of the femoral head within the acetabulum to minimize subluxation and the potential for flattening or deformity of the femoral head.

Loss of abduction and evidence of subluxation during the fragmentation stage are indications for containment therapy. This may include abduction bracing with an orthosis. A comparison of 23 patients with Legg-Calvé-Perthes disease who were braced for an average of 14 months showed no significant differences when compared with a group of 25 patients who were not braced. The authors reported that the age of the patient at disease onset and femoral head congruency at skeletal maturity were the most important features determining prognosis. A study of 74 patients with Legg-Calvé-Perthes disease who underwent progressive bilateral abduction by traction found abduction to 30° or more, which was considered necessary for containment, was obtained within 11 days.

Abduction bracing and traction, which may occur at home, and Petrie casting may all be beneficial for regaining or maintaining range of motion; however, the effectiveness of these treatment methods in influencing outcome has not been well documented in the recent literature.

Surgical Treatment

Surgical methods of containment include femoral and pelvic osteotomies. Varus intertrochanteric proximal femoral osteotomy with plate fixation is most commonly used (Figure 3, *E*), but this procedure necessitates reoperation for hardware removal and contributes to femoral shortening and persistent Trendelenburg gait in some patients. The innominate osteotomy provides good coverage, but it may cause increased femoral head pressure and exacerbate stiffness. Radiographic evidence confirming containment, often with arthrography, is necessary before performing an osteotomy.

In a landmark study, the Herring lateral pillar classification and the age at onset of the disorder were found to be the primary factors that were predictive of outcome. In patients age 8 years or older, surgical treatment was noted to have resulted in improved outcomes in patients in the Herring lateral pillar B and B/C groups when compared with patients who underwent nonsurgical management. The most severely affected patients (those in the Herring lateral pillar C group) were noted to have little benefit or improvement with surgery. Patients in the Herring lateral pillar A group and patients 8 years of age or younger in the Herring lateral pillar B group were noted to have done well regardless of therapy. The authors of this study also concluded that bracing is not effective in patients with Legg-Calvé-Perthes disease. The authors concluded that patients in the partial Herring lateral pillar C group had no improvement with surgical treatment regardless of age, and recommended finding more effective treatment alternatives for this group of patients.

Several recent studies describe distraction or arthrodiastasis as an alternative treatment for patients in the Herring lateral pillar C group, especially patients older than 9 years. The technique involves soft-tissue releases such as adductor and hip flexor tenotomy followed by articulated distraction with an external fixator spanning from ilium to femur. By distracting the joint, pressure on the vulnerable femoral head is minimized during the fragmentation phase, range of motion is facilitated (by a hinge in the external fixator), and cartilage stability and femoral head integrity are maintained. In one study of 15 patients with an average age of 10 years, the fixator was in place for 4 months; only 2 patients had a worsening in the Herring lateral pillar classification. A similar study showed favorable results for 15 patients in the Herring lateral pillar C group with improvement in radiographic parameters and in pain. Additional research may eventually validate distraction as a viable treatment option for older patients in the Herring lateral pillar group who otherwise have a poor prognosis.

Some patients with Legg-Calvé-Perthes disease will have residual deformity of the hip that often includes coxa breva, coxa plana, and poor hip congruity. Patients with severe involvement and lateral uncovering of the femoral head may benefit from coverage by a partial shelf arthroplasty. This procedure was reported in one study to have good or fair results in 86% of patients with significant incongruity. Proximal femoral valgus osteotomy is another option for patients with hinge abduction and hip joint incongruity. The Chiari pelvic osteotomy is also a treatment option in patients with femoral head enlargement and extrusion. Coxa breva with relative overgrowth of the greater trochanter and a decreased articular-trochanteric distance may result in an abductor lurch or limp. Greater trochanteric advancement may help restore the abductor mechanism to a more functional position. In patients with pain and limited range of motion caused by irregularity of the femoral head, cheilectomy or excision of abnormal bony prominence from the femoral head remains a useful salvage operation.

Summary

SCFE is a common disorder of the adolescent hip in which the diagnosis is often delayed for weeks to months. The recommended treatment of patients with stable SCFE is a single cannulated screw in situ. The development of osteonecrosis in patients with unstable SCFE remains a significant concern and a source of long-term disability.

Legg-Calvé-Perthes disease is a common cause of hip pain in children. The precise etiology is unknown, and the prognosis is determined by the age of onset, maintenance of range of hip motion, and containment of the femoral head within the acetabulum. Patients older than 9 years at the time of presentation have a guarded prognosis, and no effective treatment regimen has been identified for these patients.

Annotated Bibliography
Slipped Capital Femoral Epiphysis

Barrios C, Blasco MA, Blasco MC, Gasco J: Posterior sloping angle of the capital femoral epiphysis: A predictor of bilaterality in slipped capital femoral epiphysis. *J Pediatr Orthop* 2005;25(4):445-449.

The authors assessed the affected hip of 47 patients with unilateral SCFE and compared them with unaffected control subjects. During the 5-year follow-up, eight patients with unilateral SCFE developed contralateral SCFE. Axial radiographs showed that control subjects had a mean posterior sloping angle of 5° compared with 12° in the patients with unilateral SCFE and 18° in those who developed contralateral SCFE.

Carney BT, Birnbaum P, Minter C: Slip progression after in situ single screw fixation for stable slipped capital femoral epiphysis. *J Pediatr Orthop* 2003;23(5):584-589.

The authors of this study reviewed medical records and frog lateral radiographs of 37 children with 46 slips treated with in situ single cannulated screw fixation. Slip progression was inversely related to the number of screw threads engaging the epiphysis on the first postoperative frog lateral radiograph. Nine slips (20%) demonstrated progression of more than 10°; all nine had less than five screw threads engaging the epiphysis. None of the 24 hips with five or more threads engaging the epiphysis on the first postoperative frog lateral radiograph demonstrated progression.

Dewnany G, Radford P: Prophylactic contralateral fixation in slipped upper femoral epiphysis: Is it safe? *J Pediatr Orthop B* 2005;14(6):429-433.

The authors reviewed 65 patients (range of follow-up, 5 to 8 years) who had prophylactic fixation of the uninvolved hip at the same time as SCFE fixation. A single 7.0-mm cannulated screw was used, and average time to fusion was 18 months. Complications included a single superficial wound infection that was successfully treated with antibiotics; neither chondrolysis nor osteonecrosis was reported.

Gordon JE, Abrahams MS, Dobbs MB, Luhmann SJ, Schoenecker PL: Early reduction arthrotomy and cannulated screw fixation in unstable SCFE treatment. *J Pediatr Orthop* 2002;22(3):352-358.

The authors of this study assessed 16 consecutive patients with unstable SCFE treated with urgent reduction and in situ cannulated screw fixation with two screws. They reported generally good results, with no patients developing osteonecrosis or chondrolysis. Twelve of the 16 patients with unstable SCFE had a closed reduction with gentle manipulation, and the remaining 4 patients had an open reduction of the deformity. The authors recommended early screw fixation, arthrotomy, and gentle closed reduction (or open reduction if needed) for patients with unstable SCFE.

Kennedy JG, Hresko MT, Kasser JR, et al: Osteonecrosis of the femoral head associated with slipped capital femoral epiphysis. *J Pediatr Orthop* 2001;21(2):189-193.

The authors of this retrospective analysis of 212 patients (299 hips) with SCFE found osteonecrosis in 4 of 27 patients with unstable SCFE and 0 of 272 hips with stable SCFE. The magnitude of slip, magnitude of reduction, and chronicity of the slip were not predictive of a poorer outcome in the unstable SCFE group.

Kenny P, Higgins T, Sedhom M, Dowling F, Moore D, Fogarty E: Slipped upper epiphysis: A retrospective review. *J Pediatr Orthop B* 2003;12(2):97-99.

This is a retrospective review of the clinical and radiographic findings after single-screw fixation in 40 children with SCFE; 53 hips were followed over 2 years. The outcome showed excellent or good results in 94% of patients and a complication rate of only 5%, which validated the use of single-screw fixation for patients with SCFE.

Kocher MS, Bishop JA, Hresko MT, Millis MB, Kim YJ, Kasser JR: Prophylactic pinning of the contralateral hip after unilateral slipped capital femoral epiphysis. *J Bone Joint Surg Am* 2004;86-A(12):2658-2665.

Using an expected value decision analysis model, the optimal management strategy for management of the contralateral hip after unilateral SCFE was assessed. Twenty-five adolescent males without SCFE completed a visual analog scale to determine utility values. Following decision tree construction and one-way and two-way fold-back analysis, observation of the contralateral hip was found to be the preferred decision unless the probability of the contralateral slip exceeded 27%.

Kocher MS, Bishop JA, Weed B, et al: Delay in diagnosis of slipped capital femoral epiphysis. *Pediatrics* 2004; 113(4):e322-e325.

This is a review of 196 patients with SCFE who were referred to a tertiary care center over a 15-year period. Significant findings included a positive relationship between delay of diagnosis and severity of slip. Other factors associated with the delay in diagnosis included a history of knee pain and stable slips. The authors concluded that a longer delay in diagnosis correlated with greater slip severity.

Loder RT, Starnes T, Dikos G, Aronsson DD: Demographic predictors of severity of stable slipped capital femoral epiphyses. *J Bone Joint Surg Am* 2006;88(1):97-105.

Based on this retrospective review of 243 children (328 stable SCFEs), the authors concluded that the only two significant predictors of the severity of SCFE are age at diagnosis and symptom duration.

Mooney JF, Sanders JO, Browne RH, et al: Management of unstable/acute slipped femoral epiphysis: Results of a survey of the POSNA membership. *J Pediatr Orthop* 2005;25(2):162-166.

This survey of the Pediatric Orthopaedic Society of North America summarizes the members' use of terminology and treatment, noting that discrepancies remain in classification and fixation methods.

Poussa M, Schlenzka D, Yrjonen T: Body mass index in slipped capital femoral epiphysis. *J Pediatr Orthop B* 2003;12(6):369-371.

The authors of this article assessed 26 patients with SCFE who had complete annual height and weight measurements taken from birth to the onset of the diagnosis of SCFE. These values were compared with those of the normal adolescent population. The findings showed that patients with SCFE had a statistically higher BMI during growth than normal developing children. The results suggest that BMI may be an accurate tool for assessment of risk for SCFE.

Puylaert D, Dimeglio A, Bentahar T: Staging puberty in slipped capital femoral epiphysis: Importance of the triradiate cartilage. *J Pediatr Orthop* 2004;24(2):144-147.

The authors evaluated 83 children with SCFE to identify the stage of puberty at diagnosis. Maturity was evaluated using bone age, closure of the triradiate cartilage, the Risser sign, and the pubertal diagram of Dimeglio. Overall, SCFE occurred in 83% of girls and 95% of boys before the peak of puberty (Dimeglio stages 1 and 2). The triradiate cartilage was open in 65% of boys and 64% of girls. Once the triradiate cartilage was closed, the risk for contralateral SCFE was 4%; once the Risser sign was 1, the risk for contralateral SCFE was zero.

Sanders JO, Smith WJ, Stanley EA, Bueche MJ, Carroll LA, Chambers HG: Progressive slippage after pinning for a slipped capital femoral epiphysis. *J Pediatr Orthop* 2002;22(2):239-243.

The authors of this study assessed 7 patients with progressive SCFE after undergoing screw fixation. All patients had chronic symptoms, but five had acute exacerbation of symptoms with the appearance of acute-on-chronic SCFE. Four of the patients had single-screw fixation, whereas three had two screws placed. Progression was noted on average at 5 months after treatment. The authors recommended protected weight bearing or the addition of another screw. Neither osteonecrosis nor chondrolysis was reported in any of the patients.

Schultz W, Weinstein J, Weinstein S, Smith B: Prophylactic pinning of the contralateral hip in slipped capital femoral epiphysis. *J Bone Joint Surg Am* 2002;84-A(8): 1305-1314.

Using the model of decision analysis, evaluation of the probability of the occurrence of a contralateral slip and its clinical outcomes if undetected were evaluated using the Iowa hip score. Likewise, probabilities of complications related to prophylactic in situ screw fixation of the contralateral hip were compared with Iowa hip scores for probability of undetected slip. Based on the analysis, a higher Iowa hip score was obtained for prophylactic pinning compared with observation. Thus, this decision analysis model favored prophylactic pinning of the contralateral hip when the probabilities were held within the values defined by prior reports in the recent literature for outcomes and complications related to in situ screw fixation of the contralateral hip in children.

Tokmakova KP, Stanton RP, Mason DE: Influencing the development of osteonecrosis in patients treated for slipped capital femoral epiphysis. *J Bone Joint Surg Am* 2003;85-A(5):798-801.

This is a comprehensive review of 240 patients treated over a 35-year period at a major children's hospital with evaluation of factors that would predispose to osteonecrosis in patients with SCFE. Patients with stable SCFE were not found to be at risk for osteonecrosis, whereas osteonecrosis did occur in the patients with unstable SCFE. The authors concluded that in situ screw fixation of the unstable slips decreased the incidence of osteonecrosis in these patients.

Legg-Calvé-Perthes Disease

Aksoy MC, Caglar O, Yazici M, Alpaslan AM: Comparison between braced and non-braced Legg-Calvé-Perthes disease patients: A radiological outcome study. *J Pediatr Orthop B* 2004;13(3):153-157.

The authors of this study evaluated 23 braced and 25 non-braced patients with Legg-Calvé-Perthes disease and followed them to maturity. The findings were such that no significant differences between the groups were identified. The results also suggested that Herring lateral pillar classification was a useful outcome system for the prediction of long-term results. The nonbraced patients who received physical therapy and home traction did as well as the braced patients who received abduction orthotic devices.

Balasa VV, Gruppo RA, Glueck CJ, et al: Legg-Calvé-Perthes disease and thrombophilia. *J Bone Joint Surg Am* 2004;86-A(12):2642-2647.

The authors of this study evaluated 72 patients with Legg-Calvé-Perthes disease for the presence of factor-V Leiden, prothrombin, and plasminogen activator inhibitor-1 specific gene mutations. The homocysteine, protein C, protein S, antithrombin III, and plasminogen activator inhibitor-1 levels of these patients were compared with those of 197 healthy control subjects. Of the risk factors for thrombophilia, the factor-V Leiden mutation and anticardiolipin antibodies were found to be associated with Legg-Calvé-Perthes disease and may impact the physiology of this disorder. The significance of these findings is that the still unknown cause of Legg-Calvé-Perthes disease may be linked to a tendency for hypercoagulability or thrombophilia, and the association of these two findings may help identify which patients are at risk for Legg-Calvé-Perthes disease.

Bennett J, Stuecker R, Smith E, Winder C, Rice J: Arthrographic findings in Legg-Calvé-Perthes disease. *J Pediatr Orthop B* 2002;11(2):110-116.

The authors review the arthrographic findings in patients with Legg-Calvé-Perthes disease, including the concepts of epiphyseal extrusion and acetabular coverage. They reviewed 46 patients with Legg-Calvé-Perthes disease and developed a scheme of radiographic findings correlated with arthrographic containment. This may help better define the amount of femoral head subluxation that is clinically significant in this patient population.

Carney B, Minter C: Non surgical treatment to regain hip abduction and motion in Perthes: A retrospective review. *South Med J* 2004;97(5):485-488.

The authors of this study retrospectively assessed 74 patients with Legg-Calvé-Perthes disease who were treated with bed rest and traction to improve passive hip abduction. Skin traction with progressive bilateral abduction and physiotherapy (including swimming and biking) was also used. The authors reported that 70% of the children achieved an improvement of 10° or more of abduction by day 12 of hospitalization; however, only 7% of children achieved abduction to 45° or greater; 61% achieved abduction to 30° at a minimum and by day 11 of hospitalization. The authors concluded that these findings document one possible way to improve abduction for the containment treatment of patients with Legg-Calvé-Perthes disease.

Gigante C, Frizziero P, Turra S: Prognostic value of Catterall and Herring classification in Legg-Perthes disease: Follow-up to skeletal maturity of 32 patients. *J Pediatr Orthop* 2002;22(3):345-349.

The authors of this study followed 32 patients to skeletal maturity to assess the prognostic value of the Catterall and Herring classifications. They found that the Herring lateral pillar classification was not predictive of outcome when considered alone, but was more prognostic when related to age of onset. The Catterall classification was found to have no significant prognostic correlation with final outcome. These findings confirm that age is of significant prognostic value in determining outcome in patients with Legg-Calvé-Perthes disease.

Guille JT, Lipton GE, Tsirikos A, Bowen JR: Bilateral Legg-Perthes disease: Presentation and outcome. *J Pediatr Orthop* 2002;22(4):458-463.

The authors of this study reviewed the records and radiographs of 83 patients with bilateral Legg-Calvé-Perthes disease at a large children's hospital. When patients presented with hips in different stages or had Legg-Calvé-Perthes disease subsequently in a second hip, the level of Legg-Calvé-Perthes disease tended to be fairly mild. Approximately 22% of patients developing Legg-Calvé-Perthes disease subsequently had worse or more severe disease in the second hip. These findings support the concepts that bilateral disease is an independent event occurring separately in each hip and that the outset of the disease in one hip does not predispose patients to a more severe disease in a second hip.

Herring J, Hui K, Browne R: Legg-Calvé-Perthes disease: Part I. Classification of radiographs with use of the modified lateral pillar and Stulberg classifications. *J Bone Joint Surg Am* 2004;86-A(10):2103-2120.

This article is part of a long-awaited prospective multicenter study on Legg-Calvé-Perthes disease and includes a description of the Herring lateral pillar classification. The authors performed interobserver and intraobserver trials and found the Herring lateral pillar classification was a reliable and adequate means to assess patients with Legg-Calvé-Perthes disease. The correlation between interobserver and intraobserver reliability was good (in the mid-80% range for interobserver reliability and 77% for intraobserver reliability). These findings confirm the use and value of the Herring lateral pillar classification in assessing and staging Legg-Calvé-Perthes disease.

Herring J, Hui K, Browne R: Legg-Calvé-Perthes disease: Part II. Prospective multicenter study of the effect of the treatment on outcome. *J Bone Joint Surg Am* 2004;86-A(10):2121-2133.

The authors present the findings of a landmark multicenter study of more than 400 patients and 451 affected hips that were examined prospectively. The five treatment groups included patients who received no treatment, those who received brace treatment, those who received range-of-motion exercises, those who underwent femoral osteotomy, and those who underwent innominate osteotomy. Hips were classified based on the Herring lateral pillar and Stulberg classifications. In general, the authors found that treatment did not have a significant impact on children younger than 8 years (by chronologic age) or 6 years (by skeletal age). In the Herring lateral pillar type B group and the type B/C group (a new group midway between B and C), the outcomes of surgical treatment were found to be far more successful than nontreatment. The patients in the Herring lateral pillar type C group had no difference between surgical and nonsurgical care in outcome. The authors conclude that the Herring lateral pillar classification and age at the time of onset correlated strongly with outcome and that patients older than 8 years with involved femoral heads tend to have the poorest prognosis.

Hresko M, McDougall T, Gorlun P, et al: Prospective re-evaluation of the association between thrombotic diathesis and Legg-Perthes disease. *J Bone Joint Surg Am* 2002;84-A(9):1613-1618.

In this prospective study, 50 patients with Legg-Calvé-Perthes disease were examined for the frequency of protein C, protein S, antithrombin III, or factor-V Leiden mutations based on blood analysis. The authors found that data did not suggest that any thrombotic diatheses were caused by deficiencies of these proteins or that factor-V Leiden mutations could be correlated with causes of Legg-Legg-Calvé-Perthes disease. Based on these findings, the authors concluded that they could not support screening children with Legg-Calvé-Perthes disease for thrombophilia on a routine basis.

Kitoh H, Kitakoji T, Katoh M, Takamine Y: Delayed ossification and possible capital femoral epiphysis in Legg Calvé Perthes disease. *J Bone Joint Surg Br* 2003;85(1):121-124.

The authors studied the radiographs of 125 children and assessed the contralateral unaffected hip for maturity based on epiphyseal height and width. They found that a significant majority (approximately 90%) of these children were significantly delayed in contralateral ossification of the capital femoral epiphysis when compared with normative data of otherwise healthy normal children. This suggests that Legg-Calvé-Perthes disease may possibly be associated with a generalized constitutional disorder associated with growth disturbance of bone.

Lappin K, Kealey D, Cosgrove A: How useful is the initial radiograph in the Herring classification? *J Pediatr Orthop* 2002;22(4):479-482.

The authors assessed 275 hips treated for Legg-Calvé-Perthes disease. The initial Herring grade was recorded (as defined by Herring during the fragmentation phase) based on the initial visit and then was reevaluated on subsequent radiographs. They found that 92 hips required upgrading of the Herring classification grade from the initial radiograph; they also found that an average duration of 204 days or 7 months from the initial evaluation was the period after which no further collapse could be expected. If the Herring classification is designated before that time, the authors concluded that there is the likelihood that it is inaccurate and would need to be raised based on subsequent radiographs.

Maxwell SL, Lappin KJ, Kealey WD, McDowell BC, Cosgrove AP: Arthrodiastasis in Perthes disease. *J Bone Joint Surg Br* 2004;86(2):244-250.

The authors of this prospective study of patients with arthrodiastasis (age, > 8 years) assessed the use of a distraction technique across the hip for 4 months. The authors present a preliminary report on the outcomes of this new technique, with final outcomes pending skeletal maturity.

Segev E, Ezra E, Weintrob S, Yaniv M: Treatment of severe late onset Perthes' disease with soft tissue release and articulated hip distraction: Early results. *J Pediatr Orthop B* 2004;13(3):158-165.

In this study, 16 patients with late-onset Legg-Calvé-Perthes disease were surgically treated at an average age of 12 years with soft-tissue release and articulated distraction for 4 to 5 months. With more than a 2-year follow-up, the authors report improved range of motion and decreased pain in all patients.

Wiig O, Terjesen T, Sevenningsen S: Intraobserver reliability of radiographic classification and measurement in the assessment of Perthes. *Acta Orthop Scand* 2002; 73(5):523-530.

The authors of this study assessed the reliability of the Catterall, Salter, Thomson, and Herring lateral pillar classifications. They found that when expert examiners or experienced clinicians were doing the evaluations all the classifications were adequate for assessing the femoral head. However, with less experienced examiners, the Salter, Thomson, and the Herring lateral pillar classifications were more reliable.

Yoon TR, Rowe SM, Chung JY, Song EK, Mulyadi D, Anwar IB: A new innominate osteotomy in Perthes disease. *J Pediatr Orthop* 2003;23(3):363-367.

The authors performed a modification of a Salter innominate osteotomy in 16 hips of 15 patients with Legg-Calvé-Perthes disease. The main benefit of the osteotomy was to provide better stability by changing the direction of the osteotomy, thereby permitting improvement of the center edge angle.

Classic Bibliography

Catterall A: The natural history of Perthes' disease. *J Bone Joint Surg Br* 1971;53:37-53.

Carney BT, Weinstein SL, Noble J: Long-term follow-up with slipped capital femoral epiphysis. *J Bone Joint Surg* 1991;73:667-674.

Loder RT: Unstable slipped capital femoral epiphysis. *J Pediatr Orthop* 2001;21(5):694-699.

Maeda S, Kita A, Funayama K, Kokubun S: Vascular supply to the slipped capital femoral epiphysis. *J Pediatr Orthop* 2001;21(5):664-667.

Seller K, Raab P, Wild A, Kruspe R: Risk benefit analysis in prophylactic pinning in slipped capital femoral epiphysis. *J Pediatr Orthop B* 2001;10(3):192-196.

Chapter 14

Developmental Dysplasia of the Hip and Congenital Coxa Vara

Peter A. DeLuca, MD

Developmental Dysplasia of the Hip

Developmental dysplasia of the hip (DDH) is the most common disorder of the hip in children and remains the musculoskeletal condition that causes the highest level of concern for the pediatric practitioner. A thorough examination of the hips of newborns and infants is the mainstay of early diagnosis; the Pavlik harness is the universal method of treatment.

Terminology

Because DDH may not always be detectable at birth, it is believed that the term "developmental" rather than "congenital" dislocation best describes this condition. The physician should continually monitor the patient for DDH on repeated clinical examinations. The term DDH more accurately reflects the variable presentation of this complex disorder and is intended to encompass the entire spectrum of abnormalities from mild underdevelopment of the newborn hip to stiff nonreducible teratologic hip dislocation.

Dysplasia generally refers to a shallow or underdeveloped acetabulum, whereas subluxation refers to a hip that is not totally reduced or centered. In the perinatal period, such hips may show some degree of instability, excessive mobility, or laxity. However, acetabular dysplasia and subluxation also may be clinically undetectable during childhood and may become symptomatic during adolescence or early adulthood. A hip may be dysplastic but clinically stable, or may show early instability and acceptable acetabular development. When the femoral head is not contained in the acetabulum, it is dislocated and should be detectable in the newborn period (by age 4 to 6 weeks).

The teratologic hip has dislocated in utero and is not reducible on neonatal examination. Patients with a teratologic dislocation of the hip also may have chromosomal abnormalities or neuromuscular conditions such as myelodysplasia and arthrogryposis.

Incidence

The incidence of DDH varies with factors such as gender, age, race, and the definition of the condition. Dysplasia of the hip occurs in approximately 1 in 100 births, whereas frank dislocation is present in 1 to 2 births per 1,000. Late dislocation, subluxation, and acetabular dysplasia are reported in approximately 4 per 10,000 children.

Etiology

Genetic, hormonal, and mechanical factors have all been implicated in the etiology of DDH. It is found more commonly in whites and those of European heritage, whereas the condition is rare in blacks. DDH predominates in the left hip (60%); however, ultrasound or radiographs often confirm involvement of the contralateral hip. Girls are affected by DDH by a ratio of 6:1. Firstborn females presenting breech have the highest risk for DDH at 8%. A family history is a very strong risk factor; essentially all children with DDH share a familial ligamentous laxity. The risk for DDH in subsequent pregnancies is 6% when neither parent has the condition, 12% when one parent has hip dysplasia, and 36% with both an affected parent and child.

Other intrauterine associations appear to implicate restricted environment or abnormal intrauterine positioning as etiologic factors. These factors include being a firstborn child, prematurity, oligohydramnios, congenital recurvatum/dislocation of the knee, congenital muscular torticollis (8% to 17% coexistence), and metatarsus adductus (0 to 10% coexistence). Children with clubfeet do not warrant special screening.

Diagnosis

Neonatal Screening

The value of early diagnosis and prompt treatment of DDH is generally recognized. All infants require clinical screening; only 25% of female infants with clinically detectable hip dysplasia have risk factors. However, routine screening programs based only on clinical examination have had varied success in reducing the delay in discovery of DDH requiring treatment. In a large study, only 60% of unstable hips were clinically detectable at initial examination. Another study in South Australia found that screening infants at birth, before hospital discharge, and again at 6 weeks of age resulted in late presentation of DDH in only 2.4% of all patients. In another study, clinical screening reduced the determination of DDH in patients older than 18 months from 1.2 to 0.2 per 1,000. In a study of patients in Scotland and the Northern and Wessex regions, clinical screening before 3 months of age failed to detect DDH in 70% of patients who eventually required surgery. The literature emphasizes that successful clinical screening programs must be repetitive and continue until the child reaches walking age.

Ulstrasound screening of all newborn hips continues in many countries, although the procedure has not been shown to be cost effective; however, sufficient randomized clinical trials have not been performed. Although very sensitive for detecting abnormalities of the newborn hip, ultrasound has poor specificity in detecting DDH in patients who require treatment. A large 2003 study showed that ultrasound is the most sensitive and effective form of screening; however, it also exposes many unaffected newborns to potential adverse iatrogenic effects. Hips that are found to be unstable on ultrasound screening and in need of treatment are usually clinically evident. Neonatal hips that show immaturity or mild dysplasia but no instability do not benefit from early treatment because more than 95% of such hips spontaneously normalize. One study showed that 21% of neonatal hips (144 of 691) had ultrasound abnormalities but normal clinical examinations. After 6 months, only four infants had DDH requiring treatment, and three of these infants had associated risk factors. As long as a follow-up study is done when the clinician is presented with ultrasound evidence of immaturity or mild dysplasia, any persisting true dysplasia will still successfully respond to treatment.

Although ultrasound evaluations of infants with abnormal physical findings or risk factors have proved beneficial, screening all newborns has not significantly reduced the incidence of late diagnosis of DDH. Also, misinterpretation of ultrasound findings may result in "late" presentations of DDH in those with seemingly "normal" screening ultrasound. Other studies, however, cite a reduction in primary and late surgical procedures.

It is recommended that screening by ultrasound be delayed until age 4 to 6 weeks (or corrected age for premature infants), and performed for selected infants with risk factors for DDH based on patient history (positive family history) and clinical parameters (breech presentation, foot deformity, a persistent "click," or an otherwise asymmetric hip examination). However, in one study, the results of such a "targeted" ultrasound screening program did not reduce the risk of surgery when compared with clinical screening. After 4 to 5 months, radiographic screening replaces ultrasound in the evaluation of patients with suspected hip dysplasia. In infants

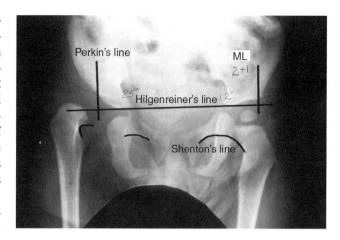

Figure 1 AP radiograph of the pelvis of an infant with a dislocation of the right hip. The ossification center is not visible. Shenton's line, which should be continual from the undersurface of the femoral neck through the upper edge of the obturator foramen (as in the left hip), is "broken" on the right side. The metaphysis lies lateral to the vertical Perkin's line (drawn at the lateral acetabular edge). In normal hips, the ossification center lies below Hilgenreiner's line.

4 to 5 months of age, the ossification center of the femoral head has generally appeared, and the acetabular parameters of importance become more readily defined. High-risk infants (breech birth) should be screened at age 4 to 6 weeks, and the hip stability of infants treated with a Pavlik harness should be followed.

Diagnostic Imaging
In the first 4 months of life, pelvic radiographs have little benefit in the evaluation of the infant with suspected DDH. Prior to ossification of the femoral epiphysis, beginning at approximately 4 months, the cartilaginous structure of the acetabulum and femoral head render radiographic evaluation unreliable in the diagnosis or exclusion of dysplasia or subluxation. Several reference lines (Shenton's, Perkin's and Hilgenreiner's) and angles (acetabular index and center-edge angle) have been shown to be helpful in evaluating the AP radiograph of the infant's pelvis and are useful in the presence of dislocation (Figure 1). Radiographic evaluation also is helpful in evaluating other suspected anomalies of the upper femur (proximal femoral focal deficiency) or spine.

It has been shown that clinically stable hips that show no radiographic subluxation but have an acetabular index higher than normal for age, spontaneously resolve without treatment.

The morphologic approach of hip ultrasonography was introduced to evaluate the infant hip and is used in children younger than 4 months to classify hips based on the degree of femoral head displacement and the degree of acetabular maldevelopment. In this technique, the angle subtended by a vertical reference line through the iliac bone and tangential to the osseous roof of the acetabulum (referred to as the α angle) represents the

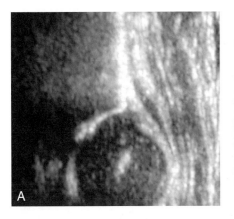 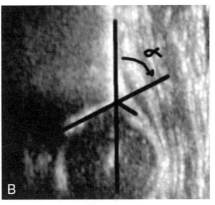 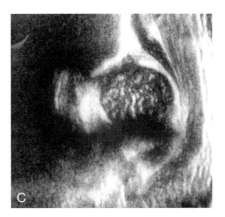

Figure 2 **A**, Hip ultrasound of a normal hip. **B**, The same ultrasound shows that the hip demonstrates greater than 50% coverage (vertical line from the iliac wing). At age 4 to 6 weeks, the α angle should be greater than 60°, and the β angle should be less than 55°. **C**, In a hip ultrasound of a dysplastic hip, the femoral head coverage is approximately 30%, the α angle is 50°, the β angle is 90°, and the labrum is excessively echogenic.

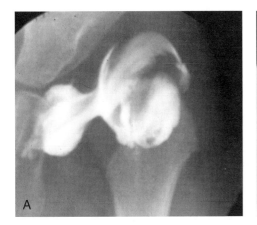 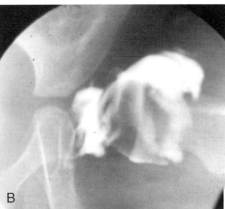

Figure 3 In these hip arthrograms demonstrating blocks to reduction, **A** demonstrates that the psoas tendon is overlying and compressing the capsule and **B** demonstrates that attempted reduction was prohibited superiorly by the thickened labrum (limbus) and inferiorly by the transverse acetabular ligament.

hard bony roof and reflects the depth of the acetabulum. The β angle, subtended by a line drawn through the labrum intersecting the iliac reference line, represents the cartilaginous roof of the acetabulum and indirectly reflects the position of the femoral head (Figure 2). At age 4 to 6 weeks, a normal α angle is ≥ 60° and a normal β angle is < 55°.

Modern ultrasound interpretation generally combines anatomic evaluation and assessment of instability (Dynamic Standard Minimum Examination). In the dynamic method, the joint is evaluated in the transverse plane while being stressed with Barlow and Ortolani maneuvers. Instability of the hip is measured by displacement of the femoral head from the acetabulum. Some physicians believe that the use of ultrasound allows for earlier diagnosis and reduction in the rate and the duration of treatment of DDH. Both techniques have a high degree of interobserver variability and excessive sensitivity may result in possible unnecessary treatment.

Arthrography performed with the patient under general anesthesia is useful in confirming the acceptability (stability and concentricity) of a closed reduction and in diagnosis of the blocks to reduction such as capsular

narrowing and labral hypertrophy (Figure 3). It is not useful in making a diagnosis, but can help in the dynamic evaluation of the hip in preparation for secondary femoral and or pelvic osteotomy performed in patients with residual dysplasia.

Neither CT nor MRI is useful in the diagnosis of DDH. CT has become a standard for confirming hip reduction for a patient in a spica cast following closed or open procedures (Figure 4). Recently, three-dimensional fluoroscopy has been used in a manner similar to CT and is performed in the operating room while the child remains under general anesthesia. After reduction of a dislocated hip and casting, multiple images are obtained using a fluoroscopy unit capable of three-dimensional reconstruction. The position of the femoral head in the acetabulum is realized with coronal images comparable to those generated by CT; the radiation exposure is comparable. Therefore, an inadequate reduction or cast position may be immediately modified without the need to return to the operating room and repeat the administration of a general anesthetic. Both MRI and CT data are useful in providing three-dimensional information for planning later reconstructive procedures such as complex pelvic osteotomy. MRI is useful in the diagnosis of labral tears in older pa-

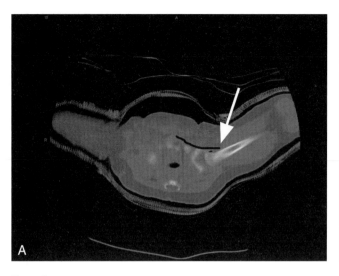

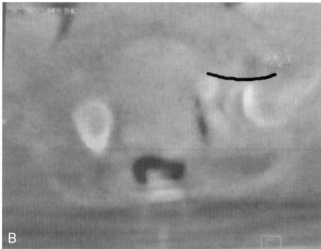

Figure 4 A, CT scan obtained with the patient in a spica cast confirms reduction. The dark line (*arrow*) represents the anterior Shenton's line, which is continual from the anterior femoral neck to the superior pubis. The amount of hip abduction in the cast can be assessed. **B,** Three-dimensional fluoroscopic image obtained with the patient in a spica cast allowed the reduction to be confirmed in the operating room. The dark line represents the anterior Shenton's line. *(Reproduced with permission from* Hip Disorders in Childhood. *London, England, MacKeith Press, 2003.)*

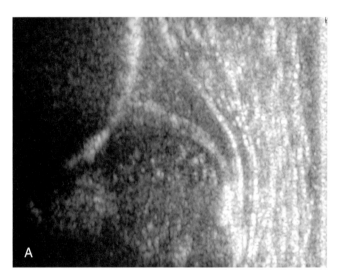

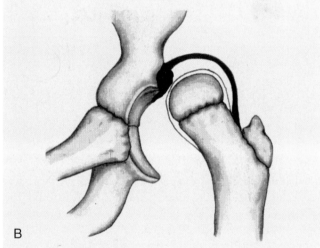

Figure 5 A, Ultrasound of a patient with hip subluxation shows that the femoral head is severely lateralized with poor coverage, the labrum is upturned, and the acetabular edge is flattened. The α and β angles are abnormal. **B,** Illustration of severe subluxation with outward flattening of the labrum and blunting of the lateral acetabular bony edge. *(B is reproduced with permission from* Hip Disorders in Childhood. *London, England, MacKeith Press, 2003.)*

tients presenting with painful dysplasia and a positive labral sign (pain with hip flexion and adduction).

Pathology

Initial instability of the hip may be the result of some combination of maternal and fetal hormonal laxity, genetic (familial) laxity, and intrauterine (and even postnatal) malpositioning. The acetabular anatomy may be normal, immature, or mildly or significantly dysplastic. The longer the femoral head remains in a subluxated or dislocated position, the more likely that progressive change in acetabular anatomy will occur.

The femoral head places pressure on the cartilaginous acetabular rim and labrum, causing it to thicken and become flattened outward. The underlying bony acetabulum also deforms under such pressure and results in an anterolateral edge that is steeper than normal. These findings are evident on ultrasound with increased echogenicity of the labrum and an increase in the α angle (representing the acetabular orientation and a blunting of the lateral edge of the bony acetabulum) (Figure 5).

With the femoral head in a more proximal and lateral position, the hip adductors shorten, producing a clinically evident limitation of hip abduction by the time the infant is approximately 3 to 4 months of age (Figure 6). The femur also assumes a foreshortened position (Galeazzi sign) (Figure 7).

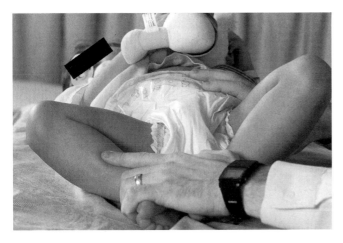

Figure 6 Photograph showing limited abduction resulting from shortening of the hip adductors in a pediatric patient with a subluxated or dislocated hip.

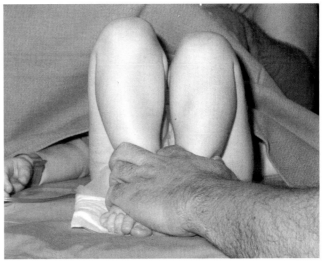

Figure 7 Photograph of a patient demonstrating the Galeazzi sign (a foreshortened left hip resulting from dislocation).

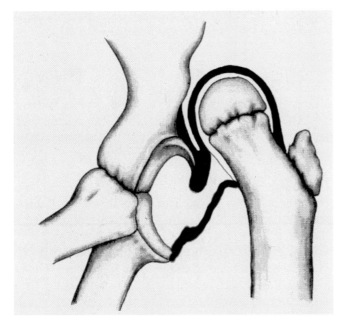

Figure 8 Illustration of dislocation with superior positioning of the femoral head, thickening and infolding of the labrum (limbus), capsular constriction, and upward pull of the transverse acetabular ligament.

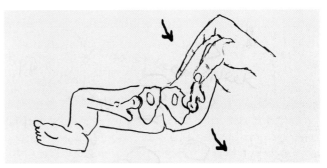

Figure 9 Illustration of the Barlow maneuver. The hip is flexed, adducted, and pushed posteriorly and laterally in the direction of the arrows. *(Adapted with permission from* Hip Disorders in Childhood. *London, England, MacKeith Press, 2003.)*

Presentation and Diagnosis

In the neonatal period (0 to 3 months), instability of the hip is the predominant feature and allows for the clinical diagnosis. A hip that is reduced at rest may be subluxated or even dislocated by the Barlow maneuver of adduction, flexion, and posterior pressure. After the force is released, the hip returns to a reduced position (Figure 9). Such a finding is described as a "Barlow positive hip." Concurrent acetabular dysplasia may or may not be present. The instability shown by these hips is the result of inherent collagen laxity in combination with maternal and fetal relaxing hormones. As the hormonal influences diminish, stability generally returns and the Barlow test becomes negative by 2 to 3 weeks of age. However, acetabular dysplasia may remain and may require treatment.

Many dislocated hips can be reduced back into the acetabulum by abducting and lifting the thigh forward (Figure 10). This maneuver elicits a clinically detectable feel of rapid acceleration and deceleration as the femoral head returns into the socket, in the sensation of a

With progression to dislocation, the labrum becomes infolded and thickened under the pressure of the femoral head, gradually closing down the superior and posterior acetabulum (Figure 8). The inferior transverse acetabular ligament pulls upward, blocking the lower opening to the acetabulum. As these two structures approximate, they create an obstacle to reduction of the femoral head back into the acetabulum. Over time, the psoas tendon presses on the underlying capsule causing it to constrict into an "hourglass" configuration (Figure 3). If treatment is begun before this occurrence, there is a high probability of achieving a successful reduction. The longer the dislocation persists, the more resistant it becomes to reduction.

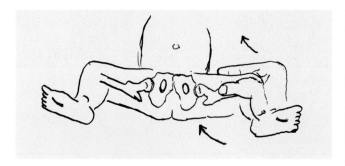

Figure 10 Illustration of the Ortolani maneuver. The dislocated hip reduces with abduction and a lifting of the proximal femur anteriorly in the direction of the arrows. *(Adapted with permission from* Hip Disorders in Childhood. *London, England, MacKeith Press, 2003.)*

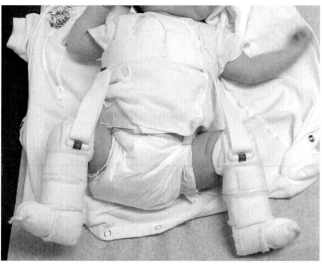

Figure 11 Photograph of a pediatric patient with a Pavlik harness in the correct position; the hips are flexed at just greater than 90°. *(Reproduced with permission from* Hip Disorders in Childhood. *London, England, MacKeith Press, 2003.)*

"clunk." This sensation has been misnamed by some examiners as a "click"; this term is actually more applicable to the benign high-pitched sounds frequently elicited at abduction. A dislocated hip that reduces is best termed an "Ortolani positive hip" and is usually accompanied by a variable degree of acetabular maldevelopment.

The Galeazzi or Allis test is positive in patients with severe subluxation or dislocation. With the hips flexed up 90°, the observer will note a decrease in height of the involved knee (Figure 7).

In the infant older than 3 months, the signs of instability become less distinct, whereas limitation of motion and apparent limb shortening predominate. The dislocated or subluxated side will develop tightness of the hip adductors and limited, asymmetric abduction. In patients with bilateral involvement, the asymmetry may be absent (including a positive Galeazzi test), and the decrease in normal spread of the hips may be the only sign. However, when present as an isolated finding, limitation of hip abduction is fairly nonspecific, with only 18% of patients positive for DDH. A recent study showed that unilateral limitation of hip abduction was more sensitive than bilateral limitation in the diagnosis of DDH requiring treatment. Parental or family reports of an infant's unusual leg positions or crawling difficulties warrant investigation.

In the toddler, restricted motion and asymmetries remain, and a Trendelenburg limp from hip abductor weakness may be evident. In patients with bilateral DDH, a waddling gait and hyperlordotic posture may be seen. Adolescents have these findings and may also report fatigue, instability, or pain in the hip, thigh, or knee.

Treatment

For the infant with a Barlow positive hip, if the ultrasound at 4 to 6 weeks is normal (α angle $\geq 60°$, β angle $< 55°$, and no evidence of instability on stress views) and the instability has resolved, the child does not require treatment or radiographic follow-up. However, serial clinical examinations of the hips should continue by the primary care physician until the child reaches walking age. The treatment of the dysplastic and unstable hip should be differentiated from that of the truly dislocated hip.

Dysplasia

From the neonatal period until 6 months of age, if ultrasound shows acetabular pathology (abnormal α or β angles) or persistent subluxation, treatment with a Pavlik harness should begin and progress should be monitored with serial ultrasound studies every 4 to 6 weeks (Figure 11). The Pavlik harness is designed to maintain hip flexion and limit adduction. The harness has anterior adjustable straps that are set to keep the hips flexed approximately 100°. Excessive flexion and tight diapering must be avoided because they may cause femoral nerve palsy. The posterior straps allow for a gentle encouragement of abduction. They should be loose enough to allow two to three finger breadths between the knees when the knees are held flexed and adducted. Prevention of forced abduction helps to minimize the complication of osteonecrosis.

When ultrasound parameters become normal, the child is weaned from the harness over a period of 3 to 4 weeks. Pavlik harness treatment of the neonate with acetabular dysplasia is more than 90% successful. After 4 to 6 months of age, follow-up is continued with AP radiographs through the growing years. There is a 10% risk of recurrence of deformity that necessitates follow-up to maturity.

In the child older than 6 months with hip subluxation, the Pavlik harness is generally not strong enough

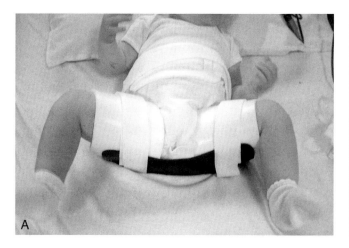 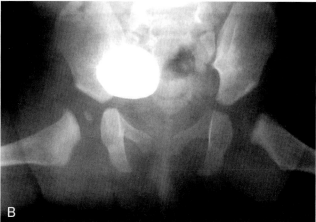

Figure 12 **A,** Photograph of a pediatric patient with a fixed hip abduction orthosis. **B,** Radiograph of the same patient in the hip abduction orthosis shows a left dysplastic hip with excellent position maintained in the brace.

to maintain hip flexion and limit adduction, and either casting or a fixed abduction orthosis is more appropriate. The later device can be used for a child of walking age as treatment for residual acetabular dysplasia (Figure 12).

Dislocaiion

The hip that is Ortolani positive (reducible dislocation) in a child younger than 2 months of age also may be treated in a Pavlik harness. However, the child should be reexamined weekly to ensure that the hip has reduced, and ultrasound should be used to confirm the clinical impression. The most common pitfall of treatment with the Pavlik harness is failure to obtain reduction, which is often compounded by nonrecognition of failure. Once the hip becomes stable, it is managed by the protocol described for treating dysplasia.

Treatment with the Pavlik harness is effective in achieving reduction of a reducible dislocation in more than 85% of patients. The incidence of osteonecrosis is low (< 5%) particularly when treatment is initiated in the first 3 months of life. Risk factors for an adverse outcome using the harness include an inability to reduce the hip (negative Ortolani dislocation) before application of the device, bilateralism, and patient age (older than 7 weeks) when treatment is started. Ultrasound results have a prognostic value because an initially irreducible hip with initial coverage of less than 20% will not be successfully treated with the Pavlik harness. After successful treatment with a Pavlik harness, 2% to 3% of hips will show evidence of persistent severe late dysplasia with a center-edge angle of less than 15°.

An Ortolani negative dislocation may be briefly treated in a Pavlik harness; however, if reduction is not achieved and confirmed by ultrasound in 2 to 3 weeks, treatment must be abandoned in favor of closed reduction or other methods. Continuation of the harness be-

yond this period increases the risk of worsening the acetabular dysplasia. The Pavlik harness is not appropriate for a teratologic dislocation.

Closed Reduction

Closed reduction is the preferred method of treatment in children 18 months of age or younger provided it can be achieved without undue force. However, treatment can be protracted in children older than 12 months of age and secondary femoral or acetabular procedures are frequently required to address residual deformity.

The use of preliminary traction for 3 to 4 weeks before attempting closed reduction is becoming less accepted. It was believed that traction diminished the incidence of osteonecrosis and increased the success of closed reduction. However, recent studies have not supported this belief. Traction did reduce the incidence of osteonecrosis in an era when forceful reduction and extreme cast positions prevailed. Education in the use of gentler reduction and casting techniques (avoiding forced abduction, excessive internal rotation and flexion, and use of adductor tenotomy) may be the actual cause of a reduction in iatrogenic complications.

Some authors have advocated delaying reduction of a dislocated hip until the ossific nucleus has appeared, to reduce the risk of osteonecrosis. However, a recent study has suggested that although waiting may result in a slight reduction in the incidence of osteonecrosis, it more than doubles the incidence for future surgery. Fewer secondary reconstructive procedures were performed on children whose hips were reduced at younger than 6 months of age.

Closed reduction of the hip should be performed with the patient under general anesthesia and with arthrographic evaluation. Closed reduction is often unsuccessful because there is a failure to recognize obstacles to reduction which may exist even when the sensation

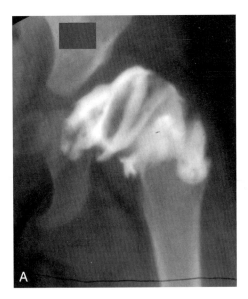
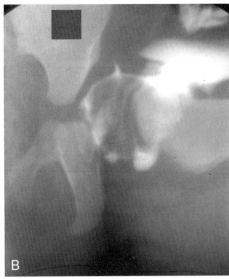

Figure 13 Hip arthrograms show the hip dislocated with excessive medial contrast pooling **(A)** and the hip reduced and mimicking the position in a cast **(B)**; no significant medial contrast pooling is evident in B, and congruous reduction was achieved without soft-tissue interposition.

of successful reduction (Ortolani sign) is present. The quality of the reduction is confirmed by arthrography and objectively defined by the width of the contrast column remaining between the femoral head and acetabulum and the status of the limbus (Figure 13). Although minimal residual contrast between the femoral head and acetabulum is desired, hips with less than 5 mm of contrast and those in which the limbus is not interposed typically have a favorable outcome. The stability of the reduction in abduction/adduction, flexion/extension, internal/external rotation (stable zone) and the safe zone are determined. The stable zone is defined as the difference between maximum abduction of the hip and the minimal amount of abduction before the hip dislocates. The safe zone is generally 15° less than the limits of the motion defined in the stable zone. In this range, the hip is safe from excessive abduction that may cause osteonecrosis and adduction that may allow dislocation. If the adductors are tight, the safe zone can be increased with percutaneous adductor longus tenotomy. With a definition of what position is both safe and stable for the particular infant being treated, the reduction is maintained in a bilateral hip spica cast. The hips are maintained in the "human position" which is considered to be flexion of 90° to 100° and abduction of less than 60° (Figure 14).

The reduction of the hip in the cast must be confirmed. Although ultrasound and MRI have been used for this purpose, the current standard is with CT, which can be performed using selective views and with radiation exposure as low as plain radiography (Figure 4, *A*). Intraoperative three-dimensional fluoroscopy has recently been used to confirm reduction (Figure 4, *B*); however, this type of fluoroscopy unit is not readily available. Cast immobilization is continued for approximately 3 to 4 months, with a cast change at approxi-

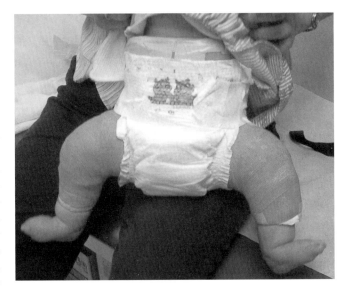

Figure 14 Photograph of a child in a fiberglass spica cast. The strength of the fiberglass obviates the need for a spreader bar. The hips are flexed at 90° and abducted at 50°.

mately 6 weeks. If the reduction is deemed stable clinically and on radiographs, removable abduction bracing is used until the acetabulum normalizes.

Open Reduction

If concentric closed reduction cannot be achieved or when excessive abduction (> 60°) is required to maintain a hip reduction, open reduction is performed. Approximately 3.6% of instances of DDH, although clinically detected before 3 months of age, will still require surgery.

The purpose of open reduction is to remove the obstacles to reduction and/or safely increase its stability. The most commonly used approaches include the anterior and some variation of a medial approach. Each ap-

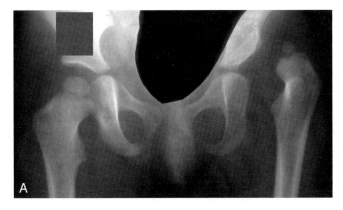
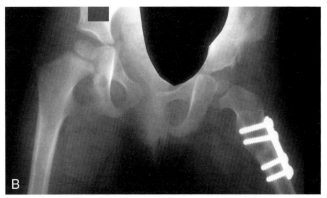

Figure 15 **A,** Preoperative radiograph of a child (age, 1 year 7 months) with a high-riding left hip dislocation. **B,** Postoperative radiograph of the same child after being treated with open reduction through an anterior approach and femoral shortening derotation osteotomy fixed with a four-hole compression plate.

proach carries its own indications, limitations, and contraindications. Intraoperative arthrography is helpful in defining the specific anatomic blocks to reduction and choosing the best approach to successful reduction.

Variations of the medial adductor approach of Ludloff are useful in children younger than 18 months and provide direct access to all of the primary obstacles to reduction of the hip except an infolded or hypertrophic labrum. In the anteromedial approach, the interval is anterior to the adductor brevis and either anterior or posterior to the pectineus, whereas in the posteromedial approach, the plane of dissection is behind the adductor brevis. The medial approach allows for release of tight adductors that limit abduction, release of the psoas tendon overlying and narrowing the capsule, and opening of a tight capsule and transaction of the transverse acetabular ligament. Attention to labral pathology and performing a capsulorrhaphy are not possible via this approach. The medial approach is generally not acceptable in the older child of walking age, and in those in whom the dislocation is believed to be high riding with a labral block to reduction. It is contraindicated in the teratologic hip and in patients in whom acetabular deformity warrants pelvic osteotomy.

The anterior approach between the sartorius and tensor fascia lata muscles is a more utilitarian approach for patients of any age and in all anatomic situations. It is preferred in children older than 18 months of age and is generally required in any dislocation in which the hip cannot be brought to the level of the acetabulum manually, such as with a long-standing or teratologic dislocation. The acetabulum is directly accessible and any blocks to concentric reduction can be removed. Capsulorrhaphy is readily achieved, thus providing more immediate stability than in the medial approach. If required, pelvic osteotomy may be done through the same incision. The risks of osteonecrosis and recurrent subluxation or dislocation do not differ significantly between the two approaches.

Femoral osteotomy is a useful adjunct to anterior open reduction, especially in the older child. In patients with a high-riding dislocation, excessive tension may be found after reducing the hip and may jeopardize stability and increase the risk of cartilage pressure and osteonecrosis. Femoral shortening subtrochanteric osteotomy (generally 1 to 2 cm) is useful in such patients to reduce soft-tissue contractures. If excessive anteversion is present and necessitates extreme internal rotation to maintain reduction, femoral derotational osteotomy is beneficial. The femur is approached through a separate lateral approach, and fixation is provided by a four-hole, one third tubular plate or phalangeal or metacarpal compression plate (Figure 15). In the older child, if coxa valga is believed to be a secondary condition, the osteotomy is performed in the intertrochanteric area and fixed with a blade plate or pediatric hip screw.

Secondary Procedures

In children older than 2 years, secondary bony femoral and/or acetabular pathology frequently demands simultaneous open reduction, femoral derotational shortening osteotomy, and redirectional osteotomy of the innominate bone to achieve and maintain concentric reduction and minimize the risk of osteonecrosis. In some studies, the risk of osteonecrosis appears to be higher when open reduction and pelvic osteotomy are performed simultaneously. Other studies, however, have determined that open reduction and concurrent innominate osteotomy can be done safely and with superior results compared with open reduction alone or open reduction followed by delayed innominate osteotomy.

Following a successful primary reduction of the hip (especially in the older child), persistent acetabular dysplasia or subluxation can occur. Biologic remodeling may be incomplete when residual bony abnormalities such as persistent femoral anteversion or significant acetabular dysplasia are present.

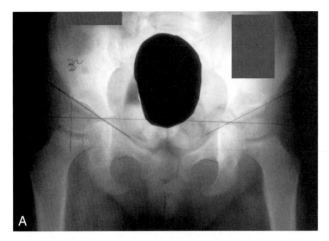

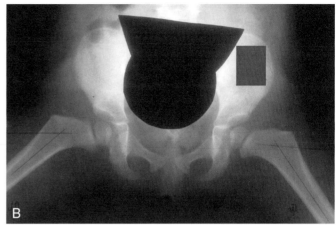

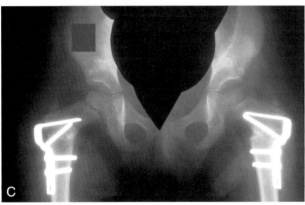

Figure 16 **A,** Preoperative radiograph of a child of walking age with persistent hip dysplasia. The right hip with more severe dysplasia with 40% has uncoverage of the femoral head. Both hips show widened medial tear drops. **B,** Abduction and internal rotation radiograph shows that the hips move to center well; the abduction shown here is much greater than what is necessary clinically. **C,** Postoperative radiograph of the same patient after bilateral varus derotation osteotomies were performed.

Acetabular remodeling is most efficient in the first 6 to 12 months following reduction of the hip; the potential for improvement depends on the amount of acetabular growth remaining. Remodeling is most predictable in children younger than 4 years of age, yet less predictable in children between 4 and 8 years. After 8 years of age, remodeling cannot be relied on and acetabular redirectional osteotomy is required. Secondary femoral and pelvic osteotomy to treat residual dysplasia should be performed before age 8 to achieve the best radiologic results with the fewest complications.

Femoral Osteotomy

Femoral derotational osteotomy is used to correct excessive femoral anteversion in conjunction with open reduction in older children if internal rotation position is found to improve hip stability. This avoids extreme casting position and removes excessive anteversion as a possible cause of delayed remodeling or subluxation. In patients younger than 4 years of age, derotation of the femur is successful in the treatment of residual acetabular dysplasia following previous successful reduction. Preoperative planning radiographs should show improvement of reduction on an abduction-internal rotation supervised view (Figure 16).

Pelvic Osteotomy

Pelvic osteotomy may be performed at the time of primary open or closed reduction of the hip to offer immediate improvement of associated acetabular dysplasia or may be done later to treat residual dysplasia. In the child older than 24 months, an isolated innominate osteotomy may be done to reduce a portion of the dysplasia and allow for the reduced hip to stimulate correction of the remainder of the deformity. The older the child is at the time of initial treatment, the less time there is for biologic factors to act and correct preexisting acetabular deformity.

There are two general types of pelvic osteotomy: reconstructive and salvage. Reconstructive osteotomies redirect or reshape the roof of the acetabulum with its normal hyaline cartilage into a more appropriate weight-bearing position. The goal of such procedures is to decrease any obliquity present in the weight-bearing portion of the acetabulum and to increase the coverage of the femoral head. In salvage procedures, weight-bearing coverage is increased by using the joint capsule as an interposition between the femoral head and bone above it.

Reconstructive Osteotomies

There are two types of reconstructive osteotomies: redirectional and reshaping. A prerequisite to a reconstruc-

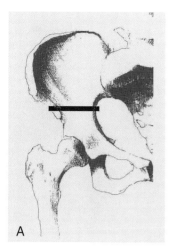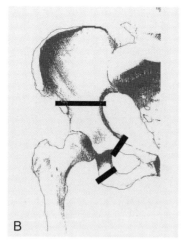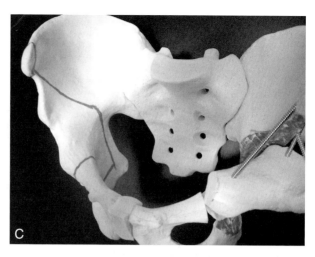

Figure 17 Illustrations of various redirectional pelvic osteotomies. **A,** Illustration of the Salter innominate osteotomy, which is an osteotomy (*bar*) through the ilium just superior to the inferior iliac spine and into the sciatic notch; the fragment rotates forward, outward, and down, hinging on the triradiate cartilage. **B,** Illustration of the Steele triple osteotomy with cuts (*bars*) as in the Salter innominate osteotomy as well as pubis and ischial cuts. Variations include inferior cuts made closer to the acetabulum (Tonnis) or a single cut made close to the symphysis (Sutherland). **C,** Model representation showing the cuts made for a Ganz periacetabular osteotomy. The pubis is cut as in the Salter innominate osteotomy and the Steele triple osteotomy, but the iliac and ischial cuts remain anterior to the sciatic notch and leave the pelvic ring intact.

tive pelvic osteotomy is that the hip must be reduced in a concentric and congruous fashion, or must be capable of reduction to a congruous state. The hip must also have a near normal range of motion. Coverage and congruence can be simulated on plain radiographs, by arthrography, or with three-dimensional CT reconstruction. CT evaluation can show abnormalities of the acetabulum such as retroversion, which may require correction. In the adolescent patient, priorities include a horizontal weight-bearing surface, adequate coverage of the weight-bearing portion of the femoral head, and maintenance of the cartilage space.

Redirectional Osteotomies

All redirectional osteotomies involve a transection of the ilium superior to the acetabulum with or without additional cuts through the pelvis depending on the type and amount of correction required. The Salter innominate osteotomy is an ideal choice when there is limited coverage of the anterolateral portion of the femoral head because of deficiency of the anterolateral acetabulum (Figure 17, *A*). The acetabulum rotates forward, outward, and down hinging on the symphysis pubis and can be expected to provide about 20° to 25° of lateral coverage and approximately 10° to 15° of anterior coverage. The Salter innominate osteotomy is also successful in adolescents and young adults. In older patients who may have limited mobility of the symphysis pubis or who need additional coverage, the Steele triple innominate osteotomy or one of the technically demanding periacetabular osteotomies may be more effective. The Steele triple innominate osteotomy involves additional osteotomies of the ischium and pubis (Figure 17, *B*). Because the sciatic notch is destabilized, the Salter

and Steele osteotomies require internal fixation of the ilium, generally with a threaded Steinmann pin or screws. The Ganz periacetabular osteotomy is the most technically demanding osteotomy of the pelvis. It involves osteotomies of the pubis, ilium, and ischium, and a vertical osteotomy of the posterior column of the acetabulum approximately 1 cm anterior to the sciatic notch, connecting the iliac and ischial cuts. This osteotomy allows for significant mobility of the acetabulum and, because the osteotomy does not violate the sciatic notch, it is quite stable. The cuts required for this osteotomy cross the triradiate cartilage, and it is contraindicated in children in whom this structure is open. In the adolescent and young adult patient this osteotomy is excellent in maximizing femoral head coverage as well as allowing medial translation of the hip joint center (Figure 17, *C*).

Reshaping Osteotomies

The Pemberton and Dega procedures involve incomplete cuts through the pericapsular portion of the innominate bone and allow for a change in the configuration of the acetabulum by hinging the periacetabular segment through the triradiate cartilage. Unlike the Salter osteotomy, these osteotomies decrease the volume of the acetabulum and are appropriate for a capacious or shallow acetabulum in children between 2 and 10 years of age. Because these osteotomies do not enter the sciatic notch, they are stable and do not require internal fixation. In the Pemberton osteotomy, the inner and outer tables of the ilium are divided, beginning laterally about one fourth inch above the joint capsule (Figure 18). By adjusting the orientation of the cuts through the inner and outer tables of the innominate

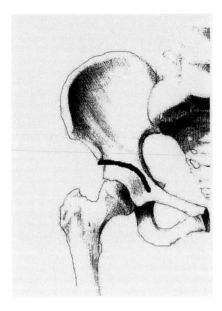

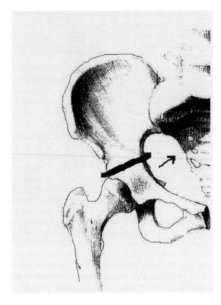

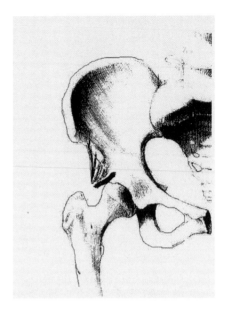

Figure 18 Illustration of the reshaping pelvic osteotomy in which the osteotomy (*curved bar*) at the level of the inferior spine is curved inferiorly toward the triradiate cartilage. (With the Pemberton variation, the cut involves both the inner and outer tables, whereas the Dega variation predominantly involves the outer table.)

Figure 19 Illustration of the Chiari osteotomy in which the iliac osteotomy (*bar*) is begun just above the acetabular margin and angled 15° upward (*arrow*) toward the sciatic notch. The distal fragment is mobilized medially, rotating on the symphysis. Frequently, anterior bone grafting is required.

Figure 20 Illustration of the shelf procedure for which various techniques have been described for adding lateral coverage over the capsule in patients with subluxation, shallow acetabulum, or coxa magna.

bone, the amount of anterior and lateral augmentation provided by the osteotomy is modified. The cut through the cancellous portion of the innominate bone is extended to a point just above the ilioischial limb of the triradiate cartilage. The posterior limb is ideally positioned halfway between the sciatic notch and the posterior margin of the acetabulum. In the Dega procedure, osteotomy is performed only through the outer table of the ilium. In both procedures, the bone inferior to the osteotomy and above the acetabulum is slowly bent downward, changing the direction of the acetabulum and decreasing its volume. The Dega procedure can correct the acetabular index by 20°. Allograft wedges can provide for successful stability and fusion and have use in limited approaches for reshaping osteotomies.

Salvage Procedures

When the hip cannot be reduced congruently and does not meet the criteria for a reconstructive osteotomy, a salvage procedure may be indicated. The intent of these osteotomies is to reduce point loading at the edge of the acetabulum by medialization of the hip center, increasing the weight-bearing surface of the hip with an extra-articular buttress of bone positioned over the subluxated femoral head, with reliance on fibrocartilaginous metaplasia of the interposed joint capsule to provide an articulating surface. In the Chiari osteotomy, the acetabulum is medially displaced along the plane of the osteotomy by abducting the hip and rotation through the pubic symphysis (Figure 19). The extent of coverage is deter-

mined by the amount of displacement of the acetabulum, which is ultimately dependent on the width of ilium at the level of the osteotomy. With stable internal fixation, spica cast immobilization can be avoided. A recent long-term study showed favorable results with the Chiari osteotomy for adults younger than 30 years of age who had low-grade osteoarthritis, a spherical or ovoid femoral head, and in whom the osteotomy provided full coverage. In the shelf procedure, augmented coverage of the femoral head is achieved by creating a buttress with strips of corticocancellous bone, which are placed in a slot created along the rim of the acetabulum and expanded in layers (Figure 20). Depending on the stability of the shelf, cast immobilization may be necessary.) When performed in patients younger than 25 years of age with acetabular dysplasia or subluxation and early osteoarthritis, a shelf procedure produced good results in 87% of patients at follow-up of more than 20 years.

Complications
Failed Reduction

Redislocation following closed reduction is not uncommon and usually can be treated by repeat closed methods or open reduction. However, redislocation following open reduction is a major complication. Factors that predispose the initial open reduction to failure are usually the result of an incomplete initial procedure and include failure to identify the true acetabulum, inadequate inferior capsular release, inadequate capsulorrhaphy, and simultaneous performance of femoral or pelvic osteotomy causing posterior subluxation or dislocation. Repeat open reduction and/or revision of the femoral or pelvic osteotomy are virtually always necessary to address this complication. A recent study reported on the successful use of the anteromedial approach to reduce recurrent hip dislocations. This approach provides access to anteromedial capsular constriction and a potentially inverted transverse acetabular ligament. The rate of osteonecrosis associated with repeat open reduction is higher, and the results of surgery are generally worse than with primary treatment.

Osteonecrosis

Osteonecrosis is a complication of the treatment of DDH and occurs with every form of treatment, including the Pavlik harness. The causes of osteonecrosis are believed to be excessive pressure on the femoral head or compression of the extrinsic blood supply of the femoral epiphysis. The prevalence of osteonecrosis is the same following open or closed reduction and ranges from 10% to 40%. Rates of osteonecrosis as high as 27% have been reported with the use of the medial approach. Treatment factors implicated in the occurrence of osteonecrosis include immobilization in excessive abduction, failure of prior closed treatment, and revision for failed reduction. Based on a recent study, there appears to be no difference in the risk of developing osteonecrosis following open or closed reduction for DDH relative to the presence or absence of the femoral ossific nucleus.

The criteria for diagnosis of osteonecrosis include failure of appearance or growth of the ossific nucleus within 1 year following reduction of the hip, broadening of the femoral neck over a similar period, increased radiographic density and subsequent fragmentation of the epiphysis, and residual deformity of the femoral head and neck after ossification is complete. The various classifications of osteonecrosis are conceptually similar in attempting to separate mild cases, which affect only a portion of the epiphysis and rarely cause clinical problems, from more severe patterns, which affect the physis, may alter growth, and often lead to severe deformity of the femoral head and neck.

The treatment of osteonecrosis is dictated by the pattern of involvement and resultant deformity of the hip. In young children with osteonecrosis, acetabular redirection should be considered at the first sign of subluxation. Proximal femoral varus osteotomy may be indicated to manage subluxation associated with coxa valga. Trochanteric epiphysiodesis (in children younger than 8 years of age) or distal lateral transfer of the greater trochanter (in children 8 years of age and older) may be necessary to correct coxa breva and the abductor insufficiency associated with elevation of the greater trochanter. Contralateral distal femoral epiphysiodesis is occasionally needed to treat limb-length inequality.

Natural History

Failure of acetabular remodeling following reduction of a congenital dislocation is a concern for the development of early osteoarthritis. In one study, an acetabular index of greater than 35° at 2 years following reduction had an 80% probability of a resultant Severin III or IV hip, which is predictive for the need for total hip arthroplasty. Persistent acetabular dysplasia alone does not correlate with later complications, but in association with hip subluxation results in an increased risk of degenerative arthritis. Subluxation, with abnormal head-acetabular forces leads to early overload of cartilage and painful osteoarthritis. Such hips may have a worse prognosis than hips that remain frankly dislocated. High-riding dislocations left untreated from birth, where the femoral head rests within a muscular bed and away from bony contact, may be well tolerated for up to 30 to 40 years before causing pain. However, such patients are affected by Trendelenburg gait with fatigue because of muscle insufficiency, increased lumbar lordosis (sometimes painful), and limitation in hip flexibility. Valgus deformity of the knee also develops. Unilateral persistent dislocations are less well tolerated because of relative limb-length inequality and pelvic obliquity. In general, successful outcome for treatment of the congenitally dislocated hip correlates with the preoperative grade of hip dislocation, the development of osteonecrosis, and the adequacy of reduction.

In young patients who have pain associated with hip dysplasia, a labral tear should be considered. Most patients with a labral tear may have a structural hip abnormality that is detectable on plain radiographs. Preparation for secondary femoral or pelvic osteotomies in such a clinical setting should include evaluation for labral tears with either arthrography or magnetic resonance arthrography.

Missed Cases of DDH

Missed cases of DDH continue to occur for several reasons. The initial signs of laxity (Ortolani, Barlow) are short lived, and in some instances may be clinically undetectable, even in the presence of dysplasia. Residual dysplasia may be present but the examinations may not show findings until the subluxation becomes pronounced. The examination may be performed in a timely fashion at each well-child visit, but the examiner may lack sufficient experience to appreciate the diagnosis. The child may not return for follow-up examinations, or examination may be sidetracked when the child is seen for episodic medical maladies. In patients referred for ultrasound, the diagnosis may be inaccurate because of a poorly performed or misinterpreted study.

Congenital Coxa Vara

Congenital coxa vara is usually present at birth; patients with congenital coxa vara typically present with a proximal femoral neck-shaft angle of less than 120°. Congenital coxa vara is believed to be the result of a primary limb bud ossification defect or an intrauterine mechanical or metabolic process affecting the physis. It has also been referred to as infantile coxa vara. Congenital coxa vara is commonly associated with a limb-length discrepancy caused by shortening or bowing of the femur.

Incidence

Congenital coxa vara occurs much less frequently than DDH, with rates of 1 per 13,000 to 25,000 persons reported. The right and left sides are equally involved in patients with congenital coxa vara, and this disorder has no gender preference. Bilateral involvement is seen in one third of patients. Congenital coxa vara may be more common in African Americans than Caucasians.

Differential Diagnosis

Other congenital conditions associated with a varus deformity of the proximal femur include proximal femoral focal deficiency, congenital short femur, and congenital bowed femur. Skeletal dysplasias include Morquio's disease, Schmid metaphyseal chondrodysplasia, cleidocranial dysostosis, and metaphyseal dysostosis and have concurrent radiographic abnormalities other than the isolated coxa vara of congenital coxa vara. Schmid metaphyseal chondrodysplasia includes coxa vara with femoral bowing, sclerosis and splaying of the ribs, diffuse metaphyseal flaring, and irregularity most pronounced at the knees. Patterson-Lowry rhizomelic dysplasia is characterized by short humeri, coxa vara with proximal femoral epiphyseal involvement, and short metacarpals, metatarsals, and phalanges.

Acquired types of coxa vara result from metabolic disturbance caused by rickets, fibrous dysplasia, or proximal physeal injury resulting from trauma or sepsis. Coxa vara from proximal femoral growth arrest has been described in a population that had neonatal extracorporeal membrane oxygenation. These patients presented with a progressive gait disturbance and pain, limb-length discrepancy, and limited abduction.

A developmental variety of isolated coxa vara has been described in two patients with normal findings on radiographs of the hips at birth and radiographic evidence of coxa vara by age 2 to 3 years.

Etiology

The most widely accepted theory concerning the etiology of congenital coxa vara is that physiologic shearing stresses (applied during weight bearing) cause fatigue of this area of dystrophic bone, resulting in progressive varus deformity. Biomechanically in patients with congenital coxa vara, the vertical orientation of the proximal femoral physis converts the normal compressive force across the physis (which is a lateral tension and medial compression force) to a greater shear force as well as increases the compressive forces across the medial femoral neck. In many patients, a separate triangular fragment involving the inferomedial aspect of the femoral neck is found and may be a response to this shift in forces. Some studies suggest that the triangular metaphyseal fragment reflects a Salter-Harris type II separation pattern through the defective femoral neck. The epiphysis and attached triangular fragment slip from the normal superoanterior portion of the femoral neck in an inferoposterior direction.

The abnormal load of the varus hip may lead to a progressive inclination of the proximal femoral epiphyseal plate, foreshortening of the neck of the femur, and associated trochanteric overgrowth. No true slippage of the epiphysis has been found. These changes may progress until surgery restores more appropriate biomechanical forces.

Clinical Presentation

Patients with congenital coxa vara usually present between walking age and 5 years of age with gait abnormalities such as limp, waddling (bilateral), or Trendelenburg gait (unilateral). They are usually pain free. Examination may show a leg-length inequality (1.5 to 4 cm) with foreshortening of the femur. Abduction strength may be decreased because of a decreased articulotrochanteric distance. Hip internal rotation may be decreased as the result of a decreased femoral anteversion or retroversion of the femoral head on the femoral neck.

Diagnostic Imaging

Radiographs demonstrate varus of the proximal femur (neck shaft angle, ≤ 90°), a shortened femoral neck, a more vertical orientation of the physis, and in some patients a triangular segment of the medial femoral metaphysis that projects with an inverted Y-shaped lucency. The femoral head may be mildly flattened, the acetabulum have an oval appearance, and some patients with severe progressive coxa vara may develop a compensatory ipsilateral genu valgum.

Radiographic evaluation of other joints (for example, the knee and the wrist) or the spine is helpful in differentiating other causes of coxa vara, such as skeletal dysplasia, fibrous dysplasia, spondyloepiphyseal dysplasia, and rickets.

CT scanning, especially with three-dimensional reconstruction, may be helpful in preoperative planning. MRI is not useful in the diagnosis of coxa vara or for surgical planning.

Surgical Indications

Measurement of the Hilgenreiner epiphyseal angle (HEA) is pivotal in the management of patients with

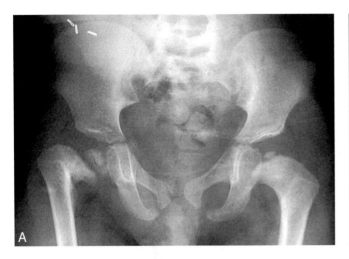 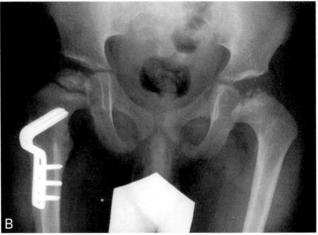

Figure 21 A, Preoperative radiograph of a pediatric patient with congenital coxa vara of the right hip shows a neck-shaft angle of 80° and a Hilgenreiner's epiphyseal angle of 60°. A small medial neck triangular region is united with the femoral neck in this patient, but is frequently a separate section. **B,** Postoperative radiograph of the same patient after undergoing valgus osteotomy fixed with a blade plate. The Hilgenreiner's epiphyseal angle is restored to within normal range.

congenital coxa vara. The HEA is the angle subtended by the horizontal Hilgenreiner's line through the triradiate cartilages and an oblique line through the proximal femoral capital physes. The HEA has been shown to have wide variation in normal patients, but in children younger than 7 years it averages 20° (range, 4° to 35°); from age 8 years to maturity it averages 8° (Figure 21, *A*).

In children with congenital coxa vara and an HEA less than 45°, the deformity frequently spontaneously resolves, whereas children with an HEA greater than 60° tend to progress and require surgery. Patients with an HEA between 45° and 60° represent a gray zone and require serial radiographic examination. If the HEA in this range progresses, surgery is indicated. It has also been suggested that rather than using Hilgenreiner's line, which can change with pelvic obliquity secondary to an associated limb-length inequality, a horizontal line parallel to the ground can be referenced. Values for congenital coxa vara average 40° to 70°, but may be as high as 70° to 90°.

Surgical Treatment

The general principles of surgery for patients with congenital coxa vara include correction of the HEA to less than 35° and restoration of the proximal femoral neck-shaft angle to a normal range (130° to 135°), correction of femoral version to a more normal range, and restoration of abduction with adductor tenotomy if needed. The goals of such correction are to restore the normal biomechanical forces across the hip to allow for healing of the abnormal inferomedial femoral neck and restoration of normal abductor strength; the latter will correct disturbances of gait. The restoration of the HEA more strongly correlates with long-term success than femoral neck-shaft angle.

As previously stated, surgery is recommended when the HEA is greater than 60° or when progression is documented in patients whose HEA is between 45° and 60°. Although it has been suggested that children older than 5 years who undergo surgery maintain correction, the femur and acetabulum have better remodeling potential in patients younger than 9 years.

The principles of correction are more important than the type of osteotomy or fixation selected. Intertrochanteric osteotomies, such as the Pauwels-Y valgus osteotomy, and subtrochanteric osteotomies have been shown to provide good results (Figure 21, *B*). A technique using multiple Kirschner wires has been described to stabilize an intertrochanteric osteotomy performed for the correction of coxa vara in small children. Multiple Kirschner wires can be used to create a custom high-angle blade plate for valgus osteotomy. A percutaneous technique with application of a low-profile Ilizarov external fixator and acute opening wedge correction also has also been described.

Results

In a large series of 130 hips, good results were reported in 80% of children who underwent correction at 2 to 9 years of age, 62% of children who underwent correction at 10 to 11 years of age, and 52% of children who underwent correction at older than 12 years of age. The younger children were more likely to have correction of the frequently associated small epiphysis, short femoral necks, and acetabular dysplasia. If the HEA is corrected and maintained before age 10 years, it has been reported that 80% of children develop excellent acetabular depth, spherical congruency, relief from pain, and correction of Trendelenburg gait.

Complications

Recurrence of varus deformity occurs in approximately 15% of patients and is typically caused by a failure to correct the HEA to less than 35°. Trochanteric overgrowth has been reported in 40% to 60% of patients at follow-up, with abductor weakness in approximately one half of these patients. Epiphysiodesis of the greater trochanter can be performed as part of the primary surgery (or later) to minimize the resultant decrease in the articulotrochanteric distance. Indications for epiphysiodesis of the greater trochanter are not clear, but sufficient growth of the trochanter mandates that the procedure be done before the patient is 10 years of age. In patients age 10 years or older, distal and lateral transfer of the greater trochanter may be useful. Premature closure of the proximal femoral physis invariably occurs in 90% to 100% of patients, even with an osteotomy. As a result, patients must be followed so that appropriate contralateral epiphysiodesis can be planned if necessary.

Summary

Current successful treatment of DDH relies on the early diagnosis of this condition by the primary care physician. Most instances of dysplasia and even dislocation are adequately treated by Pavlik harness with low morbidity rates. Follow-up through skeletal maturity is required to identify instances of recurrent dysplasia. When diagnosed, such dysplasia is amenable to correction using femoral and/or acetabular osteotomies.

Although congenital coxa vara occurs less frequently than DDH, appropriate diagnosis and early treatment based on recreation of normal proximal femoral alignment is usually successful.

Annotated Bibliography

Developmental Dysplasia of the Hip

Albinana J, Dolan LA, Spratt KF, Morcuende J, Meyer MD, Weinstein SL: Acetabular dysplasia after treatment for developmental dysplasia of the hip: Implications for secondary procedures. *J Bone Joint Surg Br* 2004;86:876-886.

This study of 72 hips followed through adulthood links early acetabular remodeling, residual dysplasia at skeletal maturity, and the long-term risk of total hip replacement The Severin grade was predictive for total hip replacement, and early measurements of the acetabular index were predictive for the Severin grade. An acetabular index of 35° or more at 2 years after reduction was associated with an 80% probability of progression to a Severin grade III/IV hip.

Alexiev VA, Harcke HT, Kumar SJ: Residual dysplasia after successful Pavlik harness treatment: Early ultrasound predictors. *J Pediatr Orthop* 2006;26(1):16-23.

The authors assessed 100 hips in 55 children with major instability on ultrasound; all patients were treated with a Pavlik

harness and followed over 4 years. Of 87 patients for whom treatment was deemed successful, 6% demonstrated late sequelae of late dysplasia and/or osteonecrosis. Initial ultrasound findings predictive of such sequelae were dynamic coverage index of 22% or less, α angle less than 43°, and abnormal echogenicity of the cartilaginous acetabulum (most specific).

Bache CE, Clegg J, Herron M: Risk factors for developmental dysplasia of the hip: Ultrasonographic findings in the neonatal period. *J Pediatr Orthop B* 2002;11:212-218.

In a large series of routine ultrasound screenings, 3 per 1,000 babies were identified as having persistent ultrasonographic abnormality at 6 weeks, yet only 20% demonstrated evidence of clinical instability on original examination. As 75% of these patients were nonbreech birth females with no family history of DDH, the authors concluded that most of the babies requiring treatment would not have been diagnosed.

Bohm P, Brzuske A: Salter innominate osteotomy for the treatment of developmental dysplasia of the hip in children: Results of seventy-three consecutive osteotomies after twenty-six to thirty-five years of follow-up. *J Bone Joint Surg Am* 2002;84-A:178-186.

In this study, 73 Salter innominate osteotomies in 61 patients were performed at mean patient age of 4.1 years (age range, 1.3 to 8.8 years). At mean 30.9-years follow-up (range, 26.2 to 35.4 years), the authors identified seven true revisions (one acetabuloplasty, one triple osteotomy, and five total hip arthroplasties), and 15 hips were considered clinical failures. The grade of the dislocation at first examination and immediately preoperatively, the grade of osteonecrosis, and the adequacy of surgical correction were cited as important prognostic factors for the long-term clinical result.

Cashman JP, Round J, Taylor G, Clarke NM: The natural history of developmental dysplasia of the hip after early supervised treatment in the Pavlik harness: A prospective, longitudinal follow-up. *J Bone Joint Surg Br* 2002; 84:418-425.

Of 546 dysplastic hips (332 pediatric patients) that were treated in a Pavlik harness, 18 hips (16 patients; 15.2% dislocations and 3.3% DDH) failed to reduce and required surgery. Of dysplastic hips that were successfully reduced in the Pavlik harness, 2.4% had persistent significant late dysplasia (center-edge angle < 20°) and 0.2% had persistent severe late dysplasia (center-edge angle < 15°). All patients could be identified by an abnormal center-edge angle (< 20°) at 5 years of age, and many could be identified from the progression of the acetabular angle by 18 months of age. The authors recommended regular radiographic surveillance up to 5 years of age for this patient population.

Castelein RM, Korte J: Limited hip abduction in the infant. *J Pediatr Orthop* 2001;21:668-670.

In a group of pediatric patients with sonographically proven hip dysplasia, 70 of 226 (31%) showed no limitation of abduction, and in a group without dysplasia, 210 of 457 (46%) showed manifest limitation of abduction. One hundred thirty-six patients with limited abduction but a normal sonographic examination were not treated and were reexamined at an average age of 5 years and 3 months (age range, 2 years to 9 years and 5 months). All had developed normally, both clinically and radiographically.

Chmielewski J, Albinana J: Failures of open reduction in developmental dislocation of the hip. *J Pediatr Orthop B* 2002;11:284-289.

Eight failures of an initial open reduction performed through an anterolateral approach were successfully treated with a new open reduction through an anteromedial approach. A constricted anteromedial capsule was found in all patients as the main precipitating factor; additionally, an inverted transverse ligament was found in three patients and a tight psoas tendon was found in another three patients.

Grudziak JS, Ward WT: Dega osteotomy for the treatment of congenital dysplasia of the hip. *J Bone Joint Surg Am* 2001;83-A:845-854.

The authors reported that the Dega osteotomy was successful at an average 55-month follow-up in 24 hips (22 children). Twenty hips (83%) had a concomitant femoral osteotomy, and 13 (54%) had an anterior open reduction of the hip. The average acetabular index changed from 33° preoperatively to 12° at the time of follow-up. The center-edge angle ranged from less than –30° to 18° preoperatively and from 18° to 40° (average, 31°) at the time of follow-up. The Shenton line was broken in 17 hips preoperatively, but in none postoperatively.

Hedequist D, Kasser J, Emans J: Use of an abduction brace for developmental dysplasia of the hip after failure of Pavlik harness use. *J Pediatr Orthop* 2003;23(2): 175-177.

In this study, 13 of 15 patients who failed treatment with a Pavlik harness (for persistent dislocation or instability) had resolution of DDH with the use of an abduction brace. The median time spent in the brace before stabilization of examination findings was 24 days; the median time in the brace before normalization of ultrasound parameters was 46 days. In these patients, persistent posterior instability may be better addressed by the fixed abduction brace.

Ito H, Matsuno T, Minami A: Chiari pelvic osteotomy for advanced osteoarthritis in patients with hip dysplasia. *J Bone Joint Surg Am* 2004;86-A(7):1439-1445.

In this study, 31 patients (32 hips) with Tonnis grade 3 osteoarthritis (large cysts, severe narrowing of the joint space, or severe deformity or necrosis of the femoral head with extensive osteophyte formation) refused total hip arthroplasty and were treated with a Chiari pelvic osteotomy at a mean age of 35.2 years and mean duration of follow-up of 11.2 years. The authors reported that although the clinical results were inferior to those of total hip arthroplasty, Chiari osteotomy may be an option for young patients with advanced osteoarthritis who prefer a joint-conserving procedure to total hip arthroplasty.

Lerman JA, Emans JB, Millis MB, Share J, Zurakowski D, Kasser JR: Early failure of Pavlik harness treatment for developmental hip dysplasia: Clinical and ultrasound predictors. *J Pediatr Orthop* 2001;21:348-353.

In 93 patients (137 hips), 17 (26 hips) failed Pavlik harness treatment. All patients with an initially irreducible hip and initial coverage of less than 20% confirmed by ultrasound (6 of 6) eventually failed treatment. The authors concluded that these patients may be candidates for alternative bracing, traction, or closed or open reduction.

Lorente Molto FJ, Gregori AM, Casas LM, Perales VM: Three-year prospective study of developmental dysplasia of the hip at birth: Should all dislocated or dislocatable hips be treated? *J Pediatr Orthop* 2002;22(5):613-621.

In this study, when instability persisted after 2 weeks and a splint was applied, the authors found no significant hip differences when comparing the treatment group of 103 consecutive patients (137 hips) with a control group of 50 patients (69 hips) who underwent treatment in the first days of life. With this approach, the authors concluded that the number of patients treated, the amount of sonographic studies, and consequently the final cost of the whole treatment could be safely reduced.

Luhmann SJ, Bassett GS, Gordon JE, Schootman M, Schoenecker PL: Reduction of a dislocation of the hip due to developmental dysplasia: Implications for the need for future surgery. *J Bone Joint Surg Am* 2003;85-A:239-243.

The authors of this study found that delaying reduction of a dislocated hip until the appearance of the ossific nucleus more than doubles the need for future surgery to make the hip as anatomically normal as possible. They report that twice as many secondary reconstructive procedures were performed on children initially treated at age 6 months or older.

Mladenov K, Dora C, Wicart P, Seringe R: Natural history of hips with borderline acetabular index and acetabular dysplasia in infants. *J Pediatr Orthop* 2002;22: 607-612.

Sixty-eight clinically stable hips with an increased age-related acetabular index were followed up for a mean of 9.5 years. Clinically stable and radiologically well-centered hips with an increased age-related acetabular index improved spontaneously without treatment. Most (37%) improved rapidly within the first 2 years.

Paton RW, Hossain S, Eccles K: Eight-year prospective targeted ultrasound screening program for instability and at-risk hip joints in developmental dysplasia of the hip. *J Pediatr Orthop* 2002;22:338-341.

In this prospective study, 1,806 infants with unstable or at-risk hips (6.3% of the birth population) underwent targeted ultrasound screening. The authors reported that this did not reduce the overall rate of surgery (0.87 per 1,000 births for dysplasia, 0.63 per 1,000 births for dislocation) compared with the best conventional clinical screening programs; therefore, they could not justify a national targeted ultrasound screening program for at-risk hips.

Roovers EA, Boere-Boonekamp MM, Mostert AK, Castelein RM, Zielhuis GA, Kerkhoff TH: The natural history of developmental dysplasia of the hip: Sonographic findings in infants of 1-3 months of age. *J Pediatr Orthop B* 2005;14(5):325-330.

The natural history of sonographic DDH was determined in this population-based study in which 5,170 infants were screened by ultrasound. Of the patients with normal hips at 1 month of age, 99.6% were still normal at 3 months. Of the patients with immature type IIa/IIa+ and type IIa– hips, if untreated, 95.3% and 84.4% had become normal, respectively. Of the patients with type IIc, type D, and type III/IV hips at 1 month of age, 70%, 58.3%, and 90.9% were treated, respectively.

Shipman SA, Helfand M, Moyer VA, Yawn BP: Screening for developmental dysplasia of the hip: A systematic literature review for the US Preventive Services Task Force. *Pediatrics* 2006;117(3):E557-E576.

The authors conducted a systematic review of the literature by using a best-evidence approach focused on screening relevant to primary care in infants from birth to 6 months of age. They found that screening with clinical examination or ultrasound can identify newborns at increased risk for DDH, but because of the high rate of spontaneous resolution of neonatal hip instability and dysplasia and the lack of evidence of the effectiveness of intervention on functional outcomes, the net benefits of screening are not clear.

Tien Y, Su JY, Lin GT, Lin SY: Ultrasonographic study of the coexistence of muscular torticollis and dysplasia of the hip. *J Pediatr Orthop* 2001;21:343-347.

In this study, 63 children (30 boys and 33 girls) younger than 6 months with torticollis underwent ultrasound scanning of both bilateral sternocleidomastoid muscle and bilateral hips. The authors reported that 47 children were confirmed to have muscular torticollis and 16 were confirmed to have postural torticollis. The coexistence rate of congenital muscular torticollis and DDH was found to be 17%. If only those dysplastic hips (type IIb, IIIa, IIIb) that required treatment were included, the coexistence rate would be lowered to 8.5%.

Vengust R, Antolic V, Srakar F: Salter osteotomy for treatment of acetabular dysplasia in developmental dys-

plasia of the hip in patients under 10 years. *J Pediatr Orthop B* 2001;10(1):30-36.

Of 44 hips in 39 patients undergoing Salter innominate osteotomy for the treatment of dysplastic acetabulum at 7 years to 13 years postoperatively, excellent or good clinical results were found in 43 hips (98%), but excellent or good radiographic results were found in only 32 hips (73%). A postoperative center-edge angle of greater than 24° correlated with significantly greater center-edge angle at follow-up.

Weinstein SL, Mubarak SJ, Wenger DR: Developmental hip dysplasia and dislocation: Part I. *Instr Course Lect* 2004;53:523-530.

The authors discuss the normal growth and development of the hip, the causes of abnormal development, and the structural and functional changes that result from DDH and dislocation. Ultrasonography, newborn screening, and radiographic evaluation are also discussed as important diagnostic tools for this patient population.

Weinstein SL, Mubarak SJ, Wenger DR: Developmental hip dysplasia and dislocation: Part II. *Instr Course Lect* 2004;53:531-542.

The authors discuss the advantages, pitfalls, and techniques for using the Pavlik harness for the treatment of patients with DDH and dislocation. Other closed and open treatments are aimed at concentric reduction and prevention of residual subluxation and dysplasia. Early diagnosis and treatment led to the best long-term results for these conditions.

Wenger DE, Kendell KR, Miner MR, Trousdale RT: Acetabular labral tears rarely occur in the absence of bony abnormalities. *Clin Orthop Relat Res* 2004;426:145-150.

In this study, 27 of 31 patients (87%) with acetabular labral tears were noted to have at least one abnormal radiographic structural finding and 35% had more than one abnormality. The authors also reported that 10 patients had a retroverted acetabulum, 16 had coxa valga, 11 had an abnormal femoral head-neck offset, and 14 had osteophytes on the femoral head.

Westberry DE, Davids JR, Pugh LI: Clubfoot and developmental dysplasia of the hip: Value of screening hip radiographs in children with clubfoot. *J Pediatr Orthop* 2003;23:503-507.

The authors report that the overall rate of DDH in the idiopathic clubfoot population in this series was less than 1.0% and conclude that screening hip radiographs in the idiopathic clubfoot population are probably not warranted.

Wirth T, Stratmann L, Hinrichs F: Evolution of late presenting developmental dysplasia of the hip and associated surgical procedures after 14 years of neonatal ultrasound screening. *J Bone Joint Surg Br* 2004;86:585-589.

The authors reported that general neonatal sonographic hip screening can significantly reduce surgical procedures, hospitalizations, and late presentation of DDH. They also found that femoral and pelvic osteotomies were almost entirely restricted to the unscreened group of patients and decreased from 6 to 10 per year in 1985 to 3 or less per year at follow-up. Late presentations of DDH were reduced to 3 or less per year from 1990 to 1994, none between 1995 and 1998, and 1 or 2 per year from 2000.

Congenital Coxa Vara

DiFazio RL, Kocher MS, Berven S, Kasser J: Coxa vara with proximal femoral growth arrest in patients who had neonatal extracorporeal membrane oxygenation. *J Pediatr Orthop* 2003;23(1):20-26.

The findings of this retrospective review of four patients suggest a correlation between neonatal extracorporeal membrane oxygenation and an unusual pattern of coxa vara with proximal femoral growth arrest.

Garrido IM, Molto FM, Lluch DB: Distal transfer of the greater trochanter in acquired coxa vara: Clinical and radiographic results. *J Pediatr Orthop B* 2003;12(1):38-43.

In this study, 10 patients (11 hips; age range, 4 to 13 years) with acquired coxa vara were retrospectively reviewed. Distal and lateral transfer of the greater trochanter was performed in all patients. At an average 42.7-month follow-up, the authors reported that radiographic assessment revealed an improvement of both the articulotrochanteric distance and the greater trochanter relative overgrowth and concluded that this simple procedure achieves good results with few complications.

Classic Bibliography

Carroll K, Coleman S, Stevens PM: Coxa vara: Surgical outcomes of valgus osteotomies. *J Pediatr Orthop* 1997; 17(2):220-224.

Cordes S, Dickens DR, et al: Correction of coxa vara in childhood: The use of Pauwels' Y-shaped osteotomy. *J Bone Joint Surg Br* 1991;73(1):3-6.

Kim HT, Chambers HG, Mubarak SJ, Wenger DR: Congenital coxa vara: Computed tomographic analysis of femoral retroversion and the triangular metaphyseal fragment. *J Pediatr Orthop* 2000;20(5):551-556.

Kutlu A, Ayata C, et al: Preliminary traction as a single determinant of avascular necrosis in developmental dislocation of the hip. *J Pediatr Orthop* 2000;20(5):579-584.

Weinstein JN, Kuo KN, Millar EA: Congenital coxa vara: A retrospective review. *J Pediatr Orthop* 1984;4(1): 70-77.

Wientroub S, Grill F: Ultrasonography in developmental dysplasia of the hip. *J Bone Joint Surg Am* 2000;82-A(7): 1004-1018.

Chapter 15

Limb-Length Discrepancy and Lower Limb Deformity

Mark J. Romness, MD

Introduction

Lower extremity deformities are usually classified as limb-length inequalities or angular deformities, but these two conditions often coincide. Defining the specific components of the deformity is essential for diagnosis and treatment. Isolated limb-length inequality is common, and angular deformities often cause a functional limb-length discrepancy without true structural length discrepancy. Congenital deficiencies, previously known as congenital amputations, may not have angular deformity, but do affect limb-length equality and have other associated anomalies.

Limb-Length Inequality

The amount of limb-length discrepancy considered significant and the effect on the patient are not well defined. Two centimeters of limb-length discrepancy at skeletal maturity is traditionally used as the threshold of significant limb-length discrepancy and is based on findings of up to 2 cm of discrepancy in two thirds of army recruits and other subjective or observational studies. A recent study found discrepancies as small as 3.2 mm can cause rear foot eversion during midstance gait, but concluded there is no absolute amount of discrepancy that can be used for treatment recommendations. Patient age, activity level, symptoms, and the duration of the deformity also need to be considered. Likewise, the size of the discrepancy did not significantly affect the quality of life in children as measured by the Child Health Questionnaire, a validated assessment tool. For discrepancies between 2 and 56 mm and an average of 21.5 mm, decreased scores were found primarily in the psychosocial domain and not in the physical domains.

Limb-length inequality has been associated with back and leg pain, osteoarthritis, stress fractures, and altered biomechanics. Simulated discrepancies have shown various changes in kinematics and kinetics of gait and posture. Increased load on the shorter limb has been consistently shown, yet severe osteoarthrosis was found in the long leg of 84% of patients with a mean discrepancy of 7.5 mm (standard deviation, 4.7 mm) and discrepancy of 7.5 mm (standard deviation, 4.7 mm) and in the short leg of only 16% of the patients with a mean discrepancy of 4.4 mm (standard deviation, 3.2 mm). Limb-length difference was found to be a significant predictor for the side that had hip arthroplasty. Limb-length inequality can also affect sitting position and other specific functional activities, but the effect of this is not well documented in the literature.

Deformity

Angular and rotational deformity have empirical and documented effects on joint function and longevity as well as distant effects, such as contributing to low back pain. The effect of malalignment is primarily biomechanical, and the long-term morbidity of malalignment in the coronal and sagittal planes has been extensively studied. There are limited studies correlating femoral rotational deformity with hip or knee arthrosis. The correction of excessive femoral anteversion and external tibial torsion has been shown to be effective for relieving anterior knee pain. Clinical and computer-generated studies of femoral shaft rotational malunions have shown difficulties with external deformity. The computer-simulated malunion model also demonstrated that isolated external rotations produce sagittal plane malalignment. Abnormal tibial rotation has been correlated with knee arthrosis in multiple studies. Long-term effects on the foot are not documented despite good correlation of tibial rotation to foot inversion and eversion.

Assessment

Accurate assessment of extremity deformity is critical to both diagnosis and treatment. All components of the deformity need to be considered, including structural or static deformity and functional or dynamic deformity. Structural deformity includes length, rotation, and angular deformity in the frontal, transverse, and sagittal planes. Functional impairments include motion, strength, and motor control problems that result in abnormal posturing and an effective deformity.

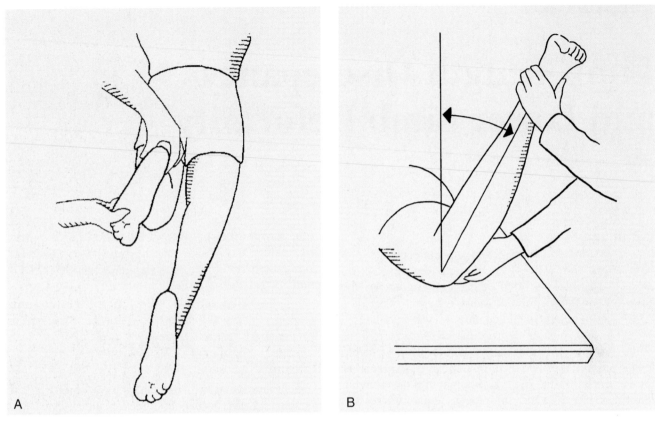

Figure 1 Illustration showing assessment of bimalleolar or thigh-foot angle **(A)** and femoral anteversion **(B)**. *(Reproduced with permission from Gage JR (ed): The Treatment of Gait Problems in Cerebral Palsy. London, England, Mac Keith Press, 2004, pp 79-81.)*

Clinical Methods

History and physical examination continue to be the most important tools for assessment. History alone can be diagnostic. Careful physical examination has been shown to be effective in isolating the deformity and directing more extensive testing.

Length measurement from the anterior-superior iliac spine to the medial or lateral malleolus provides a gross assessment of length, but does not include discrepancy in the foot and ankle or functional discrepancy from angular deformity. Use of blocks to level the pelvis includes the foot and has similar reliability to anterior-superior iliac spine measurements. None of the clinical measurements provide accuracy to within 2.0 cm, but the use of blocks is the most accurate clinical method with a 95% confidence interval of 2.2 cm. The overall effect of angular deformities can be assessed clinically, but which components make up the deformity are difficult to determine. For example, distal femoral deformity is often associated with adolescent Blount's disease, but clinically deformity of the proximal tibia predominates. The clinical techniques of palpable femoral anteversion and bimalleolar or thigh-foot angle are useful for rotational assessment despite poor sensitivity and specificity (Figure 1). Rotation through the knee or ankle joint also needs to be considered. More objective assessment

of bone rotation can be done with CT. Determining the true axis of the femoral neck is difficult even with CT, which has been reported to result in a high rate of intraobserver error. The accuracy can be improved by taking the average of two measurements, and the normal angle between the femoral neck and the posterior aspect of the femoral condyles is considered to be $17.8° \pm 8.9°$ of anteversion.

Diagnostic Imaging

Radiographic studies are important for diagnosis and definition. Standard radiographs remain the primary method of assessment. Various measurement methods have been described, including the use of orthopaedic roentgenograms, x-ray scanograms, CT scanograms, and MRI scanograms, but full-length weight-bearing radiographs (teleroentgenogram) in both the frontal and sagittal planes provide a comprehensive evaluation that includes assessment of bone and joint structure, alignment, and length (Figure 2). The advantages of this method are highlighted in Table 1.

Teleroentgenogram is also adaptable to digital capture, storage, and assessment software with only minimal additional equipment required. Digital measurements have been shown to be accurate, and specific deformity software packages have been developed.

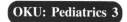

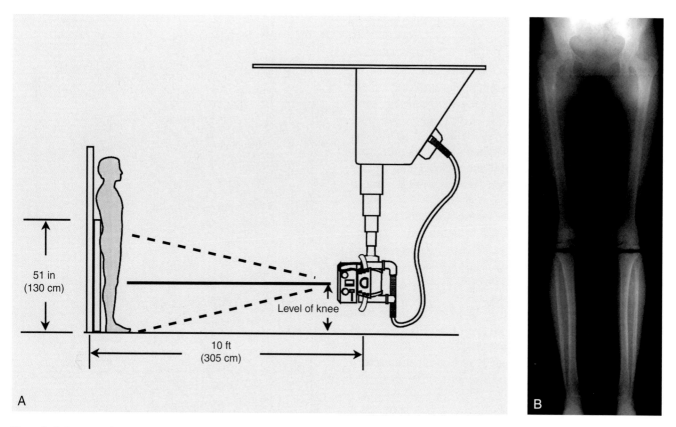

Figure 2 **A,** Illustration of the Paley x-ray technique. **B,** Radiograph obtained using the Paley x-ray technique. *(Reproduced with permission from Paley D: Principles of Deformity Correction. Berlin, Germany, Springer-Verlag, 2003, p35.)*

Table 1 | Imaging Techniques for Assessing Lower Limb Deformity

	AP Radiograph	Scanogram	CT/DLI	Microdose Digital
Weight-bearing	Yes	No	No	Yes
Foot/pelvis	Yes	No	No	Yes
Apparent length	Yes	Yes	No	Yes
True length	Yes	No	Yes	Yes
Diaphyseal deformity	Yes	No	Yes	Yes
True scale	Yes*	No	Yes	Yes
Mechanical axis	Yes	No	No	Yes
Segmental defects	Yes	No	Yes	Yes
Joint subluxation	Yes	No	No	Yes
Preoperative planning	Yes	No	No	No
Patient education	Yes	No	No	No
Parallax	Yes	No	No	No
Exposure (mrads)	42	200	60	2 (5)
Cost (US $)	95	110	100	75

CT/DLI = CT scan/digital localization image
*With radiographic magnification marker
(Reproduced with permission from Machen MS, Stevens MP: Should full-length standing anteroposterior radiographs replace the scanogram for measurement of limb-length discrepancy? J Pediatr Orthop B 2005;14(1):30-37.)

Skeletal age determination based on wrist-hand radiographs and the *Radiographic Atlas of the Skeletal Development of the Hand and Wrist* is used to predict remaining growth despite significant deficiencies in the determination that affect accuracy. More accurate skeletal age determination has not been reported, but other rarely used anatomic areas for skeletal age determination are available, including the elbow or pelvis. The usefulness of skeletal age has been brought into question and is not required for all patients. Skeletal age determination is important when there is a large discrepancy between skeletal and chronologic age.

CT remains the best diagnostic modality to assess bone structure and can be used to define bony anomalies seen on plain radiographs. MRI provides better definition of cartilage and soft-tissue structures. This makes MRI ideal for assessment of physeal deformity or arrest and joint abnormalities, especially of immature or abnormal joints whose structure is more cartilage than bone (such as in patients with infantile tibia vara). Unfortunately, MRI often requires sedation for smaller children, the risk of which needs to be individualized to the potential benefit of the information obtained.

Prediction of Progression

In the growing child, the effect of remaining growth on any existing deformity needs to be determined. The etiology, magnitude, and location of the deformity need to be considered in the context of the patient's age and remaining growth to predict deformity at skeletal maturity. The nonlinear growth rate of the various physes prevents extreme accuracy, but prediction methods have been shown to be clinically effective. Limb-length predictions have been quantified using simple methods such as growth charts and more complex measurements such as the Moseley straight-line graph and the recently described multiplier method. The Moseley straight-line graph method (Figure 3) is based on growth charts and uses skeletal age plotted against limb-length discrepancy at two or more points in time to predict mature discrepancy. The arithmetic or rule-of-thumb method of Menelaus is useful for quick calculations of simple limb-length discrepancy and has been shown to be as clinically accurate as the straight-line graph method for timing growth arrest. The rule-of-thumb method estimates growth of 10 mm/yr in the distal femur and 6 mm/yr in the proximal tibia during the last 4 years of growth, with growth completion at a chronologic age of 14 years for girls and 16 years for boys. A more accurate assessment using the multiplier method is recommended for patients with larger and more complex deformities.

The multiplier method uses simple arithmetic formulae and a multiplier table (Table 2). The multiplier (M) is an age- and gender-related coefficient that is calculated by dividing the length of a bone at maturity (Lm) by its

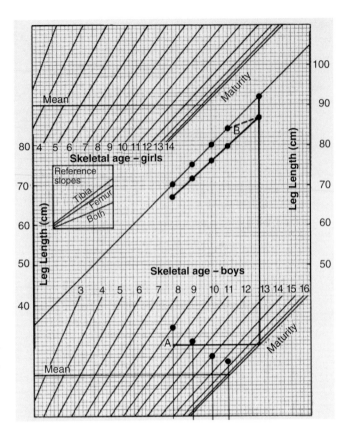

Figure 3 Moseley straight-line graph illustrating the Moseley straight-line method. The example shown is for a boy with idiopathic hemiatrophy who was observed clinically for 4 consecutive years. In 1994, the longer leg measured 70 cm, the shorter leg measured 67 cm, and bone age was 9 years. Additional scanograms and bone age radiographs are plotted as shown. Note the horizontal straight line (A) extending to the maturity line with an equal number of skeletal ages above and below line. At skeletal maturity, the longer leg is projected to measure 92 cm and the shorter leg is projected to measure 87 cm. The dotted line (B) represents the projected growth of the longer leg if epiphysiodeses of the distal femur and proximal tibia are performed when the longer leg reaches 84 cm in length, thus obtaining limb equalization by skeletal maturity. *(Reproduced with permission from Canale ST (ed): Campbell's Operative Orthopaedics, ed 9. St. Louis, MO, Mosby, 1998, p 988.)*

current length (L): M = Lm/L. The multiplier for each age and gender is a measure of the percentage of growth remaining: M × L = Lm. The multiplier is independent of growth percentile, ethnicity, and generational differences. The method does not require more than one reference point of measurement and has been validated clinically for normal and abnormal growth and timing of epiphysiodesis. Multipliers that are specific for height, femur, and tibia are also available.

Idiopathic Conditions

Generally, limb deformity is either idiopathic or the result of congenital or acquired conditions (Table 3).

Shortening

Small discrepancies in length of the lower extremities are common, and the etiology and significance of this is unknown. Classic studies have shown some degree of

Table 2 | Lower-Limb Multipliers for Boys and Girls

Age (years + months)	Multiplier	
	Boys	Girls
Birth	5.080	4.630
0 + 3	4.550	4.155
0 + 6	4.050	3.725
0 + 9	3.600	3.300
1 + 0	3.240	2.970
1 + 3	2.975	2.750
1 + 6	2.825	2.600
1 + 9	2.700	2.490
2 + 0	2.590	2.390
2 + 3	2.480	2.295
2 + 6	2.385	2.200
2 + 9	2.300	2.125
3 + 0	2.230	2.050
3 + 6	2.110	1.925
4 + 0	2.000	1.830
4 + 6	1.890	1.740
5 + 0	1.820	1.660
5 + 6	1.740	1.580
6 + 0	1.670	1.510
6 + 6	1.620	1.460
7 + 0	1.570	1.430
7 + 6	1.520	1.370
8 + 0	1.470	1.330
8 + 6	1.420	1.290
9 + 0	1.380	1.260
9 + 6	1.340	1.220
10 + 0	1.310	1.190
10 + 6	1.280	1.160
11 + 0	1.240	1.130
11 + 6	1.220	1.100
12 + 0	1.180	1.070
12 + 6	1.160	1.050
13 + 0	1.130	1.030
13 + 6	1.100	1.010
14 + 0	1.080	1.000
14 + 6	1.060	NA
15 + 0	1.040	NA
15 + 6	1.020	NA
16 + 0	1.010	NA
16 + 6	1.010	NA
17 + 0	1.000	NA

NA = not applicable
(Reproduced with permission from Paley D: Multiplier method for predicting limb length. J Bone Joint Surg Am 2000;82-A(10):1432-1446.)

Table 3 | Etiologies of Limb Deformity

Congenital
Hypoplasia syndromes
Proximal femoral focal deficiency (congenital short femur)
Tibial deficiencies
Fibular deficiencies
Hemiatrophy
Hemihypertrophy
Idiopathic
Klippel-Trenaunay-Weber syndrome
Beckwith-Wiedemann syndrome
Proteus syndrome
Skeletal dysplasia
Ollier disease
Fibrous dysplasia
Neurofibromatosis
Multiple hereditary exostoses
Acquired
Trauma
Acute bone loss
Physeal injury
Fracture healing process
Burns
Irradiation
Iatrogenic
Infection
Osteomyelitis
Septic arthritis
Purpura fulminans
Inflammation
Juvenile rheumatoid arthritis
Hemophilia
Pigmented villonodular synovitis
Neurologic
Acute brain injury
Spinal cord injury
Peripheral nerve injury
Cerebral palsy
Myelomeningocele
Poliomyelitis
Tumors
Tumor treatment
Enchondromatosis
Hemangiomas

(Adapted with permission from Finch GD, Dawe CJ: Hemiatrophy. J Pediatr Orthop 2003; 23(1):99-101 and Stanitski DF: Limb-length inequality: Assessment and treatment options. J Am Acad Orthop Surg 1999;7(3):143-153.)

discrepancy in up to 70% of the population. Limb-length discrepancies of up to 1 cm should not be considered significant and only require observation. Discrepancies of greater than 1 cm in a growing child require assessment for etiology and treatment. There is no documented benefit of using a lift on the short side; however, a lift should be considered as the first treatment option if the patient is symptomatic with any complaints such as back or leg pain.

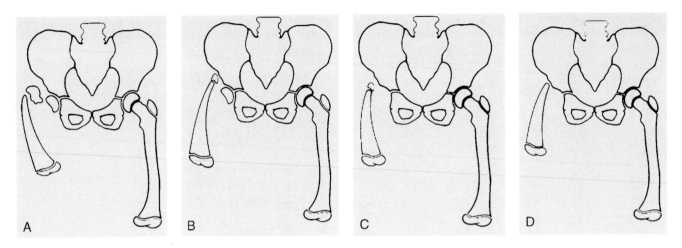

Figure 4 The Aitken classification scheme for proximal femoral focal deficiency. **A,** In class A, the hip joint appears formed, but the femoral neck is absent on early radiographs and the femur is shortened. **B,** In class B, the femoral head is more rudimentary and the deficiency of proximal femoral shaft is more significant. Pseudarthrosis between the femoral shaft and femoral head is always present. **C,** In class C, the femoral head is absent, the acetabulum is shallow, and the proximal femur is represented only by a small tuft. **D,** In class D, the femoral head and acetabulum are absent and deficiency of the femoral shaft is more significant. *(Reproduced with permission from Canale ST (ed): Campbell's Operative Orthopaedics, ed 9. St. Louis, MO, Mosby, 1998, p 978.)*

Bowing

Physiologic bowing is covered in chapter 13. Severe forms of varus and valgus deformities can occur. Bracing has been shown to be effective in young patients with genu varum and can be considered for patients with significant progressive deformity. Use of a medial upright orthosis for varus deformities and a lateral upright for valgus deformities has the potential to affect the growth of the bone, but this has not been well documented. Adherence to a bracing protocol is difficult regardless of whether this is used in the daytime or the nighttime. Surgical correction is reserved for the older patient or younger patients with severe deformities that result in major limitations on function.

Congenital Conditions

Congenital deformities are often identified at birth. This is especially true of major congenital deformities. Milder congenital deformities may not be apparent until additional growth and development uncovers the deformity. Proper diagnosis of the congenital deformity is important for genetic counseling, management, and prediction of progression.

Proximal Femoral Focal Deficiency (Congenital Short Femur)

The condition of proximal femoral focal deficiency has a spectrum of involvement as defined classically by the Aitken classification (Figure 4). Proximal femoral focal deficiency is believed to be on the severe end of the spectrum of femoral deficiency and congenital short femur is believed to be on the milder end. The important clinical aspect of the Aitken classification is the presence or absence of a hip joint and the extent of its de-

velopment if present. The absence of a hip joint results in limited reconstruction options. Various methods of femoropelvic arthrodesis and rotation of the distal limb to use the knee or ankle joint for motion have been described, but fusion has not been proved to be advantageous over leaving a flail articulation. Loss of limb length is another significant component of this condition. Limb-length correction is hampered by the deficiency of both the hip and knee joint, leading to subluxation without careful attention to these joints. Joint stability is important even when correcting small deformities in patients with congenital short femur, which is associated with anterior cruciate ligament deficiency.

Tibial Deficiencies
Bowing
Posterior medial apex bowing of the tibia is a common deformity noted at birth and is often associated with a calcaneal valgus foot. Both the tibial deformity and the foot position improve with growth and development. More severe posterior medial bowing is associated with limb-length discrepancy at maturity and can occasionally exceed 2 cm and require treatment.

Anterior lateral apex bowing is classically a concerning clinical presentation. A recently described entity, the delta tibia (Figure 5), can have spontaneous resolution as can anterior lateral apex bowing associated with duplication of the hallux. Residual limb-length discrepancy is also associated with these conditions.

Pseudarthrosis
Anterior lateral apex bowing of the tibia may be the only initial presentation of congenital pseudarthrosis of the tibia. Osteotomies to correct mild deformity have resulted in nonunions. The condition of congenital pseud-

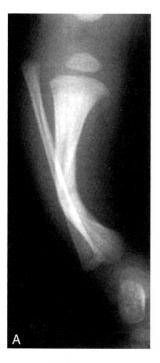
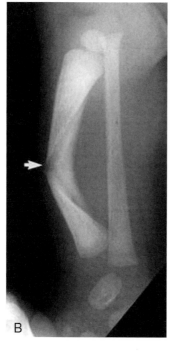
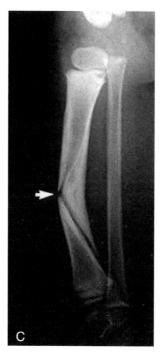

Figure 5 Congenital anterolateral bowing of the right tibia. **A,** Frontal radiograph of the right leg of a 1-month-old patient shows a marked lateral tibial bowing and a straight and elongated fibula with a lateral displacement of its proximal end. **B,** Lateral radiograph of the right leg of the same 1-month-old patient shows a prominent anterior tibial bowing, and proximal and distal tibial segments, which end in a point at the apex of the curve separated by an intervening cortical gap (*arrow*). The two tibial segments are clearly defined from the triangular osseous structure in the concavity of the curve. **C,** Lateral radiograph of the right leg at 2 years of age shows a marked improvement in the anterior tibial bowing, with fusion and partial resorption of the junction between the proximal tibial segment and the triangular osseous structure and beginning formation of the medullary cavity locally. The anterior cortical defect is still present (*arrow*). (Reproduced with permission from Currarino G, Herring JA, Johnston CE Jr, Birch JG: An unusual form of congenital anterolateral tibial angulation: The delta tibia. Pediatr Radiol 2003;33(5):346-353.)

arthrosis is not well defined pathologically, and the etiology is not known. Correction of this condition, however, is notoriously challenging. Surgical correction is not indicated until a true pseudarthrosis is established. An intact but angulated bone should be treated with a clamshell orthosis. In infants, this requires bracing above the knee, but as the patient grows, bracing below the knee is adequate. Prevention of pseudarthrosis is possible using an orthosis until skeletal maturity when the risk of fracture diminishes significantly. Current surgical treatments include intramedullary fixation and grafting for infants and either vascularized fibular graft or resection and bone transport techniques for older patients. Even in the larger series with experienced clinicians, reported success rates with these procedures are not high.

Hypoplasia

Deficiencies of the tibia can range from mild shortening to complete absence. Tibial deficiencies (previously known as tibial hemimelia) are important to distinguish from fibular deficiencies (previously known as fibular hemimelia) in that they have an autosomal dominant genetic inheritance pattern. This is especially important in patients with spontaneous mutation and lack of a previous family history. The presence or absence of a proximal tibia is an important clinical component. The lack of a proximal portion of the tibia and specifically the tibial tubercle is associated with a lack of an extension mechanism across the knee, making reconstructive procedures more challenging and resulting in less functionality. Consequently, disarticulation through the knee level is recommended in most patients. The primary reconstruc-

tive procedure is fusion of the proximal tibial remnant to the fibula with translation of the fibula to a more medial position. The fibular shaft is fitted with a below-the-knee prosthesis, but ligamentous instability, limited active motion, and contractures are common.

Fibular Deficiencies

Deformity of the fibula is variable and should be considered one aspect of a fibular deficiency syndrome. Associated anomalies can include shortening of the femur and tibia, femoral retroversion, valgus distal femur secondary to hypoplasia of the lateral femoral condyle, hypoplastic tibial spines, cruciate ligament deficiency, angular deformity of the tibia, ball-and-socket ankle, absent lateral rays, tarsal coalition, and clubfoot deformity. Even with normal fibular development, one recent study reported that two or more of these associated anomalies were found in 11% of 123 patients with limb deficiency. Treatment is based on the amount of predicted limb-length discrepancy, the status of the ankle joint, and the associated anomalies. Choice between orthosis use and lengthening versus Boyd or Syme amputation and prosthesis use is controversial. If the ankle joint can be maintained and foot development is adequate for weight bearing, lengthening procedures should be considered.

Hemihypertrophy and Hemiatrophy

Hemihypertrophy and hemiatrophy represent two different entities. Diagnosis between the two is challenging, but important because hemihypertrophy is associated with embryonal cancers (including Wilms' tumors) in up to 5.9% of patients, and recent analysis of data recommends screening abdominal ultrasounds every 3 months until age 6 years. Hemihypertrophy is also associated with more severe limb-length discrepancy than hemiatrophy. Diagnosis is based on asymmetry throughout the body, including the head, trunk, and extremities. The side with the more atypical findings of development or alignment determines the diagnosis based on its overall size to the remainder of the body. Beckwith-Wiedemann syndrome is also associated with renal tumors, is caused by mutation in the chromosome 11p15.5 region, and includes exomphalos, macroglossia, and gigantism. Jaffe-Campanacci syndrome, Klippel-Trenaunay-Weber syndrome, and McCune-Albright syndrome are additional syndromes that may develop hemihypertrophy. Treatment for hemihypertrophy and hemiatrophy follows similar principles for limb-length discrepancy. Rarely are there any angular or structural deformities, with the exception of Jaffe-Campanacci syndrome, which has structural deficiencies from the enchondromas.

Acquired Conditions

Acquired deformity of the lower extremities usually results from trauma, inflammation (including infection), and neuromuscular conditions with growth-related deformity. An accurate diagnosis is important in determining the significance of the current deformity and its potential influence with additional growth and development. Although remodeling a posttraumatic deformity is well recognized in the pediatric population, the remodeling potential varies based on patient age and location of the deformity. Specifics on remodeling have only been defined for certain fractures such as the distal radius. There are no criteria for correction of deformity in the lower extremities. It has been shown that the closer a deformity is to a joint, the more effect it has on a joint. It is also known that deformities in the plane of the local joint are more likely to correct spontaneously. In the lower extremities, this is most commonly demonstrated in the distal femur. In general, adult guidelines for posttraumatic residual deformity are used in the pediatric population as well.

Inflammatory processes can cause overgrowth of the involved extremity, which is believed to be secondary to the hyperemia. Classically, this is seen in patients with poorly controlled juvenile arthritis of the knee. This can also occur from inflammation of other processes such as trauma or infection. Angular deformity or growth arrest can occur with infection with partial or complete disruption of the physis, respectively. This is addressed in chapter 6.

Limb-length discrepancy and deformity are often observed in patients with asymmetric neuromuscular conditions. Most commonly, this condition presents as a hypoplasia of a paralytic limb, and limb-length discrepancy

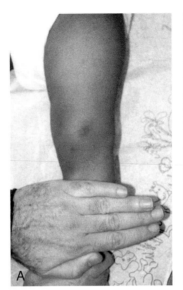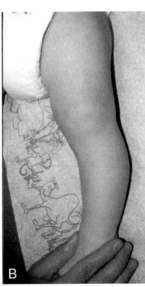

Figure 6 The cover-up test. Covering up the lower half of the tibia highlights the contribution of the proximal tibia to the bowing. **A,** If there is varus or neutral alignment, the test is positive and a radiograph should be obtained. **B,** If there is valgus, the test is negative and no radiograph is required. *(Reproduced with permission from Davids JR, Blackhurst DW, Allen BL Jr: Clinical evaluation of bowed legs in children. J Pediatr Orthop B 2000 Oct;9(4):278-284.)*

in children with spastic hemiplegic cerebral palsy of 1 cm or more is present in more than 50% of patients.

Slipped Capital Femoral Epiphysis

Slipped capital femoral epiphysis can lead to significant asymmetry about the hip, including rotational malalignment and shortening. The effect on hip motion is related to the severity of the slip, with more severe slips causing decreased flexion and internal rotation. Studies have shown that remodeling of the proximal femoral metaphysis is minimal and a corrective osteotomy is indicated for patients with significant functional problems. Osteotomy at the femoral neck and subtrochanteric level has been shown to have functional results comparable to the less technically demanding subtrochanteric osteotomy. Concern regarding osteonecrosis of the femoral head with basilar neck osteotomies has been reported, but is poorly documented.

Blount's Disease

Blount's disease is defined as asymmetric growth of the proximal tibia leading to tibia vara. The classic definition describes infantile Blount's disease, which develops shortly after the onset of ambulation. Adolescent Blount's disease is used to describe the onset of tibia vara in adolescence. Clinically, these are two distinct entities.

Infantile Blount's Disease

In the early stages, infantile Blount's disease is difficult to differentiate from physiologic genu varum. Careful clinical examination of patients between 1 and 3 years of age using the "cover-up" test (Figure 6) can be helpful, and a weight-bearing AP radiograph is indicated if the cover-up test is positive. Valgus alignment at the knee is considered a negative test and is indicative of physiologic bowing. Neutral or varus alignment is considered a positive test and suggests that the child is at greater risk for having infantile tibia vara. Radiography should also be considered if there is a family history of surgery for bowing, asymmetry in the amount of deformity, severe deformity, or height below fifth percentile for age. Internal tibial torsion often presents as genu varum; therefore, the thigh-foot angle needs to be assessed. Radiographs are not definitive in the diagnosis of Blount's disease, but help define the extent of deformity, which has been used as an indication of progression risk. The metaphyseal-diaphyseal angle has been the most evaluated measurement. An angle of 16° or more has significant risk of progression and should be treated with braces or surgery; metaphyseal-diaphyseal angles of 11° to 16° should be monitored with repeat radiographs 4 to 6 months later. Combining the metaphyseal-diaphyseal angle with other measurements such as relative tibial and femoral varus has shown that all patients with a metaphyseal-diaphyseal angle of 16° or greater and varus primarily from the tibia went on to progress.

Bracing has shown limited effectiveness in the early stages of the disease in young children, some of whom may have had physiologic bowing, and should be considered for children 3 years of age or younger and with a metaphyseal-diaphyseal angle of more than 16°. A medial upright knee-ankle-foot orthosis with an elastic calf strap is the standard brace. A more severe deformity requires surgical correction with a proximal tibial osteotomy if the physis is still open or a medial tibial plateau elevation combined with lateral physeal arrest and lengthening if the medial physis is bridged or closed.

Adolescent Blount's Disease

The etiology for adolescent Blount's disease is believed to be gender-, race- and pressure-related because more than 90% of the reported instances have occurred in male African Americans who are morbidly obese. It is usually present bilaterally, but may be asymmetric. Deformity is rarely isolated to the proximal tibia, and full assessment of alignment needs to be performed. This includes assessment of rotations clinically and a skeletal alignment radiographically. A distal femoral or distal tibial deformity is often present, but the extent varies. Bracing is not effective in this population. Hemiepiphysiodesis has been shown to be effective at correcting or preventing progression in up to 85% of patients. More severe deformity usually requires osteotomy because patients present close to skeletal maturity with the medial tibial physis near closure. Hemiepiphysiodesis cannot correct tibial torsion, which is often associated with adolescent Blount's disease.

Table 4 | Treatment Guidelines for Limb-Length Equalization

Expected Mature Discrepancy	Treatment
0 to 2 cm	Nothing unless symptomatic
2 to 5 cm	Lift, shorten, or lengthen
6 to 15 cm	Lengthen once or more
> 15 cm	Lengthen ± shorten
	Prosthesis ± amputation

Treatment

Length Equalization

Treatment guidelines for limb-length equalization have been established (Table 4). Controversy exists in the 2- to 5-cm range, and treatment tends to be individualized based on the treating physician and family preferences. The etiology of the deformity also influences treatment decisions.

Arrest (Shortening)

Premature physeal arrest (physeodesis or epiphysiodesis) has been shown to be a safe and effective way to equalize limb lengths in patients with adequate growth remaining and is generally considered for discrepancies between 2 and 5 cm. Despite the inaccuracy of skeletal bone age assessments, simple calculations with the rule-of-thumb method can accurately predict timing of arrest to obtain limb lengths within 1 cm of each other at skeletal maturity. Percutaneous arrest of the physis has been shown to be effective despite the lack of complete obliteration of the physis. Failure of arrest or angular deformity can occur with percutaneous or open techniques. Technical complications with percutaneous technique, including penetration into the knee joint or the posterior neurovascular bundle, are rare. Fibular arrest should be included with proximal tibial arrest when the patient has more than 3 years of expected remaining growth.

Acute shortening of either the femur or the tibia has been described. Most commonly, femoral shortening of 2 to 5 cm is done. The significant risks of nonunion, weakness, and compartment syndrome have kept shortening procedures from becoming popular. Loss of mature height is also not acceptable to many patients. A recent report showed 100% healing of 19 femoral shortenings ranging from 2.3 to 10.0 cm. Statistically significant quadriceps weakness was still present 2 years after surgery, and five patients were unable to stand up from squatting with the surgically treated leg, but there was no decrease or improvement of self-reported and timed functional tests.

Lengthening

Lengthening for limb-length inequality continues to evolve based on the distraction histogenesis principles of

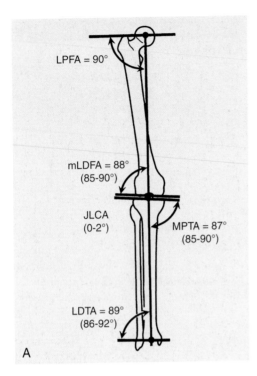

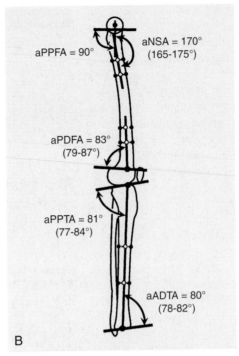

Figure 7 Normal mechanical axis joint alignment angles in the coronal **(A)** and sagittal **(B)** planes. LPFA = lateral proximal femoral angle, mLDFA = lateral distal femoral angle relative to the mechanical axis, JLCA = joint line convergence angle, MPTA = medial proximal tibial angle, LDTA = lateral distal tibial angle, aPPFA = anatomic posterior proximal femoral angle, aNSA = anatomic neck shaft angle, aPDFA = posterior distal femoral angle relative to the anatomic axis, aPPTA = posterior proximal tibial angle relative to the anatomic axis, aADTA = anterior distal tibial angle relative to the anatomic axis. *(Reproduced with permission from Paley D: Principles of Deformity Correction. Berlin, Germany, Springer-Verlag, 2003, pp 8-9.)*

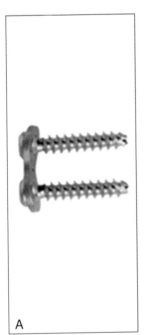

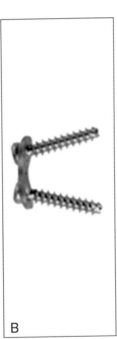

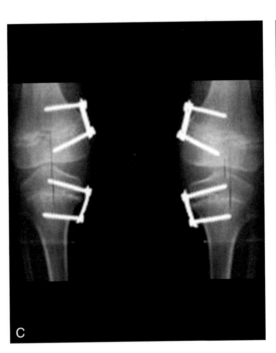

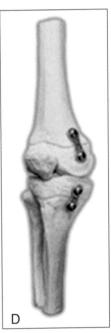

Figure 8 **A** through **D,** The diverging screws of the eight-Plate Guided Growth System (OrthoFix, McKinney, TX) function like a hinge to gently guide natural growth. The fully threaded cannulated screws resist pullout forces and allow for easy removal after treatment. *(Reproduced with permission from the OrthoFix eight-Plate Guided Growth System brochure. Available at the OrthoFix Web site: http://www.orthofix.com/ofus/PDF/EP-0404.AEightPlateSS.pdf.)*

Ilizarov. With improved success rates, the indications for lengthening include patients with 2 to 5 cm of discrepancy and up to 20% of the individual bone length for one lengthening period. Mechanical methods of lengthening include external fixation, external fixation combined with an intramedullary nail, and intramedullary distraction devices. Multiple types of external fixation

are available for correction. Lengthening with external fixation over an intramedullary rod to control angulation and allow earlier removal of the external fixation has gained popularity, and multiple recent studies show that intramedullary infection is a significant risk in patients with prior infection or open trauma, but not with primary lengthening procedures. Intramedullary distraction

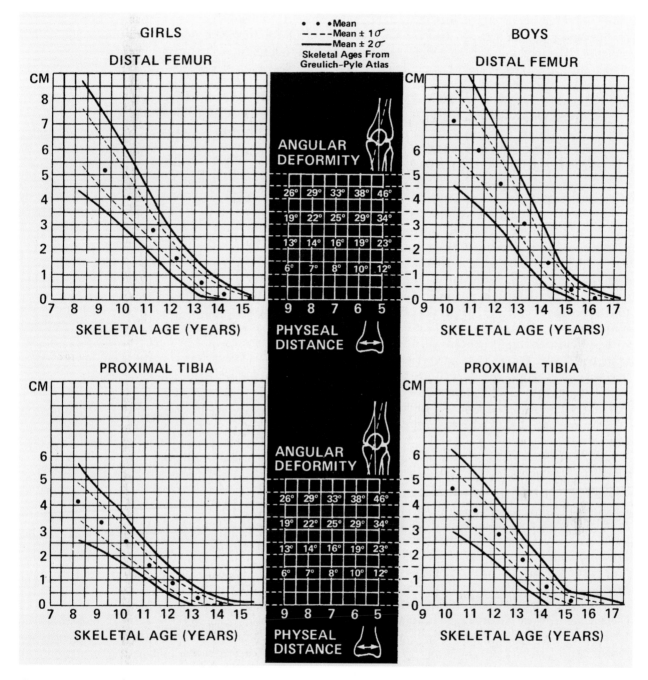

Figure 9   To appropriately time limb deformity correction, the graph quadrant that represents the patient's sex and the area (distal femur or proximal tibia) to undergo partial epiphysiodesis is chosen. Then, using the central portion of the chart, the physeal distance is located, and the angular deformity of the limb is found on the corresponding vertical line. (Note that the degree values are marked slightly above the horizontal lines that represent them.) A horizontal line is then drawn from the point identifying physeal distance and angular deformity to the patient's growth percentile on the appropriate quadrant. A vertical line is subsequently dropped from this point to identify the appropriate skeletal age at which the partial epiphysiodesis should be performed. *(Reproduced with permission from Bowen JR, Leahey JL, Zhang ZH, MacEwen GD: Partial epiphysiodesis at the knee to correct angular deformity. Clin Orthop Relat Res 1985;(198):184-190.)*

devices have been introduced, but are not widely used and currently restricted to patients with closed physes.

Limb Deformity Correction

The most important aspect of limb deformity correction is a complete assessment of all components contributing to the deformity. This includes angular, rotational, and length deformity. The goal is to restore the mechanical axis of the limb in all planes; to accomplish this goal, it is important to understand the correlation of the anatomic to the mechanical axis. Normal values are given in Figure 7. Ideally, correction should be done at the site of the primary deformity; otherwise, secondary deformities can be created with incomplete correction of the initial deformity. Methods to correct deformity include controlling remaining growth with a hemiepiphysiodesis or osteotomies. Hemiepiphysiodesis with staples is complicated by difficulty with positioning, staple breakage or back-out, and difficult removal. Single screws across a physis can tether growth and are easily removed. Recently, a plate and screw fixation combination across the physis has been shown to be simple and effective for physeal tethering (Figure 8). If timed appropriately, surgical arrest of the hemiepiphysis can be performed for a definitive correction of angular deformity. Timing is based on the skeletal age and the width of the physis, which can be plotted on a nomogram (Figure 9). Normal alignment cannot be predictably obtained with hemiepiphysiodesis in patients with severe tibia vara deformity in which the mechanical axis is more medial to the tibial plateau than the width of the medial plateau or in which the mechanical axis between the femur and the tibia is greater than 15°. Osteotomies are necessary when the deformity does not include the physeal area or when the physis has insufficient growth remaining for adequate correction. Either acute or gradual correction can be performed depending on the characteristics of the deformity and the critical structures at risk during correction. Fixation may be external or internal, each of which has advantages and disadvantages that need to be considered with each specific use.

Deficiencies (Prostheses)
Large discrepancies in limb length or alignment are often the result of congenital deficiencies or are acquired at a young age. These discrepancies usually require a combination of procedures throughout the child's lifetime. Treatment should be directed toward maintaining a functional childhood while keeping skeletal maturity in mind. The combination of procedures is often staged. When the patient is young, it is more important to maintain alignment than length, which children tend to compensate for easily. As the patient grows, length becomes more of a functional issue. Use of a prosthesis can be considered for severe discrepancies in young patients or for discrepancies that are not amenable to equalization procedures. Amputation of a nonfunctional distal appendage may be necessary for prosthetic fitting. Children tolerate prostheses well, but need careful monitoring of fit with growth to assure proper length and socket fit.

Summary
Lower extremity limb-length inequality and deformity have an influence on function and long-term morbidity, but the extent of this is not well documented except in relation to joint arthrosis. Careful and complete assessment of the lower extremity deformity is essential to appropriate diagnosis and treatment considerations. Specific causes of deformity have unique characteristics that

need to be considered for appropriate management and treatment. Treatment must be patient-specific, with the goals of each step and treatment well defined.

Annotated Bibliography
Limb-Length Inequality/Deformity
Bruce WD, Stevens PM: Surgical correction of miserable malalignment syndrome. *J Pediatr Orthop* 2004;24(4): 392-396.

The authors of this retrospective review of 14 patients who had femoral and tibial rotational osteotomies for patellofemoral pain found no patients reporting persistence of pain and 11 patients involved with organized athletic activities.

Gugenheim JJ, Probe RA, Brinker MR: The effects of femoral shaft malrotation on lower extremity anatomy. *J Orthop Trauma* 2004;18(10):658-664.

The authors found that computer simulation of malrotated femur fractures at various levels of the bone leads to deviation of the mechanical axis in both the frontal and sagittal planes. They reported that the extent of deviation varies by location, extent, and direction of the simulated deformity.

Gurney B: Leg length discrepancy. *Gait Posture* 2002; 15(2):195-206.

The author of this extensive review of the literature on all aspects of limb-length discrepancy concluded that there is no definite number that defines a significant discrepancy. The author also reported that chronic discrepancies are better tolerated than acute discrepancies and that younger persons adapt better to discrepancies than older persons.

Jaarsma RL, Pakvis DF, Verdonschot N, Biert J, van Kampen A: Rotational malalignment after intramedullary nailing of femoral fractures. *J Orthop Trauma* 2004; 18(7):403-409.

In this study, femoral malrotation of 15° or more measured by CT was found in 21 of 76 patients on recall examination of isolated femoral fractures. Certain functional scores were found to be worse in the 12 patients with external malposition, but not in those with internal malposition. Poor sensitivity and specificity of the clinical examination to assess femoral anteversion were also found.

Tallroth K, Ylikoski M, Lamminen H, Ruohonen K: Preoperative leg-length inequality and hip osteoarthrosis: A radiographic study of 100 consecutive arthroplasty patients. *Skeletal Radiol* 2005;34(3):136-139.

Leg-length inequality was found in 81 of 100 consecutive patients undergoing hip arthroplasty who were assessed using standardized weight-bearing pelvic radiographs. Leg-length difference was found to be a significant predictor for the side of surgery because arthroplasty was performed on the long side in 68 patients and on the short side in 13.

Vitale MA, Choe JC, Sesko AM, et al: The effect of limb length discrepancy on health-related quality of life: Is the "2 cm rule" appropriate? *J Pediatr Orthop B* 2006; 15(1):1-5.

Leg-length inequality of various etiologies was compared with the parent form of the Child Health Questionnaire for 76 patients. Significant negative correlation was found for the parental impact-emotional, family cohesion, and psychosocial summary score domains. A critical amount of discrepancy could not be determined with no statistical difference between the groups with more than or less than 20 mm of leg-length discrepancy.

Assessment

Aguilar JA, Paley D, Paley J, et al: Clinical validation of the multiplier method for predicting limb length at maturity: Part I. *J Pediatr Orthop* 2005;25(2):186-191.

The predicted bone lengths of the unoperated bones using the multiplier method and Anderson charts were compared with lengths at maturity in 60 patients who had epiphysiodesis of other bones. Leg length at maturity of the unoperated short lower limb was predicted by using the Moseley, Anderson, and multiplier methods. The multiplier method prediction based on a single limb measurement was found to be as accurate as the Moseley predictions based on at least three serial limb measurements.

Aguilar JA, Paley D, Paley J, et al: Clinical validation of the multiplier method for predicting limb length discrepancy and outcome of epiphysiodesis: Part II. *J Pediatr Orthop* 2005;25(2):192-196.

Data on 60 patients were evaluated with the multiplier method using chronologic and skeletal age and the Moseley method to further validate the accuracy of the multiplier method. The multiplier method was found to be significantly more accurate than the Moseley method when predicting leg-length discrepancy at maturity after epiphysiodesis. The multiplier method predictions using chronologic age were as accurate or more accurate than using skeletal age.

Machen MS, Stevens PM: Should full-length standing anteroposterior radiographs replace the scanogram for measurement of limb length discrepancy? *J Pediatr Orthop B* 2005;14(1):30-37.

Seven cases are presented that demonstrate the advantage of weight-bearing full-length AP radiographs over scanograms. The etiology of the discrepancy, angular deformities, mechanical axis, and foot or iliac discrepancy were not demonstrated on the scanogram. Other advantages are also discussed.

Paley D, Bhave A, Herzenberg JE, Bowen JR: Multiplier method for predicting limb-length discrepancy. *J Bone Joint Surg Am* 2000;82-A(10):1432-1446.

The authors provide an initial description of the multiplier method formulae derived from 20 databases of femoral, tibial, and/or limb-length measurements. They verified the accuracy of these formulae by evaluating two groups of patients with

congenital shortening who were treated with epiphysiodesis or limb-lengthening. This article includes the multiplier charts and formulae for use in patients with congenital or developmental discrepancy and for timing of the epiphysiodesis.

Terry MA, Winell JJ, Green DW, et al: Measurement variance in limb length discrepancy: Clinical and radiographic assessment of interobserver and intraobserver variability. *J Pediatr Orthop* 2005;25(2):197-201.

Measurements from the anterior-superior iliac spine to the lateral malleolus, the anterior-superior iliac spine to the medial malleolus, and for blocks to level the pelvis were compared with slit scanogram measurements for discrepancies of various etiologies in 16 patients by four examiners. Interobserver reliability of all three methods of clinical leg-length discrepancy assessment was similar, but the 95% confidence interval was smallest for block measurements. All clinical measures were considered unacceptable for clinical decision making.

Congenital Conditions

Abraham P: What is the risk of cancer in a child with hemihypertrophy? *Arch Dis Child* 2005;90(12):1312-1313.

In a literature search summary of hemihypertrophy and the risk of tumor development, the author identified two pertinent articles and concluded that the risk of tumor development is 5.9% and recommended abdominal ultrasound screening every 3 months until age 6 years.

Bressers MM, Castelein RM: Anterolateral tibial bowing and duplication of the hallux: A rare but distinct entity with good prognosis. *J Pediatr Orthop B* 2001;10(2): 153-157.

The authors provide a case report and literature review describing anterolateral tibial bowing in combination with a duplication of the hallux that spontaneously corrects. The tibial radiographs presented are similar to those of the delta tibia described by Currarino and associates (see below).

Brown KL: Resection, rotationplasty, and femoropelvic arthrodesis in severe congenital femoral deficiency: A report of the surgical technique and three cases. *J Bone Joint Surg Am* 2001;83-A(1):78-85.

Three patients and technique are described for femoral resection and pelvic arthrodesis in addition to rotation of the limb to prevent Trendelenburg lurch and prosthetic fitting versus previously described rotation procedures.

Currarino G, Herring JA, Johnston CE Jr, Birch JG: An unusual form of congenital anterolateral tibial angulation: The delta tibia. *Pediatr Radiol* 2003;33(5):346-353.

The authors discuss three cases and provide a literature review describing a specific type of anterolateral tibial bowing that tends to improve spontaneously with some residual leg-length discrepancy. They report that duplication of the hallux was present in only one of the three patients.

Finch GD, Dawe CJ: Hemiatrophy. *J Pediatr Orthop* 2003;23(1):99-101.

Seven patients with ipsilateral facial and somatic hemiatrophy are described, and the authors report that the association of facial abnormalities and clinical features were the primary features to distinguish between hemihypertrophy and hemiatrophy. Leg-length discrepancy was moderate in these patients, and surgical correction was unlikely to be necessary.

Searle CP, Hildebrand RK, Lester EL, Caskey PM: Findings of fibular hemimelia syndrome with radiographically normal fibulae. *J Pediatr Orthop B* 2004;13(3):184-188.

In this retrospective review of 16 limbs with radiographically normal fibulae that had at least two features of fibular hemimelia syndrome, the authors found absent lateral rays in 13 of 16 limbs (81%), ball-and-socket ankle joints in 14 of 16 (88%), tarsal coalitions in 15 (94%), valgus knees in five (31%), hypoplastic tibial spines in four (25%), cruciate instability in three (19%), and clubfoot in four limbs (25%). Shortening was at least 4% and occurred in 80% of unilateral cases.

Acquired Conditions

Bowen RE, Dorey FJ, Moseley CF: Relative tibial and femoral varus as a predictor of progression of varus deformities of the lower limbs in young children. *J Pediatr Orthop* 2002;22(1):105-111.

Based on a review of 173 varus limbs, the authors describe the measurement of percentage of tibial deformity that when combined with the measurement of tibial metaphyseal–diaphyseal angle was found to be more accurate at predicting the progression of infantile varus than either measurement alone.

Davids JR, Blackhurst DW, Allen BL Jr: Clinical evaluation of bowed legs in children. *J Pediatr Orthop B* 2000; 9(4):278-284.

The authors describe the cover-up test used to assess tibia vara in infants and report the accuracy of the test based on examination of 68 patients.

Navascues JA, Gonzalez-Lopez JL, Lopez-Valverde S, Soleto J, Rodriguez-Durantez JA, Garcia-Trevijano JL: Premature physeal closure after tibial diaphyseal fractures in adolescents. *J Pediatr Orthop* 2000;20(2):193-196.

The authors report on seven patients with premature closure of the distal femoral and/or proximal or distal tibia physis following diaphyseal tibia fractures. Only one patient required surgical correction.

Park SS, Gordon JE, Luhmann SJ, Dobbs MB, Schoenecker PL: Outcome of hemiepiphyseal stapling for late-onset tibia vara. *J Bone Joint Surg Am* 2005;87(10): 2259-2266.

The authors assessed 33 extremities treated by hemiepiphysiodesis with staples and found that 42% had tibial and femoral hemiepiphysiodesis and that severe deformities were less likely to correct adequately to prevent the need for osteotomy.

Westberry DE, Davids JR, Pugh LI, Blackhurst D: Tibia vara: Results of hemiepiphyseodesis. *J Pediatr Orthop B* 2004;13(6):374-378.

The authors of this study reviewed 33 extremities treated by hemiepiphysiodesis with staples or drilling and found improvement of the mechanical axis by 5° or more in 55% of the extremities and no significant change in 33%. The preoperative mechanical axis and preoperative proximal tibial articular angle were reported to be significant to the outcome.

Treatment

Barker KL, Simpson AH: Recovery of function after closed femoral shortening. *J Bone Joint Surg Br* 2004; 86(8):1182-1186.

In this prospective assessment of 19 sequential patients who had femoral shortening, the authors found that weakness continued to improve over a 2-year period. They also reported that leg extensor power persisted, but did not affect self-reported function.

Gordon JE, Goldfarb CA, Luhmann SJ, Lyons D, Schoenecker PL: Femoral lengthening over a humeral intramedullary nail in preadolescent children. *J Bone Joint Surg Am* 2002;84-A(6):930-937.

In this study, nine patients (age range, 8 to 11 years) who had femoral lengthening over a humeral nail were reviewed. The authors reported that osteomyelitis occurred in two patients, one of whom had a history of multifocal neonatal osteomyelitis and one of whom developed infection after an extensive reoperation for fracture at the end of the nail. No signs of avascular necrosis were found in any of the patients at a 2-year minimum follow-up.

Kocaoglu M, Eralp L, Kilicoglu O, Burc H, Cakmak M: Complications encountered during lengthening over an intramedullary nail. *J Bone Joint Surg Am* 2004;86-A(11):2406-2411.

The authors of this study reported that 35 femurs and 7 tibiae that were lengthened over an intramedullary nail had a complication rate of 38%, including 10 of 12 patients who required reoperation. The complication rate was significantly higher in patients whose bones were lengthened more than 21.5% of the original length.

McCarthy JJ, Burke T, McCarthy MC: Need for concomitant proximal fibular epiphysiodesis when performing a proximal tibial epiphysiodesis. *J Pediatr Orthop* 2003; 23(1):52-54.

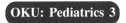

The authors conducted a retrospective review of 44 patients who underwent proximal tibial epiphysiodesis, 11 of whom underwent concomitant proximal fibular epiphysiodesis. Fibular overgrowth was reported to be more than 10 mm in patients with 3 years or more before skeletal maturity who had only tibial arrest.

Song HR, Oh CW, Mattoo R, et al: Femoral lengthening over an intramedullary nail using the external fixator: Risk of infection and knee problems in 22 patients with a follow-up of 2 years or more. *Acta Orthop* 2005;76(2): 245-252.

The authors conducted a retrospective review of femoral lengthening that was performed over an intramedullary nail in 22 patients and found that osteomyelitis occurred in 3 of 10 patients who had prior osteomyelitis or grade III open fracture before the index procedure; however, osteomyelitis did not occur in any of the 12 patients with no prior infection.

Surdam JW, Morris CD, DeWeese JD, Drvaric DM: Leg length inequality and epiphysiodesis: Review of 96 cases. *J Pediatr Orthop* 2003;23(3):381-384.

The authors conducted a retrospective comparison of 40 patients who had open Phemister-type epiphysiodesis and 56 patients who had percutaneous epiphysiodesis. They reported that one deep infection occurred in the Phemister-type epiphysiodesis group and that two complete arrest failures and one angular deformity occurred in the percutaneous epiphysiodesis group. The difference of overall complication rates and failure of closure were not statistically significant.

Watanabe K, Tsuchiya H, Sakurakichi K, Yamamoto N, Kabata T, Tomita K: Tibial lengthening over an intramedullary nail. *J Orthop Sci* 2005;10(5):480-485.

The authors of this retrospective study compared 13 tibiae with single-level lengthening over an intramedullary nail and 17 tibiae that were lengthened without an intramedullary nail and found the average fixation time per centimeter was 18 minutes with the intramedullary nail and 41 minutes without a nail. Complications were more common in the group without an intramedullary nail and included a higher infection rate.

Classic Bibliography

Anderson M, Green WT, Messner MB: Growth and predictions of growth in the lower extremities. *J Bone Joint Surg Am* 1963;45-A:1-14.

Blount WP: Tibia vara: Osteochondrosis deformans tibiae. *J Bone Joint Surg* 1937;19:1.

Blount WP, Clarke GR: The classic: Control of bone growth by epiphyseal stapling. A preliminary report. Journal of Bone and Joint Surgery, July, 1949. *Clin Orthop Relat Res* 1971;77:4-17.

Bowen JR, Leahey JL, Zhang ZH, MacEwen GD: Partial epiphysiodesis at the knee to correct angular deformity. *Clin Orthop Relat Res* 1985;198:184-190.

Boyd HB: Pathology and natural history of congenital pseudarthrosis of the tibia. *Clin Orthop Relat Res* 1982; 166:5-13.

Gabriel KR, Crawford AH, Roy DR, True MS, Sauntry S: Percutaneous epiphyseodesis. *J Pediatr Orthop* 1994; 14(3):358-362.

Greene WB: Infantile tibia vara. *J Bone Joint Surg Am* 1993;75(1):130-143.

Green WT, Anderson M: Experiences with epiphyseal arrest in correcting discrepancies in length of the lower extremities in infantile paralysis: A method of predicting the effect. *J Bone Joint Surg Am* 1947;29-A:659-675.

Greulich WW, Pyle SI: *Radiographic Atlas of Skeletal Development of the Hand and Wrist*, ed 2. Stanford, CA, Stanford University Press, 1959.

Gross RH: Leg length discrepancy: How much is too much? *Orthopedics* 1978;1(4):307-310.

Johnston CE II: Infantile tibia vara. *Clin Orthop Relat Res* 1990;255:13-23.

Jones D, Barnes J, Lloyd-Roberts GC: Congenital aplasia and dysplasia of the tibia with intact fibula: Classification and management. *J Bone Joint Surg Br* 1978; 60(1):31-39.

Kline SC, Bostrum M, Griffin PP: Femoral varus: An important component in late-onset Blount's disease. *J Pediatr Orthop* 1992;12(2):197-206.

Koman LA, Meyer LC, Warren FH: Proximal femoral focal deficiency: Natural history and treatment. *Clin Orthop Relat Res* 1982;162:135-143.

Langenskiold A: Tibia vara: Osteochondrosis deformans tibiae. Blount's disease. *Clin Orthop Relat Res* 1981;158: 77-82.

Loder RT, Herring JA: Fibular transfer for congenital absence of the tibia: A reassessment. *J Pediatr Orthop* 1987;7(1):8-13.

Maresh MM: Measurements from roentgenograms, in McCammon RW (ed): *Human Growth and Development*. Springfield, IL, Charles C. Thomas, 1970, pp 157-181.

Menelaus MB: Correction of leg length discrepancy by epiphysial arrest. *J Bone Joint Surg Br* 1966;48(2):336-339.

Moseley CF: A straight-line graph for leg-length discrepancies. *J Bone Joint Surg Am* 1977;59(2):174-179.

Paley D: *Principles of Deformity Correction.* Berlin, Germany, Springer-Verlag, 2002.

Paley D, Herzenberg JE, Tetsworth K, McKie J, Bhave A: Deformity planning for frontal and sagittal plane corrective osteotomies. *Orthop Clin North Am* 1994;25(3): 425-465.

Pritchett JW: Longitudinal growth and growth-plate activity in the lower extremity. *Clin. Orthop Relat Res* 1992;275:274-279.

Schoenecker PL, Capelli AM, Millar EA, et al: Congenital longitudinal deficiency of the tibia. *J Bone Joint Surg Am* 1989;71(2):278-287.

Schoenecker PL, Meade WC, Pierron RL, Sheridan JJ, Capelli AM: Blount's disease: A retrospective review and recommendations for treatment. *J Pediatr Orthop* 1985;5(2):181-186.

Shapiro F: Developmental patterns in lower-extremity length discrepancies. *J Bone Joint Surg Am* 1982;64(5): 639-651.

Tuncay IC, Johnston CE II, Birch JG: Spontaneous resolution of congenital anterolateral bowing of the tibia. *J Pediatr Orthop* 1994;14(5):599-602.

Chapter 16

Disorders of the Knee

Henry G. Chambers, MD

Introduction

Although congenital disorders of the knee are relatively rare in children, the incidence of injuries to the growing knee is increasing as children participate in many more activities on a year-round basis. The treatment of children with disorders of the knee, therefore, requires an understanding of normal growth and development as well as a solid understanding of sports medicine principles and procedures.

Congenital Knee Disorders

Knee Dislocation

Congenital dislocation of the knee is a rare entity (40 to 60 times less frequent than developmental dislocation of the hip). Children with this disorder usually present with a hyperextended knee that may or not be reducible. The disorder can be unilateral or bilateral. Most often subluxation is present, but a complete dislocation also can be present. When a knee dislocation is encountered, the hip must be evaluated. Severe pes calcaneovalgus also may be present. A child with a knee subluxation can be placed in a Pavlik harness in which the posterior straps are gradually pulled tighter to place the knee in increased degrees of flexion. Casting in progressing flexion can also be used. Complete dislocations may require more extensive treatment, including patellar tendon or quadriceps lengthening.

Patellar Dislocation

Congenital dislocation of the patella may not be apparent at birth because the cartilage anlage may not be palpable; in the knees of "chubby" children, it may not present until later. The patella is usually on the lateral side in patients with subluxation of the entire quadriceps mechanism. This is thought to be a failure of rotation of the quadriceps during development. It may be associated with conditions such as arthrogryposis, Larsen's syndrome, Rubinstein-Taybi syndrome, Down syndrome, and nail-patella syndrome. The patella develops later than usual in patients with congenital patellar dislocation and may not be visible on plain radiographs.

MRI usually shows evidence of a dysplastic patella and a dysplastic trochlear groove of the femur.

There are two distinct types of congenital dislocation of the patella: persistent dislocation and obligatory dislocation. Patients with persistent dislocation of the patella have lateral dislocation and knee flexion contracture that is obvious in infancy. It is frequently associated with a syndrome, nearly always results in functional disability, and usually requires early surgical correction. Patients with obligatory dislocation of the patella have a dynamic component associated with this disorder that does not present clinically until age 5 to 10 years. Patients typically report that the symptoms of obligatory dislocation of the patella may be well tolerated with little functional disability; therefore, surgical intervention may be delayed.

Reconstruction is more extensive for congenital dislocation of the patella than for acute patellar dislocation. In addition to lateral release and medial reefing, it is often necessary to extend the incision proximally to release the quadriceps up to the level of the proximal femur. The quadriceps are then rotated as a unit to medialize the entire mechanism.

Congenital Absence of the Anterior Cruciate Ligament

Congenital absence of the anterior cruciate ligament (ACL) is associated with many different entities, including congenital absence of the tibia or the fibula. In patients with this disorder, the entire knee joint is often dysplastic, and the intercondylar notch is often diminished or absent. Congenital absence of the ACL is often associated with conditions such as congenital short femur, proximal femoral focal deficiency, fibular hemimelia, congenital knee dislocation, Larsen's syndrome, or absence of the radius. There are associated intra-articular findings in the knee as well, including absent or hypoplastic menisci, discoid meniscus, and osteochondritis dissecans. There is a consistent finding of a hypertrophied ligament of Humphry in the intercondylar notch in this patient population. These patients often develop chondral changes and eventually osteoarthritis. Al-

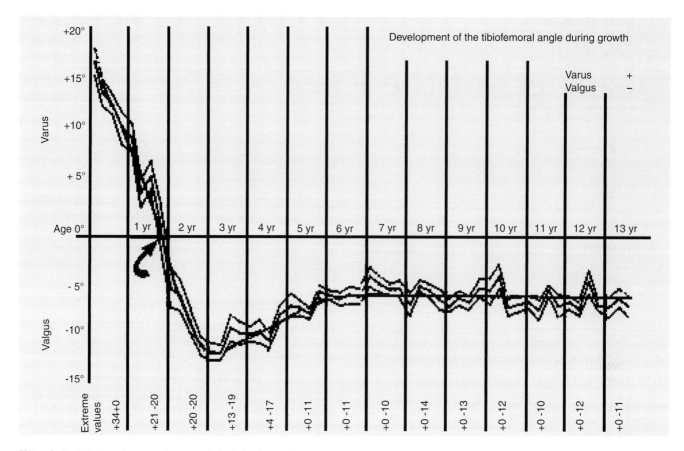

Figure 1 Graph illustrates how normal varus angulation before 2 years of age changes to valgus angulation after 2 years of age. *(Reproduced with permission from Salenius P, Vankka E: The development of the tibiofemoral angle in children. J Bone Joint Surg Am 1975;57:259-260.)*

though there are reports of reconstruction using tendon allografts, no long-term studies demonstrate their effectiveness in preventing osteoarthritis. A very narrow intercondylar notch has been reported as a challenge in performing the reconstructions as well as recurrence of bone formation within the notch after reconstruction.

Contractures About the Knee

Popliteal pterygium syndrome is a rare disorder in which webbing of the popliteal fossa occurs. The cardinal features of popliteal pterygium syndrome include popliteal webs with or without intercrural pterygia (90% of patients), cleft palate with or without cleft lip (75% of patients), genital anomalies (50% of patients), salivary pits (40% of patients), and syngnathia (oral webbing) (25% of patients). Other anomalies may also appear, such as ankyloblepharon filiforme adnatum (adhesion of the eyelids), abnormal scalp hair, inguinal hernia, hyperpigmentation around the genitals, or intraoral webbing. Associated orthopaedic findings include adactyly, syndactyly, brachydactyly, clinodactyly, toenail dysplasia, hypoplastic or absent first rays, contracted heel cords, valgus or varus foot deformities, hypoplastic patellae, scoliosis, rib anomalies, and hypoplastic tibiae. The hands and arms are usually normal in these patients.

Patients with popliteal pterygium syndrome are notoriously difficult to treat because of the shortening of the neurovascular structures in the popliteal space. MRI or magnetic resonance angiography should be performed to assess the location of the vessels prior to any treatment. Treatment should consist of soft-tissue lengthening for patients with mild deformities, with care taken to fully protect the neurovascular structures. For patients with severe deformities, gradual correction with an external fixator with or without femoral extension osteotomy is a treatment option, even though there is a high likelihood of recurrence in this patient population. Anterior staple epiphysiodesis of the distal femur may be considered in these instances.

Developmental Knee Disorders

Genu Varum

Genu varum is part of the normal development of the child (Figure 1). Most children are in mild genu varum until approximately 18 months of age. Varus may appear to be worse than it actually is because severe internal tibial torsion can present as genu varum. Genu varum disorder will resolve within a few years in most patients without treatment. The internal tibial torsion, however, may require up to 5 additional years to improve.

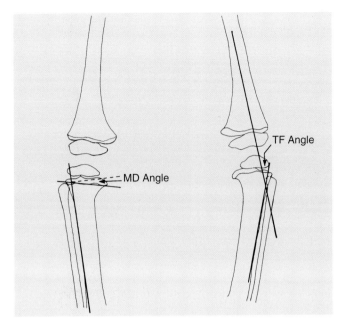

Figure 2 Illustration of the measurement of the tibial metaphyseal-diaphyseal (MD) **(A)** and tibiofemoral (TF) **(B)** angles. *(Reproduced with permission from Henderson RC, Lechner CT, DeMasi RA, Greene WB: Variability in radiographic measurement of bowleg deformity in children. J Pediatr Orthop 1990;10(4):491-494.)*

A small subset of children will not improve and varus will worsen. Tibia varum (Blount disease) is a disorder of the knee; patients typically have severe genu varum with variable effects on the physis. In juvenile Blount disease, it is unclear whether there is a primary physeal disorder or whether the malalignment leads to the characteristic changes that are visible on radiographs. The disorder has been assessed using the metaphyseal-diaphyseal angle (Figure 2). The angular deformity in both the femur and the tibia is also determined by measuring the angles between their mechanical axes and the transverse axis of the knee. Patients who have a metaphyseal-diaphyseal angle greater than 16° have been reported to experience progression of the angular deformity. Although this finding suggests that children with this type of deformity should be treated with surgical correction, treatment is controversial. Some authors have reported that early and continuous bracing in the early stages can achieve good results, whereas others believe that osteotomies must be performed to realign the lower extremity in this patient population. In two different studies, there was a 70% to 90% success rate with continuous bracing. The risk factors for failure include instability (usually a varus thrust), obesity, and bilateral involvement. Osteotomies are performed distal to the tibial physis (or proximal to the femoral physis) to avoid growth disturbance.

Adolescent Blount disease usually occurs in obese children who develop this disorder in their early teenage years. This entity is probably the result of asymmetric forces on the physis (according to the Heuter-Volkmann law), which lead to progressive varus. If adolescent Blount disease is identified before the cessation of growth, stapling of the lateral physis (often both tibia and femur) can lead to improvement of the alignment. Older children with Blount disease typically require an osteotomy of the tibia and fibula. Fixation can be done using internal plates or via external fixation. (For more on Blount disease, see chapter 15.)

Physiologic Valgus

Physiologic valgus usually occurs in children who are approximately 3½ years old whose parents report to have just recently noticed it (Figure 1). This entity is treated with observation, and most patients improve by age 7 years. Some patients, however, will experience progression of physiologic valgus or fail to improve. These children may have recurvatum of the knee as well. The indications for treatment are rather subjective and include appearance, pain, or potential for osteoarthritis. Gait studies have demonstrated correction of biomechanical axes after treatment, but there have been no long-term studies demonstrating a decrease in osteoarthritis. As with genu varum, genu valgum can be treated with physeal stapling of the femur and/or tibia, depending on where the deformity is located when the child is at the appropriate age or with tibial or femoral osteotomy when the child is older.

Discoid Meniscus

Discoid menisci typically occur in the lateral knee joint. Controversy exists about the etiology of discoid meniscus. Most authors believe discoid menisci are the result of a congenital abnormality, but some believe that the etiology of this disorder is developmental because no instances have been observed in autopsies of newborns or stillbirths. It is likely that discoid menisci develop because of a lack of peripheral attachments of the meniscotibial ligaments. Three types of discoid menisci have been described: complete, incomplete, and Wrisberg type. A complete absence of the meniscotibial ligaments with only an attachment of the ligament of Wrisberg leads to a hypermobile meniscus (Wrisberg type). A variable attachment of these ligaments and a variable extent of the meniscus from a complete discoid meniscus (a half moon) to a slightly wider meniscus may also occur.

Only children with symptoms such as popping and locking should undergo surgical treatment. If patients have adequate peripheral attachments, only the central portion of the meniscus should be removed arthroscopically (saucerization). This may be a challenging surgical procedure to perform because the knees of children are small and most arthroscopic instruments are either too large (designed for the adult knee) or not stout enough (designed for small joints). Patients with no peripheral attachments (those with Wrisberg type) are the most chal-

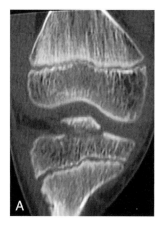 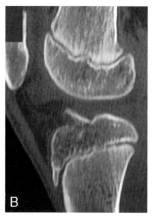 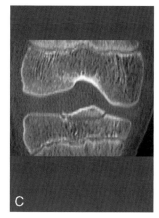 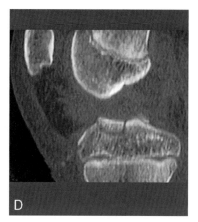

Figure 3 **A** and **B,** Preoperative CT scans of a type II intercondylar eminence fracture. **C** and **D,** Postoperative CT scans of a type II intercondylar eminence fracture after open reduction and internal fixation using suture.

lenging patients to treat. Short-term follow-up studies have suggested that repair of the distal portion of the saucerized meniscus to the capsule leads to good short-term function, but long-term outcome is unknown. A complete meniscectomy may be necessary in these patients.

Popliteal Cysts

Popliteal cysts are classified as primary or secondary cysts. The cyst is considered primary if it arises from the distension of a bursa and secondary if there is a communication between the cyst and the knee joint, indicating intra-articular pathology such as a meniscal tear, ACL deficiency, polyarthritis, villonodular synovitis, or some other connective tissue disease. In an MRI study, 6% of asymptomatic children had an incidental popliteal cyst. In children, the cyst is usually a distension of the bursa under the medial head of the gastrocnemius muscle, or it may arise from the semimembranosus muscle fascia.

In children, the clinical presentation is usually a painless mass that has been noted by the parents. Diagnostic imaging should include plain radiography, ultrasound, or MRI. Ultrasound seems to be the best diagnostic imaging modality in children in whom there is no suspicion of intra-articular pathology. Ultrasound can also distinguish between cysts and a potential solid tumor in the popliteal region.

Most popliteal cysts in children should be treated conservatively. Surgical excision should be considered if the mass becomes painful or enlarges rapidly.

Sports-Related Injuries
Tibial Eminence Fractures

The ACL is attached to the medial tibial spine, which is part of the tibial eminence. With stress, the incompletely ossified tibial eminence typically fractures through the cancellous bone of the subchondral plate before the ligament is injured. Before a tibial eminence fracture occurs, the ACL is often stretched. The fracture may extend

into the weight-bearing portion of the joint, and the meniscus or the intermeniscal ligament may be entrapped within the fracture.

Although it is generally recommended that type I and type II tibial eminence fractures should be treated conservatively in slight flexion, this may not reduce the fracture. Type III and IV tibial eminence fractures should be treated with arthroscopic or open reduction using suture, Kirschner wires, or screw fixation, with care taken to avoid injuring the tibial physis (Figure 3). Outcome studies have demonstrated that residual laxity as defined by KT1000 Knee Ligament Arthrometer (MEDmetric, San Diego, CA) testing persists, even with anatomic reduction and regardless of the technique of fixation. Most of these are asymptomatic after treatment.

ACL Injuries

The incidence of ACL injuries in children and adolescents is increasing. Some studies continue to show a female preponderance of ACL injuries. Several theories have been advanced to account for this difference, including hormonal changes, a wide pelvis with relative valgus at the knee, narrow intercondylar notches, or kinematic and kinetic differences in stopping and landing from a jump in females. Preventative plyometric exercise programs show some promise in decreasing the incidence of ACL injuries in female athletes.

There are four primary treatment options for the skeletally immature child or adolescent with an ACL tear: nonsurgical treatment, repair of the ligament tear, nonsurgical treatment until the child is near skeletal maturity (at which time ACL reconstruction is performed), or ACL reconstruction close to the time of injury regardless of age.

Nonsurgical treatment is appealing for patients with ACL tears because there is no risk of damaging the physes with surgical intervention. However, nonsurgical management can result in later meniscal tears and de-

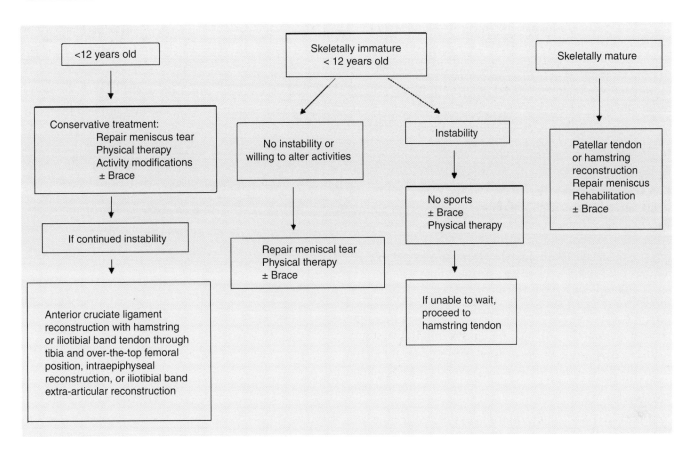

Figure 4 Algorithm for children with ACL injuries.

generative changes in most patients with ACL tears. If the patient is able to abstain from participation in cutting sports and wears a protective brace, reconstruction may not be required. Most studies demonstrate a poor long-term outcome for conservative treatment.

The main concern about ACL reconstruction in a skeletally immature athlete is the possibility of physeal damage leading to limb-length discrepancy or angular deformity. Reports have been published describing physeal damage leading to partial or complete closure of the femoral or tibial physis.

Several different methods have been cited in the literature to treat ACL injuries based on skeletal maturity and ability to cooperate with the rehabilitation and activity limitations (Figure 4). Repair of the ACL has not been proven to be effective in children or adults. Various extra-articular methods such as an iliotibial band tenodesis have been attempted, but the long-term results of this treatment have not been good. In a child whose skeletal maturity is less than 12 years (determined by chronological age, bone age, and secondary sexual characteristics), there are several treatment options. An autologous iliotibial graft placed intra-articularly has been recently described with a 5-year follow-up with no growth arrests (Figure 5). Other studies report the use of an allograft with drilling through

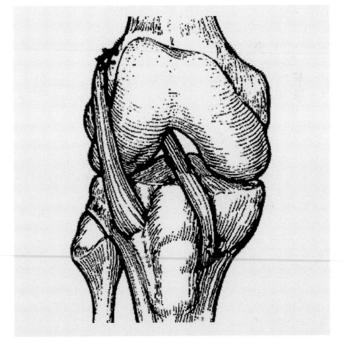

Figure 5 Illustration of physeal-sparing reconstruction of the ACL using an autologous iliotibial band graft. *(Reproduced with permission from Kocher MS, Garg S, Micheli LJ: Physeal sparing reconstruction of the anterior cruciate ligament in skeletally immature prepubescent children and adolescents. J Bone Joint Surg Am 2005;87(11): 2371-2379.)*

the tibial physes with an over-the-top femoral placement, hamstring grafts placed in the same manner as adults, and a novel intraepiphyseal graft placement (Figure 6). As children get older, hamstring (autograft or allograft) or bone-patellar tendon-bone graft may be used as in adults.

Posterior Cruciate Ligament Injuries

Posterior cruciate ligament (PCL) injuries are rare in children and are often missed during the initial evaluation of a knee injury. The mechanism of injury is usually a fall onto a flexed knee, a dashboard injury from a motor vehicle accident, or severe hyperextension. Although ACL injuries typically result in instability, PCL injuries may be associated with disability from degenerative disease of the medial joint compartment.

Children have a higher incidence of bony avulsion injuries from the tibial insertion, and they may also experience bony avulsions of the femur. Bony avulsions should be repaired with intraepiphyseal sutures or screw fixation. MRI and often arthroscopy should be performed before prone positioning of the patient because of the high incidence of associated injuries. Articular cartilage injuries may not be appreciated on MRI studies.

Combined PCL and posterolateral complex injuries are extremely difficult to treat in children. No known natural history studies in children with this injury combination have been conducted. Conservative treatment involves bracing of the patient until skeletal maturity. The most prudent surgical intervention involves procedures such as posterolateral repair or proximal advancement that do not violate the physis of the femur tibia or fibula.

Patellar Dislocation and Subluxation

Patellar dislocation and subluxation are relatively common in children, especially those who actively participate in sports. This type of injury was initially thought to occur in obese and nonactive patients, but recent findings in the literature dispute this assumption. The redislocation rate varies from 15% to 50% of patients with patellar dislocation and subluxation.

Many factors contribute to patellar dislocation and subluxation, and it is important to evaluate all of the risk factors, including generalized ligamentous laxity, increased Q angle, increased femoral anteversion and tibial external rotation, trochlear hypoplasia, and patella alta. Although no studies have confirmed that these factors are causative, each nonetheless may contribute to this type of injury.

There is controversy about the initial treatment of patellar dislocation and subluxation. Some retrospective studies recommended repair of the main stabilizer of the patella, the medial patellofemoral ligament, as initial treatment, whereas other studies have suggested that immediate casting or immobilization provides similar

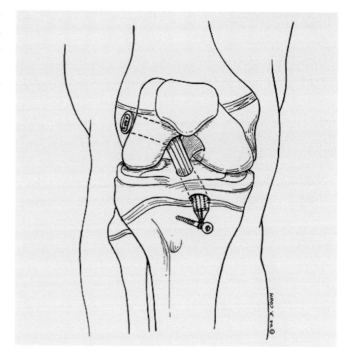

Figure 6 Illustration of transepiphyseal placement of hamstring graft. *(Reproduced with permission from Anderson, AF: Transepiphyseal replacement of the anterior cruciate ligament in skeletally immature patients: A preliminary report. J Bone Joint Surg Am 2004;86A(suppl 1):201-209.)*

results. Strengthening exercises are important after patients with patellar dislocation and subluxation undergo initial immobilization. The use of bracing is controversial in this patient population. Additionally, physicians treating these patients must be watchful for the presence of intra-articular chondral or osteochondral fractures either of the patella or the femoral condyle. Arthroscopic inspection and/or MRI evaluation of the knee should be considered if a fracture is suspected. If a patient continues to have pain and swelling after 6 to 8 weeks, there is a good chance that there is an undiagnosed chondral injury. These chondral injuries may be missed on MRI examinations.

More than 30 different procedures are available for the treatment of chronic patellar instability; therefore, clinicians face a dilemma whenever surgery is contemplated. The consensus seems to be that soft-tissue realignment, either open or arthroscopic, should be performed for chronic recurrent dislocations in skeletally immature patients. Patients with severe malalignment of their extremities may require derotational osteotomies or epiphyseal stapling; however, the literature on the indications to perform these procedures is not clear. In skeletally mature patients, studies have suggested that the Elmslie-Trillat procedure or Fulkerson procedure used to medialize the tibial tubercle may lead to improved outcomes. Osteotomies of the tibial tubercle cannot be done in children with open growth plates without significant risk of growth disturbance.

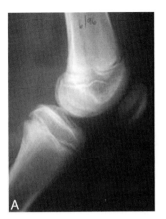
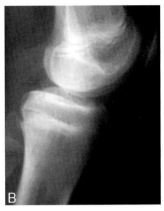

Figure 7 **A** and **B,** Lateral radiographs show osteochondritis dissecans lesion of the knee.

Osteochondral Lesions of the Knee

Osteochondritis dissecans is an osteochondral lesion of the distal femoral condyle. Although these lesions can occur on all cartilage surfaces of the knee, they most commonly occur on the lateral aspect of the medial femoral condyle. Theories about the etiology of osteochondritis dissecans of the knee range from developmental to traumatic; numerous treatment options also have been described.

Children with osteochondral lesions of the knee may present with chronic knee pain or knee pain that has occurred as the result of a single traumatic incident while participating in athletic activities. Although no effusion is typically present in these patients, when effusions do occur, clinicians should evaluate the child for the presence of a displaced fragment. Plain radiographs (including a tunnel view) can help demonstrate the presence of lesions. MRI is a helpful imaging tool that can be used to classify lesions and determine whether disruption of the cartilage surface exists.

Type I lesions (intact cartilage surface lesions) should be treated initially with activity restriction or short-term immobilization. If the lesions do not heal or are excessively large or symptomatic, then drilling of the lesions either through the joint surface or via an extra-articularly approach may reestablish the blood flow and heal the lesion. Generally, children with open femoral physes and type I lesions do well without surgical intervention. More severe lesions (large lesions that have not healed with conservative management and those with a cartilage flap [type II] or a free fragment [type III]) should have immediate arthroscopic evaluation with drilling of the lesion and possible fixation with resorbable or nonresorbable implants (Figure 7).

The treatment of displaced chondral and osteochondral injuries in children and adolescents is not clear. The goal for any reconstructive procedure is to produce a smooth gliding articular surface of hyaline or hyaline-like cartilage. Débridement, drilling, microfracture, and

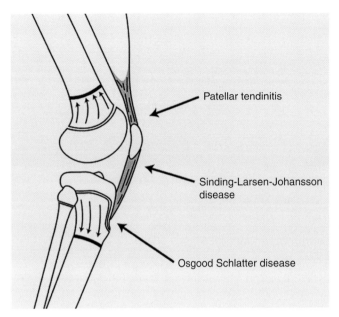

Figure 8 Illustration showing apophyseal injuries around the knee as a result of growth of the femur and tibia.

abrasion chondroplasty have been shown to result in fibrocartilage with inferior mechanical properties when compared with hyaline cartilage. Current techniques to restore the hyaline cartilage surface, including mosaicplasty, osteochondral allograft transplantation, and autologous chondrocyte transplantation, have not been extensively studied in children and adolescents.

Anterior Knee Pain

One of the most common reasons for a child to consult with a physician is anterior knee pain. Although many believe that this is a self-limited disease and that it can be treated by rest, there are many studies indicating that this entity is not as benign as once thought. Ninety percent of patients will still have pain at long-term follow-up, and 45% may eventually have a diagnosis of a systemic rheumatologic disorder. There are many different causes of anterior knee pain, but the primary etiology seems to be related to growth of the child. The weakest link in the muscle-tendon-bone interface is the cartilaginous apophysis at the proximal and distal ends of the patella. Growth often leads to mild contractures of the quadriceps and hamstrings, which leads to increased stress at these apophyses. Some anatomic variations of tendon insertion may also be present and contribute to the anterior knee pain. Tibial tubercle apophysitis (Osgood-Schlatter disease), distal pole avulsion (Sinding-Larsen-Johansson disease), and patellar tendinitis are common manifestations of this continuum. Treatment usually involves relative rest and stretching of the quadriceps and hamstring muscles. In children who have pain with rest, cast immobilization may be necessary (Figure 8).

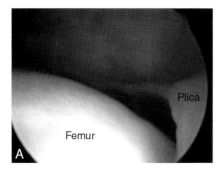
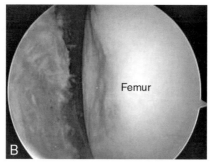
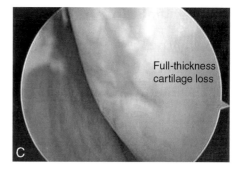

Figure 9 **A,** Arthroscopic image shows medial plica overlying the articular surface of the femur. **B** and **C,** Arthroscopic images show articular cartilage damage on the medial aspect of the femoral condyle.

Symptomatic Medial Plica

Plicae are synovial folds of the knee that are remnants of the synovial membranes present during embryologic development. Most plicae that are present in normal knees are asymptomatic. However, some, especially medial plicae, can become symptomatic after an initial traumatic event. The patient may report medial knee pain (proximal to the joint line and medial to the patella), popping, clicking, and even locking of the knee. There is usually a palpable cord that is tender and reproduces the patient's pain.

Initial treatment is rest and stretching. However, some patients may continue to have symptoms and require arthroscopic excision of the plica. There may even be erosions of the medial femoral condyle that contributes to the pain in this area (Figure 9). A prospective, randomized trial conducted in Great Britain demonstrated the efficacy of plica excision. Most patients will rapidly return to their previous sports activities.

Bipartite Patella

The bipartite patella is usually an incidental finding on a radiograph obtained to assess knee pain. This entity is most likely a failure of an accessory center of ossification to unite with the rest of the patella, but other theories such as direct trauma, stress fractures, or a traction apophysitis have been posited. A classification system has been proposed in which type I represents a lesion at the inferior pole of the patella, type II represents a lesion at the lateral margin, and type III represents a lesion at the superolateral corner of the patella—the most common and most often symptomatic type of lesion.

Patients with type III bipartite patella will exhibit tenderness at the superolateral pole and relate that this is where the pain occurs when playing sports. The treatment is rest, immobilization if significantly symptomatic, and surgery if the pain is unrelenting. Surgical procedures to treat bipartite patella vary from excision of the piece (often the articular surface is still intact), tenotomy of the vastus lateralis that attaches to the piece, or open reduction with or without internal fixation.

Summary

Disorders of the knee are an increasing problem in pediatric orthopedic surgical practices. More children are playing sports on a year-round basis, and there is an escalation in the number of significant knee injuries and reports of anterior knee pain in the adolescent age group. A careful history, physical examination, and utilization of appropriate diagnostic imaging studies will permit clinicians to diagnose disorders of the knee and develop an appropriate treatment regimen, which includes rest, physical therapy, or surgery for each of these challenging injuries.

Annotated Bibliography
General

Moti AW, Micheli LJ: Meniscal and articular cartilage injury in the skeletally immature knee. *Instr Course Lect* 2003;52:683-690.

Meniscal and articular cartilage injuries in skeletally immature patients appear to be occurring with increased frequency, particularly in athletically active children. The orthopaedic surgeon should understand the principles of diagnosis and management, as well as be aware of current surgical treatment options available.

Smith AD: The skeletally immature knee: What's new in overuse injuries. *Instr Course Lect* 2003;52:691-697.

Overuse and growth-related disorders of the knee occur frequently among children and adolescents. Most of these disorders are self-limited and respond well to a therapeutic exercise program that includes restoring or attaining normal lower extremity strength and flexibility and good dynamic lower extremity alignment. Other causes of knee pain, such as training errors and inadequate footgear, may need to be corrected. Bracing may be useful for temporary amelioration of knee pain in order to allow successful performance of the therapeutic exercise program. Surgical intervention is rarely necessary for adolescents with knee pain resulting from overuse.

Tepper KB, Ireland ML: Fracture patterns and treatment in the skeletally immature knee. *Instr Course Lect* 2003;52:667-676.

Knee injuries commonly occur in children and adolescents who participate in athletic activities. Open growth plates, apophyses, and chondroepiphyses are unique to the skeletally immature knee and account for the differences in injury patterns observed in children and adults. An understanding of anatomy and classification as related to treatment and outcome of fractures in the skeletally immature knee is important.

Congenital Knee Disorders

Gabos PG, Rassi GE, Pahys J: Knee reconstruction in syndromes with congenital absence of the anterior cruciate ligament. *J Pediatr Orthop* 2005;25:210-214.

The authors reported on four patients who underwent surgical treatment of symptomatic knee instability at a mean age of 15.8 years. All patients had other problems such as fibular hemimelia, congenital short femur, and other skeletal dysplasias. The authors found hypertrophy of the meniscofemoral ligament of Humphry in all patients. Overall, they reported improvement in function after the patients underwent ACL reconstruction.

Developmental Knee Disorders

Bowen RE, Dorey FJ, Moseley CF: Relative tibial and femoral varus as a predictor of progression of varus deformities of the lower limbs in young children. *J Pediatr Orthop* 2002;22:105-111.

The authors describe a new method of measuring tibia vara by determining the angular deformity in both the femur and tibia, which is done by measuring the angles between their mechanical axes and the transverse axis of the knee. They determined the contribution of the tibial deformity to be a percentage of the total deformity. They found that all patients with a metaphyseal diaphyseal angle of the tibia greater than 16° and a percentage of tibial deformity greater than 50% experienced progression of varus deformities; they concluded that all such patients should be treated.

Eilert RE: Congenital dislocation of the patella. *Clin Orthop Relat Res* 2001;389:22-29.

The author discusses the causes of congenital dislocation of the patella and lists two types. The first type, congenital dislocation, is fixed, often associated with syndromes, and should be treated. The second type, obligatory dislocation, requires only observation until patients are older.

Fritschy D, Fasel J, Imbert JC, Bianchi S, Verdonk R, Wirth CJ: The popliteal cyst. *Knee Surg Sports Traumatol Arthrosc* 2005;:1-6. [Epub ahead of print]

The authors of this review article examined the anatomy, diagnostic imaging, and treatment of popliteal cysts in children and adults. They report that in children, a popliteal cyst primary arises from a bursa, whereas in adults (the Baker's cyst) the cyst is associated with intra-articular pathology in most instances. Excision of the popliteal cyst in children was not advised.

Kelly BT, Green DW: Discoid lateral meniscus in children. *Curr Opin Pediatr* 2002;14:54-61.

In this review of the types and treatment of discoid menisci in children, the authors suggest that asymptomatic discoid menisci should not be treated; however, if a patient has a Wrisberg type discoid meniscus with a lack of posterior attachment, repair and saucerization should be performed.

Sports-Related Injuries

Aichroth PM, Patel DV, Zorrilla P: The natural history and treatment of rupture of the anterior cruciate ligament in children and adolescents: A prospective review. *J Bone Joint Surg Br* 2002;84:38-41.

The authors conducted a prospective review of 60 children and adolescents with ACL tears; 23 were treated conservatively, which resulted in severe instability and poor knee function. Forty-seven children subsequently underwent ACL reconstruction with a transphyseal technique. None of these children had limb-length discrepancies, and the overall results were satisfactory in 77% of patients.

Andrish JT: Anterior cruciate ligament injuries in the skeletally immature patient. *Am J Orthop* 2001;30:103-110.

The authors discuss the diagnosis, classification, anatomy, mechanism of injury, and management of ACL injuries in children and youth and present an algorithm for management.

Beasley LS, Chudik SC: Anterior cruciate ligament injury in children: Update of current treatment options. *Curr Opin Pediatr* 2003;15:45-52.

The authors describe the natural history of ACL injuries and the different treatment options available. They also provide a description of techniques for reconstruction.

Beasley LS, Vidal AF: Traumatic patellar dislocation in children and adolescents: Treatment update and literature review. *Curr Opin Pediatr* 2004;16:29-36.

The authors discuss the anatomy and physiology of patellar dislocations as well as a variety of treatment options. Although they suggest the use of conservative treatment initially, they report that repair or reconstruction of an injured ligament, such as the medial patellofemoral ligament, should be performed in instances of recurrence.

Fithian DC, Paxton EW, Stone ML, et al: Epidemiology and natural history of acute patellar dislocation. *Am J Sports Med* 2004;32:1114-1121.

The authors report the findings of a prospective study of 189 patients who were followed for 2 to 5 years. They found that the highest risk for redislocation occurred in females who were 10 to 17 years of age. Females in this age group were also found to have a greater risk for redislocation than first-time dislocators and a higher risk for dislocation of the opposite knee.

Haspl M, Cicak N, Klobucar H, Pecina M: Fully arthroscopic stabilization of the patella. *Arthroscopy* 2002;18:E2.

The authors describe a new technique for performing plication of the medial patellar retinaculum and arthroscopic release of the lateral structures. In the 17 patients for whom this technique was used, the authors reported good outcomes with no recurrences at 12- to 26-month follow-up.

Hughes JA, Cook JV, Churchill MA, Warren ME: Juvenile osteochondritis dissecans: A 5-year review of the natural history using clinical and MRI evaluation. *Pediatr Radiol* 2003;33:410-417.

The authors of this study used 5-year clinical and MRI evaluation to assess 21 knees in 19 patients with juvenile osteochondritis dissecans. Lesions were classified as either stable or unstable on MRI scans and compared with clinical and arthroscopic data. They found that despite extensive bone changes on MRI scans, 95% of patients improved with conservative treatment if the cartilage is intact.

Johnson DH: Complex issues in anterior cruciate ligament surgery: Open physes, graft selection, and revision surgery. *Arthroscopy* 2002;18(9 suppl 2):26-28.

The author discusses open physes, graft selection, and revision surgery in patients who undergo ACL surgery.

Kocher MS, Garg S, Micheli LJ: Physeal sparing reconstruction of the anterior cruciate ligament in skeletally immature prepubescent children and adolescents. *J Bone Joint Surg Am* 2005;87(11):2371-2379.

In this study, 44 skeletally immature patients underwent a physeal sparing, combined intra-articular and extra-articular reconstruction using an autogenous iliotibial band graft. Two of the patients required revision, but the rest had excellent functional outcomes, and none had growth arrest.

Kocher MS, Micheli LJ, Zurakowski D, Luke A: Partial tears of the anterior cruciate ligament in children and adolescents. *Am J Sports Med* 2002;30:697-703.

This prospective cohort study included 45 skeletally mature and skeletally immature patients (age ≤ 17 years) with an acute hemarthrosis, MRI signal changes, grade A or B Lachman and pivot shift test result, and partial ACL tears. All patients were treated without reconstruction and underwent structured rehabilitation. At a minimum 2-year follow-up, 14 patients (31%) had undergone reconstruction. Tears greater than 50%, predominantly posterolateral tears, grade B pivot shift test result, and older chronologic and skeletal patient age were significantly associated with reconstruction. Patients with tears greater than 50% or predominantly posterolateral had significantly lower Lysholm, satisfaction, and Cincinnati Knee Scale scores.

Lubowitz JH, Elson WS, Guttmann D: Part II: Arthroscopic treatment of tibial plateau fractures: Intercondylar eminence avulsion fractures. *Arthroscopy* 2005;21:86-92.

The authors describe the indications for and technique of arthroscopic fixation of type II and type III intercondylar eminence avulsion fractures.

Robertson W, Kelly BT, Green DW: Osteochondritis dissecans of the knee in children. *Curr Opin Pediatr* 2003; 15:38-44.

The authors discuss the anatomy, etiology, evaluation, classification, treatment, and expected outcome of osteochondritis dissecans lesions.

Shea KG, Apel PJ, Pfeiffer RP, et al: The tibial attachment of the anterior cruciate ligament in children and adolescents: Analysis of magnetic resonance imaging. *Knee Surg Sports Traumatol Arthrosc* 2002;10:102-108.

The authors of this study used MRI to compare the anatomy of the ACL in skeletally immature and adult subjects. They found that anatomic landmarks for the ACL were proportional in both age groups.

Stathopulu E, Baildam E: Anterior knee pain: A long-term follow-up. *Rheumatology* 2003;42:380-382.

In this study, 48 patients who were diagnosed with anterior knee pain as children were surveyed 4 to 18 years after initial presentation. The authors found that 91% of patients still had knee pain, 45% stated that it affected activities of daily living, and 36% stated that it restricted physical activities. In addition, 54% of patients reported used analgesic medications; 45% were subsequently diagnosed with other disorders such as psoriasis, arthritis, and ankylosing spondylitis; and 68% had symptoms in other joints at follow-up. The authors concluded that anterior knee pain may not be as benign as was once thought.

Classic Bibliography

Aglietti P, Buzzi R, Bassi PB, Fioriti M: Arthroscopic drilling in juvenile osteochondritis dissecans of the medial femoral condyle. *Arthroscopy* 1994;10:286-291.

Aglietti P, Bertini FA, Buzzi R, Beraldi R: Arthroscopic meniscectomy for discoid lateral meniscus in children and adolescents: 10-year follow-up. *Am J Knee Surg* 1999;12:83-87.

Clanton TO, DeLee JC, Sanders B, Neidre A: Knee ligament injuries in children. *J Bone Joint Surg Am* 1979;61: 1195-1201.

DeLee JC, Curtis R: Anterior cruciate ligament insufficiency in children. *Clin Orthop Relat Res* 1983;172:112-118.

Ehrlich MG, Strain RE Jr: Epiphyseal injuries about the knee. *Orthop Clin North Am* 1979;10:91-103.

Johnson DP, Eastwood DM, Witherow PJ: Symptomatic synovial plicae of the knee. *J Bone Joint Surg Am* 1993; 75(10):1485-1496.

Ko JY, Shih CH, Wenger DR: Congenital dislocation of the knee. *J Pediatr Orthop* 1999;19(2):252-259.

Lindholm TS, Osterman K: Treatment of juvenile osteochondritis dissecans in the knee. *Acta Orthop Belg* 1979; 45:633-640.

Lipscomb AB, Anderson AF: Tears of the anterior cruciate ligament in adolescents. *J Bone Joint Surg Am* 1986; 68:19-28.

Matelic TM, Aronsson DD, Boyd DW Jr, LaMont RL: Acute hemarthrosis of the knee in children. *Am J Sports Med* 1995;23:668-671.

Micheli LJ, Rask B, Gerberg L: Anterior cruciate ligament reconstruction in patients who are prepubescent. *Clin Orthop Relat Res* 1999;364:40-47.

Simonian PT, Metcalf MH, Larson RV: Anterior cruciate ligament injuries in the skeletally immature patient. *Am J Orthop* 1999;28:624-628.

Shelbourne KD, Patel DV, McCarroll JR: Management of anterior cruciate ligament injuries in skeletally immature adolescents. *Knee Surg Sports Traumatol Arthrosc* 1996;4:68-74.

Stanisavljevic S, Zemenick G, Miller D: Congenital, irreducible, permanent lateral dislocation of the patella. *Clin Orthop Relat Res* 1976;116:190-199.

Stanitski CL: Pediatric and adolescent sports injuries. *Clin Sports Med* 1997;16:613-633.

Stanitski CL: Patellar instability in the school age athlete. *Instr Course Lect* 1998;47:345-350.

Stanitski CL, Harvell JC, Fu F: Observations on acute knee hemarthrosis in children and adolescents. *J Pediatr Orthop* 1993;13:506-510.

Chapter 17

Idiopathic Clubfoot

John E. Herzenberg, MD

Monica Paschoal Nogueira, MD

Introduction

Clubfoot is the most common birth defect, with an incidence ranging from 1:250 to 1:1,000 live births depending on the population. For the parent of a baby with a clubfoot, some comfort may be derived from the fact that this is one of the most treatable birth defects; with modern treatment methods, children with a clubfoot are likely to lead normal, active lives and even participate in athletic activities. The etiology of clubfoot is largely unknown, but it is thought to be associated with multifactorial genetic inheritance and influenced by poorly understood environmental factors. Characterization of the precise gene that causes clubfoot remains elusive. Several studies have observed a summer seasonal peak incidence, suggesting a polio-like intrauterine enterovirus infection as the etiology. Indeed, a clubfoot resembles a foot afflicted by polio, with thin weak calf muscles, particularly the peroneal innervated muscles. More recent studies have not confirmed this seasonal variation.

The pathoanatomy of clubfoot has been well described from anatomic and radiographic perspectives. Idiopathic clubfoot can be conceptualized as an extreme position of the foot in maximum equinus, supination, and adduction (Figure 1). These movements are kinematically coupled and occur primarily around the subtalar joint and the ankle. Normal subtalar joint supination can be characterized as foot adduction, inversion, flexion, and heel varus. Subtalar pronation is foot abduction, eversion, dorsiflexion, and heel valgus. Understanding the normal pathomechanics of the subtalar joint is essential for effective manipulation of the clubfoot. As the clubfoot is manipulated, the entire foot moves obliquely around the two components of the subtalar joint: the talocalcaneal joint and the talocalcaneonavicular joint (For a discussion of vertical talus, see chapters 9 and 11.).

Prenatal Diagnosis

Routine prenatal ultrasound has been shown to be highly effective in detecting clubfoot prenatally, with virtually no false-negative predictions and a true positive

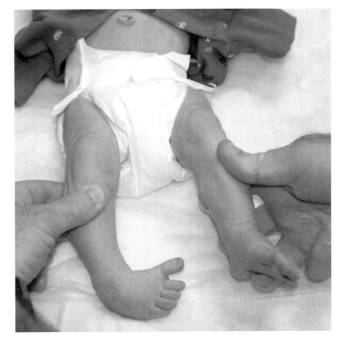

Figure 1 Photograph of a pediatric patient with an initial presentation of a moderate unilateral clubfoot.

predictive rate of 83%. In one recent study, the false-positive rate was 29% in patients with unilateral clubfoot and only 7% in those with bilateral clubfoot. Associated anomalies were more common in patients with bilateral clubfoot. Prenatal ultrasound diagnosis allows families to research the condition and prepare for the treatment. When counseling a parent with a positive prenatal ultrasound, it is worthwhile to emphasize that there may be a false-positive finding and that it may be impossible to make a determination of the severity of the clubfoot deformity until the baby is born. It is also often difficult to differentiate an idiopathic from a syndromic clubfoot in many instances until the baby can be examined after birth. Three-dimensional ultrasound provides a clearer picture of the clubfoot than standard two-dimensional ultrasound; however, studies comparing the two diagnostic modalities are lacking.

Table 1 | The Ponseti Method

Gently manipulate for approximately 30 seconds and then apply cast

First cast: raise the first metatarsal slightly to align forefoot with hindfoot and to decrease cavus

Never actively pronate the foot

Pure abduction of the forefoot with counterpressure on the neck of the talus but not the calcaneus

Long leg cast: the leg should be bent 90° at the knee and externally rotated

Weekly cast for 4 to 8 weeks (depending on severity of clubfoot)

Achilles tenotomy (90%) when foot is 70° externally rotated and heel is in valgus, then cast for 3 more weeks

Foot abduction orthosis (FAO) (Denis Browne bar) in external rotation: 70° for the clubfoot and 45° for the normal foot (in patients with unilateral clubfoot)

FAO full-time for 3 months, then nights (and naps) for 2 to 4 years

Early relapses treated with repeat casting, then resumption of FAO

Approximately 10% to 20% of patients need anterior tibialis tendon transfer with or without repeat Achilles tendon lengthening at 2 to 4 years for recurrent supination, varus, and/or equinus

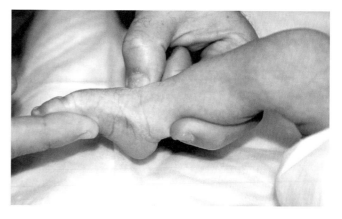

Figure 2 Photograph showing the manipulation technique (finger position); one finger pushes on the neck of the talus for counterpressure while the other abducts the forefoot, and the heel is not being touched.

Clinical Grading

There is no uniform agreement regarding the best classification system for clubfoot. The Pirani system is simple to apply, but it is not as detailed as the Dimeglio system. Recently, the International Clubfoot Study Group classification system has been shown to have good interobserver and intraobserver reliability.

Treatment

Since 2002, a veritable revolution has occurred in the treatment of idiopathic clubfoot. Whereas surgery once was the primary treatment, many pediatric orthopaedists now use the conservative method described by Ponseti. The Ponseti method has been well known in the peer-reviewed orthopaedic literature for at least four decades, but it was roundly ignored, except by Ponseti's trainees from the University of Iowa. The publication of Ponseti's monograph on idiopathic clubfoot in 1996 spurred a resurgence of interest in this largely nonsurgical method for the treatment of idiopathic clubfoot. As a result, the Ponseti method has become much more widely practiced, although with variable results. Many of the less satisfactory outcomes from this method likely result from the improper application of the technique. Because the Internet has become a major source of information on the Ponseti method for parents, orthopaedic practitioners should become well versed with the intricacies of the Ponseti method to avoid being in the position of knowing less about the Ponseti method than the parents of a child with idiopathic clubfoot.

The Ponseti Method

Table 1 lists the salient features of the Ponseti method. It should be emphasized that the Ponseti method was devised as a treatment for idiopathic clubfoot. The results have been reported as being successful in greater than 90% of patients, which obviates the need for extensive traditional open surgery. Many practitioners have successfully applied the Ponseti method to patients with selected syndromic clubfoot, but it is not always possible to avoid extensive surgery in patients with severe arthrogryposis and other teratologic foot deformities. Nonetheless, it is reasonable to attempt Ponseti manipulations in patients with nonidiopathic clubfoot as preliminary treatment before surgery. In these syndromic patients, often the forefoot deformity may correct with Ponseti manipulations, leaving only the hindfoot to be surgically corrected.

The Ponseti method calls for manipulations of the clubfoot on a weekly basis, although it has been shown to work when the casts are applied at 5-day intervals instead of 7-day intervals. The manipulations themselves are not lengthy or forceful. In the first manipulation, the first ray is gently elevated and abducted to decrease the cavus, while counterpressure is applied on the neck of the talus (Figure 2). This is counterintuitive because the forefoot is thought to already be supinated. In the classic Kite maneuver, the forefoot was treated by pronation. With the Ponseti method, pronation maneuvers are strictly prohibited because they tend to make the cavus deformity worse and lock the subtalar joint, making further correction difficult. Specifically, counterpressure should not be applied on the lateral wall of the calcaneus because this would block the external rotation correction that is desired. In this way, the Ponseti method is distinct from the Kite method. The Kite advocates firmly holding the hindfoot and abducting the forefoot against this counterforce to correct the metatarsus adductus. With the Ponseti method, the forefoot is ab-

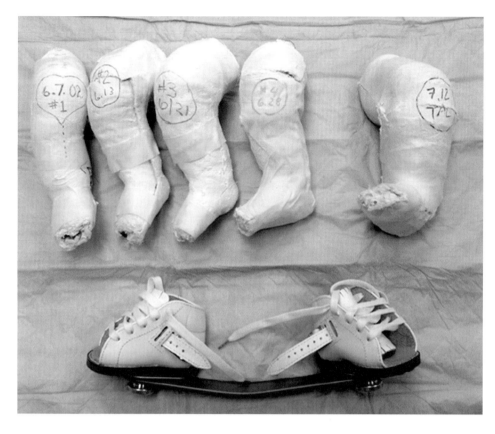

Figure 3 Photograph of casts and a brace shows how progressive correction is achieved.

ducted to not only correct the metatarsus adductus, but also to act as a force against the end of the os calcis through the calcaneocuboid joint to rotate the calcaneus externally.

The Ponseti method of casting requires two people, one to hold the foot in position and one to wrap the plaster. Some practitioners have used semirigid synthetic cast material successfully, but it is recommended to use plaster because of its superior moldability. The cast should extend beyond the toes to keep the long toe flexors stretched. On all but the tiniest of babies, the cast is applied in two parts: first, to the lower leg and foot and then, after the molding is complete, to the upper leg with the knee bent 90° (Figure 3).

With the Ponseti method, the casts are removed by soaking them briefly until softened and then cutting them off with a sharp cast knife. This is a valuable skill to acquire because it eliminates the need for the power cast saw, which can burn or scare the patient. At each additional visit, the foot is progressively abducted until the thigh-foot axis (as viewed from the foot) shows 70° of external rotation. This is critically important because stopping before 70° may eventually result in early relapse of the internal rotation deformity. Although parents may question the severe external rotation induced by the manipulations, they need to be reassured that over time the foot will gradually settle back to a more normal external rotation of about 10° to 15°.

When the foot has been externally rotated the requisite 70°, the heel will be in valgus; these are the criteria for the next step: Achilles tenotomy (Figure 4). This is done typically at age 3 months. The Ponseti is done as an outpatient office procedure using local anesthesia. In older infants, the tenotomy may be done with the patient under general anesthesia and under the supervision of a pediatric anesthesiologist. At the time of the tenotomy, the foot usually comes to neutral or about 10° above neutral. The tenotomy of the Achilles tendon adds an immediate 10° to 15° of additional dorsiflexion. The foot is then casted for the last time in maximum dorsiflexion. In approximately 10% of children, Achilles tenotomy is not needed; instead, serial casting can be done to obtain satisfactory dorsiflexion. With the Ponseti method, such decisions are made clinically, but many clinicians have been obtaining stress radiographs to determine whether there is inadvertent dorsiflexion at the midfoot (rockerbottom); if present, the foot should be recasted in plantar flexion for 1 to 2 weeks to allow the plantar ligaments to tighten, and then an Achilles tenotomy should be performed. The Ponseti Achilles tenotomy involves a complete transverse cut, not a triple cut or Z-lengthening. Complications from Achilles tenotomy are rare, but can include bleeding. One instance of pseudoaneurysm formation has been reported.

On the day of the tenotomy, measurements of the foot are made and a prescription is made for a foot ab-

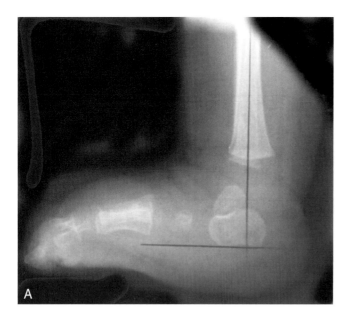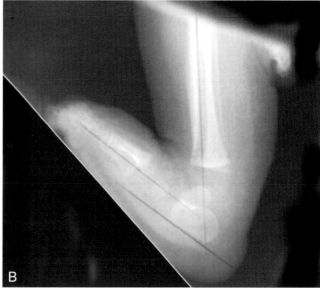

Figure 4 Radiographs obtained before **(A)** and after **(B)** tenotomy to show the improvement in dorsiflexion.

duction orthosis (FAO), which is essentially a Denis Browne bar with straight-last open-toed shoes (the Markell shoes, Yonkers, NY and the Mitchell orthosis, MD Orthopaedics, Wayland, IA). The bar is set at 75° on the clubfoot and 45° on the normal foot for patients with unilateral clubfoot, and 70° on each foot for those with bilateral clubfoot. The width of the bar should be such that the heels of the shoes are a shoulder's width apart. A small bend (concave toward the patient) ensures that the feet will be slightly dorsiflexed. The Mitchell orthosis was designed in conjunction with the Ponseti method and seems to be easier to keep on, particularly for patients with atypical clubfoot. The Steenbeck FAO was designed for inexpensive production in the developing world and has been used extensively in Uganda, South Africa.

After the Achilles tenotomy, the foot is casted in dorsiflexion for 3 weeks. During this time, the parents must obtain the FAO. When they return in 3 weeks for cast removal, the FAO is applied. It should be worn full-time (23 hours per day) for 3 months, and then part-time (at night and during naps) for 2 to 4 years. Patients with milder clubfoot require only 2 years of part-time FAO wear, and those with more severity require a full 4 years of bracing to prevent relapse.

The bracing phase can be challenging. Problems with compliance can be related to poor family cooperation and poor fitting of the orthosis. If the feet are insufficiently corrected, the orthosis will not stay on. With the Markell shoes, it may help to glue a small Plastazote bumper in the top of the heel counter to help capture the heel in the shoe. It is critical that the clinician educate the parents as to the importance of compliance. In one study, the relapse rate was 60% for noncompliant

patients and only 6% for those who were compliant with brace wear. Parent education should start when the initial castings are being done and reinforced at each visit. One study found that noncompliance and the educational level of the parents (high-school education or less) were significant risk factors for clubfoot deformity recurrence after correction with the Ponseti method.

Relapses are a common challenge when following patients treated with the Ponseti method. Early relapses are almost always the result of noncompliance with the FAO. In these instances, repeated castings are usually able to return the foot to a corrected position, and then the patient must again use the FAO with renewed vigor and cooperation. Later in the toddler phase, relapses (especially in compliant patients) can be caused by muscle imbalance. It should be stressed that the basic underlying pathology of clubfoot is not addressed by casting and bracing; the inherent muscle imbalance persists. In patients with clubfoot relapse caused by muscle imbalance, the relapse is characterized by walking on the lateral border of the foot with the heel in varus and variable degrees of inappropriate or dynamic supination of the forefoot. When assessing such children, care should be taken to watch the heel as the child walks away from the examiner and the forefoot as the child walks toward the examiner. The plantar surface of the foot should be examined after the child has been walking barefoot in the clinic. The absence of calluses under the first metatarsal head indicates dynamic supination.

For relapses that occur in patients older than 2 years, casting is required to regain correction (usually two long leg casts applied every 2 weeks). Consideration should then be made for anterior tibialis tendon transfer. Before performing an anterior tibialis tendon transfer,

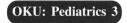

plain radiographs should be obtained to confirm that there is ossification of the lateral cuneiform. At surgery, an Achilles tendon lengthening may be performed if there is any residual tightness of the Achilles tendon. In an anterior tibialis tendon transfer, the anterior tibialis tendon is transferred from its insertion site subcutaneously to the new insertion in a drill hole through the middle of the lateral cuneiform. It may be held in place with a pullout button and a bioabsorbable screw for additional security. After 6 weeks, the cast is removed. The FAO is generally not required after an anterior tibialis tendon transfer.

Long-term results of the Ponseti method have been published and show superior functional results compared with extensive posteromedial release surgery. The Ponseti method requires great attention to detail and the cooperation of the patient's family. Despite best efforts, some patients with clubfoot may not respond to this type of treatment, and some families may not comply with the bracing protocol. For these reasons, orthopaedic surgeons who treat patients with clubfoot must maintain their surgical skills for open posteromedial release. Most patients with idiopathic clubfoot, however, are amenable to excellent outcomes using a strict Ponseti protocol.

Summary

A major paradigm shift has taken place in the management of idiopathic clubfoot. Whereas extensive posteromedial release surgery was the gold standard, the clinical pendulum has swung strongly toward the nonsurgical approach of Ponseti. However, clinicians must follow Ponseti's detailed method closely in order to reproduce his excellent short- and long-term results.

Annotated Bibliography

General

Carney BT, Coburn TR: Demographics of idiopathic clubfoot: Is there a seasonal variation? *J Pediatr Orthop* 2005;25:351-352.

In a group of 245 babies with clubfoot, no seasonal variation in incidence was found.

Dietz F: The genetics of idiopathic clubfoot. *Clin Orthop Relat Res* 2002;401:39-48.

The complex inheritance pattern for clubfoot may be caused by etiologic/genetic heterogeneity with possible environmental influences.

Prenatal Diagnosis

Barker SL, Macnicol MF: Seasonal distribution of idiopathic congenital talipes equinovarus in Scotland. *J Pediatr Orthop* 2002;11:129-133.

According to this study, the incidence of clubfoot in Scotland is highest in March and April.

Bar-On E, Mashiach R, Inbar O, Weigl D, Katz K, Meizner I: Prenatal ultrasound diagnosis of club foot: Outcome and recommendations for counselling and follow-up. *J Bone Joint Surg Br* 2005;87:990-993.

Clubfoot was diagnosed on prenatal ultrasound in 91 feet, but at birth, only 79 feet were truly clubbed. The positive predictive value was 83%. All inaccuracies were overdiagnoses.

Mammen L, Benson CB: Outcome of fetuses with clubfeet diagnosed by prenatal sonography. *J Ultrasound Med* 2004;23:497-500.

According to this study, the false positive rate is higher in unilateral than bilateral clubfeet. Associated anomalies were more common in bilateral clubfeet.

Clinical Grading

Celebi L, Muratli HH, Aksahin E, Yagmurlu MF, Bicimoglu A: Bensahel et al. and International Clubfoot Study Group evaluation of treated clubfoot: Assessment of interobserver and intraobserver reliability. *J Pediatr Orthop B* 2006;15:34-36.

Using the International Clubfoot Study Group outcome evaluation system, interobserver and intraobserver reliability were good.

Treatment

David RH, Packard DS Jr, Levinsohn EM, Berkowitz SA, Aronsson DD, Crider RJ Jr: Ischemic necrosis following clubfoot surgery: The purple hallux sign. *J Pediatr Orthop B* 2004;13:315-322.

This article discusses seven patients with with clubfeet with deficient anterior tibialis and dorsal pedal arteries in whom massive ischemic necrosis developed after clubfoot surgery.

Heilig MR, Matern RV, Rosenzweig SD, Bennett JT: Current management of idiopathic clubfoot questionnaire: A multicentric study. *J Pediatr Orthop* 2003;23:780-787.

A survey of the membership of Pediatric Orthopaedic Society of North America confirms the renewed interest in the Ponseti method.

Huber H, Dutoit M: Dynamic foot-pressure measurement in the assessment of operatively treated clubfeet. *J Bone Joint Surg Am* 2004;86-A:1203-1210.

It is important to preserve hindfoot pronation and subtalar mobility in clubfeet, for the best possibility of a painless long-term outcome.

Richards BS, Johnston CE, Wilson H: Nonoperative clubfoot treatment using the French physical therapy method. *J Pediatr Orthop* 2005;25:98-102.

Ninety-eight patients (142 clubfeet) were treated with the French method; 42% needed no surgery, 9% required heel cord tenotomies, 29% required posterior release, and 20% needed comprehensive release.

Souchet P, Bensahel H, Themar-Noel C, Pennecot G, Csukonyi Z: Functional treatment of clubfoot: A new series of 350 idiopathic clubfeet with long-term follow-up. *J Pediatr Orthop B* 2004;13:189-196.

The originators of the French method of conservative/ physiotherapy management report their most recent series of 350 clubfeet. At average 14-year follow-up, 77% had good results.

The Ponseti Method

Bor N, Herzenberg JE, Frick SL: Ponseti management of clubfoot in older infants. *Clin Orthop Relat Res* 2006 Jan 26;Publish Ahead of Print [Epub ahead of print].

The Ponseti method was successfully applied in 23 infants (36 feet) who were 3 to 6 months of age at presentation after failed non-Ponseti treatment. Posteromedial release was performed on one foot.

Dobbs MB, Gordon JE, Walton T, Schoenecker PL: Bleeding complications following percutaneous tendoachilles tenotomy in the treatment of clubfoot deformity. *J Pediatr Orthop* 2004;24:353-357.

In 4 of 200 feet undergoing Ponseti percutaneous tenotomy, serious bleeding developed at the surgical site.

Dobbs MB, Rudzki JR, Purcell DB, Walton T, Porter KR, Gurnett CA: Factors predictive of outcome after use of the Ponseti method for the treatment of idiopathic clubfeet. *J Bone Joint Surg Am* 2004;86-A:22-27.

Noncompliance with bracing was the most important factor predicting relapse. Parental educational level (high school or less) was also an associated independent risk factor.

Herzenberg JE, Radler C, Bor N: Ponseti versus traditional methods of casting for idiopathic clubfoot. *J Pediatr Orthop* 2002;22:517-521.

In this study, 27 patients (34 feet) were treated using Ponseti protocol. Only one foot required posteromedial release. This is one of the first studies outside of Iowa to confirm the Ponseti method.

Ippolito E, Fraracci L, Farsetti P, Di Mario M, Caterini R: The influence of treatment on the pathology of club foot: CT study at maturity. *J Bone Joint Surg Br* 2004;86: 574-580.

The authors conducted a CT study of feet treated by posterior release or Ponseti tenotomy. Heel varus was better correlated in the Ponseti group, as were cavus, supination, and adductus.

Morcuende JA, Abbasi D, Dolan LA, Ponseti IV: Results of an accelerated Ponseti protocol for clubfoot. *J Pediatr Orthop* 2005;25:623-626.

The Ponseti method was shown to work as well if casts were changed every 5 days versus every 7 days.

Morcuende JA, Dolan LA, Dietz FR, Ponseti IV: Radical reduction in the rate of extensive corrective surgery for clubfoot using the Ponseti method. *Pediatrics* 2004; 113:376-380.

From 1991 to 2001, the authors treated 157 babies (256 clubfeet) with the Ponseti method. Only 4 patients required extensive release surgery. There were 17 relapses, mostly related to bracing noncompliance. Four patients required anterior tibialis transfers.

Pirani S, Zeznik L, Hodges D: Magnetic resonance imaging study of the congenital clubfoot treated with the Ponseti method. *J Pediatr Orthop* 2001;21:719-726.

This article discusses MRI documentation of the morphologic improvements in osseous and articular pathology that take place with Ponseti casting.

Scher DM, Feldman DS, van Bosse HJ, Sala DA, Lehman WB: Predicting the need for tenotomy in the Ponseti method for correction of clubfeet. *J Pediatr Orthop* 2004;24:349-352.

According to this study, babies with initial Pironi scores ≥ 5.0 or Dimeglio grade IV feet are likely to need tenotomy.

Tindall AJ, Steinlechner CW, Lavy CB, Mannion S, Mkandawire N: Results of manipulation of idiopathic clubfoot deformity in Malawi by orthopaedic clinical officers using the Ponseti method: A realistic alternative for the developing world? *J Pediatr Orthop* 2005;25:627-629.

The authors show that a well-trained group of nonphysician orthorpaedic technicians can obtain excellent results using the Ponseti method. Of 100 clubfeet, 57 were treated with manipulation; 41 of these required percutaneous tenotomy and 2 required extensive surgery.

Classic Bibliography

Abrams RC: Relapsed club foot: The early results of an evaluation of Dillwyn Evans' operation. *J Bone Joint Surg Am* 1969;51(2):270-282.

Bensahel H, Csukonyi Z, Desgrippes Y, Chaumien JP: Surgery in residual clubfoot: One-stage medioposterior release "a la carte". *J Pediatr Orthop* 1987;7(2):145-148.

Carroll NC: Pathoanatomy and surgical treatment of the resistant clubfoot. *Instr Course Lect* 1988;37:93-106.

Cooper DM, Dietz FR: Treatment of idiopathic clubfoot: A thirty-year follow-up note. *J Bone Joint Surg Am* 1995;77(10):1477-1489.

Crawford AH, Marxen JL, Osterfeld DL: The Cincinnati incision: A comprehensive approach for surgical procedures of the foot and ankle in childhood. *J Bone Joint Surg Am* 1982;64(9):1355-1358.

Garceau GJ, Palmer RM: Transfer of the anterior tibial tendon for recurrent club foot: A long-term follow-up. *J Bone Joint Surg Am* 1967;49(2):207-231.

Kite JH: Nonoperative treatment of congenital clubfoot. *Clin Orthop Relat Res* 1972;84:29-38.

Laaveg SJ, Ponseti IV: Long-term results of treatment of congenital club foot. *J Bone Joint Surg Am* 1980;62(1):23-31.

Lichtblau S: A medial and lateral release operation for club foot: A preliminary report. *J Bone Joint Surg Am* 1973;55(7):1377-1384.

McKay DW: Surgical correction of clubfoot. *Instr Course Lect* 1988;37:87-92.

Ponseti IV: Treatment of congenital club foot. *J Bone Joint Surg Am* 1992;74(3):448-454.

Ponseti IV: *Congenital Clubfoot: Fundamentals of Treatment.* Oxford, England, Oxford University Press, 1996.

Pryor GA, Villar RN, Ronen A, Scott PM: Seasonal variation in the incidence of congenital talipes equinovarus. *J Bone Joint Surg Br* 1991;73:632-634.

Robertson WW, Corbett D: Congenital clubfoot: Month of conception. *Clin Orthop Relat Res* 1997;338:14-18.

Simons GW: The complete subtalar release in clubfeet. *Orthop Clin North Am* 1987;18(4):667-688.

Turco VJ: Resistant congenital club foot: One-stage posteromedial release with internal fixation. A follow-up report of a fifteen-year experience. *J Bone Joint Surg Am* 1979;61(6A):805-814.

Chapter 18

Conditions of the Foot

Bradford W. Olney, MD

Calcaneovalgus Deformity

Positional calcaneovalgus deformity, also called talipes calcaneal valgus, is the most common foot deformity noted at birth. It is characterized by dorsiflexion of the entire foot at the ankle joint with associated lesser degrees of hindfoot eversion and forefoot abduction. Although this is a common deformity, the exact incidence is unknown primarily because of the variability of the severity of this condition. It is more common in females than males and in first-born children. It is generally agreed that the etiology of this condition is the result of intrauterine positioning. The clinical features of calcaneovalgus deformity are consistent, but they present to varying degrees. The most noticeable finding on physical examination is typically a flexible dorsiflexion of the ankle (Figure 1) with abduction and eversion of the foot. Although calcaneovalgus deformity is a flexible deformity, there may be some mild tightness of the dorsal structures of the ankle. The physical examination should be able to differentiate a calcaneovalgus deformity from a congenital vertical talus deformity, which shows a fixed hindfoot equinus and valgus along with rigid dorsiflexion through the midfoot (for a discussion of vertical talus, see chapters 9 and 11). A severe calcaneovalgus posture may also be noted with posteromedial bowing of the tibia, but physical examination and radiographs should help diagnose the condition of posteromedial bowing of the tibia. Radiographs are generally not necessary for patients with the typical flexible calcaneovalgus deformity.

Because calcaneovalgus deformity is caused by intrauterine positioning, the natural history of the disorder is gradual resolution. Mild to moderate deformities require nothing more than observation, whereas severe deformities may improve more quickly with passive stretching exercises performed by the parents of the affected child. Serial casting can be done, and surgery is not required. Some studies have noted a relationship between positional calcaneovalgus deformities in the infant and flexible flatfoot deformities in the older child.

Congenital Overriding Fifth Toe

Congenital overriding of the fifth toe is a condition in which there is dorsomedial subluxation of the metatarsophalangeal (MTP) joint of the fifth toe that results in the toe being dorsiflexed and adducted, causing it to overlap the fourth toe. The fifth toe also rotates so that the nail bed tends to lie laterally. This condition is also known as congenital digitus minimus varus or varus fifth toe. The deformity is present at birth and, although common, the exact incidence is unknown. There is bilateral involvement in 20% to 30% of patients, and there is often a familial tendency.

Physical examination typically shows normal interphalangeal joints and a contracture at the MTP joint (Figure 2). The skin web between the fourth and fifth toes is usually out of alignment with the other web spaces, but there is no contracture of the skin. There is contracture of the dorsomedial capsule of the fifth MTP joint and shortening of the extensor tendon. Younger children are typically asymptomatic, but approximately 50% will develop symptoms over time, consisting of

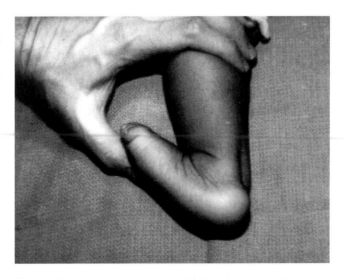

Figure 1 Photograph of a calcaneovalgus deformity of the foot in an infant demonstrating increased dorsiflexion of the ankle.

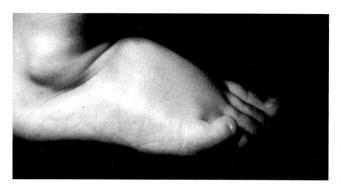

Figure 2 Photograph of congenital overriding fifth toe in a young child.

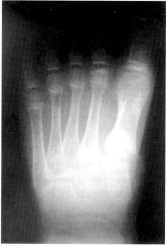

Figure 3 Radiograph of the foot of a child with Freiberg's disease of the second metatarsal head. Note the sclerosis of the metatarsal head with flattening of the articular surface.

pain over the dorsum of the fifth toe caused by irritation from shoe wear.

Radiographs are generally not helpful initially, but they should be obtained prior to surgical correction to exclude the presence of structural anomalies. The primary indication for surgical treatment of this condition is pain with shoe wear, although many parents elect to have the deformity corrected, even in asymptomatic children. Conservative treatments such as taping and splinting have not been found to be effective. Surgical correction is generally delayed until the patient is at least 3 or 4 years of age. Numerous surgical procedures have been proposed, but two procedures provide the most predictable outcome: the Butler procedure and the McFarland procedure. The Butler procedure involves a double racket-handle incision with release of the extensor digitorum longus tendon and dorsal capsule of the MTP joint. The toe is then translated to the plantar aspect of the incision before closure of the skin. This procedure generally provides good results, but care must be taken not to compromise the neurovascular status of the toe with the circumferential incision. The McFarland procedure consists of release of the MTP joint and extensor tendon as well as excision of the proximal phalanx and partial syndactylism of the fourth and fifth toes. This procedure is more involved than the Butler procedure and can result in secondary deformities. Amputation of the fifth toe is considered a salvage procedure that should be performed only in rare circumstances.

Freiberg's Disease

Freiberg's disease, occasionally called Köhler's second disease (Köhler's first disease, an osteochondrosis of the tarsal navicular, is discussed later in this chapter), is an osteochondrosis of the metatarsal head. This condition is characterized radiographically by flattening of the articular surface of the metatarsal head with occasional fragmentation of the metatarsal head and loose bodies. The second metatarsal is the most commonly affected metatarsal, followed by the third metatarsal. The other metatarsal heads are rarely involved, and approximately 10% of patients have bilateral involvement. The condition is more common in girls than boys and generally occurs between the ages of 10 and 18 years. The exact etiology of this disorder is unknown, but it is thought to be caused by osteonecrosis of the metatarsal head. It has been postulated that repetitive stress, such as that which occurs during athletic activities, contributes to the onset of osteonecrosis.

The typical pediatric patient with Freiberg's disease is an adolescent girl, approximately 13 years of age, who presents with a vague history of forefoot pain that is often exacerbated by athletic activity and relieved by rest. The patient usually reports pain around the affected metatarsal head and has an antalgic limp. The physical findings are normally limited to the area of involvement with associated swelling. If the area of tenderness is more proximal, then a stress fracture of the metatarsal needs to be excluded. Changes in the metatarsal head are usually evident on plain radiographs and can be highly variable. Symptoms do not correlate with the extent of findings on plain radiographs. Radiographs typically show an area of lucency and collapse of the metatarsal head with loss of normal shape (Figure 3). Early in the course of the disease, there may be flattening of the metatarsal head with a subchondral fracture line noted. In patients with severe disease, the affected metatarsal head can demonstrate collapse, fragmentation, and osteophyte formation.

The natural history of this condition is variable. It can lead to significant fragmentation and ultimately severe arthrosis of the joint or can be less severe with early healing of the subchondral bone. Treatment is nonsurgical in the early stages of this condition and includes restriction or modification of athletic activity as well as use of a stiffer sole shoe. Cast immobilization or avoiding weight bearing may be indicated in patients with more severe disease. Surgical treatments are considered earlier in patients with severe Freiberg's disease or when prolonged attempts at nonsurgical treatment fail to alleviate symptoms. There is no general consensus as to the best surgical treatment for patients with Freiberg's disease. Surgical treatment consists of débridement and possible bone grafting of the metatarsal head or metatarsal excision osteotomy to relieve the pressure on the metatarsal head. Other procedures such as excision of the metatarsal head, excision of the proximal portion of the proximal phalanx, or joint arthroplasty are considered salvage procedures.

Juvenile Hallux Valgus (Bunion)

Juvenile hallux valgus deformity (bunion), which typically occurs in the preteen or teenage years, is an enlargement of the medial aspect of the first MTP joint that is associated with an increase in the hallux valgus angle. By definition, the deformity is present when the growth plates of the first metatarsal and proximal phalanx are still open. The exact incidence of juvenile hallux valgus is unknown, but there is a strong female preponderance, with more than 80% of patients with this deformity being girls. Because of a strong positive family history of hallux valgus in female ancestors, it has been suggested there is a possible sex-linked dominant trait with variable penetrance. The exact etiology of juvenile hallux valgus deformity remains controversial. Numerous causes have been suggested, including genetics, improperly fitting shoes, ligamentous laxity, and varus angulation of the first metatarsal-cuneiform joint with obliquity of this joint. Anatomic variations that may predispose the patient to hallux valgus deformity are hypermobility of the first metatarsal-cuneiform joint, lateral deviation of the articular surface of the first metatarsal head, and a flexible flatfoot.

Many adolescents with hallux valgus deformity are asymptomatic but dissatisfied with the appearance of the foot. Other children may report pain, which generally occurs in the soft tissues on the medial aspect of the first metatarsal head. In patients with milder deformities, pain may be relieved by modifying shoe wear. In patients with more severe deformity, pain may be reported with any type of shoe. There may also be symptoms related to the second toe if it overlaps with the first toe. Unlike adult bunions, there is rarely intra-articular pain with joint motion or restriction of first MTP joint range of motion in juvenile hallux valgus deformity. The entire foot should be evaluated for a possible contributing factor, such as hypermobility of the first metatarsal-cuneiform joint, flexible flatfoot deformity, and secondary contracture of the Achilles tendon. The exact natural history of juvenile hallux valgus deformity is unknown. It has been suggested that a congruous first MTP joint may be more stable and less likely to progress. Conversely, it has been suggested that joint in-

congruity can lead to a progressive deformity, but at an unpredictable rate. In most patients with juvenile hallux valgus deformity, it is difficult to predict whether a deformity will progress and at what rate.

Radiographic evaluation is particularly important in patients for whom surgical treatment is being considered. Evaluation generally includes weight-bearing AP and lateral radiographs of the foot. The orientation and congruity of the first MTP joint should be evaluated as well as the orientation of the first metatarsal-cuneiform joint. It is important to determine whether the first MTP joint is subluxated or congruous (Figure 4, *A*). Important radiographic measurements include the hallux valgus angle, the first and second intermetatarsal angle (Figure 4, *B*), and the distal metatarsal articular angle (Figure 4, *C*). In addition, the relative length of the first metatarsal compared with the second metatarsal should be evaluated. Using the hallux valgus angle as a general guide, bunions with angles less than 25° are considered mild deformities, those between 25° and 40° are considered moderate deformities, and those greater than 40° are considered severe deformities.

Treatment of hallux valgus deformities in children or adolescents should start with reassurance and shoe wear modification. Patients should be instructed to find shoes that look like the foot, which generally entails buying shoes that have a wide toe box and avoiding shoes with high heels. Bunion splints and foot orthotics to control flatfoot may be of limited benefit. Surgery should be considered for patients who experience significant pain with normal activities and have not responded to orthotics and shoe modification. It is generally better to wait until skeletal maturity before attempting surgical correction because once skeletal maturity is reached there is less likelihood of recurrence. Surgery for purely cosmetic considerations is contraindicated because of the risk of postoperative pain and/or stiffness in a previously asymptomatic foot.

Once the decision to treat a juvenile hallux valgus deformity with surgery has been made, all components and elements of the deformity must be analyzed both clinically and radiographically. There is no one surgical procedure that is suitable for all patients with juvenile hallux valgus deformity. All elements of the deformity should be addressed and corrected without creating secondary deformities. Surgical treatment is generally broken down into four basic components: distal soft-tissue realignment, distal metatarsal osteotomy, proximal first metatarsal osteotomy, and correction of deformity at the metatarsal-cuneiform joint. The surgical procedures used are based on the clinical and radiographic analysis of each patient. If the hallux valgus deformity consists of a subluxated and incongruous MTP joint with an increased first and second intermetatarsal angle (Figure 5, *A*), surgical treatment generally consists of a distal soft-tissue realignment combined with a proximal first meta-

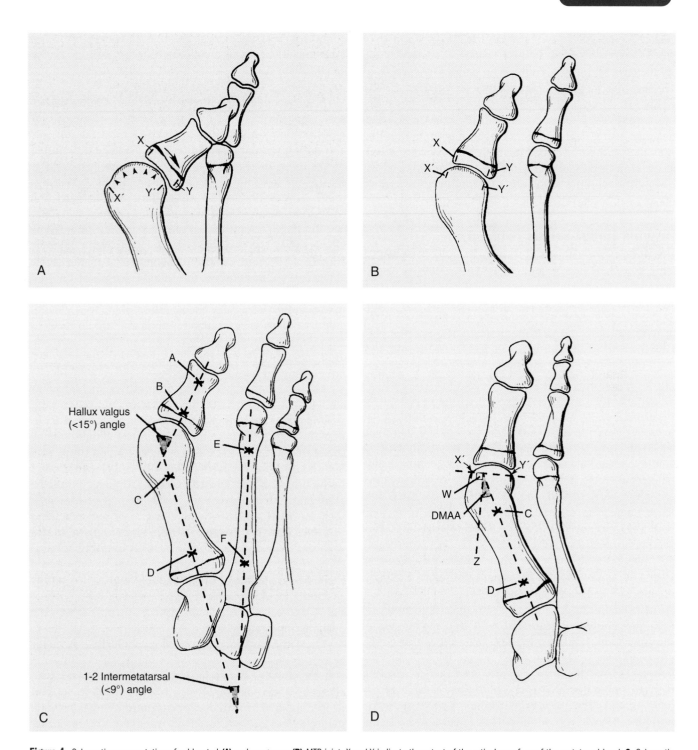

Figure 4 Schematic representation of subluxated **(A)** and congruous **(B)** MTP joint; X and Y indicate the extent of the articular surface of the metatarsal head. **C,** Schematic representation of the hallux valgus angle (normally < 15°) and the first and second intermetatarsal angle (normally < 9°). A, B, C, D, E, and F represent index points for the various lines that need to be drawn to calculate these angles. **D,** Schematic representation of the distal metatarsal articular angle (DMAA), which shows the relationship between a line (Z) drawn perpendicular (W) to the articular surface (X-Y) and a line drawn down the center of the first metatarsal shaft (**C-D**). *(Reproduced with permission from Coughlin M: Juvenile hallux valgus, in Coughlin M, Mann R (eds): Surgery of the Foot and Ankle, ed 7. St. Louis, MO, Mosby, 1999, p 270.)*

tarsal osteotomy. The physeal plate of the first metatarsal is located proximally; therefore, osteotomies done proximally are more likely to damage this growth plate and result in a shorter and possibly deviated first metatarsal. Caution must be exercised to assure that osteoto-mies are done away from an open growth plate. If the increased first and second metatarsal angle is the result of marked obliquity of the metatarsal-cuneiform joint, then an opening wedge osteotomy of the medial cunei-form can be used in place of the basilar first metatarsal

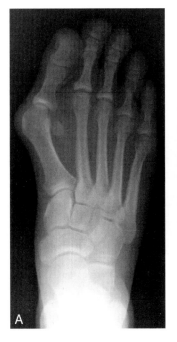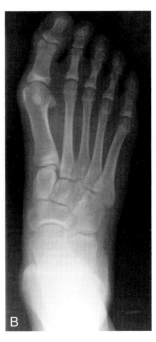

Figure 5 **A,** Radiograph of the foot of a 15-year-old girl with a juvenile hallux valgus deformity and subluxation of the MTP joint. Note the increased first and second inter-metatarsal angle and oblique orientation of the first metatarsal cuneiform joint. **B,** Radiograph of the foot of an adolescent girl with juvenile hallux valgus deformity associated with a congruous MTP joint and a laterally directed distal metatarsal articular angle.

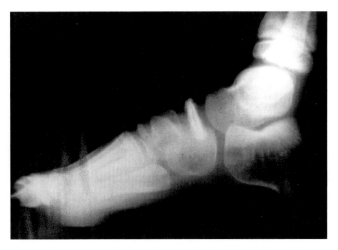

Figure 6 Lateral radiograph of the foot of a child with Köhler's disease. Note the sclerosis and flattening of the navicular bone.

osteotomy. In patients with severe hypermobility of the metatarsal-cuneiform joint resulting in varus of the first metatarsal, consideration should be given to a first metatarsal-cuneiform fusion. In patients with a hallux valgus deformity with a congruous MTP joint and a laterally deviated articular surface (Figure 5, *B*), a distal metatarsal osteotomy is a better choice. The distal metatarsal osteotomy needs to realign the articular surface with a simple closing wedge procedure or a Mitchell osteotomy. The standard chevron osteotomy does not correct the distal metatarsal articular angle. In the rare patient with lateral deviation of the distal articular surface and an increase in the first and second intermetatarsal angle, a double osteotomy may be necessary, including a distal articular realignment osteotomy combined with a proximal first metatarsal osteotomy or medial opening cuneiform osteotomy. In the patient in whom a significant portion of the overall hallux valgus deformity is caused by valgus at the interphalangeal joint, an additional osteotomy of the proximal phalanx may need to be performed.

Postoperative complications after juvenile hallux valgus deformity treatment include recurrence, overcorrection, undercorrection, joint stiffness, metatarsalgia, physeal injury of the first metatarsal, and osteonecrosis of the metatarsal head. Because of these possible complications, the most reasonable approach to juvenile hallux valgus deformity is to exhaust all forms of conserva-

tive management. The risk of complications can also be decreased by carefully choosing the appropriate surgical procedure based on clinical and radiographic evaluations to correct all of the deformities and not create secondary deformities.

Köhler's Disease
Köhler's disease, an osteochondrosis of the tarsal navicular, is a painful condition of the midfoot in young children with characteristic radiographic changes of sclerosis and flattening of the tarsal navicular. The etiology of Köhler's disease is unknown, but it has been suggested that later ossification of the navicular in relation to the other tarsal bones renders it more vulnerable to mechanical compression injury. In addition to the mechanical compression theory, another possible etiology is that the periodic compression of the bone leads to intermittent disruption of the blood supply to the navicular and leads to osteonecrosis. Köhler's disease is four times more common in boys than girls, and most patients present between the ages of 2 and 7 years. Children with Köhler's disease usually have an antalgic limp and may bear weight on the lateral aspect of the foot. The pain is usually located over the dorsomedial aspect of the midfoot. These symptoms may be associated with swelling, redness, and increased warmth, which can result in Köhler's disease being confused with infection or inflammatory arthropathy. The diagnosis is confirmed by plain radiographs that reveal the characteristic findings of sclerosis, fragmentation, and flattening of the navicular bone (Figure 6). The tarsal navicular bone is the last bone of the foot to ossify; this generally occurs between the ages of 18 and 24 months in girls and 30 and 36 months in boys. Irregular or multiple ossification centers of the navicular are common when the tarsal bone first starts to ossify and should not be mistaken for Köhler's disease.

Köhler's disease is a self-limiting condition in which the navicular reconstitutes over 6 months to several years. The symptoms of Köhler's disease typically resolve within 7 to 15 months. No residual deformity or disability is typically noted in older children or adults with this condition. Several studies have shown that a treatment of 6 to 8 weeks in a short leg walking cast can decrease the duration of symptoms. Except for the duration of symptoms, treatment has no effect on the final outcome of Köhler's disease. For milder symptoms that do not warrant a short leg walking cast, over-the-counter arch supports may help relieve symptoms. There is no role for surgery in the treatment of Köhler's disease.

Metatarsus Adductus

Metatarsus adductus is defined as medial deviation of the forefoot with a normal hindfoot. It is one of the more common congenital foot deformities. The terminology for this deformity is often confusing because the terms metatarsus varus, hook-foot, bean-shaped foot, and skewfoot are often used to describe the same condition; however, skewfoot generally refers to a foot that has severe metatarsus adductus in association with fixed hindfoot valgus or eversion. The incidence of metatarsus adductus has been estimated to be between 0.1% and 12% of full-term births. The exact etiology of this condition is not known, but it has long been thought to be caused by intrauterine positioning of the foot. One study showed there may be some abnormality of the medial cuneiform, resulting in the bone being trapezoid-shaped and causing the first metatarsal to tilt into its varus position.

Clinical features of metatarsus adductus are usually apparent at birth and include medial deviation of the forefoot in relation to the hindfoot. The hindfoot demonstrates full range of motion at the ankle and subtalar joints, with a neutral to slight valgus position of the hindfoot. When viewed from the plantar surface, the foot is often described as being bean-shaped (Figure 7). The severity of the metatarsus adductus can be determined using the heel bisector method (Figure 8) or by accessing the flexibility of the foot with manipulation. Flexibility can generally be estimated by maintaining the hindfoot in a neutral position and gently pushing the head of the first metatarsal laterally to determine the degree of force required to correct the forefoot to realign with the heel. More rigid deformities will often have a medial soft-tissue crease at the level of the tarsometatarsal joint. Many children will also have associated internal tibial torsion that makes the metatarsus adductus appear worse.

Radiographs are not generally necessary when evaluating a newborn or infant with metatarsus adductus; they are, however generally indicated for older children

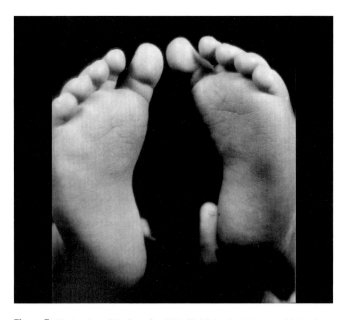

Figure 7 Plantar view of the feet of a child with bilateral metatarsus adductus demonstrating the classic bean-shaped foot.

with significant residual deformity or pain. Radiographs typically show medial deviation of all the metatarsals at the tarsometatarsal joint with normal alignment of the hindfoot.

The natural history of metatarsus adductus is benign. Studies show that most patients resolve spontaneously or have only mild deformity. Few patients have long-term disability or pain from this condition; however, a small percentage of patients with a more rigid deformity may require treatment. Treatment of the mild to moderate deformities usually involves observation with possible passive stretching exercises, although the efficacy of this has not yet been documented. Numerous types of shoes, braces, and splints have been suggested for this deformity. For moderate to severe deformities in children younger than 1 year, serial casting can be effective in correcting this deformity. An above-the-knee cast is traditionally used, although one study suggested that a below-the-knee cast may also be effective in treating metatarsus adductus. Whichever type of cast is used, care must be taken not to place excessive valgus force on the hindfoot, especially if heel eversion or valgus (skewfoot) already exists. After a short period of corrective casting, splints or shoes are often recommended to maintain the correction. Surgery is rarely indicated in this patient population because resolution of this deformity usually occurs by 4 years of age. Older children with severe deformities who have problems with shoe wear or pain with activity can be considered for surgical intervention. In patients with more severe deformities who do not respond to serial casting, a medial soft-tissue release (capsulotomy of the naviculocuneiform and first metatarsal-cuneiform joints with abductor hallucis

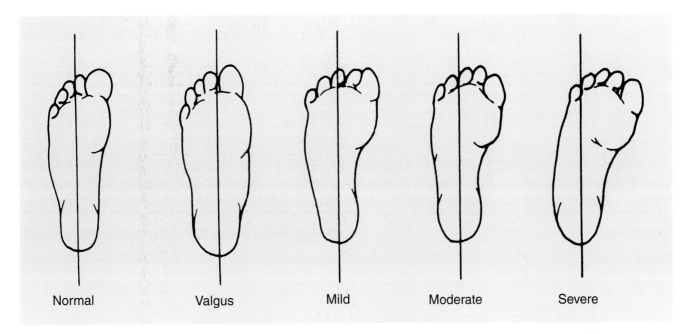

Normal   Valgus   Mild   Moderate   Severe

Figure 8 Schematic representation of the heel bisector method for grading the severity of metatarsus adductus. *(Reproduced with permission from Mosca VS: The foot, in Morrissy RT, Weinstein SL (eds): Lovell & Winter's Pediatric Orthopaedics. Philadelphia, PA, Lippincott, Williams & Wilkins, 2001, p 1163.)*

lengthening) followed by several corrective casts has been reported to provide results in children age 1 to 5 years. Although rare in children older than 5 years, surgical treatment of symptomatic severe metatarsus adductus becomes more difficult. Two surgical procedures described for these older patients have included multiple tarsometatarsal capsular releases and multiple osteotomies at the base of all the metatarsals. These two procedures are difficult to perform, however, and have been shown to have significant failure rates and complications. If surgery is indicated in older patients, medial soft-tissue releases combined with an opening wedge osteotomy of the first cuneiform and a closing wedge osteotomy of the cuboid has been shown to have good results with fewer complications.

Polydactyly

Polydactyly is the most common congenital toe deformity, with an incidence of approximately 1 to 1.5 instances per 1,000 live births. This condition occurs more frequently in blacks, with about 50% of the instances being bilateral and approximately 30% of patients having a positive family history of polydactyly. Polydactyly has an autosomal dominant inheritance pattern with variable expressivity. Polydactyly is most often an isolated trait.

The fifth toe is the most frequently duplicated digit, accounting for approximately 80% of polydactyly in the foot. Duplication of the fifth toe is called postaxial polydactyly (Figure 9, *A*). Preaxial polydactyly involves duplication of the great toe and is the second most common type of polydactyly (Figure 9, *B*). The central toes

are occasionally duplicated, but this is rare. Polydactyly can be further subdivided into two basic types. Patients with type A polydactyly have a well-formed digit with normal articulation. Patients with type B polydactyly have rudimentary or vestibular digits that are nonfunctional. The toenails may be separate or conjoined in patients with polydactyly.

Clinical and radiographic evaluation is necessary to help determine the proper treatment of each individual patient with polydactyly. Clinical examination can show which toe has normal alignment and size. Radiographic evaluation is mandatory to determine which bony structures are duplicated. The phalanges are often not ossified at birth; therefore, radiography should be delayed until after 6 months of age. Radiographs are necessary before surgical treatment to help with the surgical planing and generally show duplication of the phalanges, although the duplicated proximal phalanges may be connected at the base with either a cartilaginous or bony connection. The associated metatarsal may show a wide variety of abnormalities ranging from complete duplication of the metatarsal to a Y- or T-shaped metatarsal or single widened metatarsal. Surgery is generally performed when patients are approximately 1 year of age to improve cosmesis of the foot and, more importantly, to facilitate normal shoe fitting. Preoperative plain radiographs and physical examination are used to determine the most normal-looking digit to retain and also how much bony resection is necessary. In most patients, the most malaligned toe is resected, which is usually the most medial digit in patients with preaxial polydactyly and the most lateral digit in those with postaxial poly-

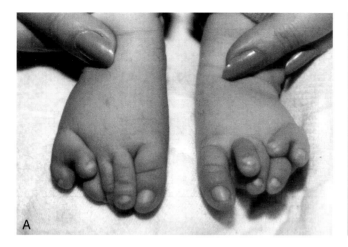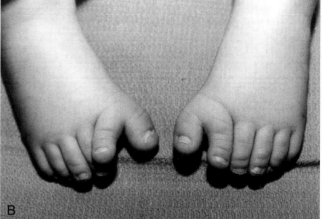

Figure 9 **A,** Photograph of the feet of a child with duplication of the fifth toe (postaxial polydactyly). **B,** Photograph of the feet of a child with duplication of the first toe (preaxial polydactyly).

dactyly. Division of the synchondrosis at the base of the duplicated proximal phalanx is often necessary as well as division of the nail bed if the toenail is conjoined. The nail fold must be carefully reconstructed to prevent chronic nail growth problems. In some patients, the outer toe is the most normal, in which instance the inner toe needs to be removed. If this is the case, then capsular and intermetatarsal ligament repair is important to prevent deviation of the remaining digit. If there is complete duplication of the metatarsal, then it should be completely removed with the extra digit. If there is a Y- or T-shaped metatarsal, the removal of the extra portion of the metatarsal head can be performed at the time the extra digit is removed. In patients with a widened metatarsal, any prominence of the metatarsal head can be removed. Generally, all procedures are done through a dorsal lateral or dorsal medial racket-shaped incision, depending on whether the condition is preaxial or postaxial. In the rare patient with central polydactyly, amputation consists of a ray amputation with care taken to repair the intermetatarsal ligament.

Sever's Disease
Sever's disease, an apophysitis of the calcaneus, is the most common cause of heel pain in skeletally immature patients. It is believed that overuse or repetitive microtrauma results in apophysitis of the calcaneus. Sever's disease is more common in boys than girls and is often related to physical activity. Most patients are between the ages of 10 and 12 years, and more than 50% of instances of Sever's disease are bilateral.

Physical examination generally demonstrates tenderness to palpation at the insertion of the Achilles tendon. The classic finding is pain to compression of the calcaneal apophysitis. Generally, there are no signs of swelling, redness, or warmth. If these signs are present, then other diagnoses such as infection, tumor, or fracture should be considered. The differential diagnosis also includes Achilles tendinitis, stress fracture of the calcaneus, plantar fasciitis, and unicameral bone cyst of the calcaneus.

There is no pathognomonic radiographic feature for this condition, and radiographs are not necessary if the history and physical examination are consistent with the diagnosis. The normal apophysis of the calcaneus often has sclerosis and fragmentation of the ossification center. Radiographs are generally obtained to rule out other causes of heel pain, particularly if there are physical findings such as swelling or erythema. Sever's disease is also generally associated with activity; therefore, a history of night pain is also an indication for radiographs.

Treatment of Sever's disease is purely symptomatic because the natural history shows that it is a self-limiting and age-limited condition that does not occur after skeletal maturity. Treatment options include rest, ice, and activity restrictions for patients with acute symptoms. Anti-inflammatory medications and cast immobilization can be used for a short period if the symptoms are severe. Heel cord stretching exercises and cushion heel inserts may also lessen the severity of symptoms. Generally, patients are allowed to participate in athletic activity as their symptoms permit.

Curly Toe
Curly toe is a congenital deformity of the lesser toes in which there is flexion and varus of the interphalangeal joints that causes the toe to curl underneath the adjacent medial toe (Figure 10). This is a common deformity, with a high familial incidence and a suspected autosomal dominant inheritance pattern. The deformity is often bilateral, and the third toe is most often involved, followed by the fourth toe. The deformity itself is caused by contracture of the flexor digitorum longus tendon.

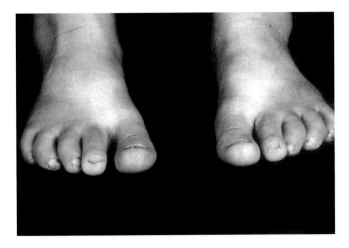

Figure 10 Photograph of the feet of a young child with bilateral curly toe deformities primarily of the third and fourth digits.

This toe deformity is often asymptomatic and does not interfere with the toddler's ability to walk. Symptoms can occasionally develop from abnormal pressure on the tip of the underlying toe or rubbing of the elevated medial toe on the shoe. Approximately 25% of these deformities will resolve spontaneously. Taping or splinting of the affected toe does not seem to be effective treatment, and radiographs are not usually indicated for this patient population.

Surgical treatment is indicated if the deformity persists and causes symptoms. Occasionally, abnormal growth or deformity of the nail can occur, which is another indication for surgical treatment. Flexor-to-extensor tendon transfers and simple open flexor tenotomy have both been shown to be effective treatment of the persistently symptomatic curly toe. One study comparing these two treatments showed that similar results were obtained with both; however, open flexor tenotomy is an easier procedure to perform and is generally the preferred treatment of the persistently symptomatic curly toe. No consensus exists as to whether both flexor tendons need to be released or just the flexor digitorum longus. It seems reasonable, however, to release the long toe flexor first and then release the flexor digitorum brevis tendon if it is tight or causing any residual deformity.

Annotated Bibliography
Congenital Overriding Fifth Toe

Thordarson DB: Congenital crossover fifth toe correction with soft tissue release and cutaneous Z-plasty. *Foot Ankle Int* 2001;22(6):511-512.

The author describes a new procedure to correct an overriding fifth toe deformity using a lateral Z-plasty of the skin combined with a dorsal and medial MTP capsule release and an oblique lengthening of the extensor tendon. The procedure is similar to the Butler procedure, but uses a lateral Z-plasty

of the skin instead of a circumferential racket incision. The author reports no recurrence in three patients at an average 33-month follow-up and concludes that this procedure is simpler than the Butler procedure.

Freiberg's Disease

Gong HS, Baek GH, Jung JM, Kim JH, Chung MS: Technique tip: Fixation of dorsal wedge osteotomy for Freiberg's disease using bioabsorbable pins. *Foot Ankle Int* 2003;24(11):876-877.

In this technique article, the authors describe the use of multiple bioabsorbable (polyglycolide) pins for fixation of dorsal wedge metatarsal osteotomies for the treatment of Freiberg's disease. They report early gradual weight bearing in a short leg walking cast, but do not report their series of patients.

Juvenile Hallux Valgus (Bunion)

Andreacchio A, Origo C, Rocca G: Early results of the modified Simmonds-Menelaus procedure for adolescent hallux valgus. *J Pediatr Orthop* 2002;22:375-379.

The authors report the outcome of surgical treatment of 11 patients (20 feet) with adolescent hallux valgus using a distal soft-tissue procedure combined with a proximal first metatarsal osteotomy. The osteotomy was an incomplete, medial opening wedge procedure using the exostosis bone for a graft and no fixation. The average decrease of the hallux valgus angle was 13.4°, but only an average 2.2° decrease in the first and second intermetatarsal angle. Outcome assessment showed 4 excellent and 16 good results at an average follow-up of 2.9 years.

Aronson J, Nguyen LL, Aronson EA: Early results of the modified Peterson bunion procedure for adolescent hallux valgus. *J Pediatr Orthop* 2001;21:65-69.

The authors report the results of correction of 16 patients (18 feet) with adolescent hallux valgus using a modification of the Petersen double metatarsal osteotomy procedure. The modifications to the original procedure included fixation of both osteotomies with a single medial plate and use of an osteoperiosteal distally based flap to correct MTP joint subluxation. At an average follow-up of 23.4 months, all osteotomies healed primarily. There was recurrence of the deformity in three feet (16%), which the authors believe was caused by undercorrection at the time of surgery. No patients required the removal of the hardware.

Johnson AE, Georgopoulos G, Erickson MA, Eilert R: Treatment of adolescent hallux valgus with metatarsal double osteotomy: The Denver experience. *J Pediatr Orthop* 2004;24:358-362.

In this article, the authors reviewed nine patients (14 feet) with adolescent hallux valgus deformities treated with double first metatarsal osteotomies. At an average 27-month follow-up, the authors reported good correction of the hallux valgus angles with this procedure and two surgical complications (one nonunion and one infection). Functional outcome studies showed that 90% of patients reported good or excellent results. Three patients (three feet) reported significant first MTP joint stiffness, two of which led to unsatisfactory results.

Talab YA: Hallux valgus in children: A 5-14 year follow-up study of 30 feet treated with a modified Mitchell osteotomy. *Acta Orthop Scand* 2002;73:195-198.

The author reports on 18 patients (30 feet) with adolescent hallux valgus who were treated with a modified Mitchell osteotomy. At an average follow-up of 8 years, the author reported satisfactory results in all patients and only occasional pain noted in two feet. The modifications to the procedure included divergent osteotomy cuts, release of the lateral MTP ligament and adductor insertion, plantar displacement of the metatarsal head, and Kirschner wire fixation of the osteotomy.

Köhler's Disease

Sharp RJ, Calder JD, Saxby TS: Osteochondritis of the navicular: A case report. *Foot Ankle Int* 2003;24(6):509-513.

This is a case report of a 12-year-old boy who developed bilateral osteochondritis of the navicular with symptoms and radiographic changes that persisted into adulthood. This patient is out of the typical age range of patients with Köhler's disease, but does demonstrate that an atypical instance of Köhler's disease can develop in an older child with symptoms that may persist.

Metatarsus Adductus

Gordon JE, Luhmann SJ, Dobbs MB, et al: Combined midfoot osteotomy for severe forefoot adductus. *J Pediatr Orthop* 2003;23:74-78.

The authors report on the treatment of the older pediatric patient with severe, symptomatic metatarsus adductus using a combined opening wedge osteotomy of the medial cuneiform and a closing wedge osteotomy of the cuboid. The study included 33 patients (50 feet) with a mean age at surgery of 5.5 years. At minimum follow-up of 2 years, clinical and radiographic improvement was seen in 90% of patients. There was an increased risk of medial graft extrusion (with loss of correction) in children younger than five years without a well-defined medial cuneiform ossific nucleus. The authors concluded that this procedure provides good correction in older pediatric patients with severe metatarsus adductus, but cautioned that it should be reserved for patients older than 5 years.

Polydactyly

Morley SE, Smith PJ: Polydactyly of the feet in children: Suggestions for surgical treatment. *Br J Plast Surg* 2001; 54(1):34-38.

The authors report on a consecutive series of 34 instances of polydactyly of the foot in 25 patients who were treated surgically and classified according to the protocol described by Blauth and Olason. Although reports in the literature advocate that in patients with polydactyly of the fifth ray of the foot the most lateral digit should be excised regardless of

whether it is the more fully formed digit, the authors conclude that this should not always be the case and describe two instances of polysyndactyly in which the more medial element of a fifth ray polydactyly was excised to allow for better maintenance of the contour of the foot.

Uda H, Sugawara Y, Niu A, Sarukawa S: Treatment of lateral ray polydactyly of the foot: Focusing on the selection of the toe to be excised. *Plast Reconstr Surg* 2002;109(5):1581-1591.

The authors report the results of a study of 25 feet that were surgically treated for lateral ray polydactyly and describe an algorithm that was developed for selection of the toe to be excised. Because the most common problem with medial toe excision is valgus deformity and the most common problem noted with lateral toe excision is postoperative pain, to help avoid these problems, the patients in this study were divided into two groups for treatment recommendations. In feet with duplication of both the metatarsal and phalanges, the toe with a radiographically dominant metatarsus was retained. In the feet with only duplication of the phalanges, the morphologically smaller toe was excised independent of the radiographic appearance of the bones. If the medial and lateral toes were equal in size in the latter group, the authors recommended excision of the lateral toe.

Sever's Disease

Volpon JB, de Carvalho Filho G: Calcaneal apophysitis: A quantitative radiographic evaluation of the secondary ossification center. *Arch Orthop Trauma Surg* 2002;122: 338-341.

The authors studied the foot radiographs of 392 children with no apophysitis and 69 children with calcaneal apophysitis to assess bone density as well as determine the time of appearance and the number of fragments of the secondary nucleus. The authors noted that sclerosis of the secondary nucleus is a normal feature, but the apophysitis group seemed to have a more fragmented appearance of the secondary nucleus. The primary ossific nucleus and secondary ossific nucleus were both less dense in the apophysitis group. From these findings, the authors suggested a mechanical etiology of Sever's disease.

Classic Bibliography

Asirvatham R, Stevens PM: Idiopathic forefoot-adduction deformity: Medial capsulotomy and abductor hallucis lengthening for resistant and severe deformities. *J Pediatr Orthop* 1997;17:496-500.

Black GB, Grogan DP, Bobechko WP: Butler arthroplasty for correction of the adducted fifth toe: A retrospective study of 36 operations between 1968 and 1982. *J Pediatr Orthop* 1985;5:439-441.

Bleck EE: Metatarsus adductus: Classification and relationship to outcomes of treatment. *J Pediatr Orthop* 1983;3:2-9.

Borges J, Guille J, Bowen J: Kohler's bone disease of the tarsal navicular. *J Pediatr Orthop* 1995;15:596-598.

Canale PB, Aronson DD, Lamont RL, Manoli A: The Mitchell procedure for the treatment of adolescent hallux valgus: A long-term study. *J Bone Joint Surg Am* 1993;75:1610-1618.

Coughlin MJ: Juvenile hallux valgus: Etiology and treatment. *Foot Ankle Int* 1995;16:682-697.

Hamer AJ, Stanley D, Smith TW: Surgery for curly toe deformity: A double-blind, randomized, prospective trial. *J Bone Joint Surg Br* 1993;75:662-663.

Katcherian DA: Treatment of Freiberg's disease. *Orthop Clin North Am* 1994;25:69-81.

Katz K, David R, Soudry M: Below-knee plaster cast for the treatment of metatarsus adductus. *J Pediatr Orthop* 1999;19:49-50.

Kilmartin TE, Barrington RL, Wallace WA: A controlled prospective trial of a foot orthosis for juvenile hallux valgus. *J Bone Joint Surg Br* 1994;76:210-214.

Kinnard P, Lirette R: Dorsiflexion osteotomy in Freiberg's disease. *Foot Ankle* 1989;9:226-231.

Liberson A, Lieberson S, Mendes DG, Shajrawi I, Ben Haim Y, Boss JH: Remodeling of the calcaneus apophysis in the growing child. *J Pediatr Orthop B* 1995;4:74-79.

Micheli LJ, Lloyd Ireland M: Prevention and management of calcaneal apophysitis in children: An overuse syndrome. *J Pediatr Orthop* 1987;7:34-38.

Nogami H: Polydactyly and polysyndactyly of the fifth toe. *Clin Orthop Relat Res* 1986;204:261-265.

Peterson HA, Newman SR: Adolescent bunion deformity treated with double osteotomy and longitudinal fixation of the first ray. *J Pediatr Orthop* 1993;13:80-84.

Phelps D, Grogan D: Polydactyly of the foot. *J Pediatr Orthop* 1985;5:446-451.

Ponseti IV, Becker JR: Congenital metatarsus adductus: the results of treatment. *J Bone Joint Surg Am* 1966;48:702.

Rushforth GF: The natural history of hooked forefoot. *J Bone Joint Surg Br* 1978;60:530.

Venn-Watson EA: Problems in polydactyly of the foot. *Orthop Clin North Am* 1976;7:909-927.

Weiner BK, Weiner DS, Mirkopulos N: Mitchell osteotomy for adolescent hallux valgus. *J Pediatr Orthop* 1997; 17:781-784.

Section 4

Pediatric Trauma

Section Editor:
Paul D. Sponseller, MD, MBA

Chapter 19

Principles of Trauma Management in the Pediatric Patient

Keisha M. DePass, MD

Introduction

Traumatic injury, the leading cause of death in childhood and adolescence, accounts for 16 million emergency department visits, 600,000 hospitalizations, and 20,000 deaths per year in the United States. The direct cost of pediatric trauma exceeds $8 billion annually. Most injuries are the result of accidents. However, intentional injuries also occur and must be recognized on presentation. In this chapter, management of the multiply injured pediatric patient is reviewed. Child abuse and injury prevention are also discussed. The appropriate and timely management of musculoskeletal injuries in coordination with the management of life-threatening injuries will help to minimize long-term morbidity and dysfunction in pediatric patients. Orthopaedists must be aware that pediatric patients are not just little adults and that anatomic and physiologic differences make the management of pediatric trauma different from that of adults.

The Multiply Injured Pediatric Patient

The management of the multiply injured pediatric patient begins before the patient arrives at the hospital. First responders and emergency medical technicians are trained in basic trauma life support and are responsible for prehospital extrication, resuscitation, spinal protection and immobilization, splinting, control of external hemorrhage, and transport. These first responders are the first medical professionals to interact with the patient and help to prevent additional injury. In addition, first responders and emergency medical technicians also assess and maintain airway, breathing, and circulation during transport to the closest level I facility. Once at the hospital, the primary survey is repeated, and the secondary survey occurs once the patient has been stabilized.

The anatomy and physiology of pediatric patients provide unique challenges in both the prehospital and hospital settings (Figure 1). To establish and maintain the airway of children can be difficult because of their unique anatomic features. Compared with adults, pediat-

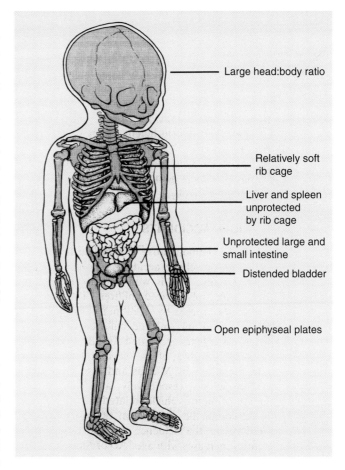

Figure 1 Schematic representation of the anatomic differences in children that require a different approach in the management of trauma. *(Reproduced with permission from Browner BD, Jupiter JB, Levine AM, Trafton PG (eds): Skeletal Trauma: Basic Science, Management, and Reconstruction, ed 3. New York, NY: WB Saunders, 2003.)*

- Large head:body ratio
- Relatively soft rib cage
- Liver and spleen unprotected by rib cage
- Unprotected large and small intestine
- Distended bladder
- Open epiphyseal plates

ric patients have relatively large tongues and small mouths. The larynx of a child is also small, and it is located more anterior and caudal than in adults. The trachea of a child is soft and short, and failure to recognize this can lead to bronchial intubation and/or perforation. The head of a child is proportionately larger and has weaker cervical muscles than in adults, which leads to a higher frequency of head injuries in pediatric patients.

Table 1 | The Modified Injury Severity Scale for Multiply Injured Children

Body Area	1-Minor	2-Minor	3-Severe but not life-threatening	4-Severe and life threatening	5-Critical and survival uncertain
Neural	Glasgow Coma Score: 13-14	Glasgow Coma Score: 9-12	Glasgow Coma Score: 9-12	Glasgow Coma Score: 5-8	Glasgow Coma Score: 4
Face and neck	Abrasion or contusions of the ocular apparatus or lid	Nondisplaced facial bone fracture	Loss of an eye, avulsion of the optic nerve	Bone or soft-tissue injury with minor destruction	Injuries with airway obstruction
	Vitreous or conjunctival hemorrhage	Laceration of the eye, disfiguring laceration	Displaced facial fracture		
	Fractured teeth	Retinal detachment	Blowout fracture of the orbit		
Chest	Muscle ache or chest wall stiffness	Simple rib or sternal fracture	Multiple rib fractures	Open chest wounds	Lacerations, tracheal hemomediastinum
			Hemothorax or pneumothorax	Pneumomediastinum	Aortic laceration
			Diaphragmatic rupture	Myocardial contusion	Myocardial laceration or rupture
			Pulmonary contusion		
Abdomen	Muscle ache, seat belt abrasion	Major abdominal wall contusion	Contusion of abdominal organs	Minor laceration of abdominal organs	Rupture or severe laceration of abdominal vessels or organs
			Retroperitoneal hematoma	Intraperitoneal bladder rupture	
			Extraperitoneal bladder rupture	Spine fractures with paraplegia	
Extremities and pelvic girdle	Minor sprains	Open fractures of digits	Thoracic or lumbar spine fractures	Multiple closed long bone fractures	Multiple open long bone fractures
	Simple fractures and dislocations	Nondisplaced long bone or pelvic fractures	Displaced long bone or multiple hand or foot fractures	Amputation of limbs	
			Single open long bone fractures		
			Pelvic fractures with displacement		
			Laceration of major nerves or vessels		

Adapted with permission from Mayer T, Matlak ME, Johnson DG, Walker ML: The modified injury severity scale in pediatric multiple trauma patients. J Pediatr Surg 1980;15:719-726.

In addition, because of the size of a child's head, immobilization on a standard adult backboard will flex a child's neck and can worsen a cervical spine injury. The mediastinum is mobile in children; therefore, intramediastinal injuries more readily compromise venous return than in adults. The protuberant abdomen of a child receives less protection from either the rib cage or the pelvis, consequently pediatric patients have a higher incidence of intra-abdominal injuries.

Physiologic differences between pediatric and adult patients include the response to hypovolemia. In the pediatric population, decreased blood pressure is often a late sign of hypovolemic shock. Blood loss is followed by immediate constriction of small- and medium-sized arteries to maintain blood pressure. Tachycardia, tachypnea, and changes in the level of consciousness are earlier indicators of shock. Hypothermia is also more prevalent in pediatric patients because of the large ratio of surface area to body weight. Unidentified hypothermia can induce pulmonary hypotension, increase hypoxia, and worsen metabolic acidosis, rendering the child unresponsive to resuscitation.

Injury Assessment

Injury severity scales, which provide a valuable method of assessing and triaging patients who experience multi-

Table 2	Pediatric Trauma Score			
Category	**+2**	**+1**	**-1**
Weight	> 20 kg	10 to 20 kg	< 10 kg
Airway	Normal	Maintainable	Not maintainable
Systolic blood pressure	> 90 mm Hg	50 to 90 mm Hg	< 50 mm Hg
Central nervous system	Awake	Obtunded	Comatose
Open wound	None	Minor	Major
Skeletal	None	Closed fracture	Open or multiple fracture(s)
Prognosis			
Score > 8		Predicts < 1% mortality	
Score < 8		Suggests need for treatment at trauma center	
Score = 4		Predicts 50% mortality	
Score < 1		Predicts > 98% mortality	

Adapted with permission from Tepas JJ, Alexander RH, Campbell JD, et al: An improved scoring system for assessment of the injured child. J Trauma 1985;25:720.

system trauma, have been reliably proven to aid in the triage of patients to hospitals that specialize in pediatric trauma and critical care. Emergency medical personnel should be familiar with the injury severity scales to ensure that patients are transported to facilities that are capable of treating each patient's injuries. Outcomes have been shown to be worsened by a delay in arrival to these centers. The multiple scoring systems used today are based on either the anatomic distribution of injury, the physiologic response to injury, or a combination of the two. An example of an injury severity scale with anatomic classification is the Injury Severity Score. The Injury Severity Score identifies the three most severely injured body parts (anatomic region) and grades them on a scale of 0 to 5, 5 representing a life-threatening injury. The scores are then squared to give a maximum of 75 points. An example of an injury severity scale based on physiologic parameters is the Trauma Score, which evaluates a patient's response to injury by scoring capillary refill, respiratory effort, systolic blood pressure, and level of arousal. The Modified Injury Severity Score and the Pediatric Trauma Score, which combine both anatomic and physiologic criteria, are widely used. In the Modified Injury Severity Score, the three most severely injured areas are squared and the results are summed. A score of 25 or more is associated with increased risk of permanent disability, and a score of greater than 40 is associated with a higher risk of mortality (Table 1). In the Pediatric Trauma Score, respiration, body weight, blood pressure, level of arousal, soft-tissue injury, and the presence of fractures are graded. A score of 9 or less is associated with a higher risk of mortality (Table 2).

Central Nervous System Injuries
Head injury is the leading cause of death and disability in pediatric patients who experience trauma injuries.

Head injuries occur most commonly as a result of motor vehicle collisions and falls. The primary insult occurs at the time of injury; however, secondary insults may occur as a result of hypoxia, hypotension, and intracranial hypertension. Prompt reestablishment of an airway and adequate resuscitation can help to prevent secondary injuries and improve long-term outcomes.

Pediatric patients are more prone than adults to develop intracranial hypertension after injury. Methods that combat hypertension include elevation of the head, sedation, pain control, hyperventilation, and the use of osmotic agents to decrease brain edema. Initial evaluation of the child with a head injury should include assessment with the Glasgow Coma Scale, which measures motor, verbal, and eye opening responses to verbal cues and noxious stimuli to assess impairment of consciousness on presentation. The Glasgow Coma Scale has been modified for the pediatric population to account for children who are extremely young and preverbal (Table 3). Assessment with the Glasgow Coma Scale is usually followed by CT and inpatient observation if there is a history of loss of consciousness for more than 5 minutes, seizure, or neurologic deficit.

Spinal cord injuries are rare in the pediatric population; when they do occur, they are often difficult to diagnose because many anatomic variations of the immature spine make evaluation by an inexperienced medical provider challenging. The presence of multiple ossification centers in the vertebrae can lead to the overdiagnosis of spinal fractures. Spinal injuries are more common in the cervical spine because of the large head size, weak muscles, and loose ligaments of children. Damage to the spinal cord has been reported to occur in children even though there are no radiographic signs of injury. This phenomenon is known as spinal cord injury without radiographic abnormality, and it is discussed in more de-

Table 3 | Pediatric Glasgow Coma Scale

Score	Patient Age		
	> 5 Years	**1 to 5 Years**	**Younger than Age 1 Year**
Best Motor Response (of 6)			**(of 5)**
6	Obeys commands	Obeys commands	
5	Localizes pain	Localizes pain	Localizes pain
4	Withdrawal	Withdrawal	Withdrawal
3	Flexion to pain	Flexion to pain	Flexion to pain
2	Extensor rigidity	Extensor rigidity	Extensor rigidity
1	None	None	None
Best Verbal Response			
5	Oriented	Appropriate words	Smiles/cries appropriately
4	Confused	Inappropriate words	Cries
3	Inappropriate words	Cries/screams	Cries inappropriately
2	Incomprehensible	Grunts	Grunts
1	None	None	None
Eye Opening			
4	Spontaneous	Spontaneous	Spontaneous
3	To speech	To speech	To speech
2	To pain	To pain	To pain
1	None	None	None

Reproduced from Sponseller PD, Paidas C: Management of the pediatric trauma patient, in Sponseller PD (ed): Orthopaedic Knowledge Update: Pediatrics 2. Rosemont, IL, American Academy of Orthopaedic Surgeons, 2002, p 75.

tail in chapter 26. With the identification of a spinal fracture at one level, there is a 5% to 10% risk of fracture at other levels of the spine. Appropriate immobilization in the field and subsequent clinical evaluation with examination and radiographs are needed to ensure the proper management of spinal injuries in children.

Abdominal Injuries

The spleen and the liver are injured in approximately equal frequency in children who experience blunt trauma; together spleen and liver injuries account for approximately 75% of all childhood abdominal injuries. Injuries to the hollow viscus are less common in the pediatric population than in adults. Nonsurgical management of these injuries is preferred to avoid serious complications. The incidence of postsplenectomy sepsis is higher in patients who are younger at the time of splenectomy. Indications for surgical exploration of an abdominal injury include a pneumoperitoneum and fluid in the abdomen without solid organ injury.

Specific findings on physical examination, including lap belt marks, ecchymosis, lacerations, and evidence of abdominal guarding, should prompt physicians to investigate abdominal injuries further with diagnostic imaging studies. CT of the abdomen with intravenous contrast is the preferred diagnostic imaging modality for the assessment of the hemodynamically stable patient. In patients who are hemodynamically unstable, focused

abdominal sonography can quickly identify fluid in the abdomen without the delay introduced by CT. CT can also be used for serial examination of hematomas in patients with solid organ injury. Physicians must be aware of an association among seat belt injuries, flexion-distraction vertebral fractures, traumatic pancreatitis, and bowel injuries in children following motor vehicle accidents; if one of these injuries is found, then the patient should be assessed for the others as well.

Thoracic Injuries

Thoracic injures are associated with an overall mortality rate of 25% in children younger than 5 years. Because of the compliance of the chest wall in children, a pulmonary contusion may occur without much external evidence of injury. Rib fractures are less common in children because of their intrinsic flexibility, and the presence of a rib fracture may serve as a marker of severe trauma. Rib fractures are also frequently seen with child abuse and their presence should alert the physician to the possibility of child abuse. Because of the compliant chest walls of children, hemothoraces and pneumothoraces can also lead to hypotension by decreasing the venous return to the heart; therefore, they should be managed appropriately and quickly because children proceed to hypovolemic shock after the loss of a smaller blood volume than adults.

Table 4 | Guidelines to Help Determine When Surgical Intervention for a Fracture Should Occur in Multiply Injured Pediatric Patients

Make sure that any child with a long bone fracture does not have any other significant injuries.

Early fracture care should be compatible with the general care of the patient.

Fracture care should consider the need for early mobilization of the child.

Fractures care should facilitate the management of associated soft-tissue injuries.

The initial method of fracture management should be the definitive method whenever possible.

Fracture care should be carefully individualized.

All children should be treated as if they are going to survive; in the management of femur fractures in children who also had closed head injuries, early versus late fixation has been reported to lead to similar long-term results; however, early fixation decreased the length of hospital stay and decreased the number of nonorthopaedic and nonneurologic complications.

Adapted with permission from Armstrong P, Smith J: Initial management of the multiply injured child, in Letts RM (ed): Management of Pediatric Fracture. New York, NY, Churchill Livingstone, 1994, p 27.

Musculoskeletal Injuries

The management of fractures in multiply injured patients must be prioritized to accommodate for the treatment of other injuries. Traumatic musculoskeletal injuries can lead to the loss of a limb, growth arrest, angular deformities, arthritis, and chronic pain. The frequency of musculoskeletal injury in pediatric patients is bimodal with peaks in both the toddler and adolescent years. The most important decision is when to surgically intervene for the treatment of a fracture. A series of guidelines designed to assist in the decision-making process is listed in Table 4. The blood loss associated with bony injuries, especially in the pelvis, is proportionately greater in children than in adults; therefore, because hypovolemic shock may follow after multiple long bone fractures, urgent stabilization is indicated.

Social Implications of Traumatic Injuries

Traumatic injuries affect much more than the physical well-being of a child; they carry psychosocial and emotional ramifications that extend beyond the departure from the acute care setting. Traumatic injuries affect not only the patients themselves, but also their families. In patients with traumatic brain injuries, negative social outcomes have been associated with lower socioeconomic status, fewer family resources, and poorer family functioning. Interpersonal resources such as supportive family members and friends can help attenuate the long-term burden and cost associated with the care of pediatric patients with traumatic injury.

Isolated Orthopaedic Trauma

Isolated orthopaedic trauma injuries again illustrate how the anatomic and physiologic variations between children and adults affect management decisions. Because of persistent growth, bone remodeling potential, elastic bone, open physes, thick periosteum, and smaller structures in children, the same mechanism of injury may produce different injury patterns in children and adults. Closed management with casting results in good outcomes in pediatric patients without adding the potential complications associated with surgery. In the pediatric patients who require surgical intervention, it is important for the health care provider to know when and how to intervene.

Femur fractures are the most frequent major orthopaedic injury in children, accounting for approximately 18,000 fractures annually. This is followed by tibial, humeral, radial/ulnar, and vertebral fractures (Figure 2). Males have a higher injury rate than females for most fracture types (between 56% and 78% of all fractures), which is thought to be the result of more males participating in contact sports such as football and hockey. The only type of fracture that has been reported to be more prevalent in females is pelvic fractures, but the difference is slight.

Mechanism of Injury

Motor vehicle accidents account for a large proportion of the injuries sustained by children. After being hit by a motor vehicle, the incidence of severe trauma is approximately 11% (as defined by an Injury Severity Score of > 15 in children 14 years and younger). Thirty-nine percent of these injuries represent trauma to the musculoskeletal system, particularly the femur, tibia, pelvis, and spine. Of the patients who require surgical intervention, 67% require orthopaedic surgery. Fractures of the pelvis, spine, and tibia are more common in the adult population, whereas fractures of the femur are more common in children, which is thought to be associated with the height of car bumpers.

Other causes of unintentional childhood injuries include drowning, burns, choking, firearms, falls, poisonings, and athletic participation. The use of all-terrain vehicles is becoming another source of major injuries in the pediatric population. The average Injury Severity Score for patients injured as a result of all-terrain vehicle accidents is 9 on presentation to the emergency department; the most common of these injuries are orthopaedic, representing about 60% of the total injuries, followed by head trauma and facial injuries.

Open Fractures

Timely management of soft-tissue injuries associated with open fractures, including surgical débridement and perioperative antibiotic therapy, has decreased morbid-

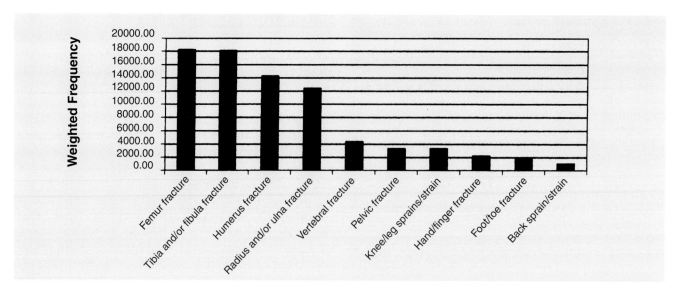

Figure 2 Bar graph showing the 10 pediatric orthopaedic injuries that most often require hospitalization. *(Reproduced with permission from Galano GJ, Vitale MA, Kessler MW, Hyman JE, Vitale MG: The most frequent traumatic orthopaedic injuries from a national pediatric inpatient population. J Pediatr Orthop 2005;25(1):39-44.)*

ity and mortality rates. Open fractures are treated as surgical emergencies in the adult population and the pediatric population.

Gustilo and associates described the most widely used classification system for open fractures in 1984 (Table 5). This classification system quantifies the amount of soft-tissue damage and the level of contamination with these injuries and has been used to standardize treatment based on the grade of injury. Initial management, no matter what Gustilo grade, should consist of tetanus prophylaxis, a sterile dressing, splinting, and intravenous antibiotics. With the current schedule of immunizations required in the United States, most children are up to date on their immunizations and do not require dosing for tetanus prophylaxis. However, any patient who has not completed a series of toxoid immunizations or who has not received a booster dose in 5 years should receive the tetanus toxoid. If the wound is highly contaminated, then tetanus human immunoglobulin can also be given to provide passive immunization for up to 3 weeks.

Antibiotics have been shown to decrease the long-term morbidity associated with open fractures. Gustilo grade I injuries require intravenous antibiotic therapy with a first-generation cephalosporin for 24 hours. A Gustilo grade II injury is treated with a first-generation cephalosporin, with or without an aminoglycoside, depending on the level of contamination. Aminoglycosides are ototoxic and nephrotoxic and should be used carefully. Gustilo grade III injuries are treated with a cephalosporin and an aminoglycoside. For farm injuries, penicillin is added to cover for *Clostridium* and other anaerobes.

Lawn mower accidents create a dilemma in the management of open fractures, primarily because of the ex-

Table 5	Gustilo Classification of Open Fractures
I	Low-energy mechanism, wound < 2 cm, minimal muscle contusion
II	Wound between 2 and 10 cm with moderate soft-tissue damage
III	High-energy mechanism, wound > 10 cm with extensive soft-tissue damage
	A Adequate soft-tissue cover
	B Inadequate soft-tissue cover
	C Associated with arterial injury

Adapted with permission from Gustilo R, Mendoza R, Williams D: Problems in the management of type III open fractures: A new classification. J Trauma 1984;24:742.

tensive soft-tissue and vascular damage. The Mangled Extremity Severity Score, which uses readily available and quantifiable parameters, was designed to help surgeons decide whether amputation or reconstruction of the injured limb should be done. Scores of 7 or higher predict the need for initial amputation.

Compartment Syndrome

Compartment syndrome, which occurs when there is a sustained elevation of intracompartmental pressures and can result in muscle necrosis and neurovascular compromise, represents an orthopaedic emergency. The diagnosis is made primarily on clinical findings, the most important of which is pain out of proportion to the injury. Paresthesias, pain with passive stretching, and loss of motor function are also signs of compartment syndrome, although some of these symptoms occur after permanent muscle damage has occurred. In children who are extremely young, it is difficult to interpret the symptoms because they cannot verbalize what they are feeling. Most patients are crying on approach and are difficult to examine. If compartment syndrome is suspected, then measurement of pressures is indicated. It is likely that some sort of sedation will be required to perform this procedure.

Elevated intracompartmental pressures can be measured with an electronic monitor. Although the pressure threshold for fasciotomy is not clearly established, values between 30 and 40 mm Hg or within 30 mm Hg of the diastolic blood pressure are dangerous and used as surgical criteria for compartment release. The first step in the management of compartment syndrome is the release of any tight or compressive dressings. A circumferential cast may provoke compartment syndrome in an injured extremity. Surgical management includes fasciotomy of all affected compartments. The fasciotomies are often left open at the index procedure and undergo delayed primary closure or skin grafting.

Emergency Department Management

The emergency department physician acts as a gatekeeper and is often the first medical subspecialist to interact with a traumatically injured child. Identification and triage of orthopaedic injuries must be performed in a timely manner. Most orthopaedic injuries can be treated closed because of the enormous potential for bone remodeling in children. Conscious sedation, dissociative anesthesia, and regional anesthesia can be used to facilitate reduction. Conscious sedation is defined as a level of consciousness that maintains protective reflexes and retains the patient's ability to control the airway independently. Patients under conscious sedation can follow commands and respond to physical stimulation. Agents used for conscious sedation include opioids and benzodiazepines such as fentanyl, Demerol, morphine, and midazolam; these agents may be used in a variety of combinations. Patients are monitored during the procedure to ensure that they do not pass into deep sedation (a level of sedation similar to that achieved using general anesthesia) and lose control of the protective reflexes. Dissociative anesthesia induces a trance-like state that combines sedation, analgesia, and amnesia. The most common agent used to induce dissociative anesthesia is ketamine, which increases upper airway secretions and is often used in combination with atropine. Caution should be used when using this agent with older children because it may induce hallucinations. Regional anesthesia can be achieved using hematoma and nerve blocks, both of which work well in providing anesthesia for the reduction but do little to reduce patient anxiety. In some patients, propofol (an induction agent) has been used in the emergency department setting without need of assisted ventilation.

Child Abuse

An estimated 2 million children experience child abuse annually, with over 150,000 being seriously injured or impaired. Child abuse was initially defined as physical injury inflicted on children by their caregivers, but the definition has since been expanded to include emotional neglect, psychologic abuse, and sexual abuse. Approximately 60% of the perpetrators of child abuse are male and are the child's father, stepfather, or the male partner of the child's mother. The clinical presentation of children who have experienced child abuse includes injuries to the soft tissue, head, and musculoskeletal system. Soft-tissue injuries include burns, welts, lacerations, and ecchymosis. The health care provider must be aware of typical patterns that are made by common objects. Bruising on the buttocks, trunk, and back of the legs all suggest intentional injury. In addition, burns that are symmetric and have sharp lines of demarcation suggest intentional injury. Fractures sustained from physical abuse can take on any pattern; however, a few patterns should raise suspicion of child abuse at the time of initial evaluation, including skull fractures, rib fractures, metaphyseal corner fractures and long bone fractures in nonambulatory patients with minor trauma. In addition, the presence of multiple long bone fractures of varying ages should raise suspicion of child abuse. Osteogenesis imperfecta can also cause long bone fractures and must be considered, especially in the presence of a positive family history of this disorder or other clinical findings.

Children who have experienced child abuse are initially evaluated by the trauma team. The age distribution of children who have intentional injury differs from those whose injuries are unintentional. Fifty-seven percent of all the children who are abused are younger than 1 year, whereas 66% of patient who experience unintentional trauma are older than 5 years. If child abuse is suspected, hospital admission is mandatory. Skeletal surveys may uncover evidence of other fractures. Medical therapy is provided, and the process of legal and social protection is initiated. The basis of notification of these protective agencies is a reasonable suspicion or belief. Therefore, a medical provider is mandated by law to report any possible instances of child abuse.

Injury Prevention

The institution of laws to regulate the seating of children within passenger vehicles has helped to decrease the incidence of fatal injuries in motor vehicle collisions. However, more children are still killed as passengers in motor vehicle collisions than as a result of any other type of injury because of a failure of education and compliance with these laws. A total of 62% of children 4 to 8 years of age are inappropriately restrained in motor vehicles by adult seat belts. Health care providers should play a role in the education of parents as to the

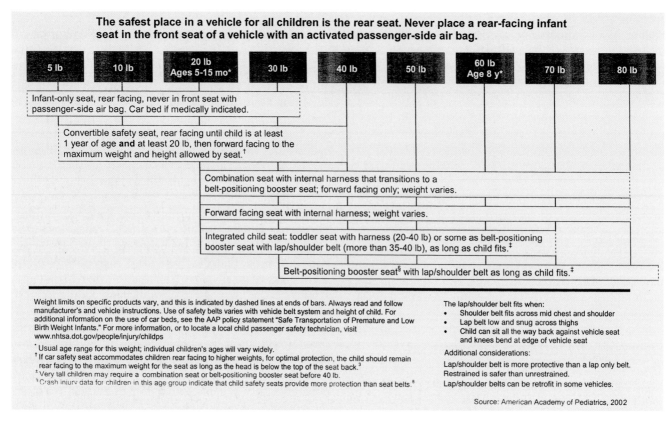

The safest place in a vehicle for all children is the rear seat. Never place a rear-facing infant seat in the front seat of a vehicle with an activated passenger-side air bag.

Figure 3 A summary of the current recommendations for car safety seating as recommended by the American Academy of Pediatrics. *(Reproduced with permission from The American Academy of Pediatrics: Committee on Injury and Poison Prevention: Selecting and using the most appropriate car safety seats for growing children: Guidelines for counseling parents. Pediatrics 2002;109(3):550-553.)*

current safety recommendations. The American Academy of Pediatrics published recommendations for the selection of car safety seats based on the weight of the child (Figure 3).

The cooperation of parents, safety seat manufacturers, regulatory agencies, and health care professionals is needed to decrease the rate of morbidity and mortality in a primarily pediatric population. The strategies for the prevention of orthopaedic injuries can be organized into broad categories: engineering, enforcement, education, and economics. These areas address the potential for injury from the time of a product's initial design to its implementation and use. Prevention also requires education of the public, legislation, and enforcement of laws to ensure large scale compliance.

Annotated Bibliography
General
Gladden PB, Wilson CH, Suk M: Pediatric orthopedic trauma: Principles of management. *Semin Pediatr Surg* 2004;13:119-125.

In this review of musculoskeletal injuries in pediatric trauma patients, the authors give special consideration to the long-term consequences of fractures and emphasize multidisciplinary evaluation and treatment of children with these injuries.

The Multiply Injured Pediatric Patient
Mendelson SA, Dominick TS, Tyler-Kabara E, Moreland MS, Adelson PD: Early versus late femoral fracture stabilization in the multiply injured pediatric patient. *J Pediatr Orthop* 2001;21:594-599.

The purpose of this study was to analyze whether time to fixation of fracture adversely affected outcomes in patients with head injury. The authors found that early and late fixation led to similar long-term results, but early fixation decreased the length of hospital stay and decreased the number of nonorthopaedic and nonneurologic complications.

Isolated Orthopaedic Trauma
Galano GJ, Vitale MA, Kessler MW, Hyman JE, Vitale MG: The most frequent traumatic orthopedic injuries from a national pediatric inpatient population. *J Pediatr Orthop* 2005;25:39-44.

This article was a retrospective review of patients with traumatic orthopaedic conditions as the principal diagnosis. Patients were identified using the 1997 National Pediatric Inpatient Database to evaluate the incidence of fractures requiring hospitalization. The authors then used these data to compile a list of common fractures, management methods, and length and cost of hospital stay.

Emergency Department Management

Molczan KA: Triaging pediatric orthopedic injuries. *J Emerg Nurs* 2001;27:297-300.

The author reports that triaging patients appropriately in the emergency department can decrease the morbidity associated with a delay in treatment and presents special challenges for emergency department nurses and physicians. The author discusses major concepts in triage and summarizes the major differences between adult and pediatric fractures.

Child Abuse

Chang DC, Knight V, Ziegfeld S, Haider A, Warfield D, Paidas C: The tip of the iceberg for child abuse: The critical roles of pediatric trauma service and its registry. *J Trauma* 2004;57:1189-1198.

The authors report that the significant characteristics of abused children include higher Injury Severity Scores (especially in the head and integument), longer hospital stays, and a risk of mortality that is approximately 10 times higher than that of the emergency department population. The authors propose the use of the Diagnostic Index for Physical Child Abuse to assist physicians in identifying child abuse in pediatric trauma patients.

Johnson K, Chapman S, Hall CM: Skeletal injuries associated with sexual abuse. *Pediatr Radiol* 2004;34:620-623.

The authors used radiography to evaluate three patients who had been sexually abused and concluded that the presence of pelvic fractures of varying ages can assist in the confirmation of the diagnosis of abuse.

Injury Prevention

Demetriades D, Murray J, Martin M, Velmahos G, Salin A, Alo K: Pedestrian injured by automobiles: Relationship of age to injury type and severity. *J Am Coll Surg* 2004;199:382-387.

The authors of this study conducted a retrospective review of 5,838 trauma patients from a registry of patients who were injured by automobiles and treated at a level I trauma center. Injury Severity Score as well as other parameters were calculated according to four age groups ($\leq$ 14 years, 15 to 55 years, 56 to 65 years, and > 65 years). Results showed that age plays a significant role in the anatomic distribution of injuries and Injury Severity Scores.

Mace SE, Gerardi MJ, Dietrich AM, et al: Injury prevention and control in children. *Ann Emerg Med* 2001; 38:405-414.

The authors discuss the formulation and application of injury prevention strategies in an emergency department setting.

Winston FK, Chen IG, Elliot MR, Arbogast KB, Burbin DR: Recent trends in child restraint practices in the United States. *Pediatrics* 2004;113:e458-e464.

The authors conducted a cross-sectional study of children younger than 9 years who were involved in motor vehicle collisions between 1998 and 2002. Data were collected from insurance claims and telephone surveys and showed that although regulations are in place, inappropriate restraint of children in motor vehicles is still commonplace.

Classic Bibliography

Armstrong P, Smith J: Initial Management of the multiply injured child, in Letts RM (ed): *Management of Pediatric Fracture.* New York, NY, Churchill Livingstone, 1994, p 27.

Bond SJ, Eichelberger MR, Gotschall CS, Sivit CJ, Randolph JG: Nonoperative management of blunt hepatic and splenic injury in children. *Ann Surg* 1996;223:286-289.

Eichelberger MR, Randolph JG: Pediatric trauma: An algorithm for diagnosis and therapy. *J Trauma* 1983;23: 91-97.

Gustilo RB, Mendoza RM, Williams DN: Problems in the management of type III open fractures a new classification. *J Trauma* 1984;24:742-746.

Kocher MS, Kasser JR: Orthopaedic aspects of child abuse. *J Am Acad Orthop Surg* 2000;8:10-20.

Loder RT, Bookout C: Fracture patterns in battered children. *J Orthop Trauma* 1991;5:428-433.

Loder RT: Pediatric polytrauma: Orthopedic care in hospital course. *J Orthop Trauma* 1987;1:48-54.

Maksoud JG, Moront ML, Eichelberger MR: Resuscitation of the injured child. *Semin Pediatr Surg* 1995;4: 93-99.

Matsen FA 3rd, Veith RG: Compartmental syndromes in children. *J Pediatr Orthop* 1981;1:33-41.

Mayer T, Matlak ME, Johnson DG, Walker ML: The modified injury severity scale in pediatric multiple trauma patients. *J Pediatr Surg* 1980;15:719-726.

McCarty EC, Mencio GA, Walker LA, Green NE: Ketamine sedation for the reduction of children's fractures in the emergency department. *J Bone Joint Surg Am* 2000;82:912-918.

Tepas JJ, Alexander RH, Campbell JD, et al: An improved scoring system for assessment of the injured child. *J Trauma* 1985;25:720.

Chapter 20

Fractures of the Hip and Pelvis

Michael G. Vitale, MD, MPH

Benjamin D. Roye, MD, MPH

Introduction

Pelvic and hip fractures are uncommon injuries in the pediatric population, accounting for fewer than 1% of all childhood fractures. These injuries, frequently a result of high-energy trauma, can have devastating complications; therefore, immediate and appropriate management is critical to optimizing outcomes. There are many treatment strategies available for pediatric patients with pelvic and hip fractures that range from the timing of surgery to the type of implant (if any) and the rehabilitation protocol. The low incidence of hip fractures in the pediatric population has resulted in limited consensus regarding the treatment of these injuries and associated complications. Working within these limitations, this chapter reviews the recent literature to discuss how to make the best, evidence-based decisions based on the age of the patient, the injury pattern, and other factors.

Fractures of the Pelvis

Pelvic fractures in children differ significantly from those in adults. The pediatric pelvis is plastic and deformable and will absorb significant energy before failure. Overall mortality from pelvic fractures in children is only one third the rate reported for adults. Furthermore, injuries to the pediatric growth plate may result in progressive deformity. Conversely, remodeling may occur during growth, leading some orthopaedic surgeons to opt for nonsurgical treatment of injuries that would require open reduction and internal fixation in an adult population. Closure of the triradiate cartilage has been suggested to be a convenient marker for differentiating pediatric from adult fracture types.

A displaced pediatric pelvic fracture in a child is indicative of a high-energy injury (Figure 1). With regard to injury, the pediatric pelvis has been described as a suit of armor; there is more concern about the contents than about the structure itself. Associated injuries, including abdominal, genitourinary, and head trauma, are common and contribute significantly to morbidity and mortality. Children who present with a pelvic fracture and additional bony fractures are much more likely to have head and abdominal injuries and have twice the mortality risk of those presenting without concomitant skeletal injuries.

Improved understanding of important issues in the early management of these injuries has resulted in a marked improvement in short-term outcomes, including mortality and early complications. Initial management of a pediatric pelvic fracture demands a multidisciplinary approach. Although the trauma team most often performs the initial survey and resuscitation, the orthopaedic surgeon may be called on for urgent consultation in patients with hemodynamic instability. Children are much less likely to have life-threatening exsanguination as a result of pelvic fracture, and there has been an increased awareness that hemodynamic instability in this patient population demands an aggressive search for other sources of bleeding.

Rectal examination, inspection of the perineum and genitourinary systems, and a careful neurologic examination are essential parts of the evaluation of a patient with a pelvic fracture. Destot sign (inguinal or scrotal hematoma), Earle sign (mass on digital rectal examination), and Morel-Lavalle injury (a closed degloving injury over the greater trochanter) have all been described as indicators of more severe trauma. Lacerations to the perineum or rectum should be regarded as possible sites of open fracture and managed accordingly.

Radiographic evaluation classically includes multiple views of the pelvis. Inlet views can demonstrate injuries to the posterior ring and anterior-posterior displacement, whereas outlet views can better show injuries to the anterior ring and vertical displacement. CT, which is routinely performed in trauma patients and provides detailed information about bony and visceral injuries, has increasingly supplanted radiography as the primary imaging tool for assessing patients with this type of injury.

Types of Fractures

The AO/ASIF system, based on the Tile classification system, provides information about the mechanism of

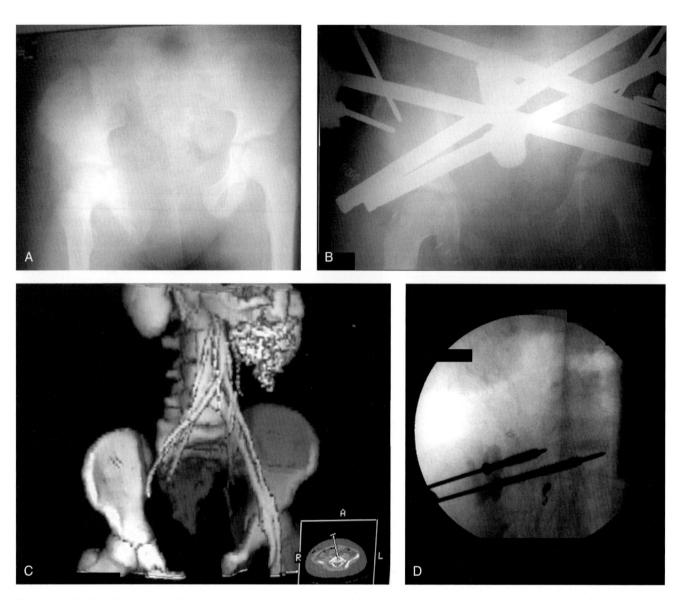

Figure 1 **A,** AP pelvis radiograph obtained in the emergency department of a 12-year-old boy who was struck by a car showing unstable displaced pubic diaphyseal disruption and a posterior sacroiliac joint injury. **B,** Radiograph showing a rare example of hemodynamic instability secondary to pelvic fracture that responded to emergent application of an external fixator. **C,** Subsequent CT scan of the same patient better delineates the fracture pattern and demonstrates disrupted external iliac vessels by the sacroiliac joint disruption. **D,** Arthroscopic view of the patient as he underwent angiographic embolization (note angiographic coils) and percutaneous sacroiliac joint fixation with screws 72 hours after injury.

injury. Type A injuries are stable fractures that include avulsions or isolated fractures of the iliac wing or pubic ramus. Type B fractures are caused by lateral compression and result in rotationally unstable injuries, including diastasis of the pubic symphysis (open book fractures). Lateral compression, often arising after a pedestrian is struck by a car, is the most common mechanism of pelvic injury in children. Type C injuries are related to vertical shear (caused by falls) and usually involve combined anterior (symphysis disruption or bilateral rami fractures) and posterior (disruption of the sacroiliac joint) injuries.

The fracture classification system of Torode and Zieg has been shown to be an accurate predictor of blood loss, associated injuries, and expected outcomes and is the most widely used system of classification for patients with pelvic injuries. Type I fractures are simple avulsion injuries. Type II fractures are fractures of the iliac wing, most often caused by a lateral compression force. Type III fractures are simple ring fractures (ramus or symphyseal disruption without other pelvic injuries) and are also relatively more common in children than in adults. Type IV injuries are unstable injuries that are the result of combined anterior and posterior injuries.

In contrast to adults, children can experience a single break to the pelvic ring. Although an isolated fracture to the pubic ring is stable, it is important to perform diagnostic imaging to assess patients for the presence of possible occult posterior injuries; moreover, pediatric patients should be thoroughly evaluated for an injury to the genitourinary system. Most pelvic injuries in children occur as a result of being struck by a car. Thus, lateral compression injuries are relatively more common in children and have a relatively high risk of concomitant head injury, but a lower risk of an open book fracture pattern with its associated risk of hemorrhage.

Treatment

The paucity of data describing long-term outcomes of pediatric patients with pelvic fractures has led to some controversy regarding the appropriate treatment of these uncommon but potentially devastating injuries. Generally speaking, bed rest and protected weight bearing can be used to treat patients with stable fractures. Greater controversy exists regarding the treatment of unstable fractures.

Long-term morbidity has been thought to be related to associated injuries, most notably head injury, rather than bony injury. Significantly high rates of psychiatric complaints and genitourinary problems have been reported in patients after pelvic fracture with no real disability attributable to pelvic ring disruption.

Traditionally, management of all but the most unstable fractures has been nonsurgical, based on the concept that remodeling will correct pelvic asymmetry over time. However, several reports of both adults and children have suggested that the quality of the reduction may in fact correlate with outcome. Bony asymmetry and malposition have been found to result in low back pain and functional impairment. In an attempt to improve anatomic reduction of the pediatric pelvis, treatment recommendations of pediatric pelvic fracture over the past decade have evolved toward more aggressive surgical treatment.

External fixation has been advocated as a means to decrease blood loss and control unstable fractures during the acute period and as a means of definitive treatment. In contrast to adults, urgent external fixation is rarely needed to control hemorrhage in pediatric patients with pelvic injuries, especially in those who present before triradiate closure has occurred. Although the appropriate indications for its use in children are still evolving, external fixation should be considered in patients with displaced open book injuries with more than 3.0 mm of diastasis, in those with open fractures, and in those with multiple trauma. External fixation is generally contraindicated in patients with unstable iliac wing fractures. In patients who will require laparotomy for abdominal injuries and those with associated posterior injuries, open reduction and internal fixation with a reconstruction plate allows anatomic reduction and can greatly simplify management.

Traction is sometimes used to control vertically unstable fractures. Traction can also be an appropriate technique to control the fracture pending more definitive treatment, which may be delayed for several days to fully stabilize and evaluate the patient. Either anterior plating or posterior compression screws can be used to stabilize a disrupted sacroiliac joint. Vertically unstable fractures that involve combined injuries to the anterior and posterior pelvis are rare in children, but recent studies have recommended a more aggressive approach using sacroiliac screws as in adult fractures. Acetabular fractures with more than 2 mm of displacement warrant reduction and fixation and may lead to early closure of the triradiate cartilage.

It is possible that discrepancies between historical and more recent long-term functional results in children with pediatric pelvic fracture reflect a greater proportion of children with high-energy, displaced fractures surviving initial evaluation and management. At the present time, treatment options for children with an unstable pelvic fracture should be considered on a patient-by-patient basis, with consideration given to the age of the child, the fracture pattern, and associated injuries.

Hip Fractures
Proximal Femur Fractures

As with pelvic fractures, hip fractures are nearly always the result of high-energy trauma, such as a motor vehicle accident or a fall from a height, placing children with these injuries at risk for multiple injuries. Associated injuries include head trauma, multiple fractures, and visceral injuries.

Children presenting with a hip fracture typically adopt a flexed, abducted, externally rotated posture. Intracapsular femoral neck fractures represent an orthopaedic emergency. Urgent, anatomic reduction is critical to restore blood flow to the femoral head that may have been disrupted by fracture displacement or occluded by fracture hematoma. Treatment of the hip fracture should be superseded only by treatment of life-threatening injuries or grossly contaminated open fractures.

The reason for this urgency is the high complication rate seen in skeletally immature patients with hip fractures, which is related to the high energy of the injury and to the unique vascular anatomy of the hip in the growing child. The metaphyseal branches of the medial and lateral circumflex arteries supply the proximal femur at birth, but they begin to decrease in importance as the proximal femoral physis develops. After the age of 4 years, the blood supply to the hip is derived almost entirely from the posterosuperior and posteroinferior retinacular branches of the medial circumflex artery. The femoral head is essentially an end organ supplied almost exclusively by the lateral epiphyseal vessels, making it susceptible to injury.

Types of Fractures

Femoral neck fractures are classified using the system developed by Delbet (Figure 2). The relative rarity of these injuries has made the development of a standard treatment protocol or algorithm difficult, but attempts to do so have been made based on the aggregate of information in the literature (Figure 3).

Diagnosis and Treatment

Type I fractures (transphyseal fractures) are the least common, accounting for less than 10% of all hip fractures. They also carry the highest morbidity of all hip fractures, frequently complicated by osteonecrosis and premature growth arrest. The diagnosis of this fracture is usually evident on AP and lateral radiographs of the hip (Figure 4), but a CT scan may provide more detailed information.

The type I fractures in particular should be reduced as quickly as possible to minimize the rate of osteonecrosis. Only one attempt at gentle closed reduction with traction and internal rotation is recommended; multiple attempts may increase the risk of osteonecrosis or premature physeal closure. When any concern exists about the quality of the reduction, the fracture site should be exposed through an anterior approach to visually confirm the reduction. A stable closed reduction may be obtained in children younger than 2 years, but there should be a low threshold for the use of internal fixation.

Approximately 50% of type I fractures are dislocated; along with otherwise irreducible type I fractures, dislocated type I fractures require open reduction. In general, the approach should be anterior, although when

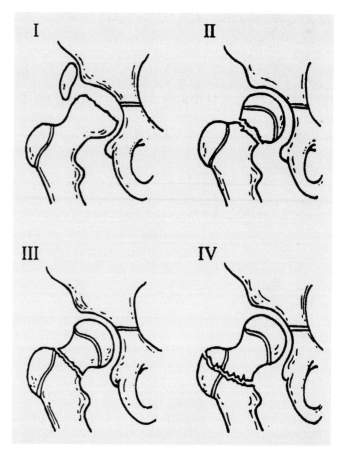

Figure 2 Schematic representation of the hip fracture classification system of Delbet for children. Type I is a transepiphyseal separation with or without dislocation of the femoral head from the acetabulum. Type II is a transcervical fracture. Type III is a cervicotrochanteric fracture. Type IV is an intertrochanteric fracture. *(Reproduced with permission from Hughes LO, Beaty JH: Fractures of the head and neck of the femur in children. J Bone Joint Surg Am 1994;76:283-292.)*

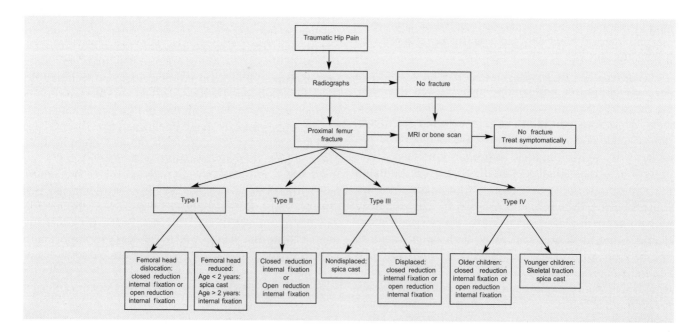

Figure 3 Algorithm for the treatment of pediatric hip fractures. *(Reproduced with permission from Shah AK, Eissler J, Radomisli T: Algorithms for the treatment of femoral neck fractures. Clin Orthop Relat Res 2002;399:28-34.)*

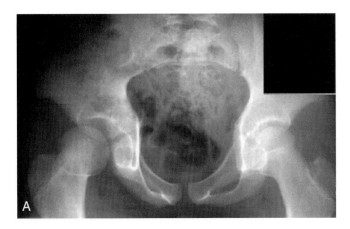
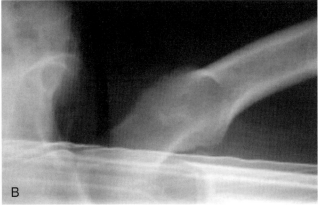

Figure 4 Standard AP **(A)** and lateral **(B)** radiographs of a posteriorly displaced type I transphyseal hip fracture. *(Reproduced with permission from Totterman A, Madsen JE, Naess CE, Roise O: Initially neglected tissue interposition after reduction of posterior hip dislocation in a child: A case report. Acta Orthop Scand 2004;75(2):221-224.)*

the femoral head is dislocated, the approach should be directed toward the side of the dislocation (an anterior approach for an anterior dislocation and a posterior approach for a posterior dislocation).

To obtain stable fixation in a patient with a transphyseal fracture, the physis needs to be crossed. The use of two or three smooth pins is recommended to reduce the risk of premature growth arrest in young children. However, there is general consensus that stable fixation should take priority over preservation of the physis. The stability of the reduction and the years of growth remaining should both be considered when determining the appropriate type of fixation. The proximal femoral physis contributes only 13% to 15% of the total length of the femur (about 3 to 4 mm/yr). Therefore, premature physeal closure in a child with as many as 8 years of growth remaining could result in a limb-length discrepancy of less than 1 inch, which is a manageable deficit and preferable to other complications such as malunion, nonunion, or osteonecrosis. Children younger than 10 years should be protected postoperatively with a one and one-half hip spica cast.

Delbet type II (transcervical) and type III (basocervical or cervicotrochanteric) fractures are the most common types of hip fractures in children. These two injuries differ primarily in their associated complication rates, with type II fractures having approximately twice the rate of osteonecrosis as type III fractures. The diagnosis is usually evident on routine radiographs (Figure 5). As with type I fractures, type II and type III fractures should be treated with an urgent reduction within 24 hours of injury.

Spica casting as a definitive treatment can be considered for nondisplaced type III fractures in children younger than 6 years. However, percutaneous internal fixation is preferable to reduce the risk of a varus malunion. All displaced type II and type III fractures that are amenable to a closed anatomic reduction

should be protected with percutaneous internal fixation. The importance of an anatomic reduction cannot be overstated. Cannulated screws or pins should pass from the metaphysis toward, but not across, the proximal femoral physis. If the growth plate must be crossed to provide adequate stability, a minimal number of smooth pins should be used to reduce the risk of a growth disturbance.

Fractures requiring open reduction are exposed through an anterior or anterolateral approach to minimize the risk of injury to the blood supply of the hip. To visualize the femoral neck, the joint capsule should be incised longitudinally away from the cervicotrochanteric line to avoid compromising the blood supply to the hip. Some current theories attribute declining rates of osteonecrosis to this arthrotomy, which is believed to increase blood flow by reducing intracapsular pressure from the fracture hematoma. The fracture is then anatomically reduced and fixed with cannulated screws that should not cross the physis. If transphyseal fixation is required for stability, smooth pins are recommended. Most type II and type III fractures are protected postoperatively with a spica cast. The exception would be the adolescent patient who is close to skeletal maturity in whom screw fixation across the physis is possible.

Delbet type IV fractures (intertrochanteric fractures) are extracapsular and have the most favorable prognosis of all hip fractures in children. They are typically diagnosed with plain radiographs (Figure 6). Because the blood supply to the proximal femur is preserved, the rate of osteonecrosis is low (less than 10%). Other complications include varus malunion and nonunion.

Children 6 years of age and younger with type IV fractures can usually be treated with closed reduction and spica casting. Casting can be immediate after closed reduction or after a period of skeletal traction. Percutaneous internal fixation with pins or screws is an option for older children after a closed reduction or for

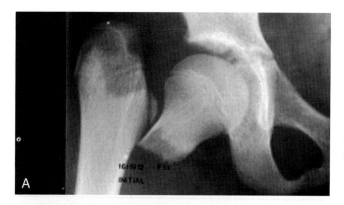

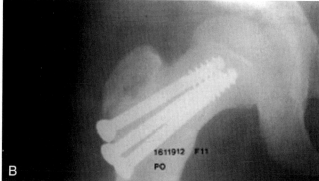

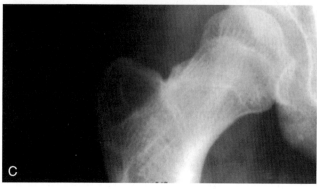

Figure 5 Initial **(A)**, 24-hour postoperative **(B)**, and 2-year postoperative **(C)** radiographs of an 11-year-old girl with a type III basocervical fracture that was treated with open reduction and internal fixation. *(Reproduced with permission from: Song KS, Kim YS, Sohn SW, Ogden JA: Arthrotomy and open reduction of the displaced fracture of the femoral neck in children. J Pediatr Orthop B 2001;10(3):205-210.)*

younger children when the reduction cannot be maintained with a spica cast. However, for large children or when a closed reduction is not possible, open reduction and internal fixation is necessary. The goal is anatomic reduction that will help reduce the rate of coxa vara postoperatively. A lateral approach usually provides adequate exposure for this procedure. A variety of pediatric-sized blade plates as well as screw and side plates can be used. Rigid internal fixation should also be a primary treatment option in polytrauma patients. Whichever implant is used, fixation should never cross the proximal femoral physis. When pins or screws are used, supplemental protection with a one and one-half spica cast or fracture brace (hip-knee-ankle-foot orthosis) should be strongly considered. The blade plate and screw and side plate do not usually require this supplemental reinforcement.

Complications

Osteonecrosis, the most frequent and devastating complication of hip fractures, is most common in patients with Delbet type I and II fractures. Osteonecrosis usually develops in the first 6 months, but it can develop as late as 2 years after injury. The exact incidence of osteonecrosis is difficult to pinpoint. Rates of osteonecrosis in patients with type II and type III fractures vary from 0 to more than 50%, whereas a rate of osteonecrosis in those with type I fractures has been reported to be as high as 100%. The factors that lead to the development of osteonecrosis include initial fracture displace-

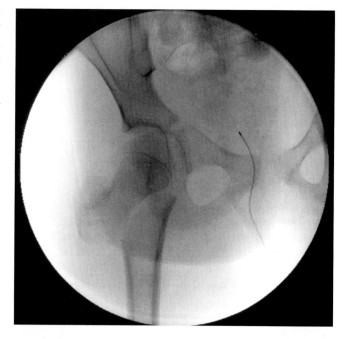

Figure 6 Fluoroscopic view of a type IV intertrochanteric hip fracture in 12-year-old boy. This fracture has a reverse obliquity pattern that is quite unusual in pediatric patients.

ment, time to reduction, and the quality of the reduction. Although the relative importance of these factors is still under debate, greater awareness of these issues appears to be contributing to the reduced rates of osteonecrosis reported in the recent literature. Most re-

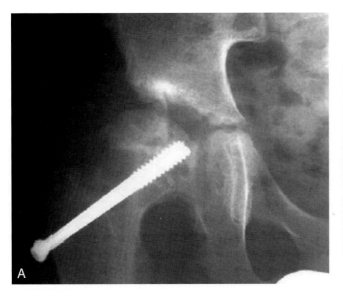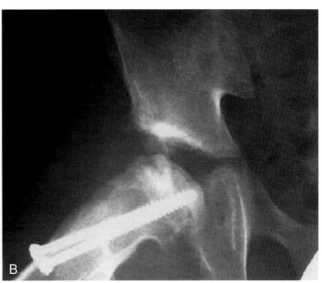

Figure 7 AP **(A)** and frog lateral **(B)** radiographs of the right hip of a patient obtained 11 months after open reduction and internal fixation of displaced type I fracture shows evidence of osteonecrosis. *(Reproduced with permission from Tsirikos AI, Shah SA, Riddle E, Stanton RP: Transphyseal fracture-dislocation of the femoral neck: A case report and review of the literature.* J Orthop Trauma 2003;17(9):648-653.)

cently, open arthrotomy for all displaced type II and type III fractures has been advocated to decompress the fracture hematoma. This may improve blood flow to the femoral head, and several studies have documented reduced rates of osteonecrosis using this technique.

Plain radiographs will typically document osteonecrosis as the weakened femoral head begins to collapse (Figure 7). The use of MRI or bone scintigraphy to detect early osteonecrosis has not yet been shown to be effective or practical; therefore, their routine use has not been recommended in this patient population.

The treatment of osteonecrosis is challenging. After the onset of osteonecrosis, the femoral head can rapidly collapse over a 6- to 12-month period. In the early stages, evidence suggests that no weight bearing for 1 year may help avoid severe collapse of the femoral head. Similarly, arthrodiastasis, in which a joint-spanning external fixator is used to reduce forces across the hip, has shown promising results in minimizing the sequelae of osteonecrosis in skeletally immature patients. Proximal femoral osteotomies have been used to direct intact portions of the femoral head into the weight-bearing zone. Because of limited experience using vascularized free-fibula grafting to treat osteonecrosis in skeletally immature patients, this technique is still considered experimental. Salvage procedures for patients with unremitting pain and stiffness include fusion and joint arthroplasty.

Deformity of the femoral neck as a result of malunion or growth disturbances (coxa vara and coxa valga) is the second most common complication, with an incidence of 20% to 30% of patients; however, reported incidences range widely from 10% to 50% of patients.

The patients at greatest risk include those with type II, type III, or type IV fractures with inadequate fixation, a nonanatomic reduction, or transphyseal fixation. Coxa vara is best prevented with an anatomic reduction and rigid fixation. Although spontaneous improvement can occur in the growing child, a subtrochanteric valgus osteotomy has been shown to be effective for children with a persistent deformity.

Nonunion and delayed union are associated complications in 5% to 10% of pediatric patients with hip fractures, although rates as high as 46% have been reported. Although nonunion and delayed union are most common in patients with displaced type II fractures, they can occur in all fracture types. The risk for nonunion and delayed union is greatest when an anatomic reduction is not achieved or when osteonecrosis develops. The traditional treatment consists of valgus intertrochanteric osteotomy with bone grafting. More recently, some success has been reported using free vascularized fibular grafts in skeletally immature patients.

Premature physeal closure occurs most frequently in pediatric patients with type I injuries, although it can occur in association with any intracapsular fracture, especially in patients with osteonecrosis or with implants crossing the growth plate. This complication, associated with osteonecrosis and transphyseal fixation, has been reported to range from 5% to 65% of patients. Anatomic reductions and avoidance of the physis seem to minimize the risk. When a growth disturbance causes a clinically significant limb-length inequality, it can often be treated with a contralateral epiphysiodesis. When clinically significant trochanteric overgrowth occurs, it can be treated with epiphysiodesis or advancement of the greater trochanter. Other reported complications include sciatic nerve injury, chondrolysis, and heterotopic ossification, especially in children with a closed head injury.

Proximal Femoral Epiphysiolysis

Separation of the femoral head from the femoral neck can occur in the infant. This injury is analogous to Delbet type I hip fractures, but it has a much better prognosis in the newborn infant than in the older child. This injury can complicate a difficult vaginal delivery and has been described as a complication of closed reduction of a congenitally dislocated hip. Children with this injury typically present with pseudoparalysis of the leg; therefore, a septic hip should be ruled out. Although plain radiographs may not be diagnostically useful in this patient population because the femoral head is not yet ossified, ultrasonography or arthrography can help make a diagnosis.

When the diagnosis is made early, the fracture usually can be reduced with gentle skin traction. If the diagnosis is delayed and fracture healing has already begun, observation is indicated. The remodeling potential is tremendous in newborn patients, and outcomes are favorable provided physeal growth arrest does not occur.

Stress Fractures of the Proximal Femur

Stress fractures of the hip have rarely been reported in skeletally immature patients, but the incidence of such fractures seems to be increasing. Pediatric patients with stress fractures of the proximal femur usually present with groin pain and often provide a history of a recent significant increase in activity, such as running. The diagnosis of this injury can be challenging because radiographs are often normal. Although technetium bone scanning will usually demonstrate evidence of a lesion, it is nonspecific; consequently, it can be difficult to differentiate a stress fracture of the proximal femur from an early slipped capital femoral epiphysis or to tell which side of the femoral neck the fracture is on. MRI may be the most useful diagnostic imaging modality to help confirm the diagnosis and provide anatomic information on the location of the fracture (Figure 8). As with adults, these are most commonly found on the compression (inferior) side of the femoral neck in pediatric patients, and they can usually be treated by limiting weight bearing and activity restriction. However, tension-sided fractures have been described in skeletally immature adolescents, which have been treated with percutaneous cannulated screws placed up the femoral neck up to but not beyond the proximal femoral physis.

Traumatic Hip Dislocation

As with hip and pelvic fractures, hip dislocations are rare in the pediatric population; only 5% of all trau-

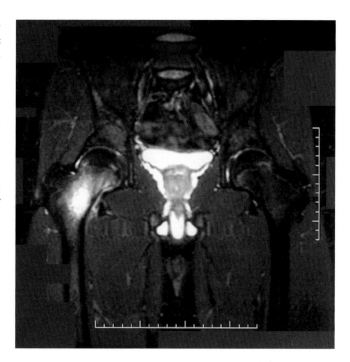

Figure 8 T2-weighted MRI scan of a femoral neck stress fracture. *(Reproduced with permission from Lehman RA Jr, Shah SA: Tension-sided femoral neck stress fracture in a skeletally immature patient: A case report. J Bone Joint Surg Am 2004;86-A(6): 1292-1295.)*

matic hip dislocations occur in patients younger than 14 years. Males account for approximately two thirds to three fourths of all patients with traumatic hip dislocation, and more than 99% of these dislocations are unilateral. Interestingly, the mechanism of injury for hip dislocations is classified as low energy in approximately two thirds of patients. This seems to be particularly true for young children. For example, hip dislocations frequently occur as the result of sports injuries or falls from relatively low heights. Children entering adolescence more closely resemble adults, however, in that higher energies are required to dislocate the hip.

Types of Hip Dislocations

The diagnosis of hip dislocations is usually suggested by the history and initial presentation. Patients with posterior dislocations, which account for approximately 90% to 95% of all dislocations, typically present with the leg flexed, adducted, and internally rotated. Anteriorly dislocated hips are extended, abducted, and externally rotated. Obturator dislocations are characterized by wide abduction of the hip. The diagnosis is usually obvious based on the clinical presentation and radiographs. When the diagnosis is questionable or if there is a possibility of an ipsilateral pelvic injury, CT can be helpful. Some patients present with normal radiographs and a history consistent with a hip dislocation or subluxation. Hip dislocations can spontaneously reduce, but there are many reports of soft-tissue interposition in these patients. There must be a high index of suspicion and a critical evaluation of the radiographs to confirm whether a concentric reduction exists. If there is any doubt, CT or MRI can be helpful to better visualize the joint.

A traumatic hip dislocation should not be confused with a habitual hip dislocation. Children with this rare disorder usually present between the ages of 3 and 6 years with an atraumatic, painless posterior hip dislocation that may be voluntary. Associated factors include generalized ligamentous laxity, osteocartilaginous defects or deformation of the posterior acetabulum, excessive femoral anteversion, and psychiatric problems. The dislocations usually cease spontaneously with observation or psychiatric counseling when indicated. If the dislocations persist for more than 3 years or if they become involuntary and painful, surgical stabilization may be indicated.

Treatment

Traumatic hip dislocations must be treated as a true emergency. Reduction within the first 6 hours seems critical to minimize the risk of osteonecrosis. Most pediatric patients with traumatic hip dislocation can be treated with closed reduction in the emergency department under intravenous sedation. If this attempt fails, closed reduction should be reattempted in the operating room with the patient under general anesthesia. Postreduction radiographs should be critically assessed for joint symmetry because soft-tissue interposition can lead to an eccentric reduction (Figure 9). However, it is important to distinguish interposed tissue from a hematoma, which can cause an increase in the apparent joint space but does not need to be treated. CT or MRI can help clarify the clinical picture when uncertainty exists.

Open reduction is indicated when closed reduction fails after two or three attempts or when there is soft-tissue or bony fragment interposition between the femoral head and acetabulum. CT is sensitive in detecting subtle widening and finding small bone fragments that may be difficult if not impossible to detect using routine radiography. The surgical approach to the hip should be on the side of the dislocation; an anterior approach for anterior dislocations and a posterior approach for posterior dislocations should be used. The acetabulum should be cleared of debris, and the capsular tear should be repaired once the hip is reduced. When osteochondral fractures occur in children, small fragments can be excised, but larger fragments should be repaired. It can be a challenge to obtain stable fixation of these articular fractures while keeping hardware out of the joint space. Options for fixation include headless screws sunk to the subchondral bone or headed screws in a nonarticular

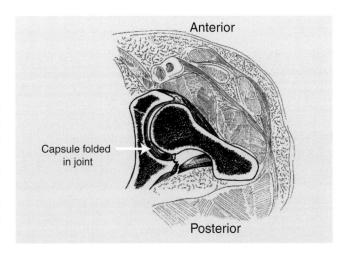

Figure 9 Schematic representation of soft-tissue interposition that can lead to a nonconcentric reduction of a hip dislocation. *(Reproduced with permission from Price CT, Pyevich MT, Knapp DR, Phillips JH, Hawker JJ: Traumatic hip dislocation with spontaneous incomplete reduction: a diagnostic trap. J Orthop Trauma 2002;16(10):730-735.)*

portion of the proximal femur that lag the fragment down to the head.

There is considerable variety in methods of postreduction care. Children younger than 10 years are generally placed in a spica cast to allow the soft tissues to heal for a period of 3 to 6 weeks. Older children are typically prescribed bed rest or instructed not to bear weight for 2 to 3 weeks followed by another 3 weeks of protected weight bearing.

Complications

Osteonecrosis usually occurs within the first year and should be monitored with serial radiographs. Bone scintigraphy has not been shown to be helpful in assessing this patient population and is therefore not recommended as a routine diagnostic study. The incidence of osteonecrosis has been reported to be between 5% and 58% of patients, but it is probably between 5% to 15% of patients. The incidence increases by as much as 20-fold if the time from injury to reduction is greater than 6 hours. Tension on the posterior blood vessels supplying the head almost certainly is the cause of this complication. Evacuation of the intracapsular hematoma has not been shown to change the rate of osteonecrosis as has been reported to occur in patients with intracapsular hip fractures.

Sciatic nerve palsies complicate approximately 5% of pediatric hip dislocations and have a fair prognosis; 60% to 70% of patients can expect full to partial recovery of nerve function. Reported indications for nerve exploration range from immediate exploration and neurolysis to waiting a few weeks or a few months or never exploring the nerve. Other reported complications include coxa magna, heterotopic ossification, and recurrent dislocations.

Summary

Although relatively uncommon, fractures of the hip and pelvis in children require prompt diagnosis and appropriate treatment that acknowledge the unique anatomic and physiologic aspects of children. Outcomes after pelvic fracture are more commonly related to concomitant injury, including head trauma. Although treatment of the pelvic ring disruption has historically allowed for remodeling, recent reports suggest that more anatomic reduction may in fact be warranted, especially in somewhat older children after the closure of the triradiate cartilage. Outcomes and treatment of hip fracture are determined by the proximity of the fracture to the growth plate. Unfortunately, even with appropriate and prompt treatment, complications after hip fracture, including osteonecrosis, nonunion, and malunion, are not uncommon.

Annotated Bibliography

Fractures of the Pelvis

Karunakar MA, Goulet JA, Mueller KL, Bedi A, Le TT: Operative treatment of unstable pediatric pelvis and acetabular fractures. *J Pediatr Orthop* 2005;25:34-38.

This report demonstrates satisfactory outcomes following open reduction and internal fixation of 18 children with unstable pelvic fractures. The authors advocate for a more surgical approach to the treatment of pelvic asymmetry and periarticular congruity in children.

Silber JS, Flynn JM: Changing patterns of pediatric pelvic fractures with skeletal maturation: Implications for classification and management. *J Pediatr Orthop* 2002; 22:22-26.

In a retrospective review of 166 children with pelvic fracture, the authors noted that closure of the triradiate cartilage differentiates between adult and pediatric fracture types. Although patients with open triradiate cartilage demonstrated associated injuries, all patients requiring open reduction and internal fixation had closed physes.

Smith WR, Oakley M, Morgan SJ: Pediatric pelvic fractures. *J Pediatr Orthop* 2004;24:130-135.

This comprehensive review summarizes the controversy surrounding the appropriate indications for surgical treatment of pediatric pelvic fractures. The authors conclude that surgical treatment is appropriate for a subset of patients with unstable fractures.

Hip Fractures

Lehman RA Jr, Shah SA: Tension-sided femoral neck stress fracture in a skeletally immature patient: A case report. *J Bone Joint Surg Am* 2004;86-A:1292-1295.

This is the first case reported in the English literature of a tension-sided femoral neck stress fracture in a skeletally immature patient. The authors discuss the diagnostic workup and

suggest that MRI may be the best diagnostic imaging tool for this injury.

Maeda S, Kita A, Fujii G, Funayama K, Yamada N, Kokubun S: Avascular necrosis associated with fractures of the femoral neck in children: Histological evaluation of core biopsies of the femoral head. *Injury* 2003;34:283-286.

The authors obtained core biopsies in patients with osteonecrosis after experiencing femoral neck fractures. Only biopsies obtained more than 1 year after the onset of osteonecrosis demonstrated any healing. The authors recommend at least 1 year of not bearing weight to minimize femoral head collapse.

Morsy HA: Complications of fracture of the neck of the femur in children: A long-term follow-up study. *Injury* 2001;32:45-51.

The authors of this retrospective study followed 53 pediatric femoral neck fractures for an average of 9.4 years. They found that the onset of osteonecrosis correlated with greater initial fracture displacement and with the quality of the surgical reduction. Growth arrest was closely correlated to the onset of osteonecrosis.

Song KS, Kim YS, Sohn SW, Ogden JA: Arthrotomy and open reduction of the displaced fracture of the femoral neck in children. *J Pediatr Orthop B* 2001;10:205-210.

The authors of this retrospective review of intracapsular femoral neck fractures in children followed 13 children (average follow-up, 2.7 years) who were treated with anatomic open reduction, internal fixation, and decompression of the fracture hematoma. They reported no instances of osteonecrosis, coxa vara, nonunion, or growth arrest.

Stress Fractures of the Proximal Femur

Maezawa K, Nozawa M, Sugimoto M, Sano M, Shitoto K, Kurosawa H: Stress fractures of the femoral neck in child with open capital femoral epiphysis. *J Pediatr Orthop B* 2004;13:407-411.

Stress fractures of the femoral neck in pediatric patients are rare. This report presents two such instances and summarizes the reported literature, which contains 11 reports of such fractures. In all patients, the fracture healed with conservative therapy.

Traumatic Hip Dislocation

Song KS, Choi IH, Sohn YJ, Shin HD, Leem HS: Habitual dislocation of the hip in children: Report of eight additional cases and literature review. *J Pediatr Orthop* 2003;23:178-183.

The authors of this article reviewed the rare diagnosis of habitual dislocation of the hip and in so doing increased the total number of described instances by 50%. They recommended a conservative approach to all patients with habitual dislocation of the hip and suggested that surgical stabilization should be reserved for patients whose dislocation of the hip persists for 3 or more years or those who develop involuntary, painful dislocations.

Classic Bibliography

Barquet A: Natural history of avascular necrosis following traumatic hip-dislocation in childhood: A review of 145 cases. *Acta Orthop Scand* 1982;53:815-820.

Blasier RD, McAtee J, White R, Mitchell DT: Disruption of the pelvic ring in pediatric patients. *Clin Orthop Relat Res* 2000;376:87-95.

Forlin E, Guille JT, Kumar SJ, Rhee KJ: Complications associated with fracture of the neck of the femur in children. *J Pediatr Orthop* 1992;12:503-509.

Forlin E, Guille JT, Kumar SJ, Rhee KJ: Transepiphyseal fractures of the neck of the femur in very young children. *J Pediatr Orthop* 1992;12:164-168.

Hamilton P, Broughton NS: Traumatic hip dislocation in childhood. *J Pediatr Orthop* 1998;18:691-694.

Hughes LO, Beaty JH: Fractures of the head and neck of the femur in children. *J Bone Joint Surg Am* 1994;76: 283-292.

Mehlman CT, Hubbard GW, Crawford AH, Roy DR, Wall EJ: Traumatic hip dislocation in children: Long-term followup of 42 patients. *Clin Orthop Relat Res* 2000;376:68-79.

Rieger H, Brug E: Fractures of the pelvis in children. *Clin Orthop Relat Res* 1997;336:226-239.

Schwarz N, Posch E, Mayr J, Fischmeister FM, Schwarz AF, Ohner T: Long-term results of unstable pelvic ring fractures in children. *Injury* 1998;29:431-433.

Torode I, Zieg D: Pelvic fractures in children. *J Pediatr Orthop* 1985;5:76-84.

Chapter 21

Pediatric Fractures of the Femur

John M. Flynn, MD

Pediatric Diaphyseal Femoral Fractures

Pediatric fractures of the femoral shaft are relatively common injuries that usually occur as a result of high-energy impact trauma, such as a child being struck by a car, or low-energy playground trauma, usually in toddlers. For children younger than 1 year, 40% of femoral diaphyseal fractures are a result of nonaccidental injury. If a child who is not yet walking presents with a femoral fracture, orthopaedists should be highly suspicious of a nonaccidental injury and enlist the assistance of experts in this area.

A variety of treatment options exist for pediatric femoral shaft fractures: spica casting, traction followed by spica casting, external fixation, flexible intramedullary nailing, rigid intramedullary nailing, and compression plate fixation (Figure 1). The choice of treatment depends on many different factors, the most important of which are age of the patient, location and fracture pattern, and experience of the surgeon with the proposed treatment method.

Treatment Options

Casting

Casting is an ideal method for managing femoral shaft fractures in infants and toddlers because angulation and shortening remodels extensively in this patient population. For infants up to 6 months of age, the Pavlik harness (sometimes supplemented with a simple splint) is used for the treatment of proximal and middle-third shaft fractures; this device obviates skin problems usually associated with spica casting. In a recent study, the clinical and radiographic outcomes of 24 patients treated in a Pavlik harness were compared with 16 patients treated in a spica cast. The average age and weight of the two groups were significantly different, but there were no differences in radiographic outcomes between the Pavlik and spica cast groups. Approximately one third of all spica cast patients had skin complications that contributed additional risk. There were no similar complications in the Pavlik harness group. There were no differences in the outcome of the frac-

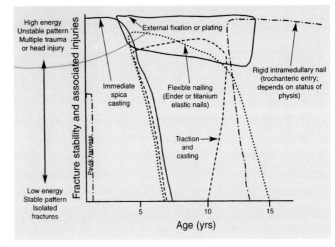

Figure 1 Schematic representation of treatment options for pediatric femoral fractures based on type of injury and patient age. *(Reproduced from Flynn JM, Schwend RM: Management of pediatric femoral shaft fractures. J Am Acad Orthop Surg 2004; 12:347-359.)*

tures in the two groups. The authors concluded that all children younger than 1 year with femoral shaft fractures are candidates for treatment with a Pavlik harness.

For children between the ages of 1 and 6 years, early spica casting is recommended for all but the most unstable, high-energy fractures. Only in rare circumstances is internal fixation recommended for children younger than 6 years. For children 2 to 10 years of age, acceptable fracture alignment at union is ≤ 15° of varus or valgus, ≤ 20° of anterior or posterior angulation, and ≤ 30° of malrotation.

If the cast is not applied immediately after an injury, a few days of traction or splinting can be used before spica cast application. Although simple, low-energy fractures can be casted with the patient under conscious sedation, reduction and casting in the operating room with the patient under general anesthesia provides several advantages. Examination under anesthesia is useful to determine fracture stability. Fluoroscopic evaluation of the fracture can allow adjustments before the cast has hardened. Casting should be done with the hip and knee

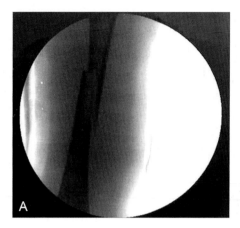

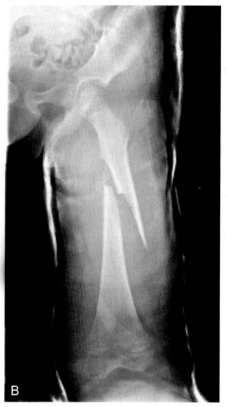

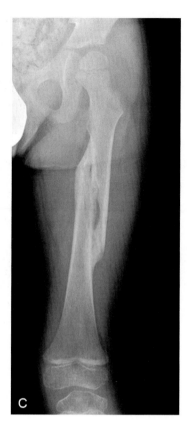

Figure 2 **A,** Fluoroscopic image obtained immediately after reduction and spica casting of a proximal third femoral shaft fracture in a 5-year-old boy. There is near-anatomic alignment. **B,** Radiograph of the same patient obtained 10 days postoperatively. The femur is in 15° of varus. The surgeon wedged the cast to correct angulation and shortening and to prevent further displacement. **C,** Radiograph obtained at the time of cast removal, 6 weeks after injury, shows that the fracture is healed and in satisfactory alignment. The child's injured femur was 1 cm shorter; this amount of shortening typically corrects with overgrowth in the first year after injury.

each flexed to 90°. A Gortex liner (W.L. Gore and Associates, Flagstaff, AZ), although expensive, may decrease skin problems. After a folded sheet is temporarily placed over the entire abdomen, the cast is applied in sections. First, a long leg cast is applied to the injured side. Then, with the child securely on the spica table, the fracture is reduced, a valgus mold is applied at the fracture, and the rest of the cast is applied up to the nipple line. The surgeon should not apply excessive force to the posterior calf or the popliteal area because this contributes to compartment syndrome of the leg, which has recently been reported to occur after spica cast application. Reinforcing the cast with splints in either the anterior or posterior groin crease may obviate the need for a bar and allow parents to carry the child close. Follow-up radiographs should be obtained within the first 10 days (Figure 2).

A reclining wheelchair with elevated leg rests facilitates mobility in the cast, and a beanbag on the floor provides for secure and comfortable sitting. When mature callus is present, the cast can be removed, typically in 6 to 8 weeks. For most children, no special therapy is needed after cast removal. A limp may be apparent for several months, so the patient's family should be forewarned.

Traction Followed by Casting

Traction followed by casting is a traditional method that is preferred for the treatment of femoral shaft fractures in children older than 6 years or children with high-energy fractures in whom surgical procedures are not appropriate. Traction is also indicated in patients in whom there is a high risk of unacceptable shortening with immediate casting, as in patients with many comminuted fractures. The telescope test is recommended to evaluate this risk. In this test, if the patient's leg shows 3 cm or more of shortening with gentle force, there is a much greater chance of unacceptable shortening. Relative contraindications to traction and casting include obesity, multiple trauma, significant head injury, floating knee injury, and distal fractures that compromise traction pin placement. The traction pin is placed in the distal femur, generally with the patient under conscious sedation or general anesthesia. The largest threaded Steinmann pin is drilled medially to laterally, its position is confirmed radiographically, any areas of tented skin are released, and the child is placed in 90/90 traction (90° of hip flexion and 90° of knee flexion). Radiographs in traction are obtained periodically to ensure that the fracture is out to length and in satisfactory alignment. When radiographs show callus and there is no tenderness at the fracture site (typically in 17 to 21 days), the pin is removed and a spica cast is applied.

External Fixation

External fixation can be thought of as a form of portable traction for pediatric femoral fractures. This treatment method has often been used to manage open frac-

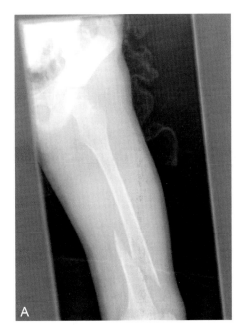
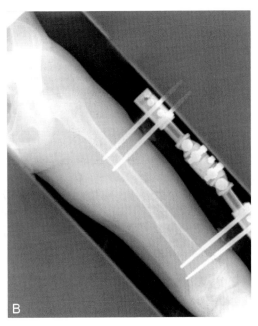

Figure 3 **A,** Preoperative AP radiograph of a distal, short oblique fracture through a nonossifying fibroma in a 9-year-old boy. Fixation can be compromised in such fractures treated with flexible nailing. The surgeon chose to use an external fixation as "portable traction." **B,** Postoperative AP radiograph of the same patient shows anatomic alignment and no shortening. The fixator was used for 6 weeks; after fixator removal, the patient was placed in a long leg cast with a pelvic band and allowed to bear weight as tolerated until union was complete and the fixator pin holes had filled in.

tures, fractures associated with severe soft-tissue injury, patients with head or vascular injuries, or patients with complex fracture patterns that are less amenable to flexible intramedullary nailing. Such fractures include subtrochanteric fractures and fractures of the distal diaphyseal-metaphyseal junction, where the proximity of the fracture to the insertion site for the intramedullary nail makes nailing technically difficult and nail fixation less reliable (Figure 3).

The benefits of external fixation include the avoidance of long incisions, exposure of the fracture site, and significant blood loss as well as minimization of the risk of physeal injury or osteonecrosis. However, complications associated with external fixation have been discouraging for many surgeons and families, particularly delayed union and refracture after the removal of the device resulting from unsatisfactory development of the fracture callus. Both dynamic and static fixation devices have been used in correcting femoral fractures in children, but a recent study demonstrated that no significant difference in time to healing and frequency of complications exists between the two methods. Four 4- or 5-mm pins are sufficient to achieve stability in children, and compared with longitudinal incisions, transverse skin incisions for pin insertion lessen scarring and soft-tissue irritation. Patients are typically allowed unrestricted weight bearing and may simply use soap and water for pin site care.

Flexible Nail Fixation
Flexible intramedullary nailing has gained widespread popularity in the past decade for treating pediatric femoral fractures, and it has replaced external fixation and spica casting as the preferred method of treatment of

most femoral fractures in school-aged children. Flexible intramedullary nails are ideal for skeletally immature children older than 5 years with transverse fractures in the middle 60% of the femoral diaphysis. For more proximal or distal fractures, and fractures with comminution or spiral patterns, flexible intramedullary nail fixation may be more tenuous; supplemental immobilization, perhaps using a single-leg walking spica cast for 4 to 6 weeks may be helpful in maintaining reduction in some patients.

Flexible intramedullary nailing offers several benefits over other surgical methods used to treat pediatric femoral fractures. Flexible intramedullary nailing is load-sharing fixation that does not disturb the fracture hematoma or periosteal blood supply. Motion at the fracture site leads to abundant external callus. With flexible intramedullary nailing, children usually have short hospital stays, good early knee motion, rapid mobilization on crutches, and low risk of malunion or refracture. Two studies compared flexible intramedullary nailing with other treatment methods, and one such study found it to be more effective than external fixation. A recent prospective trial showed that recovery milestones were reached sooner and with a lower complication rate with flexible intramedullary nailing than with traditional traction and casting. The most commonly reported complication from titanium elastic nailing is tissue irritation by the extraosseous portion of the nail tip at the insertion site. Refracture has also been reported after premature intramedullary nail removal. As flexible intramedullary nailing has become more popular, surgeons have tested the limits of the device, finding that titanium elastic nails can sometimes lead to angular or axial deformity, particularly in oblique, spiral, and comminuted femoral fractures, and in bigger, older children and adolescents. A recent study reported a relationship between the prominence of the titanium elastic nails and pain at the nail tip or skin erosion. Of 43 femoral fractures, two major complications occurred: one instance of septic arthritis after nail removal and one instance of hypertrophic nonunion. The authors concluded that fracture angulation and outcome were associated with the weight of the patient and the size of the intramedullary nails implanted. They recommended leaving less than 2.5 cm of the intramedullary nail out of the femur and using the largest intramedullary nail sizes possible.

Two types of intramedullary nails are commonly used for intramedullary fixation: stainless steel Ender nails and titanium elastic nails. The stainless steel Ender nails are stiffer than titanium nails, and their stability is based on the bend placed in the nail as well as on the stacking of the nails to increase the canal fill. Stacking is not part of the classic titanium nail technique as described by the French innovators. Instead, the elastic nail technique involves balancing the forces of two opposing implants. For both titanium and Ender nails, the entry site, nail size, and nail length should be symmetric.

Preoperative planning for titanium elastic nailing includes measuring the narrowest diameter of the femoral canal and multiplying by 0.4 to determine nail size; for example, if the minimum canal diameter is 10 mm, two 4.0-mm nails are used. In the standard technique, the nails should enter the bone about 2.5 cm proximal to the distal femoral physis. An incision is made from this point and extends distally approximately 2 to 3 cm. Great care should be taken to avoid any deep dissection in the area of the distal femoral physis. An appropriately sized drill (such as a 4.5-mm drill for the 4.0-mm nails) is used to broach the cortex of the femur at the same distance from the physis on the medial and lateral sides. The drill should be angled obliquely within the medullary canal and aimed proximally to create a sharply angled distal-to-proximal track for the nail to follow. Nails are then bent with a gentle contour such that the apex of the convexity will be at the level of the fracture. Both nails are tapped up to the fracture site. The nail that will improve the alignment is advanced across the fracture site and into the proximal fragment. Often, it is helpful to rotate the nail tip up to 180° to facilitate passage. The second nail is then passed into the proximal fragment. The nails are then tapped distal to proximal until the nail that entered laterally has its distal tip at the level of the greater trochanteric apophysis, and the nail that entered medially has its tip at the same level near the medial femoral neck. When the nail has reached its final position, each nail is backed out slightly, cut at the skin, and then tapped back in so that only 1 cm to 1.5 cm of nail lies in the soft tissues. The nail can be bent slightly away from the femur to facilitate later removal, but it should not be sharply bent because this will cause soft-tissue irritation. Postoperative

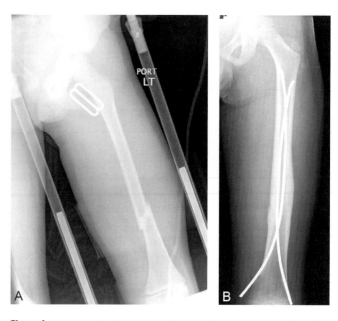

Figure 4 **A,** Preoperative AP radiograph of a femoral fracture in a 9-year-old boy. This short oblique fracture at the junction of the middle and distal thirds of the femur can be managed with flexible intramedullary nails. **B,** AP radiograph obtained 7 months after fixation with titanium elastic nails shows a healed fracture in perfect alignment. Ideally, the proximal end of the intramedullary nails should extend to the intertrochanteric metaphyseal bone to ensure optimal fixation.

immobilization is based on the fracture pattern. In patients with stable, transverse fractures, a knee immobilizer is used for 6 weeks with partial weight bearing. Immobilization is stopped once callus is noted at the fracture site (in 4 to 6 weeks in most patients). Nail removal is done once the fracture line is no longer visible—usually 4 to 12 months after injury (Figure 4).

Alternatively, the Ender nail technique uses either proximal or distal starting points; the nails are bent in either a C or an S shape to gain cortical contact at the fracture site. A third nail is added if more canal fill is needed for stability. The eyelet near the end of an Ender nail can be used to secure the nail to the femur with a screw; however, nail backout is rare because pediatric metaphyseal bone is dense, so screw fixation is not generally used.

Either titanium elastic nails or stainless steel Ender nails can be inserted in an anterograde fashion. The advantages of proximal entry include elimination of knee irritation from the nail tip (the most common complaint in children treated with the retrograde technique) and better stability for certain fracture patterns. A disadvantage of proximal entry is the lack of a safe medial and lateral starting point, resulting in unbalanced, asymmetric implants. Also, nail removal sometimes leaves a stress riser in the proximal femur, which is a more difficult area to protect. The transtrochanteric approach eliminates the concern about a stress riser but introduces the possibility of trochanteric apophyseal damage, which might lead to coxa valga (Figure 5).

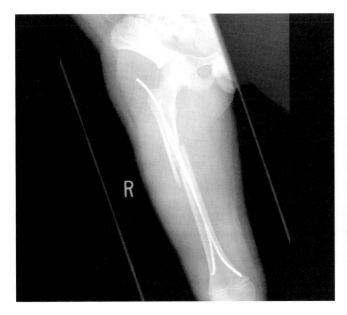

Figure 5 AP radiograph of a long oblique proximal femoral fracture that was managed with an anterograde transtrochanteric titanium elastic nail and a retrograde nail through the distal medial metaphysis. This technique allows the surgeon to get good spread of the nails at the fracture site and good fixation on both fragments.

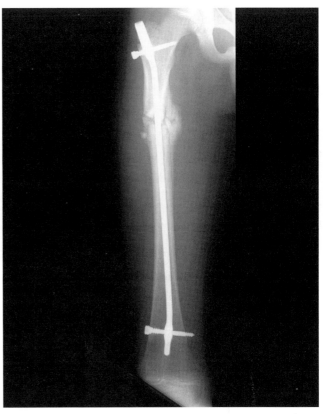

Figure 6 AP radiograph of a proximal third femoral fracture that was managed with a new small-diameter interlocking nail designed for anterograde insertion. *(Courtesy of Jonathan Philips, MD.)*

When fixation is complete, traction is released and the fracture can be gently impacted through manipulation so that it is not fixed in distraction. Normal rotation should be ensured before the patient leaves the operating room. Postoperative immobilization is based on the fracture pattern. For patients with stable transverse fractures, a knee immobilizer may be used with partial weight bearing. Immobilization is stopped when callus is noted at the fracture site, usually in 4 to 6 weeks.

Rigid Intramedullary Nail Fixation

Rigid intramedullary nail fixation is the treatment of choice for displaced femoral shaft fractures in skeletally mature adolescents. Positive results have been reported with its use. Several studies extend the indications for this method to children with open proximal femoral physes, but this use of rigid nailing remains controversial. The benefits of rigid intramedullary nail fixation are clear from the successful results of its use: rigid intramedullary rods prevent problems with angular malalignment and limb-length discrepancy. They also offer increased stability of the leg and rapid mobilization.

The major reported complication associated with the use of rigid intramedullary nailing is osteonecrosis of the capital femoral epiphysis. Insertion of rigid intramedullary nails through the piriformis fossa disrupts the lateral ascending cervical branches of the medial circumflex artery, which serve as the blood supply to the head of the femur. There is also a documented potential for trochanteric growth arrest with subsequent coxa valga when this method is used in children who are not skeletally mature. Using the greater trochanter as the

nail entry site instead of the piriformis fossa can avoid femoral head osteonecrosis, but intraoperative trochanteric fracture and varus deformity at the fracture site can occur. Furthermore, growth disturbance of the proximal femur is known to occur from rigid nailing through both the piriformis fossa and the greater trochanter. To avoid these problems, several centers are exploring innovative rigid nail designs and techniques (Figure 6).

A recent series reported the outcomes of 15 children and adolescents with displaced femoral diaphyseal fractures and open physes stabilized who were treated using a modified humeral intramedullary nail placed through the lateral aspect of the greater trochanter. At a minimum follow-up of 16 months, no patient had developed osteonecrosis, femoral neck valgus, femoral neck narrowing, or other complications.

Plate Compression

Traditional plate compression, which was popular at some centers in the past, is used much less frequently now that flexible nailing has become the most effective treatment for most femoral fractures in school-age children. Traditional plating indications included children younger than 12 years with multiple trauma, open fractures, head injuries, or compartment syndrome. Plate fixation has also

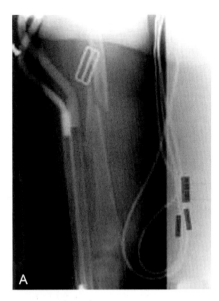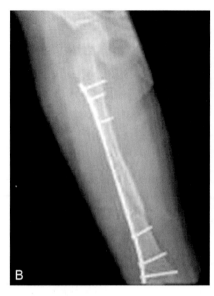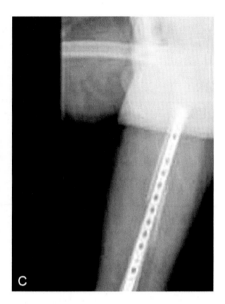

Figure 7 **A,** Radiograph of a comminuted femoral shaft fracture in a 10-year-old boy. The surgeon chose the submuscular bridge plating technique for repair of this difficult length-unstable fracture. Postoperative AP **(B)** and lateral **(C)** radiographs of the same patient after submuscular bridge plating. The fracture is out to length, and there is more early callous than would be expected using traditional fully open plating techniques (in which instance the fracture site would be exposed and fragments stripped, thereby compromising vascularity and healing). *(Courtesy of Ernest Sink, MD.)*

been used for proximal (subtrochanteric area) or distal (near the diaphyseal metaphyseal junction) fractures. Traditional plating of femoral fractures provides excellent stability and bone alignment at the fracture site, but there has been a high incidence of hardware failure and a nonunion rate approaching 10% in one study.

Submuscular bridge plating has also become popular in some centers. This technique uses longer plates with fewer screws, percutaneous plate placement with indirect reduction, and less soft-tissue stripping. No cast, brace, or traction is necessary after surgery. Six to 12 weeks of protected weight bearing after surgery is recommended. A prospective study on this method showed a 4% rate of significant complications, including the fracture of one 3.5-mm plate and the refracture of a pathologic fracture after early plate removal. Malrotation and limb-length discrepancy were minimal. The published results of larger series will likely establish the role of submuscular plating in the management of pediatric femoral fractures (Figure 7).

Pediatric Subtrochanteric Femoral Fractures

Fractures of the subtrochanteric femur are particularly difficult to manage. As in adults, the proximal fragment is flexed, abducted, and externally rotated and the cortical bone is not as vascularized and, thus, heals more slowly than metaphyseal bone. In addition, the proximal femoral physis in children may limit proximal fixation, and the medullary canal can be narrow proximally, precluding the use of devices used to treat similar fractures in adults. Treatment techniques for pediatric subtrochanteric femoral fractures vary depending on the type

and severity of the fracture, but in general nonsurgical techniques are associated with high nonunion, delayed union, and malunion rates.

Flexible intramedullary nails can be used successfully to treat these fractures. The technique can be modified by using one proximal and one distal entry site. If there is sufficient room for two pins in the proximal fragment, external fixation can be used as a form of portable traction, in which instance the device is left in place until callus is formed; it is subsequently removed and a single-leg spica cast is applied until the external fixator pin holes have filled in and fracture healing is complete. Some fractures are so proximal that the best or only treatment option is screw and side-plate fixation (Figure 8).

Pediatric Supracondylar Femoral Fractures

Supracondylar fractures represent approximately 12% of femoral fractures in children. Traditional traction and casting is a challenge because of the deforming force of the gastrocnemius and adductor muscles on the distal femur. Two-pin epiphyseal-metaphyseal traction has been used, which has the added benefit of controlling sagittal rotation. As with subtrochanteric fractures, external fixation can be used as a form of portable traction as long as there is sufficient room between the physis and the fracture to place two distal pins (Figure 8).

Closed reduction and percutaneous fixation with crossed wires can be valuable, especially in younger children who will heal rapidly and can tolerate cast protection until union. Plate fixation allows for anatomic reduction of the fracture site, but it is challenging because of the adjacent physis.

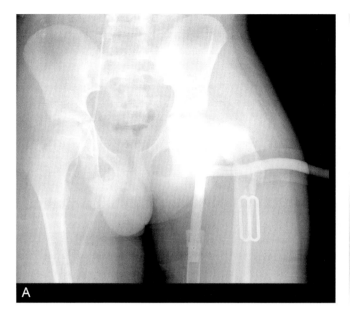
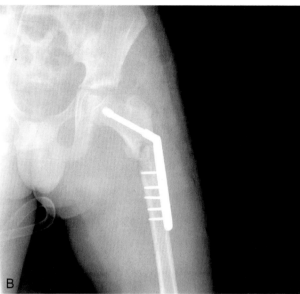

Figure 8 **A,** Preoperative AP pelvis radiograph of an 11-year-old boy with a subtrochanteric femoral fracture and a severe closed head injury from being struck by a van. The proximal location of this fracture limits the surgeon's options. **B,** Postoperative AP radiograph of the same patient after fixation with a hip screw and side plate. Rapid formation of abundant callus would be anticipated because of the patient's severe head injury.

Summary

In evaluating a child with a femoral fracture, management is based on the risks and benefits of each treatment method and the goal of mobilizing the child as quickly and safely as possible. The possibility of abuse must be considered, especially in children who are not yet walking. Fractures in young infants can be managed with splints or a Pavlik harness. Older infants and preschool-age children may be best treated with an early spica cast. For school-age children, especially those with high-energy trauma or associated injuries, internal or external fixation is now the standard of care. When making treatment recommendations, surgeons should consider the presence of associated injuries or multiple trauma, the personality of the fracture, the acceptable age-appropriate reduction, family issues, and cost. Complications of all treatments include limb-length discrepancy, angular deformity, rotational malunion, delayed union, nonunion, and compartment syndrome.

Annotated Bibliography
Pediatric Diaphyseal Femoral Fractures

Buechsenschuetz KE, Mehlman CT, Shaw KJ, Crawford AH, Immerman EB: Femoral shaft fractures in children: Traction and casting versus elastic stable intramedullary nailing. *J Trauma* 2002;53:914-921.

The authors found no difference in the clinical results of 68 children (71 femoral fractures) who underwent either traction and casting or elastic stable intramedullary nailing. They did, however, report that elastic stable intramedullary nailing was associated with lower cost.

Caird MS, Mueller KA, Puryear A, Farley FA: Compression plating of pediatric femoral shaft fractures. *J Pediatr Orthop* 2003;23:448-452.

This retrospective review examined 60 children younger than 16 years with femoral shaft fractures that were treated with compression plate fixation. The reported union rate was 100%, and the complication rate was low compared with published data on other treatment options. The authors suggested that this method is effective for children with isolated femoral shaft fractures and associated injuries.

Domb BG, Sponseller PD, Ain M, Miller NH: Comparison of dynamic versus static external fixation for pediatric femur fractures. *J Pediatr Orthop* 2002;22:428-430.

The authors of this randomized controlled trial found that axial dynamization had no effect on time to healing or frequency of complications.

Flynn JM, Hresko T, Reynolds RA, Blasier RD, Davidson R, Kasser J: Titanium elastic nails for pediatric femur fractures: A multicenter study of early results with analysis of complications. *J Pediatr Orthop* 2001;21:4-8.

In a multicenter trial that was conducted before the general release of titanium elastic nails, 57 of 58 patients had a satisfactory or excellent result. Soft-tissue irritation by the nail tip was the most frequent complication.

Flynn JM, Luedtke LM, Ganley TJ, et al: Comparison of titanium elastic nails with traction and a spica cast to treat femoral fractures in children. *J Bone Joint Surg Am* 2004;86-A:770-777.

In this study, 83 children with femoral fractures were assessed prospectively, 35 of which were treated with traction and spica casting, and 48 with titanium elastic nails. All fractures healed, but three patients treated with the spica cast had unsatisfactory alignment; 34% of patients treated with traction and casting had complications compared with 22% of those treated with intramedullary nail fixation. The authors concluded that flexible intramedullary nailing leads to faster recovery with a more favorable complication rate than traction and application of the spica cast; however, the hospital charges for both methods are similar.

Flynn JM, Schwend RM: Management of pediatric femoral shaft fractures. *J Am Acad Orthop Surg* 2004;12: 347-359.

The authors discuss the current concepts in pediatric femur fracture treatment, with a focus on sound decision making and avoidance of complications.

Gordon JE, Khanna N, Luhmann SJ, Dobbs MB, Ortman MR, Schoenecker PL: Intramedullary nailing of femoral fractures in children through the lateral aspect of the greater trochanter using a modified rigid humeral intramedullary nail: Preliminary results of a new technique in 15 children. *J Orthop Trauma* 2004;18:416-422.

This retrospective study evaluated the clinical results of rigid intramedullary nailing of femoral shaft fractures with entry points through the lateral aspect of the greater trochanter in older children and adolescents. Fifteen children were evaluated to determine time to union, final fracture alignment, length of hospital stay, complications, clinical outcome, and proximal femoral changes, including osteonecrosis or proximal valgus with femoral neck narrowing. The average hospital stay for patients was 2.8 days, and after an average follow-up of 141 weeks, no patient had developed osteonecrosis, femoral neck valgus, femoral neck narrowing, or other complications. The authors concluded that this method of rigid nailing is effective for patients in this age group.

Gordon JE, Swenning TA, Burd TA, Szymanski DA, Schoenecker PL: Proximal femoral radiographic changes after lateral transtrochanteric intramedullary nail placement in children. *J Bone Joint Surg Am* 2003; 85-A:1295-1301.

This retrospective review was conducted to assess changes in the proximal femur after rigid intramedullary nailing through the lateral trochanteric area in children with a mean age of 10 years and 6 months. No patient exhibited osteonecrosis or clinically important femoral neck narrowing or valgus deformity. The authors thus concluded that lateral transtrochanteric intramedullary nailing in children 9 years of age or older is safer than nailing through the piriformis fossa and the tip of the greater trochanter.

Hedin H, Larsson S: Technique and considerations when using external fixation as a standard treatment of femoral fractures in children. *Injury* 2004;35:1255-1263.

This prospective study examined techniques for external fixation in 98 femoral fractures of children 3 to 15 years of age. The authors recommended surgery on a traction table, which can aid in avoiding malrotation and facilitate reduction prior to insertion of the pins. They also recommended transverse skin incisions and the use of 4- or 5-mm pins. Most fractures healed effectively within a relatively short period.

Kanlic EM, Anglen JO, Smith DG, Morgan SJ, Pesantez RF: Advantages of submuscular bridge plating for complex pediatric femur fractures. *Clin Orthop Relat Res* 2004;426:244-251.

Minimally invasive submuscular bridge plating was evaluated as a technique that avoids the complications of traditional compression plating in this prospective study. Fifty-one children were treated, and all fractures healed with excellent clinical results. Two significant complications occurred: fracture of the plate and refracture after early plate removal. Four patients had limb-length discrepancies. The authors concluded that this technique offers predictable healing while maintaining length and alignment for all pediatric femoral shaft fractures.

Large TM, Frick SL: Compartment syndrome of the leg after treatment of a femoral fracture with an early sitting spica cast: A report of two cases. *J Bone Joint Surg Am* 2003;85-A:2207-2210.

Two cases are presented in which compartment syndrome developed after a low-energy fracture of the femoral shaft was treated with an early sitting spica cast. The authors describe the diagnosis of compartment syndrome and examine the factors associated with this treatment that could contribute to compartment syndrome. They also describe a modification of the cast-application technique in which an above-the-knee cast is applied first.

Luhmann SJ, Schootman M, Schoenecker PL, Dobbs MB, Gordon JE: Complications of titanium elastic nails for pediatric femoral shaft fractures. *J Pediatr Orthop* 2003;23:443-447.

The authors identified 39 patients with femoral shaft fractures who were managed using titanium elastic nailing. The average patient age was 6.0 years. Twenty-one complications were reported, two of which were major postoperative complications (one septic arthritis after nail removal and one hypertrophic nonunion). Minor complications included pain at the nails, nail erosion through the skin, and one delayed union. Fracture angulation was associated with patient weight and nail size. The authors suggested using large nails and leaving less than 2.5 cm of the nail out of the femur to minimize technical pitfalls.

Mendelson SA, Dominick TS, Tyler-Kabara E, Moreland MS, Adelson PD: Early versus late femoral fracture stabilization in multiply injured pediatric patients with closed head injury. *J Pediatr Orthop* 2001;21:594-599.

This retrospective study analyzed 25 patients with femoral fractures and associated head injuries to determine whether time to fracture fixation affects central nervous system, ortho-

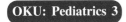

paedic, or other complications. The group of patients that underwent early femoral fracture stabilization had an average time to treatment of 10.5 days, and the group that underwent late femoral fracture stabilization had an average time to treatment of 18.5 days. Orthopaedic and central nervous system complications were similar in the two groups, but significantly more additional complications occurred in the late femoral fracture stabilization group. The authors concluded that early femoral fracture fixation decreases the length of hospital stay and the number of associated complications.

Narayanan UG, Hyman JE, Wainwright AM, Rang M, Alman BA: Complications of elastic stable intramedullary nail fixation of pediatric femoral fractures, and how to avoid them. *J Pediatr Orthop* 2004;24:363-369.

Complications of flexible intramedullary nailing were studied prospectively in 78 children. The reported complications included irritation at the insertion site, malunion, refracture, transient neurologic deficit, and superficial wound infection. The authors maintained that most complications are preventable and advised surgeons to ensure that nail ends lie against the supracondylar flare of the femur to avoid symptoms at the insertion site; the authors also suggested avoiding the use of nails of different diameters.

Podeszwa DA, Mooney JF 3rd, Cramer KE, Mendelow MJ: Comparison of Pavlik harness application and immediate spica casting for femur fractures in infants. *J Pediatr Orthop* 2004;24:460-462.

The authors retrospectively compared Pavlik harness use (24 patients) versus spica casting (16 patients) for the treatment of femoral shaft fractures in children younger than 1 year. There were no reported differences in the radiographic or clinical outcomes between these groups. One third of the patients who underwent spica casting had a skin complication that contributed to the overall risk. No similar complications existed in the Pavlik harness group. The authors suggested using a Pavlik harness in children younger than 1 year.

Pediatric Subtrochanteric Femoral Fractures

Bedi A, Toan Le T: Subtrochanteric femur fractures. *Orthop Clin North Am* 2004;35:473-483.

In this article, the authors reviewed the types of subtrochanteric fractures and the relevant techniques for management, including the use of intramedullary devices, fixed-angle devices, and the compression hip screw.

Pediatric Supracondylar Femoral Fractures

Smith NC, Parker D, McNicol D: Supracondylar fractures of the femur in children. *J Pediatr Orthop* 2001;21: 600-603.

In this retrospective review, the authors studied 102 femoral fractures, in which there was a 12% incidence of supracondylar fractures. Seven of these fractures were displaced and required surgical intervention. The authors also review the literature and classification systems for supracondylar fractures and discuss treatment options.

Classic Bibliography

Bar-On E, Sagiv S, Porat S: External fixation or flexible intramedullary nailing for femoral shaft fractures in children: A prospective, randomised study. *J Bone Joint Surg Br* 1997;79:975-978.

Beaty JH, Austin SM, Warner WC, Canale ST, Nichols L: Interlocking intramedullary nailing of femoral-shaft fractures in adolescents: Preliminary results and complications. *J Pediatr Orthop* 1994;14:178-183.

Heinrich SD, Drvaric DM, Darr K, MacEwen GD: The operative stabilization of pediatric diaphyseal femur fractures with flexible intramedullary nails: A prospective analysis. *J Pediatr Orthop* 1994;14:501-507.

Hutchins CM, Sponseller PD, Sturm P, Mosquero R: Open femur fractures in children: Treatment, complications, and results. *J Pediatr Orthop* 2000;20:183-188.

Illgen R II, Rodgers WB, Hresko MT, Waters PM, Zurakowski D, Kasser JR: Femur fractures in children: Treatment with early sitting spica casting. *J Pediatr Orthop* 1998;18:481-487.

Infante AF Jr, Albert MC, Jennings WB, Lehner JT: Immediate hip spica casting for femur fractures in pediatric patients: A review of 175 patients. *Clin Orthop Relat Res* 2000;376:106-112.

Linhart WE, Roposch A: Elastic stable intramedullary nailing for unstable femoral fractures in children: Preliminary results of a new method. *J Trauma* 1999;47:372-378.

O'Malley DE, Mazur JM, Cummings RJ: Femoral head avascular necrosis associated with intramedullary nailing in an adolescent. *J Pediatr Orthop* 1995;15:21-23.

Sanders JO, Browne RH, Mooney JF, et al: Treatment of femoral fractures in children by pediatric orthopedists: Results of a 1998 survey. *J Pediatr Orthop* 2001;21:436-441.

Schwend RM, Werth C, Johnston A: Femur shaft fractures in toddlers and young children: Rarely from child abuse. *J Pediatr Orthop* 2000;20:475-481.

Shapiro F: Fractures of the femoral shaft in children: The overgrowth phenomenon. *Acta Orthop Scand* 1981; 52:649-655.

Stans AA, Morrissy RT, Renwick SE: Femoral shaft fracture treatment in patients age 6 to 16 years. *J Pediatr Orthop* 1999;19:222-228.

Townsend DR, Hoffinger S: Intramedullary nailing of femoral shaft fractures in children via the trochanter tip. *Clin Orthop Relat Res* 2000;376:113-118.

Chapter 22

Pediatric Injuries About the Knee

Paul D. Sponseller, MD, MBA

Introduction

Fractures about the knee have important implications for growth and require accurate reduction; even minor degrees of angulation about the knee can produce visible deformity. Stiffness and articular degeneration may eventually occur if chondral or significant muscle damage has occurred. Surgeons should also be aware that ligament injuries may coexist with physeal fractures about the knee.

Relevant Anatomy and Principles

The growth occurring at the distal femoral physis is approximately 10 to 11 mm/yr; growth at the proximal tibial physis is approximately 6 to 7 mm/yr. The knee joint capsule and collateral ligaments originate just distal to the distal femoral physis and thereby concentrate any regional stress on this vulnerable growth cartilage. Injuries to the distal femoral physis are approximately twice as common as those of the proximal tibia. The growth plate of the distal femur has a complex, undulating shape, forming four depressions into which four matching mammillary processes of the distal femoral metaphysis fit. This shape provides some degree of resistance to shear. However, it also may decrease the odds of a "clean" cleavage plane along the physis and therefore increase the risk of focal damage to the physis. In contrast, the proximal tibial epiphysis is spanned by and protected by the collateral ligaments. Its physis is continuous with that of the tibial tubercle, which ossifies in preadolescence. The neurovascular structures about the knee are at some risk with any injury to the knee region, but this risk is greatest for injury to the proximal tibia because of tethering of the popliteal artery at its trifurcation, the peroneal nerve around the proximal fibula, and the tibial nerve at the proximal interosseous membrane. The results of a neurovascular examination should be documented for pediatric patients with injuries about the knee, and an arteriogram is not routinely needed in displaced fractures if the examination is normal.

Knee dislocations are extremely rare in skeletally immature patients. When they do occur, at least some of the injury typically occurs through the relatively weaker bone and cartilage around the growth plate. However, intra-articular injury to cruciate ligaments and menisci may coexist with osteocartilaginous injury.

Distal Femoral Epiphyseal Injuries
Mechanism and Classification

Description of an injury should take into account the direction and degree of displacement, physeal injury pattern, and age of the patient. The most common displacements of the region about the knee are into valgus or hyperextension. The direction of displacement influences the method of reduction and immobilization. In addition, a hyperextension pattern carries a greater risk of neurovascular injury, and a varus displacement, although rare, increases the risk of peroneal nerve injury. Highly displaced fractures are more unstable, even after reduction. Nondisplaced physeal fractures may require stress radiographs to visualize the extent of the injury (Figure 1), but clinical examination can provide an accurate explanation for swelling about the knee in some injured adolescents. The Salter-Harris pattern of physeal injury does not predict the risk of growth disturbance in the knee region as well as it does in injuries to other areas. All physeal injuries of the distal femur carry a significant risk of growth disturbance because of their complex shapes and because of the forces involved. Growth disturbance is somewhat less common in young patients than in adolescents, but its implications are far greater. CT with reconstruction is helpful to assess some complex Salter-Harris type IV fractures.

Treatment

Treatment in a cast is appropriate for all nondisplaced fractures. Closed reduction should also be attempted for all minimally to moderately displaced Salter-Harris type I and type II fractures. This may be accomplished after administering adequate sedation and analgesia to the patient in the emergency department. For patients with

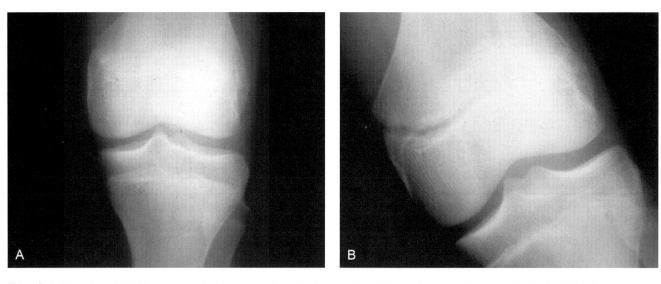

Figure 1 **A,** Knee radiograph of a 14-year-old boy who felt a pop while twisting his knee. **B,** Stress radiograph of the same patient demonstrates physeal widening.

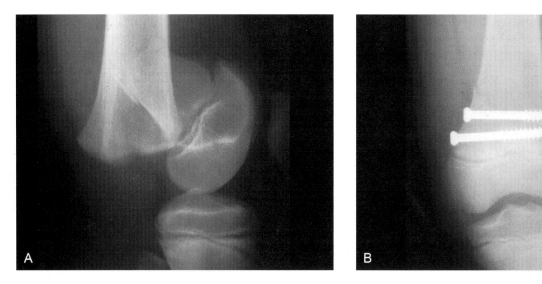

Figure 2 **A,** Preoperative radiograph of a type II fracture of the distal femoral physis with a large metaphyseal fragment displaced into hyperextension. **B,** Postoperative radiograph after the patient underwent closed reduction and fixation of the fracture with percutaneous cannulated screws.

severe displacement, especially those with a hyperextension pattern, the risk of redisplacement is increased, and the surgeon may elect to follow these injuries more closely or stabilize them with percutaneous fixation. An additional factor to consider is the shape of the thigh; patients with "ample" thigh girth are more difficult to immobilize with a cast. For fractures that do not reduce well in the emergency department or appear to be unstable, closed (or open) reduction followed by internal fixation should be performed. Percutaneous screws are the preferred method of fixation if they can be inserted without crossing the physis. Salter-Harris type II fractures can be stabilized using fixation across the metaphyseal "spike" if it is large enough (Figure 2). If stability cannot be obtained by fixation across the metaphysis, Salter-Harris type I and type II fractures

can be stabilized using one or two smooth Steinmann pins from epiphysis to metaphysis or metaphysis to epiphysis (Figure 3). If retrograde pinning is performed, it is recommended that these pins are left buried under the skin and removed later. If left outside the skin, they can cause significant irritation, which may lead to joint infection because fixation pins entering the epiphysis will often cross the joint as described previously.

Complex displaced transphyseal fractures may result from crushing or sharp object injuries. These require open anatomic reduction and internal fixation. Alignment can be difficult to assess because once the fragments are reassembled, only the periphery of the growth plate can be seen. Bone and growth plate may also be missing. In this instance, secondary markers for alignment should be used, such as the articular surface

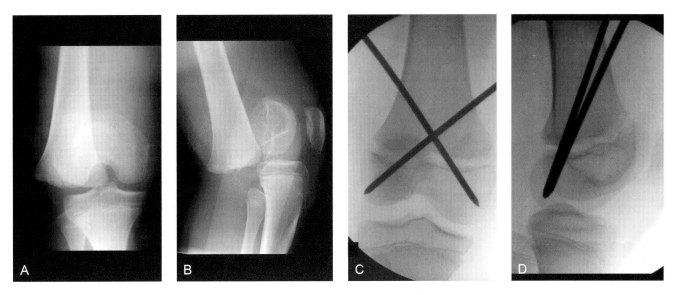

Figure 3 AP **(A)** and lateral **(B)** radiographs showing displaced hyperextension type II fracture of the distal femoral physis with a small metaphyseal fragment. Postoperative AP **(C)** and lateral **(D)** fluoroscopic views showing that closed reduction of the fracture was achieved with percutaneous stabilization using two smooth Steinmann pins retrograde to avoid the joint.

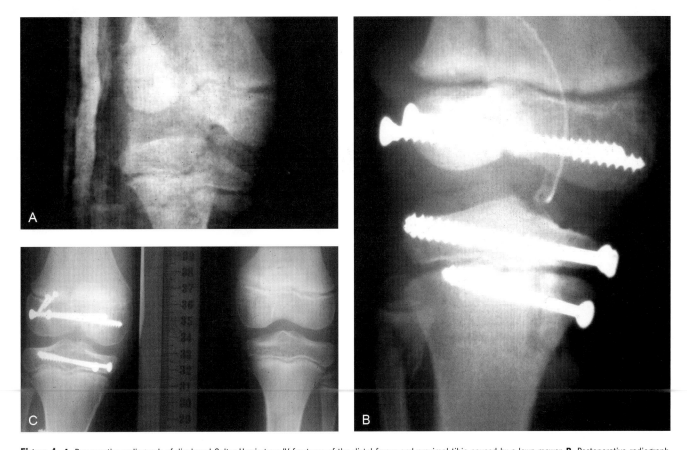

Figure 4 **A,** Preoperative radiograph of displaced Salter-Harris type IV fractures of the distal femur and proximal tibia caused by a lawn mower. **B,** Postoperative radiograph obtained after open reduction and internal fixation with realignment of physes. **C,** Radiograph obtained 2 years after open reduction and internal fixation shows normal growth occurring.

and metaphyseal fracture line (Figure 4). Cannulated screws are helpful in this situation as well to place the fixation away from both the joint surface and the growth plate in small epiphyses. Usually 4.5-mm or 6.5-mm screws are appropriate. In very young patients, smaller screws or headless screws may be useful.

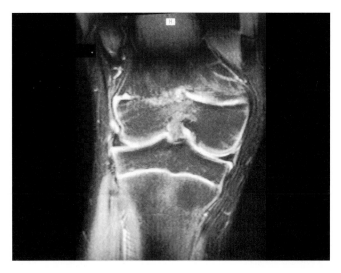

Figure 5 Partial physeal arrest shown on an MRI scan with gradient echo sequence.

Follow-up and Complications

Joint movement should be started as stability dictates, but usually by 6 weeks after injury at the latest. Growth should be assessed carefully approximately 6 months after injury. This can be done by using radiographs that are coned and centered on the physis to examine the appearance of the physis and the Park-Harris growth lines parallel to it. The distance to these lines in the femur should be greater than the distance of the lines from the adjacent proximal tibial physis because of the greater growth rate. MRI with gradient echo sequence may be used to assess the physis if there is a concern, provided there is no implant in the region (Figure 5). These diagnostic imaging tools are of limited clinical utility within the first 3 months after injury because of the changes of fracture healing. Long radiographs of

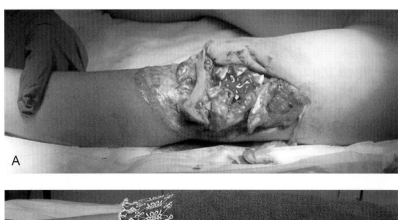

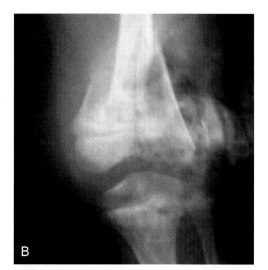

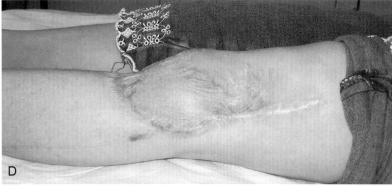

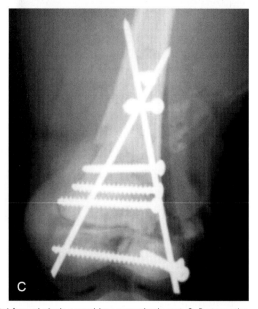

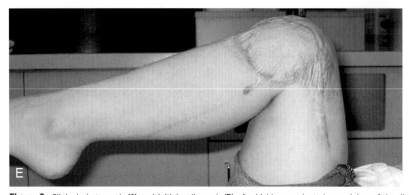

Figure 6 Clinical photograph **(A)** and initial radiograph **(B)** of a highly comminuted open injury of the distal femoral physis caused by a power implement. **C,** Postoperative radiograph shows that stable internal fixation was performed to facilitate early range of motion; lateral gastrocnemius flap coverage was performed. **D** and **E,** Postoperative clinical photographs show that the patient eventually recovered flexion from 0° to 105°. The patient developed a physeal arrest.

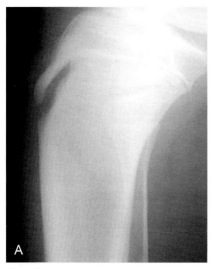
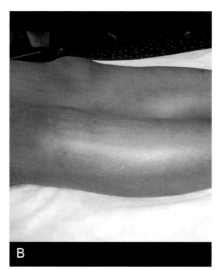
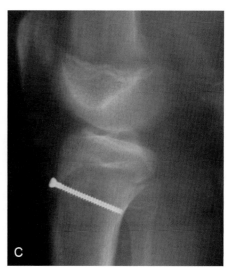

Figure 7 **A,** Radiograph of a Salter-Harris type I injury to the proximal tibial epiphysis. **B,** Clinical photograph shows significant swelling associated with compartment pressures of 45 mm Hg. **C,** Postoperative radiograph shows that reduction and internal fixation was performed along with fasciotomy.

both limbs are also useful to assess length and angulation if any noticeable angulation appears, usually more than 6 months after the fracture. If an injury to the growth plate is identified, options include bar resection, completion of the epiphysiodesis, contralateral epiphysiodesis, and corrective osteotomy with or without lengthening.

Stiffness is rare in children, but it may develop if there is significant associated injury to the quadriceps or the articular surface. To prevent this from occurring, optimal internal fixation to allow early motion is recommended (Figure 6). If loss of motion is severe despite conservative therapy, care should be taken to avoid the temptation to manipulate the knee in a child with widely open physes because separation may occur through the growth plate instead of movement at the joint. Quadricepsplasty and/or lysis of adhesions are a safer treatment option if a plateau of motion has been reached. Continuous passive motion after surgery may help to maintain the gains.

Proximal Tibial Epiphyseal Injuries
Mechanism and Classification
Injuries to this region are uncommon and most often the result of force applied to the planted leg. Displacement is similar to that of the distal femur, usually in the direction of hyperextension or valgus. Neurovascular damage is present in up to 10% of patients with proximal tibial epiphyseal injuries, especially those with an apex posterior angulation.

Treatment
The circulation of patients with proximal tibial epiphyseal injuries should be carefully assessed clinically, and an arteriogram should be obtained for those in whom vascular

injury is suspected. Compartment syndrome should be ruled out clinically (Figure 7). Fractures that can be reduced using closed methods can usually be aligned with a long leg cast. The cast should be bivalved and the patient should be observed overnight for vascular complications if displacement was significant. Because of the shape of the epiphysis, the Salter-Harris type III pattern of injury is rare in the proximal tibia, except as a pattern of tibial tubercle avulsion. Unstable fractures of any pattern and all displaced Salter-Harris type III and type IV fractures should be reduced and stabilized with internal fixation such as smooth Steinmann pins.

Tibial Spine Avulsion
Mechanism and Classification
Tibial spine avulsions can occur as a result of athletic activity or trauma. Because of the decreased resistance to tensile stress of the bone and cartilage of the tibial spine compared with that of the anterior cruciate ligament, the spine is more likely than the ligament to fail during twisting injuries in young children. However, there is significant overlap between the anterior cruciate ligament injuries and tibial spine avulsions. Anterior cruciate ligament injuries are being recognized more frequently in preadolescents. In addition, some stretch of the ligament and associated stabilizers seems to occur in patients who sustain tibial spine avulsions, leading to mild residual laxity, even in patients who have had anatomic reduction of the tibial spine. Meyers and McKeever have classified these injuries into three types: type I (nondisplaced), type II (hinged), and type III (completely displaced).

Treatment
Nondisplaced fractures are treated in a long leg cast, and hinged fractures can usually be reduced with exten-

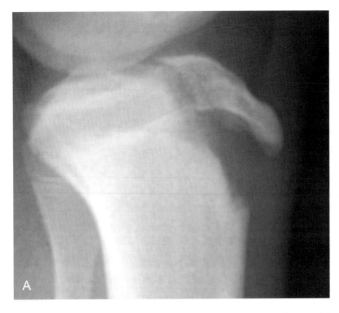
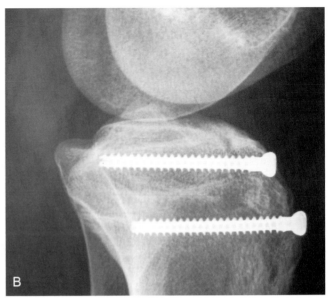

Figure 8 **A,** Preoperative radiograph shows an Ogden type III avulsion fracture of the tibial tubercle in a 13-year-old boy. **B,** Postoperative radiograph obtained after closed reduction and internal fixation.

sion of the knee and held in a cast for 6 weeks. Although some authors advise attempting to reduce completely displaced fractures by extending the knee, these fractures often will not reduce or will redisplace. Open or arthroscopic reduction and internal fixation is the most effective treatment in patients with completely displaced fractures. The knee should be inspected for meniscal entrapment under the cartilaginous flaps of the tibial spine. Internal fixation may be achieved using peripheral sutures, a transepiphyseal pull-out suture, or an intraepiphyseal screw (in patients who are near skeletal maturity).

Complications
Although most patients have some residual laxity on clinical examination, it is rarely symptomatic. A block to extension of the knee may occur if the fragment heals with excessive proximal displacement.

Tibial Tubercle Avulsion
Mechanism and Classification
Tibial tubercle avulsions occur through the physis of the tubercle and vary in the degree of propagation proximally. Ogden has classified these into three types: type I is an avulsion of only the distal part of the tubercle, type II is a fracture that propagates to the junction of the tubercle with the transverse portion of the proximal tibial epiphysis, and type III propagates into the proximal tibial epiphysis and crosses into the joint itself (Figure 8). Type III tibial tubercle avulsions occur when patients are near skeletal maturity and when the posterior portion of the physis has already started to close (analogous to the Tillaux fracture of the ankle). All types of tibial tubercle

avulsion are caused by the pull of the quadriceps against the fixed knee and usually occur during jumping or landing. These injuries are to be distinguished from Osgood-Schlatter lesions, which are stress avulsions of the insertion of the patellar tendon into the superficial surface of the tubercle, usually at the microscopic level. A small number of patients with tibial tubercle avulsions report preexisting Osgood-Schlatter disease symptoms.

Treatment
Small, nondisplaced avulsions may be treated with a cast in extension. If the fracture is displaced, the tubercle should be replaced anatomically. Interposed periosteal fragments should be removed. Small (type I) avulsion fragments may be anchored using Krackow tendon-holding sutures in the patellar tendon that are anchored into the bone around a screw or buried wire. Large (type II and type III) avulsion fragments may be held with screws into the metaphysis. Growth disturbance will not typically occur in children older than 11 years. Most of these injuries occur when patients are near skeletal maturity. If the child is more than 3 years from skeletal maturity, fixation should be removed.

Complications
Most patients with tibial tubercle avulsions heal uneventfully. Genu recurvatum may occur in the rare tubercle fractures in patients younger than 11 years. Although not typical in such a location, compartment syndrome has been reported in several patients with type III tibial tubercle avulsions, presumably because of bleeding into the leg from the anterior tibial recurrent arteries.

Patellar Fractures

Patellar fractures are rare in children, presumably because of decreased body mass and increased resistance to impact. One unique feature in this age group is the relatively thick layer of unossified cartilage on the undersurface and distal rims (the patella is entirely made up of cartilage until approximately age 4 years); therefore, a small rim of bone avulsed from the inferior pole of the patella in a young child may signal a larger cartilaginous injury. This pattern has been termed a "sleeve" fracture. Patients with spasticity or other neuromuscular disorders causing knee stiffness may have notable prolongation or even discontinuity in the distal pole of the patella that can be mistaken for a fracture.

For a nondisplaced patellar fracture, treatment in a cylinder cast for 6 weeks is recommended, and there is usually no problem regaining motion. For fractures that are displaced more than 2 to 3 mm, open reduction and internal fixation with a modified tension band technique (a wire loop or figure-of-8 around parallel Kirschner wires) is recommended.

Patellar Dislocations

Patellar dislocations are the most common cause of a knee effusion in the skeletally immature child. Patients may feel a "pop" or describe the knee giving out. The examiner should assess the contralateral knee for predisposing factors such as ligamentous laxity, valgus, or underdevelopment of the lateral condyle or vastus medialis obliquus. Tenderness is common along the medial patellar border or the femoral origin of the medial patellofemoral ligament. Radiographs should be obtained to assess for the presence of osseous fragments. Many orthopaedic surgeons elect to inspect the knee arthroscopically in any child with a significant effusion or osseous fragment. Small fragments may be removed, whereas large fragments should be reattached. The knee should be immobilized for 1 to 3 weeks, followed by a rehabilitation program to decrease the risk of recurrence. About 15% to 20% of patients will have recurrent episodes of instability. Factors that predispose patients to recurrence include valgus alignment, ligamentous laxity, hypoplasia of the lateral femoral condyle, and a shallow femoral sulcus. The natural history of patellar instability is usually one of decreasing frequency during the third decade of life. Conservative treatment is the mainstay and includes strengthening of the vastus medialis obliquus, hamstring stretching, proprioceptive training, and patellar bracing or taping. Surgical reconstruction to reduce the risk of these episodes depends on the impact of such recurrences on athletic activity and lifestyle.

Components of a surgical reconstruction may include a lateral release, a vastus medialis advancement, and a medial subperiosteal transfer of the lateral portion of the patellar tendon (Roux-Goldthwaite procedure) or tenodesis using the semitendinosus tendon (Galeazzi procedure). In teenage patients nearing skeletal maturity, a tibial tubercle transfer is an option. Surgical results are less predictable in patients with ligamentous laxity, such as those with Ehlers-Danlos syndrome or Down syndrome.

Ligament Injuries

Physeal injuries and osseous avulsions are the equivalent of ligament injuries in many children. It is being increasingly recognized, however, that ligament injuries do occur in association with fractures in children.

Medial Collateral Ligament Injuries

Medial collateral ligament injuries may result in medial laxity similar to that caused by physeal disruption. Stress radiographs may differentiate the two types of injury. Medial collateral ligament injuries are more common in skeletally mature teenagers. These injuries, if occurring in isolation, heal well with a period of immobilization for 1 to 3 weeks followed by rehabilitation, possibly with a brace. If the medial collateral ligament injury occurs in association with a cruciate ligament injury, the latter injury dictates the treatment.

Anterior Cruciate Ligament Injuries

Anterior cruciate ligament injuries occur with increasing frequency as children get older. Patients with a narrower femoral notch are more prone to ligament tear, whereas those with a wider notch are more likely to sustain a tibial spine avulsion. Hearing a "pop" is usually reported by the patient, and a hemarthrosis is evident. The most common cause of these findings in children is a patellar dislocation followed by a tibial tubercle avulsion, and these must be ruled out. The Lachman test is the most sensitive test for diagnosis. MRI or diagnostic arthroscopy is used for confirmation. The sensitivity and specificity of MRI are not as high in children as in adults.

For a complete anterior cruciate ligament injury, nonsurgical treatment yields no better results in children than it does in adults. Surgical reconstruction provides superior results if the child desires to continue an active lifestyle. Direct repair and extra-articular reconstruction, however, do not yield good results. Intra-articular reconstruction using bone tunnels may be performed on boys who have achieved skeletal maturity and are at least 15 years of age or on girls who are at least 14 years of age. In younger children with anterior cruciate ligament injuries, controversy exists regarding treatment. Rehabilitation, bracing, and activity modification will suffice for a certain subset of children. For those who continue to experience instability, however, the anterior cruciate ligament may be reconstructed using the hamstring tendons or the medial one third of the patellar tendon with or without physeal-sparing tunnels. During reconstruction, the tendons are detached proximally at their musculotendinous junctions and passed over a groove or through a tunnel on the anterior aspect of the tibial epiphysis.

Posterior Cruciate Ligament Injuries

Posterior cruciate ligament injuries are rare in children. Because the tendon is extrasynovial, no effusion may be present. Diagnosis is made by noting a posterior displacement of the proximal tibia or by the quadriceps active drawer test. In this test, the patient is positioned supine on the examination table, the knee is flexed to 70°, and the foot is flat on the table. As the patient contracts the quadriceps, the tibial plateau moves anteriorly if there is posterior cruciate ligament insufficiency. On radiographs, an avulsion may be heralded by a fleck of bone posteriorly at the site of the posterior cruciate ligament insertion.

Displaced avulsion fractures are best treated by open reduction and internal fixation using intraepiphyseal sutures or screws. Tears within the substance of the ligament are best treated nonsurgically. If necessary, reconstructive surgery for patients with symptomatic knees may be performed after skeletal maturity is achieved.

Meniscal Injuries

Meniscal injuries are uncommon in children and usually occur as a result of a traumatic episode. Pain, giving way, locking, and joint line tenderness are common symptoms. Differential diagnosis includes patellar instability, osteochondritis dissecans, inflammatory arthropathies, and hip pathology such as slipped capital femoral epiphysis. Initial evaluation should include plain radiographs with tunnel and patellar views. Although MRI is commonly used to assess patients with meniscal injuries, normal menisci in children often have increased signal on T1-weighted images, and the diagnostic utility, therefore, is not superior to that of clinical examination. For patients being considered for a possible diagnosis of isolated medial meniscus tear, serial examinations over a short period are appropriate to rule out minor injuries that can spontaneously resolve.

Meniscal tears in children have superior healing potential compared with those in older patients. Meniscal repair should be attempted whenever possible in children, including tears in the white-white region in children who are 12 years of age or younger. Skeletally mature adolescents should be managed using the same guidelines as adults. Total meniscectomy should be avoided whenever possible. A partial meniscectomy should be used for patients with irreparable tears. Meniscal repairs that occur in association with anterior cruciate ligament disruption should be repaired regardless of whether the anterior cruciate ligament is being repaired at the time.

Summary

Injuries about the knee demand accurate reduction and close follow-up for physeal and osteochondral injuries. The families of patients should be made aware of these issues from the initial contact. Fractures of the proximal tibia merit close examination for neurologic or vascular injury, with diagnostic imaging if necessary. Compartment syndrome may also occur with fractures in this region. Advanced diagnostic imaging and newer fixation techniques promise improved range of movement and outcomes. Fortunately, most children with fractures about the knee can expect return to a high level of function.

Annotated Bibliography

Relevant Anatomy and Principles

Tepper KB, Ireland ML: Fracture patterns and treatment in the skeletally immature knee. *Instr Course Lect* 2003;52:667-676.

The authors of this article discuss the anatomy and classification as related to the treatment and outcome of fractures in the skeletally immature knee.

Wessel LM, Scholz S, Ruch M, et al: Hemarthrosis after trauma to the pediatric knee joint: What is the value of magnetic resonance imaging in the diagnostic algorithm? *J Pediatr Orthop* 2001;21:338-342.

The authors of this study reported that although MRI and arthroscopy are highly useful in determining the diagnosis of hemarthrosis in children, each diagnostic modality was unable to detect 4% of these injuries.

Zionts LE: Fractures around the knee in children. *J Am Acad Orthop Surg* 2002;10:345-355.

The author discusses diagnosis and treatment for fractures around the knee in children.

Distal Femoral Epiphyseal Injuries

Butcher CC, Hoffman EB: Supracondylar fractures of the femur in children: Closed reduction and percutaneous pinning of displaced fractures. *J Pediatr Orthop* 2005;25:145-148.

The authors of this study reported good results from the retrograde pinning of 10 supracondylar fractures of the femur in children.

Proximal Tibial Epiphyseal Injuries

Muller I, Muschol M, Mann M, Hassenpflug J: Results of proximal metaphyseal fractures in children. *Arch Orthop Trauma Surg* 2002;122(6):331-333.

This retrospective study was conducted to determine the extent of the two typical outcomes (valgus deformity and leg overgrowth) in seven children (age range, 1 year 10 months to 10 years 2 months) with proximal metaphyseal fractures. At an average 34-month follow-up, all patients had subjective recovery; one patient, however, had minor functional problems. All patients were able to move their knee joint freely. Six patients

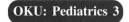

developed a genu valgum (proximal tibia angle, 6° to 16°), and conservative therapy was instituted. Only two patients (both younger than 5 years) had a partial spontaneous correction. Overgrowth on the side of the fracture (range, 0.5 to 1.5 cm) was reported in four patients. The authors recommended surgical correction and osteosynthesis as the preferred method of treatment, even with the increased likelihood of overgrowth.

Tibial Spine Avulsion

Hunter RE, Willis JA: Arthroscopic fixation of avulsion fractures of the tibial eminence: Technique and outcome. *Arthroscopy* 2004;20(2):113-121.

The authors of this study reported that suture and screw fixation had equal results in the arthroscopic fixation of avulsion fractures of the tibial eminence.

Kocher MS, Forman ES, Micheli L: Laxity and functional outcome after arthroscopic reduction and internal fixation of displaced tibial spine fractures in children. *Arthroscopy* 2003;19:1085-1090.

The authors of this study reported that children had persistent laxity but excellent function after undergoing internal fixation of a displaced tibial spine with a cannulated screw.

Tibial Tubercle Avulsion

Mosier SM, Stanitski CL: Acute tibial tubercle avulsion fractures. *J Pediatr Orthop* 2004;24:181-184.

The authors conducted a retrospective analysis of 18 patients (19 acute tibial tubercle avulsion fractures); the mean patient age at injury was 13 years 8 months. Mean follow-up time was 2 years 8 months. Four preadolescent patients (age range, 9 to 12 years) at injury were identified. Athletic participation resulted in 77% of fractures. Fifteen fractures were treated with open reduction and internal fixation, four were treated with closed reduction and cylinder cast immobilization. Final outcome was good in all patients regardless of fracture type or treatment, and no complications were reported.

Patellar Fractures

Hunt DM, Somashekar N: A review of sleeve fractures of the patella in children. *Knee* 2005;12(1):3-7.

Fractures of the patella in children differ from avulsions because of the "sleeve" of periosteum which is pulled off the patella and will continue to form bone if not treated. Treatment typically involves prompt reduction and internal fixation of the disrupted patella tendon.

Patellar Dislocations

Luhmann SJ: Acute traumatic knee effusions in children and adolescents. *J Pediatr Orthop* 2003;23:199-202.

The author reported that anterior cruciate ligament injuries, meniscal injuries, and patellofemoral injuries were the most common causes of hemarthrosis in children; females were far more likely to have patellofemoral injuries, and males were more likely to have anterior cruciate ligament injuries.

Ligament Injuries

Aichroth PM, Patel DM, Zorilla P: The natural history and treatment of rupture of the anterior cruciate ligament in children and adolescents: A prospective review. *J Bone Joint Surg Br* 2002;84:38-41.

The authors of this study reported that the results of conservative treatment for anterior cruciate ligament ruptures were poor, a trend that was reversed by surgical treatment with transphyseal graft. Good results were seen postoperatively in 77% of patients, which is not as high as the rate of good outcomes in adults who undergo this procedure.

Kocher MS, Mandinga R, Klingele K, Bley L, Micheli L: Anterior cruciate ligament injury versus tibial spine fracture in the skeletally immature knee: A comparison of skeletal maturation and notch width index. *J Pediatr Orthop* 2004;24:185-188.

The authors of this study reported that in an age- and weight-matched comparison, children with anterior cruciate ligament injury had narrower intercondylar notches than those with tibial spine avulsion.

Classic Bibliography

Gomes LS, Volpon JB: Experimental physeal fracture-separations treated with rigid internal fixation. *J Bone Joint Surg Am* 1993;75:1756-1763.

Grogan DP, Carey TP, Leffers D, Ogden JA: Avulsion fractures of the patella. *J Pediatr Orthop* 1990;10:721-730.

Lombardo SJ, Harvey JP Jr: Fractures of the distal femoral epiphyses: Factors influencing prognosis. *J Bone Joint Surg Am* 1977;59:742-751.

Riseborough EJ, Barrett IR, Shapiro F: Growth disturbances following distal femoral physeal fracture-separations. *J Bone Joint Surg Am* 1983;65:885-893.

Wroble RR, Henderson RC, Campion ER, El-Khoury DY, Albright JP: Meniscectomy in children and adolescents: A long-term follow-up study. *Clin Orthop Relat Res* 1992;279:180-188.

Chapter 23

Tibial and Ankle Fractures

Daniel G. Hoernschemeyer, MD

Eric S. Moghadamian, MD

Tibial Fractures

Proximal Tibial Metaphyseal Fractures

First described in 1953, proximal tibial metaphyseal fractures are rare (incidence, 5.6 per 100,000 persons) and occur most commonly in children age 3 to 6 years as a nondisplaced greenstick fracture of the proximal tibial metaphysis. The medial cortex is usually fractured when valgus or torsional stress is applied to the proximal tibia, whereas the lateral cortex of the proximal tibia and the fibula usually remains intact. The child may present with pain at the proximal tibia, minimal soft-tissue swelling, and little or no clinical evidence of deformity. Radiographs will show either a nondisplaced torus, greenstick, or complete fracture of the proximal tibia.

Valgus deformity of the affected leg, the most common complication, typically develops within 12 to 18 months after the initial injury despite radiographic evidence of union of the initial fracture. Although a torus fracture is unlikely to result in a progressive deformity, a valgus tibial deformity can result from a gap in the medial cortex that develops thickening and sclerosis (Figure 1, A). The possible development of this deformity should be discussed at the time of injury with the family of the patient. There is controversy regarding the cause of the valgus deformity; therefore, conflicting treatments have been proposed. Proposed theories suggest that the valgus deformity is caused by early weight bearing; tethering of the iliotibial tract, soft-tissue interposition (specifically, pes anserinus, periosteum, and medial collateral ligament), tethering by intact fibula, asymmetric growth of proximal tibial epiphysis, injury to the lateral proximal tibial physis, or asymmetric growth of the medial proximal tibia caused by an asymmetric vascular response.

Much of the literature supports nonsurgical treatment of both the initial fracture and the subsequent valgus deformity (Figure 1, B). Restoring normal limb alignment while the patient is in a cast is extremely important. With the patient under conscious sedation at the time of initial presentation, gentle manipulation of the fracture may be required to close down any medial

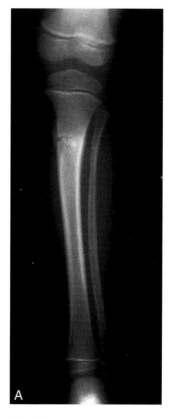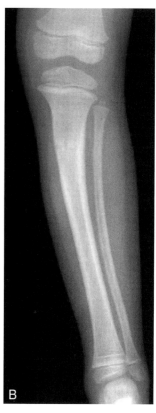

Figure 1 **A,** Radiograph of a proximal tibial metaphyseal fracture showing a gap and sclerosis of the medial cortex. **B,** Radiograph showing a valgus tibial deformity that developed 18 months after this proximal tibial metaphyseal fracture occurred.

gapping. Resolution of any valgus deformity that may develop typically occurs gradually and may take as long as 3 years after the initial injury to resolve.

Surgical treatment is considered necessary when soft tissues are blocking reduction of the fracture. This includes interposition of either the pes anserinus or the medial collateral ligament at the fracture site. Surgical treatment of the residual deformity using proximal tibial osteotomies and medial tibial hemiepiphysiodesis has been recommended for symptomatic patients and those with a valgus deformity greater than 15°. Surgical correction, particularly when performing a proximal tibial

Table 1 | Tibial Shaft Fractures

Pattern of Fracture	Force	Incidence	Comments
Spiral/oblique	Torsional forces from indirect trauma	48%	Most commonly seen in tibial fractures with an intact fibula; likely to drift into varus; toddler fractures
Transverse	Direct trauma	20%	Occur in older children
Comminuted	High-energy trauma	31%	Tend to show the most growth acceleration and may result in overgrowth
Open	Most commonly from high-energy trauma	< 5%	Motor vehicle-pedestrian injuries account for 80% of open tibial fractures

osteotomy, can be complicated by recurrence of the deformity and compartment syndrome.

In addition to the development of a valgus deformity, overgrowth of the injured tibia may occur. In long-term follow up studies, this has been reported to average approximately 1 cm. Despite the angular deformity and overgrowth that may occur after proximal tibial metaphyseal fractures, patients with these injuries have an overall good functional outcome and are usually asymptomatic when treated nonsurgically.

Tibial Shaft Fractures

Tibial shaft fractures account for 5% of all pediatric fractures and are the third most common type of long bone fracture in children (Table 1). About 70% of pediatric tibial shaft fractures have an intact fibula (Figure 2). These fractures have a bimodal frequency and occur more commonly in boys, with the incidence peaking at 3 to 4 years and 15 to 16 years of age. The incidence in girls remains fairly constant until age 12 years, at which time it begins to decrease.

The mechanism of injury for pediatric tibial shaft fractures can be fairly predictable based on the age of the patient. In younger children, tibial shaft fractures are the result of indirect trauma from a torsional force placed on the tibia, which can occur when a child stumbles while running, falls from a standing height, or catches and twists a foot in a moving object, resulting in a toddler fracture (Figure 3). In older adolescents, direct trauma from being struck by a motor vehicle, athletic injuries, and falls account for most of these fractures. When this type of injury is classified by athletic activity, the highest number of tibial shaft fractures occurs while playing soccer. Motor vehicle accidents account for 72% of all open tibial shaft fractures in children.

After obtaining the patient's history to determine the mechanism of injury, a thorough evaluation of the child's leg should be performed to assess for clinical deformity, soft-tissue injury, and integrity of the skin. An open fracture will typically have venous drainage from the wound. After initial inspection, a sterile dressing should be applied to the wound, and intravenous antibiotics should be administered. If significant soft-tissue

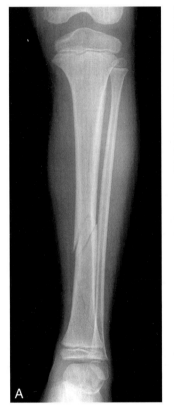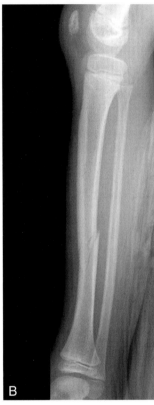

Figure 2 AP **(A)** and lateral **(B)** radiographs of a stable tibial shaft fracture with an intact fibula.

swelling is present, the injury is likely the result of high-energy trauma. If the patient is unconscious at the time of presentation, the patient should be monitored for the development of compartment syndrome. Compartment syndrome has been reported in 5% to 10% of all pediatric patients with tibial shaft fractures and may still be present despite the patient having an open fracture. Although vascular injury is uncommon in children with tibial shaft fractures, distal pulses in the injured limb should be evaluated and monitored for change.

Radiographic evaluation of the patient should begin with AP and lateral views of the injured tibia and fibula that include both the knee and ankle joints. Again, most patients with these fractures will have an intact fibula.

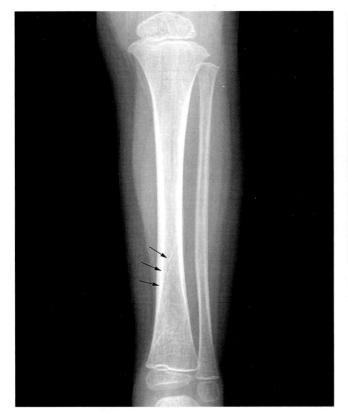

Figure 3 Radiograph of a toddler fracture (arrows) in a 4-year-old patient who was unable to bear weight after tripping and falling.

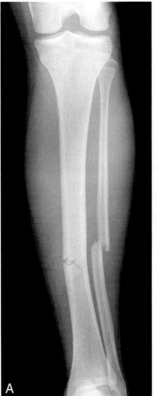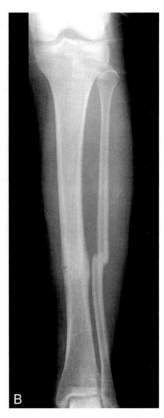

Figure 4 A, Radiograph of a pediatric tibial shaft fracture with 12° of valgus angulation. **B,** Radiograph showing that the fracture healed after being treated with closed manipulation and casting.

When evaluating younger children for a tibial fracture after a fall, standard radiographs can often show no evidence of injury. In these patients, an oblique radiograph may be needed to identify tibial shaft fractures. When evaluating a preschool-aged child for an occult fracture, bone scanning, which has high sensitivity and specificity, can often be helpful. A bone scan can also help evaluate the patient for other possible causes for the pain that may not otherwise be present on plain radiographs, such as osteomyelitis, septic arthritis, or a primary or secondary bone tumor.

In the management of all pediatric tibial shaft fractures, the goal is complete union with satisfactory alignment, avoidance of any limb-length discrepancy, and good functional outcome with little cosmetic deformity.

Most pediatric tibial shaft fractures can be managed with closed treatment in a long leg cast and may require reduction depending on the amount of angulation of the fracture at the time of presentation (Figure 4). Coronal and sagittal angulation of less than 5° to 10° and less than 10° to 15° of rotation are considered acceptable. Younger children will have greater remodeling in the sagittal plane, especially when the fracture is close to the proximal or distal physis; less remodeling will occur in the coronal and rotational alignment of the fracture. Rotational alignment is difficult to assess radiographi-

cally; therefore, clinical judgment is critical, especially when applying the cast. Assessment of the thigh-foot angle can be helpful when determining rotation. A small amount of shortening is acceptable, but anything greater than 1 cm may be of concern in older adolescent patients. Forty percent of all tibial shaft fractures will have some amount of shortening. Although overgrowth after a fracture of the tibia has been reported, it is quite variable.

The indications for the surgical treatment of a tibial shaft fracture include the presence of open fractures, unstable closed fractures, fractures in a polytrauma patient, or fractures with a concomitant severe soft-tissue injury or compartment syndrome. The criteria for an acceptable reduction of a tibial shaft fracture become more stringent in patients older than 10 years; as a result, many older children may need surgical stabilization. The surgical treatment options differ in a child because of the risk of physeal injury with the use of a locked reamed intramedullary nail; therefore, treatment options include external fixation, intramedullary flexible nail fixation, and percutaneous pinning with casting.

Percutaneous pinning and casting does not provide the same rigidity as other methods of fixation. The pins should be viewed as a supplement to the cast to allow for better control at the fracture site. This technique may be more useful in younger patients when a closed reduction cannot be maintained. Typically, one or two smooth Kirschner wires are placed across the fracture site, with the size of the pin varying with the size and age of the patient. These pins are incorporated into a long leg cast and removed 4 weeks later or once callus is seen on radiographs. The presence of percutaneous pins does not allow for the patient to be treated in a short leg cast. Severe comminution and shortening or obesity would be contraindications to using this technique. Pin-tract infections may result as a complication of this technique.

External fixation can provide fairly rigid fixation of a tibial shaft fracture and provide orthopaedic surgeons with the ability to restore length when comminution and shortening are present. Use of an external fixator can also allow for care of significant soft-tissue injuries and open tibial fractures. Although simple monolateral fixators are being used more routinely for pediatric tibial shaft fractures, ring fixators may be beneficial in treating fractures closer to the physis or when postoperative correction of residual deformity is necessary. Placement of pins should be considered preoperatively with the awareness that medially placed pins may protrude and hinder the contralateral leg while walking. Laterally placed pins pierce more muscle and soft tissues and may result in more drainage. Two bicortical half pins above and below the fracture site are usually satisfactory (Figure 5), but in larger patients, three pins are necessary. Although weight-bearing status is dictated by the fracture pattern, type of construct, and soft-tissue concerns, most pediatric patients can achieve full weight bearing within 3 to 4 weeks. Dynamization of the external fixator may be necessary if a delayed union is suspected postoperatively. Pin-tract infections are a known complication when using an external fixator, and daily cleaning of the pins with warm soap and water has been found to be effective in preventing infection.

Flexible intramedullary nailing can be an excellent alternative to external fixation for pediatric tibial shaft fractures, depending on the fracture pattern. A displaced diaphyseal fracture of the tibia with minimal comminution and shortening would be ideal for intramedullary fixation. This method of fixation has a lower refracture rate and a shorter time to union when compared with external fixation. Properly placed, flexible nails typically avoid injury to the proximal tibial physis and are placed antegrade through one incision medially or through two incisions by adding a second incision laterally. Two flexible nailing constructs have been described and compared recently in the literature: a double-C construct and a C and S construct for the nails. Although the C and S construct was found to have greater biomechanical strength in the laboratory, the divergent, double-C construct remained clinically superior at maintaining tibial alignment. A cast or splint should be ap-

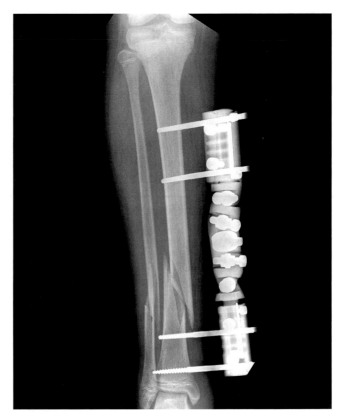

Figure 5 AP radiograph of a tibial fracture treated with external fixation.

plied after fixation with the flexible nails. The flexible nails may be left proud beneath the skin or left outside the skin for early removal in the clinic. Patients with unstable fractures should not bear weight until callus is present, whereas those with stable fractures may begin to bear partial weight after surgery.

Floating Knee

The floating knee refers to a concomitant fracture of the ipsilateral femur and tibia that is rare in children. This complex fracture is most often the result of a high-velocity injury, typically involving a child as a pedestrian or bicyclist who is struck by a motor vehicle. This mechanism of injury may result in an open fracture of at least one of the fractures or significant soft-tissue injury. The incidence of open injury has been reported in the literature to be approximately 50%.

Age has been reported to be the determining factor for treatment guidance and clinical course for floating knee injuries. In patients younger than 10 years, most fractures can be managed with closed treatment. Treatment consisting of 90-90 traction (90° of hip flexion and 90° of knee flexion) for 4 weeks followed by a one and one-half spica cast until union is achieved is recommended. While the patient is in traction, the tibial fracture should be immobilized with a short cast or splint. Open or closed reduction and internal fixation of at least the femoral fracture is recommended for children older than 10 years. Surgical treatment of the femur fractures in this age group has been shown to have fewer associated complications and better functional results. Rigid fixation of at least one of the two fractures has also been recommended to avoid complications.

Surgical stabilization of the floating knee is recommended for patients with severe head trauma, for those with severe soft-tissue injury, and when a satisfactory closed reduction of the femur or tibia cannot be achieved regardless of the patient's age.

Follow-up should continue until 18 months after the initial injury and until after skeletal maturity in younger children. Short-term and long-term complications may include peroneal nerve palsy, pin-tract infection, osteomyelitis, malunion, nonunion, ligamentous laxity of the involved knee, and limb-length discrepancies resulting from overgrowth of the bone after fracture and ipsilateral physeal arrest.

Ankle Fractures

Fractures about the ankle are relatively common injuries in children. These injuries are seen more frequently in males and most commonly occur in patients between the ages of 8 and 15 years. Pediatric ankle fractures are usually a result of indirect trauma from a twisting mechanism, although direct trauma associated with falls, contact sports, or motor vehicle collisions is not an uncommon mechanism of injury. The relative frequency of these injuries is a result, in part, to the constrained anatomic relationships and limited freedom of motion of the ankle mortise combined with the relative weakness of the physis in relationship to the strength of the surrounding ligaments. The overall prognosis of an ankle fracture in the pediatric population depends on many factors, including patient age, fracture type, overall severity of the injury, and adequacy and maintenance of reduction. Although most of these injuries are easily treated and portend a benign prognosis, certain fracture patterns, if treated improperly, may result in growth disturbances and/or long-term functional impairment.

An understanding of physeal anatomy and closure is important in the diagnosis and treatment of pediatric ankle injuries. The distal tibial physis provides 3 to 4 mm of growth annually and contributes approximately 35% to 45% of overall tibial length. Fusion of the distal tibial physis generally begins at approximately age 12 years in females and 13 years in males. This closure of the physis does not proceed uniformly, but starts centrally in the physis then proceeds in a medial to posterior direction, with the anterolateral portion of the physis being the last area to close. This process generally occurs over a period of approximately 18 months, and it is during this transitional period that certain unfused areas of the physis represent areas of relative weakness

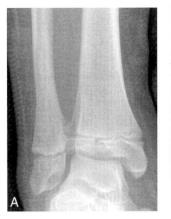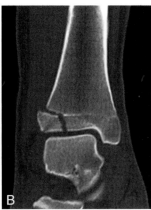

Figure 6 A, Mortise radiograph of an ankle with a transitional Tillaux fracture. **B,** Coronal CT scan of the same fracture showing intra-articular displacement.

and are prone to fracture. The anterior tibiofibular ligament can play an important role in the pathomechanics of certain fractures that occur during this adolescent transitional period.

Initial diagnostic imaging should always consist of AP, lateral, and mortise radiographs of the affected ankle. The mortise radiograph is especially important because many fractures (such as Tillaux fractures) may not be readily visualized on simple AP and lateral radiographs. In pediatric patients, accessory ossification centers are often noted on routine diagnostic imaging of the ankle, usually appear between the ages of 7 and 10 years, and eventually fuse with the secondary ossification center at skeletal maturity. On the medial side, this ossicle (the os subtibiale) can be seen in up to 20% of patients. On the lateral side, the os subfibulare is seen in approximately 1% of patients. Physical examination, contralateral radiographs, and in certain instances, bone scanning will help distinguish acute fractures from these normal anatomic variants. CT is recommended when plain radiographs show intra-articular fractures with displacement greater than 2 mm. CT allows for more accurate estimation of articular displacement, fracture mapping, and surgical planning, especially with transitional fractures (Figure 6).

Distal Tibial Fractures
Salter-Harris Type I Fractures
Salter-Harris type I fractures of the distal tibia occur through the zone of hypertrophy of the distal tibial physis. Many of these injuries are misdiagnosed as ankle sprains because no evidence of a fracture is visible on radiographs. Produced by a variety of mechanisms, these physeal injuries are more common than ligamentous injuries of the ankle because of a weaker physes and stronger surrounding ligaments (Figure 7, *A*). Although most of these fractures are usually nondisplaced, Salter-Harris type I fractures may show slight displacement of

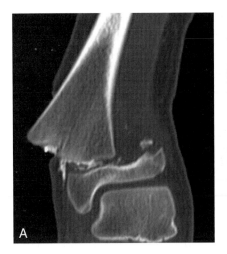
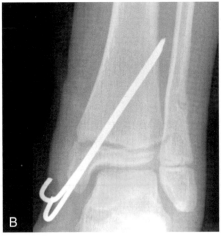
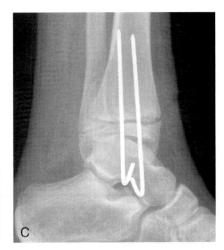

Figure 7 **A,** Radiograph of an open Salter-Harris type I fracture of the distal tibia. Postoperative AP **(B)** and lateral **(C)** radiographs of the same fracture after irrigation and débridement with open reduction and internal fixation.

the tibial epiphysis or slight widening of the tibial physis when compared with the contralateral side.

Fractures with physeal widening greater than 3 mm have been recognized to have a higher incidence of premature physeal closure. Gentle closed reduction or open reduction may be necessary for these displaced fractures, especially when the periosteum and soft tissues are interposed in the fracture and prevent anatomic reduction (Figure 7, *B* and *C*). Adequate sedation is imperative during attempted reduction to minimize any further trauma to the physis. At this point, reduced fractures should be treated in a long leg cast for 4 weeks followed by a short leg walking cast for an additional 2 weeks. Nondisplaced fractures can be treated in a short leg cast. Follow-up radiographs at 6 or 12 months should be obtained to evaluate for premature physeal closure.

Salter-Harris Type II Fractures
Salter-Harris type II fractures are the most common distal tibial physeal injuries in children. Supination with external rotation has been found to be the most common mechanism of injury. In Salter-Harris type II fractures, the fracture line extends through the physis and exits into the metaphyseal portion of the distal tibia (Figure 8), creating a metaphyseal spike of bone known as a Thurston-Holland fragment. Treatment of nondisplaced Salter-Harris type II fractures consists of immobilization in a long leg cast for 4 weeks followed by a short leg walking cast for an additional 2 weeks. Displaced Salter-Harris type II fractures require closed reduction under sedation. Flexion of the knee and plantar flexion of the ankle can be helpful when trying to reduce these fractures. In most instances, reduction with the patient under general anesthesia is preferred to ensure adequate relaxation. Any fracture that does not reduce by closed means or has more than 3 mm of physeal widening

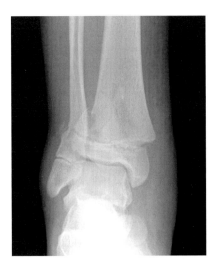

Figure 8 Radiograph of a Salter-Harris type II fracture of the distal tibia demonstrating a metaphyseal spike.

should be reduced by open means to remove any soft-tissue interposition. Once reduction has been achieved, good results can be achieved with immobilization of the fracture in a long leg cast for 4 weeks followed by an additional 2 to 3 weeks in a short leg walking cast.

Salter-Harris Type III Fractures
Salter-Harris type III fractures of the distal tibia are almost always the result of a supination inversion injury. In these injuries, the distal fibula epiphysis is avulsed as a result of the inversion stress, and the talus is then driven into the medial aspect of the distal tibial epiphysis, creating a fracture from the articular surface into the physis (Figure 9, *A*). These fractures are distinguished from Tillaux fractures by the location of the epiphyseal fragment always being medial to the midline. Nondisplaced fractures are treated similarly to Salter-Harris type I and type II fractures with long leg cast immobilization and the foot held in slight eversion for 4 weeks followed by 2 weeks in a short leg cast.

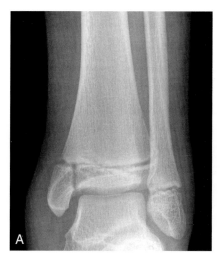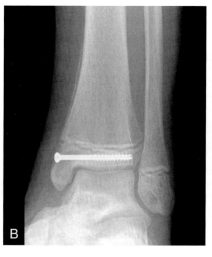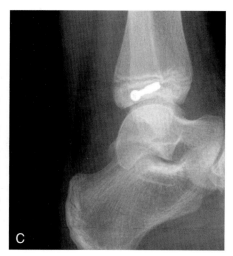

Figure 9 **A,** Preoperative mortise radiograph of a Salter-Harris type III distal tibia fracture. Postoperative mortise **(B)** and lateral **(C)** radiographs of the same Salter-Harris type III fracture treated with a compression screw.

If articular displacement is greater than 2 to 3 mm, however, the patient should be taken to the operating room for either closed or open reduction followed by screw fixation. Fixation is generally accomplished with interfragmentary compression screws placed parallel to the physis using a standard anterior or anteromedial approach to the ankle joint for direct visualization of the articular surface (Figure 9, *B* and *C*). At this point, the patient is generally placed in a short leg cast for a period of 4 to 6 weeks. In general, patients treated with open and anatomic reduction heal well, with lower incidences of angular deformity or traumatic arthritis. Nonetheless, some series have reported up to a 15% incidence of partial physeal arrest and angular deformity despite open reduction and internal fixation of these fractures.

Salter-Harris Type IV Fractures
Salter-Harris type IV fractures of the distal tibial epiphysis are extremely rare. The mechanism for Salter-Harris type IV injuries is supination and inversion (as in Salter-Harris type III fractures). Open reduction and internal fixation is the treatment of choice for all Salter-Harris type IV fractures and is generally accomplished with a standard anterior or anteromedial approach to the ankle joint. Anatomic reduction of the fracture may often be limited by the metaphyseal fragment. Anatomic reduction is essential for preventing formation of a bony bridge. After treatment of Salter-Harris type IV fractures, serial imaging of the distal tibial physis should be undertaken at 6 month intervals to evaluate for premature arrest.

Salter-Harris Type V Fractures
Salter-Harris type V fractures are extremely rare and are usually diagnosed retrospectively after the onset of

physeal arrest following trauma to the ankle with seemingly normal-appearing radiographs. Controversy exists as to whether these injuries are caused by direct axial compression of the physis or are secondary to physeal ischemia as a result of prolonged immobilization. Regardless, once diagnosed, these injuries should be further analyzed and treated in a manner similar to any other physeal arrest injury.

Transitional Fractures
Triplane Fractures
Triplane fractures are uncommon injuries that can be challenging to identify and treat. These fractures comprise less than 8% of all distal tibial physeal injuries. Triplane fractures represent external rotation injuries that occur in patients during their early adolescence.

Plain radiographs in multiple views may be necessary to identify all three fracture planes. A Salter-Harris type III fracture may be noted on the AP and mortise views of the ankle (Figure 10, *A*), whereas a Salter-Harris type II fracture may be noted on the lateral view (Figure 10, *B*). In actuality, an initial sagittal fracture line extends from the articular surface and extends into the physis. The fracture then runs transversely through the physis and eventually exits the physis by creating a coronal fracture line from the physis and out of the metaphyseal portion of the distal tibia. These resultant fracture lines generally result in either a two-part or three-part triplane fracture.

In two-part triplane fractures, the proximal tibia, medial malleolus, and anteromedial aspect of the distal tibial epiphysis form a large medial fragment, and a second lateral fragment is composed of the posterior aspect of the tibial metaphysis and the remaining anterolateral portion of the distal tibial epiphysis. In three-part triplane fractures, the medial fragment is the same as in

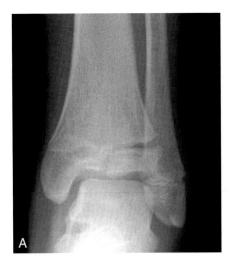
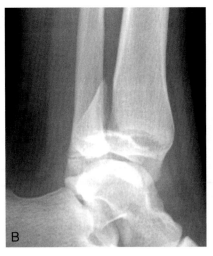
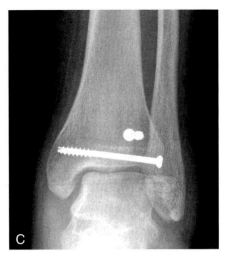

Figure 10 **A,** AP view of a triplane ankle fracture that has the appearance of a Salter-Harris type III fracture. **B,** The same triplane ankle fracture that has the appearance of a Salter-Harris type II fracture on the lateral radiograph. **C,** Postoperative AP radiograph of a triplane ankle fracture treated with open reduction and internal fixation.

a two-part triplane fracture; however, the lateral fragment is further fractioned into separate anterolateral Tillaux fragments and posterior metaphyseal fragments. Because these fractures can be difficult to diagnose and to assess three-dimensionally, CT with sagittal and coronal reconstruction images is usually indicated in any patient suspected of having a triplane fracture.

The primary goal of treatment in all triplane fractures is anatomic reduction of the articular surface. In reporting short-term and long-term follow-up on a series of triplane fractures, one study found that patients in whom less than anatomic reduction was achieved significant arthritis resulted. This was especially evident in patients with greater than 1 mm of articular displacement. The same study also reported that fractures with initial displacement greater than 3 mm were not amenable to successful closed reduction. Other studies have shown that acceptable results can be achieved if the reduction is less than 2 mm at the articular surface.

When a closed reduction is needed, the mechanism of injury should be reversed with pronation and internal rotation of the foot with the patient under adequate sedation. This is followed by immobilization in a long leg cast and no weight bearing for 4 weeks followed by a short leg cast for an additional 2 weeks. After closed reduction, CT should be performed to confirm adequate reduction of the articular surface to within 2 mm.

If an open reduction is necessary, it can be accomplished by first reducing the anterolateral epiphyseal fragment under direct visualization followed by closed manipulation of the posterior metaphyseal fragment. If this is unsuccessful, open reduction of the posterior metaphyseal fracture should be performed either through posteromedial or posterolateral exposure. Internal fixation can be performed with compression screws placed from anterior to posterior in the metaphysis, lateral to medial, and parallel to the physis in the epiphyseal fragment (Figure 10, *C*). A non–weight-bearing cast should be applied for a total of 6 weeks.

Juvenile Tillaux Fracture

The juvenile Tillaux fracture is an isolated fracture of the anterolateral epiphysis. These fractures account for approximately 3% to 5% of pediatric ankle fractures. Juvenile Tillaux fractures, in the truest sense, are Salter-Harris type III fractures. This transitional fracture occurs later in adolescence after the medial and posterior physis has closed but the anterolateral portion of the physis remains open. During this period, an external rotation applied to a supinated foot can cause an avulsion of this anterolateral fragment as the anterior tibiofibular ligament pulls on this fragment. Diagnosis is generally confirmed with standard radiography, although CT should be performed to assess intra-articular displacement (Figure 11, *A*).

Nondisplaced fractures with less than 2 mm of articular displacement can be treated with immobilization in a long leg cast for 4 weeks followed by an additional 2 weeks in a short leg cast. If this fracture is displaced more than 2 mm, closed reduction and percutaneous fixation or open reduction and internal fixation is recommended. Reduction can be accomplished by internally rotating the foot while applying direct digital pressure on the Tillaux fragment to reduce it to its original position. An open reduction, when necessary, should be performed using an anterior or anterolateral approach to the ankle joint. Fixation is accomplished with compression screws placed parallel to the physis (Figure 11, *B*); however, avoidance of the physis is not mandatory as the growth plate is essentially closed in these patients. Open reduction should be followed with a period of cast immobilization. Outcomes after treatment of juvenile

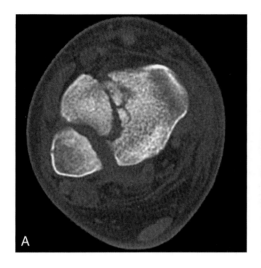

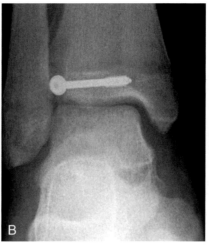

Figure 11 A, Preoperative axial CT scan of a Tillaux fracture showing intra-articular displacement. **B,** Postoperative AP radiograph of a Tillaux fracture treated with open reduction and internal fixation with a compression screw.

Tillaux fractures are generally good, and patients with anatomic reductions should be expected to have satisfactory results.

Distal Fibula Fractures

One of the most common ankle injuries in children is the isolated Salter-Harris fracture of the distal fibula. Displacement in these injuries is usually minimal, and these injuries are also often misdiagnosed as ankle sprains. Patients typically report lateral ankle pain, and examination reveals point tenderness, often with significant swelling directly overlying the physis. Distal fibula fractures are fairly simple to treat. Once diagnosed, treatment consists of a short leg cast for 3 to 4 weeks until pain in the area is relieved. These fractures typically heal uneventfully.

Occasionally, small chip or avulsion fractures may occur at the distal tip of the fibula. Although these injuries are often initially diagnosed as ankle sprains as well, when the patient returns with continued pain about the ankle, a small rounded ossicle distal to the epiphysis may be observed. Also known as an os subfibulare, in this situation the os is posttraumatic and should not be considered a normal variant. Immobilization often resolves the pain, but the ossicle rarely proceeds to union with the remainder of the distal fibula. For patients with persistently painful os subfibulare, treatment involves excision of the ossicle with ligamentous repair.

Annotated Bibliography
Tibial Fractures

Goodwin R, Gaynor T, Mahar A, Oka R, Lalonde F: Intramedullary flexible nail fixation of unstable pediatric tibial diaphyseal fractures. *J Pediatr Orthop* 2005;25(5): 570-576.

In this retrospective review of 19 patients with unstable or open tibial shaft fractures, all patients were treated with flexible intramedullary nailing using one of two implant configura-

tions (a medially inserted C and S construct or a divergent, double-C construct). Although the C and S construct was found to have greater biomechanical strength when tested in the laboratory, the divergent, double-C construct was clinically superior in maintaining tibial alignment.

Johner R, Staubli HU, Gunst M, Cordey J: The point of view of the clinician: A prospective study of the mechanism of accidents and the morphology of tibial and fibular shaft fractures. *Injury* 2000;31(suppl 3):C45-C49.

This prospective study of 210 tibial shaft fractures was designed to evaluate the biomechanics involved in the initial traumatic injury and the resultant tibial and fibular shaft fracture morphology. Twenty-two of the 210 fractures were in pediatric patients; 86 of the fractures were caused by indirect impact and had few associated soft-tissue injuries; 124 of the fractures were the result of direct impact and had a large number of associated soft-tissue injuries. In the indirect impact group, the fracture morphology consisted of short and long spiral fractures with few fibular fractures noted at a different level than the tibial fracture. Transverse or oblique segmental (or crush) fractures with a large number of fibular fractures at the level of the tibial impact were observed.

Kubiak EN, Egol K, Scher D, Wasserman B, Feldman D, Koval K: Operative treatment of tibial fractures in children: Are elastic stable intramedullary nails an improvement over external fixation? *J Bone Joint Surg Am* 2005;87(8):1761-1768.

In this retrospective review of 31 patients with surgically treated tibial shaft fractures, flexible intramedullary nailing was compared with treatment using external fixation. Patients treated with flexible nailing had better functional results than those treated with external fixation. A shorter time to union with fewer complications were reported in the patients who were treated with flexible intramedullary nailing. In this series, two patients had a delayed union, two patients developed a malunion, and three patients developed a nonunion. All seven of these patients were treated with external fixation. These authors concluded that flexible intramedullary fixation is the preferred method of fixation for this patient population.

Muller I, Muschol M, Mann M, Hassenpflug J: Results of proximal metaphyseal fractures in children. *Arch Orthop Trauma Surg* 2002;122(6):331-333.

In this retrospective review of seven children with proximal metaphyseal fractures, the authors evaluated typical treatment outcomes, valgus deformity, and leg overgrowth. They also examined spontaneous corrections and compared surgical and conservative treatments. The authors recommended open surgical treatment of children older than 5 years because of the high incidence of valgus deformity in the conservatively treated patients. For pediatric patients age 5 years and younger, they concluded that conservative treatment is acceptable because spontaneous correction of the posttraumatic angulatory deformity was found to have occurred in this age group.

Pill SG, Hamilton W, Dormans JP: Percutaneous toggle technique for manipulating displaced, unstable, and nonreducible proximal tibial fractures in children. *Am J Orthop* 2003;32(3):156-157.

A percutaneous technique to stabilize and reduce a pediatric proximal tibial metaphyseal fracture is explained. The toggle technique offers a simple, percutaneous approach using a Kirschner wire to lever the proximal and distal fragments; thereby decreasing the need for open reduction. The opposing fragments are aligned by inserting a guide pin percutaneously to manipulate the proximal and distal segments in preparation for percutaneous Kirschner-wire stabilization. A long leg cast is applied. The authors report that this approach provides a much lower risk of physis damage in this pediatric population.

Yue JJ, Churchill RS, Cooperman DR, et al: The floating knee in the pediatric patient: Nonoperative versus operative stabilization. *Clin Orthop Relat Res* 2000;376:124-136.

The authors conducted a retrospective review of 29 pediatric patients who were treated for ipsilateral femur and tibia fractures. Sixteen patients were treated nonsurgically with traction and spica casting, and 13 were treated surgically with fixation of both fractures. The surgical patients were found to have a decreased length of stay in the hospital and a decreased time to unassisted weight bearing on the injured leg. The younger patients in this study (those younger than 9 years) were found to have an increased rate of angular malunion and limb-length discrepancy and required second surgery when treated nonsurgically. Based on these findings, the authors recommended surgical stabilization of both fractures in these patients.

Ankle Fractures

Barmada A, Gaynor T, Mubarak SJ: Premature physeal closure following distal tibia physeal fractures: A new radiographic predictor. *J Pediatr Orthop* 2003;23(6):733-739.

In this study, 44 Salter-Harris type I and type II fractures occurring between 1991 and 2000 were retrospectively reviewed with at least 1 year of follow-up or until physiologic closure of the growth plates. Postreduction radiographs of Salter-Harris type I and type II distal tibial physeal fractures were reviewed, and the amount of residual physeal widening or gapping was recorded. In fractures with more than 3 mm of physeal widening postreduction, the incidence of premature physeal closure increased to 60%; if no gap was present, the incidence decreased to 17%. Open reduction was performed in nine Salter-Harris type II fractures that had a residual gap. Five of these patients had interposed periosteum removed from the physis at the time of surgery. None of these five patients developed premature physeal closure. The authors concluded that anatomic reduction appears to decrease the incidence of physeal closure and interposed periosteum or soft tissue appears to play an important role in preventing reduction and subsequent premature physeal closure.

Brown SD, Kasser JR, Zurakowski D, Jaramillo D: Analysis of 51 tibial triplane fractures using CT with multiplanar reconstruction. *AJR Am J Roentgenol* 2004;183:1489-1495.

The authors of this article reviewed 51 children with triplane ankle fractures who underwent CT and multiplanar reconstruction of the fracture. The classic two-part triplane fracture was found to be the most common fracture pattern in the series. Fractures involving the medial malleolus and distal fibula were found to occur more commonly than had previously been recognized in patients with triplane fractures. The authors concluded that CT with reconstruction greatly facilitates in the assessment of the pattern of injury in triplane fractures.

Jones S, Phillips N, Ali F, Fernandes JA, Flowers MJ, Smith TWD: Triplane fractures of the distal tibia requiring open reduction and internal fixation: Pre-operative planning using computer tomography. *Injury* 2003;34:293-298.

In this study, 10 orthopaedic surgeons were given conventional radiographs of displaced triplane fractures and asked to plan the appropriate position and direction of interfragmentary compression screws. They were later provided with CT scans of the same fracture and asked to again plan the placement and direction of similar screws. The authors found that all surgeons polled changed the position and direction of their proposed compression screws after reviewing the CT scans, thus underscoring the importance of prereduction CT scans for fracture mapping and surgical planning in an attempt to achieve a more anatomic reduction.

Lohman M, Kivisaari A, Kallio P, Puntila J, Vehmas T, Kivisaari L: Acute paediatric ankle trauma: MRI versus plain radiology. *Skeletal Radiol* 2001;30(9):504-511.

Over a 3-year period, 60 consecutive children (age 8 to 16 years) who were evaluated and diagnosed with either an acute lateral ligament tear or a physeal fracture were subsequently evaluated with plain radiography and MRI (MRI was used as the gold standard for radiographic diagnosis). All radiographic images were then reviewed by three blinded radiologists, and the fracture classification and diagnosis obtained from plain radiographs and MRI scans were then compared. Although a small percentage of minor injuries were misdiagnosed using conventional radiography, the authors were unable to identify any instance in which the treatment or prognosis based on plain radiographs should have been significantly altered after having done a routine MRI examination.

Classic Bibliography

Blake R, McBryde AM Jr: The floating knee: Ipsilateral fractures of the femur and tibia. *South Med J* 1975; 68(1):13-16.

Bohn WW, Durbin MD: Ipsilateral fractures of the femur and tibia in children and adolescents. *J Bone Joint Surg Am* 1991;73(3):429-439.

Briggs TW, Orr MM, Lightowler CD: Isolated tibial fractures in children. *Injury* 1992;23(5):308-310.

Buckley SL, Smith G, Sponseller PD, Thompson JD, Griffin PP: Open fractures of the tibia in children. *J Bone Joint Surg Am* 1990;72(10):1462-1469.

Caterini R, Farsetti P, Ippolito E: Long-term followup of physeal injury to the ankle. *Foot Ankle* 1991;11(6):372-383.

Cullen MC, Roy DR, Crawford AH, Assenmacher J, Levy MS, Wen D: Open fracture of the tibia in children. *J Bone Joint Surg Am* 1996;78(7):1039-1047.

de Sanctis N, Della Corte S, Pempinello C: Distal tibial and fibular epiphyseal fractures in children: Prognostic criteria and long-term results in 158 patients. *J Pediatr Orthop B* 2000;9(1):40-44.

Ertl JP, Barrack RL, Alexander AH, VanBuecken K: Triplane fracture of the distal tibial epiphysis: Long-term follow-up. *J Bone Joint Surg Am* 1988;70(7):967-976.

Hope PG, Cole WG: Open fractures of the tibia in children. *J Bone Joint Surg Br* 1992;74(4):546-553.

Jackson DW, Cozen L: Genu valgum as a complication of proximal tibial metaphyseal fractures in children. *J Bone Joint Surg Am* 1971;53(8):1571-1578.

Karrholm J, Hansson LI, Selvik G: Changes in tibiofibular relationships due to growth disturbances after ankle fractures in children. *J Bone Joint Surg Am* 1984;66(8):1198-1210.

Karrholm J, Hansson LI, Svensson K: Incidence of tibiofibular shaft and ankle fractures in children. *J Pediatr Orthop* 1982;2(4):386-396.

Kling TF Jr, Bright RW, Hensinger RN: Distal tibial physeal fractures in children that may require open reduction. *J Bone Joint Surg Am* 1984;66(5):647-657.

Kreder HJ, Armstrong P: The review of open tibia fractures in children. *J Pediatr Orthop* 1995;15(4):482-488.

Letts M, Vincent N, Gouw G: The "floating knee" in children. *J Bone Joint Surg Br* 1986;68(3):442-446.

McCarthy JJ, Kim DH, Eilert RE: Posttraumatic genu valgum: Operative versus nonoperative treatment. *J Pediatr Orthop* 1998;18(4):518-521.

Ogden JA, Ogden DA, Pugh L, Raney EM, Guidera KJ: Tibia valga after proximal metaphyseal fractures in childhood: A normal biologic response. *J Pediatr Orthop* 1995;15(4):489-494.

Robert M, Khouri N, Carlioz H, Alain JL: Fractures of the proximal tibial metaphysis in children: Review of a series of 25 cases. *J Pediatr Orthop* 1987;7(4):444-449.

Robertson P, Karol LA, Rab GT: Open fractures of the tibia and femur in children. *J Pediatr Orthop* 1996;16(5):621-626.

Salter RB, Best TN: Pathogenesis of progressive valgus deformity following fractures of the proximal metaphyseal region of the tibia in young children. *Instr Course Lect* 1992;41:409-411.

Shannak AO: Tibial fractures in children: Follow-up study. *J Pediatr Orthop* 1988;8(3):306-310.

Song KM, Sangeorzan B, Benirschke S, Browne R: Open fractures of the tibia in children. *J Pediatr Orthop* 1996;16(5):635-639.

Stefanich RJ, Lozman J: The juvenile fracture of Tillaux. *Clin Orthop Relat Res* 1986;210:219-227.

Templeton PA, Farrar MJ, Williams HR, Bruguera J, Smith RM: Complications of tibial shaft soccer fractures. *Injury* 2000;31:415-419.

Tuten HR, Keeler KA, Gabos PG, Zionts LE, Mackenzie WG: Posttraumatic tibia valga in children: A long-term follow-up note. *J Bone Joint Surg Am* 1999;81(6):799-810.

Yang JP, Letts RM: Isolated fractures of the tibia with intact fibula in children: A review of 95 patients. *J Pediatr Orthop* 1997;17(3):347-351.

Chapter 24

Injuries of the Shoulder, Elbow, and Forearm

Peter M. Waters, MD

Upper extremity injuries are commonplace in skeletally immature children. Upper extremity injuries predominantly occur secondary to a fall onto an outstretched arm and most commonly in the supracondylar region of the distal humerus. Other elbow region injuries are less common, but still require anatomic, stable reduction. Forearm fractures occur frequently in growing children; proximal forearm injuries are less common but often problematic. This chapter reviews the principles of treatment of injuries from the shoulder region to the elbow and provides an update on clinical information.

Shoulder Injuries

Clavicular Fractures and Dislocations

Sternoclavicular dislocations and medial clavicular fractures are rare. Posterior fractures or dislocations are of concern for associated tracheal, esophageal, and/or major vessel compression in the mediastinum. In patients with these injuries, plain radiographs are often difficult to interpret; therefore, CT scans are recommended for diagnosis (Figure 1). Closed reduction under careful scrutiny for vascular compromise has been traditionally recommended. Because of concerns about recurrent instability after closed reduction, open reduction of these injuries has recently been advised. A direct anterior approach is used, and reduction of the posteriorly displaced fracture or dislocation is performed under direct visualization. Open suture repair of the medial clavicle to the sternum provides an anatomic, stable reduction (Figure 2).

Diaphyseal clavicle fractures are the most common injury to the clavicle. Standard treatment is brief immobilization in a sling or figure-of-8 dressing. Rapid healing in 3 to 6 weeks is expected with restoration of full motion, function, and strength in most pediatric patients. Remodeling of the malunited fracture is anticipated if there is sufficient growth remaining. In adults, the concerns regarding malunion, nonunion, and refracture has led to recent enthusiasm for open reduction and internal fixation for comminuted or markedly displaced fractures. Techniques include standard compres-

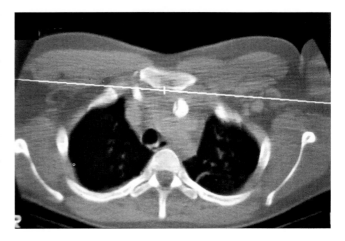

Figure 1 CT scan showing posterior dislocation with a posterior dislocation of the medial clavicle compressing the mediastinal structures.

sion plating and intraosseous screw fixation. Early results are promising, but precise indications and long-term results are still unknown. The applicability of these techniques to adolescent patients is still unclear, but there may be a role for open treatment of severe fractures in older adolescents.

Shoulder Region and Humeral Shaft Injuries

Proximal humerus fractures are either physeal or metaphyseal injuries. Most commonly, Salter-Harris type I and type II injuries occur, predominantly in adolescents. Physeal separations have been described in neonates, and ultrasound or MRI is usually diagnostic. Up to 80% of the growth of the humerus comes from the proximal physeal region. The glenohumeral joint has near universal motion, which leads to tremendous remodeling potential in any physeal fracture if there is sufficient growth remaining. Thus, closed treatment in a sling and swathe is recommended for nearly all pediatric patients with metaphyseal and physeal fractures of the proximal humerus. Malunions are rare and generally secondary to markedly displaced fractures in the near skeletally mature adolescent. Closed reduction and pin fixation is

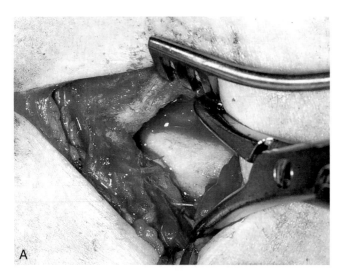

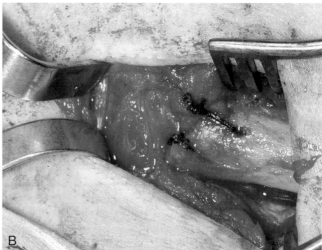

Figure 2 **A,** Intraoperative photograph of a posterior sternoclavicular fracture-dislocation. **B,** Intraoperative photograph showing open reduction of transosseous suture repair of the same patient.

usually not recommended unless there is greater than 40° of malalignment, expected acromial impingement with combined abduction-forward flexion, and insufficient growth remaining to remodel the malunion. Techniques for fixation include percutaneous fixation (Figure 3), retrograde flexible intramedullary nail fixation, or open reduction and internal fixation. A clear indication for open reduction and internal fixation is an entrapped biceps tendon in the fracture site.

Humeral shaft fractures in children are rarely treated with open reduction. Shoulder and elbow function does not appear to be affected by up to 40° of malalignment in this patient population. Because remodeling occurs in pediatric patients, the standard treatment is immobilization in a sling and swathe, hanging cast, or compressive brace. These fractures generally heal without complication. Open reduction is reserved for the rare polytrauma patient, patients with open injuries, or those with a neurovascularly compromised limb. The two remaining issues that should be considered in pediatric patients with humeral shaft fractures are the possibility of child abuse and treatment of associated radial nerve injuries. Child abuse is an unfortunate reality, and humerus fractures in children younger than 3 years may be associated with abuse. If there is an inconsistent history of injury, delay in presentation for care, or associated injuries in children younger than 3 years with a humerus fracture, additional investigation into possible abuse is warranted. Most radial nerve injuries associated with a humerus fracture are secondary to contusion from the displaced fracture. Patients with fractures at the junction of the middle and distal third (Holstein-Lewis fractures) are more likely to have an associated radial nerve injury. Entrapment of the radial nerve in the fracture is rare. Almost all associated radial nerve injuries in pediatric patients can be treated conserva-

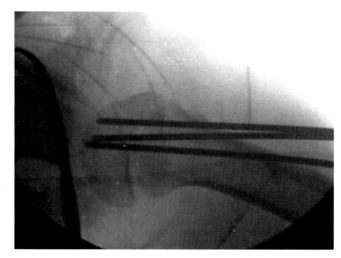

Figure 3 Radiograph of the percutaneous pinning technique of a displaced proximal humerus physeal fracture.

tively with observation, and full recovery should be expected. If the radial nerve fails to recover within 3 to 4 months, electrodiagnostic studies and surgical exploration are warranted.

Elbow Injuries

Fractures about the elbow require precise evaluation and treatment. Knowledge of the sequence, timing, and appearance of the secondary ossification centers about the elbow is imperative for proper diagnosis of any injury about the elbow. The order of ossification may be abbreviated as CRMTOL, which stands for capitellum, radial head, medial epicondyle, trochlea, olecranon, and lateral epicondyle. If it is difficult to distinguish a secondary center of ossification or vagaries of ossification from a fracture, contralateral radiographs of the elbow, ultrasound, arthrography, or MRI may be necessary to avoid missing a displaced articular fracture.

Lateral Condylar Fractures

Lateral condylar fractures of the distal humerus involve the physis and the articular surface. Anatomic alignment and healing should be the goal of treatment of all lateral condyle fractures. Truly nondisplaced fractures are at low risk for displacement in a cast; however, even minimally displaced (< 2 mm) fractures can progress to wider diastasis at the fracture site and result in a nonunion. Any nondisplaced or minimally displaced lateral condylar fracture treated in a cast must be carefully monitored to avoid loss of articular and physeal alignment.

Most lateral condylar fractures require surgical reduction and stabilization. These fractures are classified by degree of displacement in terms of malangulation, malrotation and the site of fracture propagation through the distal humeral articular surface (medial or lateral to capitellar trochlear groove). Fractures with more than 2 mm of displacement but no malrotation can be treated with closed reduction and percutaneous pin fixation. Arthrography can be used to confirm articular congruity with reduction and pinning. However, most lateral condylar fractures require open reduction and internal fixation. Surgical dissection is a direct lateral approach over the fracture. The subcutaneous dissection to the fracture is made by following the fracture hematoma and disrupted soft tissues. Care is taken to avoid posterior or distal soft-tissue dissection that would disrupt the blood supply to the lateral crista of the trochlea. Careful anterior exposure of the joint and fracture site is used to assess anatomic reduction. Two or three lateral entry pins are used to maintain reduction until healing. The pins are generally removed at 3 to 6 weeks when the fracture is healed (Figure 4).

Growth arrest or joint degeneration is unexpected with anatomic reduction. Lateral spur formation is commonplace and usually remodels over time. The lateral spur can give the appearance of an apparent malunion. Cubitus varus can occur with malunion, lateral column overgrowth, or trochlear osteonecrosis and undergrowth. The most common severe complication is nonunion from a displaced fracture that is not adequately reduced and stabilized. Delayed unions are treated with reduction, pin fixation, and bone grafting if necessary. Late presenting nonunions are more problematic, particularly if there is marked displacement. Treatment of this problem is controversial, but it usually involves in situ fixation and bone grafting to avoid osteonecrosis of the lateral condylar fragment. Secondary osteotomy to correct a valgus deformity is performed only if necessary and usually requires concomitant transposition of

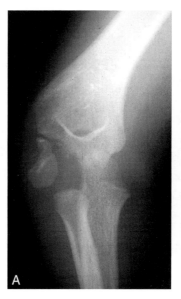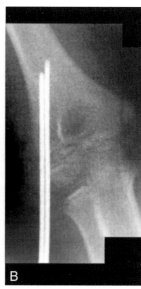

Figure 4 A, Radiograph of a displaced lateral condyle fracture that requires open reduction and internal fixation. **B,** Postoperative radiograph shows that reduction and pinning has been performed.

the ulnar nerve. Ideally, these complications are avoided by accurate diagnosis, anatomic reduction, and stabilization.

Medial Epicondyle Fractures and Elbow Dislocations

Medial epicondylar fractures are usually secondary to excessive valgus stress, which can be caused by a fall on an outstretched arm in valgus or an avulsion fracture from a baseball pitcher throwing hard. The flexor-pronator muscle mass of the forearm and wrist originates in part from the medial epicondyle and is a factor in fracture displacement and affects methods of closed reduction. A high incidence of medial epicondylar fractures has been reported in association with elbow dislocations (60% of patients). The major concern in patients with this type of injury is entrapment of the medial epicondyle in the joint. This potential complication needs to be assessed in all elbow dislocations.

Surgical treatment of medial epicondylar fractures is controversial (Figure 5). Nondisplaced fractures can be treated with immobilization until healed, followed by rehabilitation until patients regain full motion and strength. Care should be taken to avoid prolonged immobilization because of the risk of elbow flexion contracture. Pitchers with avulsion injuries require restoration of full strength and may need to alter pitching techniques to avoid recurrent valgus overload problems at the elbow. Patients with isolated displaced fractures, even those with more than 5 mm of displacement, may be functional long-term with a fibrous union or nonunion. Thus, the only clear indication for surgical treatment of a displaced medial epicondylar fracture is entrapment in the joint. The medial epicondylar fragment

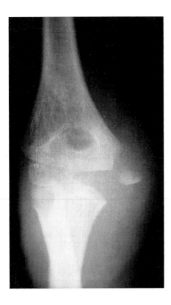

Figure 5 Radiograph of a displaced medial epicondylar fracture. Treatment for this injury is nonsurgical unless repetitive stress is anticipated.

is carefully extracted from the joint while protecting the ulnar nerve. Fixation is with smooth pins or compressive screw depending on the patient's age. Protected early mobilization is used to avoid long-term contracture problems.

Fractures with more than 5 mm of displacement in patients who participate in repetitive valgus stress activities (gymnastics and pitching) may be treated with open reduction and internal fixation. Again, care must be taken to protect the ulnar nerve with exposure. Anatomic reduction in the sulcus is necessary to avoid loss of motion postoperatively. Rigid internal fixation with a compression screw is used to allow early protected mobilization. When the medial epicondylar fragment is small, screw fixation needs to be of appropriate size so as to not break the fragment or smooth, smaller pins are necessary for fixation.

Elbow dislocations occur with a hyperextension force at the elbow. Associated fractures include not only the medial epicondyle, but also the radial head, lateral condyle, olecranon, and coronoid process. These fractures must be identified and treated appropriately. Missed displaced intra-articular chondral or osteochondral fractures can lead to long-term complications and poor outcomes. Congruency of the joint must be ensured with reduction. If there is doubt, MRI or arthrography is necessary to evaluate joint and bony alignment. Prompt treatment of any associated displaced fractures or entrapped chondral or bony fragments is necessary for successful treatment of complex fracture-dislocations about the elbow.

Elbow dislocations are classified by the direction of displacement. Most are posterolateral. Closed reduction with the patient under sedation is the treatment of choice. Hyperextension must not occur with reduction to avoid entrapment of the median nerve and/or brachial artery. Longitudinal traction and flexion will reduce the uncomplicated dislocation. Early protected motion is recommended to prevent long-term stiffness.

Ulnar neuropathy occurs in approximately 10% of patients with dislocations and commonly resolves spontaneously. Although entrapment of the nerve in the joint is rare, it can occur with an entrapped medial epicondylar fragment. Persistent median neuropathy can be indicative of an entrapped median nerve. Marked loss of motion, severe pain, and median neuropathy almost always indicate an entrapped nerve. The sooner the entrapped nerve is recognized and surgically treated, the better the long-term outcome. Marked delay in treatment requires resection of the fibrotic segment of the nerve and grafting.

Heterotopic ossification and a minor loss of motion are common. Flexion contractures beyond 30° are uncommon. Marked loss of motion may require a secondary surgical release if therapy and bracing fail to improve the range of motion. The best results for improved range of motion have occurred with highly motivated patients, extensive surgical release, and extensive rehabilitation, including the use of continuous passive motion.

Late instability is rare. In children, most late instability is the result of nonunion of chondral attachment of the posterolateral ligamentous complex. Soft-tissue laxity is also rare. In either instance, repair of the posterolateral complex is appropriate.

Supracondylar Humerus Fractures

Supracondylar fractures of the humerus have a relatively high rate of complications compared with other pediatric fractures. Precise treatment is necessary to prevent malunions and permanent neurovascular injuries, especially Volkmann's ischemic necrosis and contracture. Simple nondisplaced fractures may be diagnosed by local tenderness on clinical examination and radiographically by an elevated posterior fat pad sign. Displaced fractures are typically apparent on radiographs and are classified by the direction and degree of displacement. Most fractures displace in extension, either posterolaterally or posteromedially. Flexion injuries are far less common. The degree of displacement often indicates the risk of neurovascular compromise and the amount of instability requiring specific pin fixation. Type I supracondylar humerus fractures are nondisplaced and stable and are treated with short-term immobilization. Type II fractures are displaced with an intact cortical hinge and are treated with closed reduction and lateral pin fixation. Type III fractures are completely displaced and have a high rate of neurovascular compromise. Open fractures occur rarely in this subgroup. These fractures need to be treated urgently with closed reduction and either medial and lateral or widely divergent lateral pin fixation. Emergent treatment is necessary for any fracture with vascular compromise, open fractures, patients with worsening pain, or those with neurologic status that is indicative of a pending compartment syndrome.

Prereduction clinical examination in this patient population requires a thorough neurologic examination and documentation of results. Although these patients experience pain and anxiety as a result of the injury, it is usually possible, even in young children, to conduct an accurate motor function examination. Testing of the median nerve function is by thenar opposition for intrinsic innervation, and flexor pollicus longus and flexor digitorum profundus to the index finger is used to assess anterior interosseous function. Radial nerve extrinsic motor function is evident by metacarpophalangeal joint extension, wrist extension, and thumb interphalangeal joint extension. Ulnar nerve extrinsic motor function is assessed by testing the patient's ability to move the flexor digitorum profundus to the small finger, and intrinsic function is assessed by testing abduction of the index finger by the first dorsal interosseous muscle. It is imperative to accurately assess and record neurologic function preoperatively and postoperatively. The inability to obtain an accurate examination should be recorded as such in the patient's chart. The clinical dilemma of treatment of a postoperative nerve injury is made more challenging by inadequate or inaccurate preoperative nerve examination. Most nerve injuries are secondary to contusion and traction ischemia from the displaced fracture. The nerve injury, therefore, correlates with the direction and degree of displacement. Radial nerve injuries are associated with posteromedial displacement. Median nerve injuries, especially those of the anterior interosseous nerve, are associated with posterolateral displacement. Ulnar nerve injuries are associated with flexion type fractures. Assessment of vascular integrity is critical for all displaced fractures. An avascular limb is a surgical emergency. Many type III supracondylar humerus fractures will tent the anterior skin and have associated bruising and ecchymosis. However, approximately 1% of fractures will be open, and it is critical to make this diagnosis acutely and treat such injuries emergently.

Radiographs of nondisplaced supracondylar humerus fractures usually reveal a positive posterior fat pad sign. Displaced fractures will have an altered relationship between the capitellar secondary center of ossification and the distal humerus above the fracture. On the AP radiograph, this will be an altered Baumann's angle (between the lateral condylar physis and the long axis of the distal humerus) (Figure 6). On the lateral radiograph, the anterior humeral line will no longer pass through the middle region of the capitellum. With marked displacement, the fracture becomes obvious, although at times the radiographs may be suboptimal be-

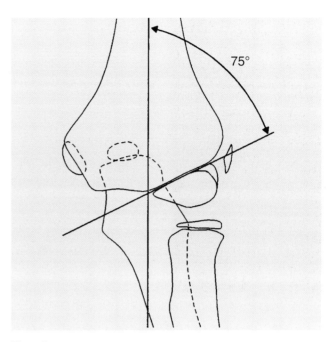

Figure 6 Schematic representation of the measurement of Baumann's angle to assess alignment for displaced supracondylar humerus fractures. *(Reproduced with permission from Lins RE, Waters PM: Fractures and dislocations about the elbow, in Gupta A, Kay S, Schemer LR: The Growing Hand: Diagnosis and Management of the Upper Extremity in Children. St. Louis, MO, Mosby, 2000, p 547.)*

cause of the inability to obtain true AP and lateral views. More accurate preoperative plain radiographs or intraoperative fluoroscopic images should be obtained before reduction attempts to assess fracture type, degree of comminution, extension of fracture lines into the joint, or associated fractures.

Any displaced supracondylar humerus fracture requires surgical reduction and stabilization with pin fixation. Cast immobilization or hospital traction is rarely used to treat these injuries because of the increased associated risk of malunion, neurovascular compromise, and the high cost of traction. Reductions are done in the operating room with the patient under anesthesia. Reduction of the common extension fracture is performed by distraction in slight flexion followed by correction of the varus or valgus malalignment and flexion with pronation and pressure on the olecranon process to correct the extension deformity. Some posterolaterally displaced fractures require supination for reduction and stability. Some fractures have entrapped brachialis musculature preventing reduction. Usually the skin is puckered over the fracture site. Manipulating the brachialis by "milking" it distally is usually successful in extracting it away from the metaphyseal spike. Reduction is maintained for lateral pin fixation with greater than 120° of flexion and appropriate forearm rotation. Anatomic reduction is required before pin fixation.

Pin fixation for type II supracondylar humerus fractures is usually done with two lateral pins. Entry is percutaneous in the lateral condylar region. Ideally, the

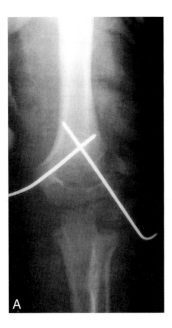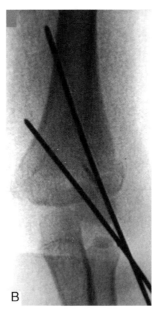

Figure 7 Radiographs of a crossed medial and lateral pin technique **(A)** and a lateral pin divergent pin technique **(B)** for the treatment of a displaced type II supracondylar fracture.

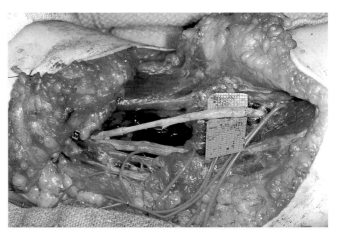

Figure 8 Intraoperative photograph of a vein graft repair of disrupted brachial artery associated with a type III displaced supracondylar fracture.

pins are placed divergently from distal to proximal. Bicortical fixation of each pin is desired for stability. Pins crossing the olecranon fossa provide more rotational stability and do not appear to result in long-term elbow stiffness. In type III supracondylar humerus fractures, there is debate regarding the use of lateral entry pins and crossed medial and lateral pins (Figure 7). Laboratory data indicate that crossed medial and lateral pins are more stable. Clinical data indicate that two or three lateral entry divergently placed pins may provide equivalent stability to medially and laterally crossed pins and do not pose the risk of ulnar nerve injury associated with medial pin placement. If medial pins are used, they should be placed after lateral pin placement with the elbow at 90° of flexion or less to reduce the risk of injury to a subluxatable or dislocatable nerve in pediatric patients. A recent prospective, randomized single-center clinical trial did not reveal any differences in outcome with medial and lateral pins versus lateral entry divergently placed pin fixation. Additionally, no ulnar nerve injuries occurred with the use medial pins.

Splint or cast immobilization is used in patients who undergo pinning for 3 to 4 weeks. The pins are removed on an outpatient basis without the use of anesthesia. Long-term motion and function is usually normal in patients without complications.

A child with an avascular limb represents a surgical emergency. The site of vascular impairment is typically at the site of the displaced fracture. The brachial artery is usually tented over the metaphyseal fragment and tethered by the supratrochlear branch. Most of the fractures with vascular impairment are posterolaterally dis-

placed and associated with median neuropathy. Immediate reduction of the fracture is necessary to lessen the risk of a compartment syndrome. In most fractures (80% to 90%), the vascularity to the hand will be restored by reduction; however, some limbs may still be without arterial flow after reduction. In such situations, there is typically persistent kinking of the artery or fascial or bony entrapment. Immediate surgical exploration is necessary. An extended Henry approach can be used, or experienced surgeons can use a transverse medial incision directly over the fracture. Once the site of impairment is identified, restoration of vascularity may require vein grafting of an entrapped damaged vessel (Figure 8).

Most nerve injuries noted associated with the fracture recover spontaneously within 6 to 12 weeks. Complete recovery is expected within 3 to 6 months. Nerve entrapment in the fracture site is rare, but nerves that do not show signs of significant recovery by 3 months are at risk for permanent loss of function because of entrapment. Pediatric patients with these symptoms should be referred at 3 months for consultation regarding nerve exploration, decompression, and possible nerve grafting.

Patients with ulnar nerve injuries associated with medial pinning (approximately 3% of patients) or those with nerves that were clearly functional preoperatively and nonfunctional postoperatively require immediate exploration. The ulnar nerve is explored, and the site of impairment from the medial pin is resolved, which usually requires pin removal and replacement with a new medial or lateral pin. Emergent exploration of a median or radial nerve requires accurate comparative clinical examinations preoperatively and postoperatively. The preoperative examination, however, is often too substandard to define the nerve that is truly entrapped by reduction maneuvers.

Malunion still occurs in association with this type of fracture, most commonly because of inadequate reduction and/or stabilization. True growth arrest is reportable. Corrective osteotomy for the marked cubitus varus deformity is performed in the supracondylar region with a lateral closing wedge or dome technique. As with acute fractures, stable fixation postoperatively is necessary for a successful outcome.

T Condylar Fractures

Intra-articular fractures of the distal humerus commonly occur in adolescents as the result of a fall. The fracture patterns are similar to those in adults, with T or Y intercondylar displacement; however, there usually is less articular comminution. Open fractures occur more commonly with intra-articular fractures of the distal humerus than with supracondylar fractures, with a peak incidence in patients 5 to 7 years of age. Most of these fractures, regardless of patient age, have articular displacement and require reduction and stabilization. Rarely, the patient is young enough and the displacement mild enough that closed reduction and percutaneous pin fixation can be used. Most patients require open reduction and internal fixation. Surgical approaches include triceps splitting, Bryan-Morrey elevation of the triceps mechanism off the olecranon, or an olecranon osteotomy. Because there is limited articular comminution in this patient population, triceps splitting and the Bryan-Morrey elevation provide adequate visualization for joint reduction and stabilization. Each technique resulted in similar triceps strength and range-of-motion outcomes in published studies. Olecranon osteotomy is reserved generally for more patients with severe articular injuries (or for surgeon preference). In all three types of exposure, the ulnar nerve is decompressed and transposed if necessary for fixation methods. Transarticular screw fixation is used to reduce and stabilize the joint. Bicolumn fixation is necessary for rotational control of fracture (Figure 9). In younger children, smaller plates may be required. The adult principles of anatomic joint reduction and stabilization with an intercondylar screw followed by reduction and stabilization of the columns are adhered to in the treatment of these fractures in adolescent patients. Postoperative rehabilitation is essential to a successful outcome. Continuous passive motion machines have been used successfully to maximize outcomes.

Although ulnar neuropathy is not unusual in patients with this type of fracture, it generally resolves spontaneously. In patients with a preoperative ulnar neuropathy, decompression and transposition is recommended to avoid further traction on the nerve during surgery. Long-term loss of motion, usually minor (< 30°), is the most common complication; however, more marked contractures may require hardware re-

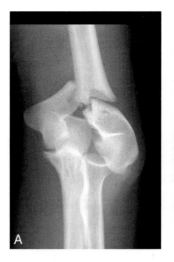
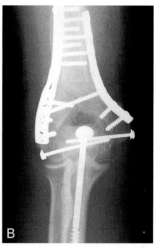

Figure 9 **A,** Preoperative radiograph of a displaced T condylar humerus fracture. **B,** Postoperative radiograph shows that the fracture was treated with open reduction and internal fixation of both columns and a transarticular screw. In this patient, an olecranon osteotomy was used for surgical exposure.

moval and extensive elbow contracture releases. Careful patient selection and postoperative rehabilitation are important for this procedure. In one series, the average improvement in postoperative flexion-extension gain with extensive contracture release and postoperative continuous passive motion was 53°.

Proximal Radius and Ulna Fractures

The elbow joint consists of the radiocapitellar, ulnotrochlear, and radioulnar articulations. Maintaining the congruency and stability of these articular surfaces and joints is paramount to the treatment of any fracture in this region. The annular ligament provides stability to the radioulnar joint, the radiocapitellar joint, and the lateral collateral ligamentous complex. Maintaining and/or restoring the integrity of the annular ligament is key to the treatment of proximal radial fracture-dislocations. The radial neck in young children has a normal valgus alignment, which is important to understand in the interpretation of acceptable fracture reductions of the head and neck of the radius in the pediatric population.

Forearm Injuries

Radial Head and Neck Fractures

Fractures of the proximal radius are usually either metaphyseal or physeal (Salter-Harris type II) fractures of the neck. Intra-articular fractures are rare in skeletally immature patients, but they can occur in adolescents. These fractures are usually secondary to a valgus stress fall. Associated injuries, such as an elbow dislocation, olecranon fracture, or medial epicondylar fracture, may occur that affect treatment decisions. Controversy exists regarding the acceptable alignment of a radial head or neck fracture. Most authors agree, however, that up to 30° of malalignment and one third displacement may be acceptable in a radial neck fracture. Ultimately, the restoration of forearm rotation, elbow flexion-extension arc without pain, and joint congruency with healing are the determinants of an acceptable reduction. Fortunately, most fractures with less than 30° malalignment and sufficient growth remaining will remodel. Fractures with greater than 30° of malalignment should be reduced. This may be done in the emergency setting with the patient under conscious sedation or in the operating room with the patient under general anesthesia.

Several methods of closed reduction are used to treat this type of fracture. In extension, varus stress is applied to disengage the fracture. Lateral thumb pressure is then applied to the displaced head and neck fragments. Forearm rotation is used to maneuver the fragment into alignment. In flexion, thumb pressure is applied anteriorly over the displaced proximal radius. Pronation of the forearm reduces the fragment. When the fracture is too displaced, impacted, or unstable for these closed maneuvers, percutaneous reduction should be performed. Fluoroscopy is used to isolate the fracture, and a smooth pin is placed against the radial head to push it back into place. The pin entry should be posterior enough to avoid injury to the posterior interosseous nerve. If the fracture is impacted, the pin can be placed into the fracture site to lever the reduction. Forearm rotation aids in the reduction and allows the surgeon to assess alignment and stability after reduction.

Another percutaneous treatment method is the intramedullary method advocated by Metaizeau. A thin (1.4- to 1.8-mm) smooth wire with a curved tip is placed from the distal radial metaphysis proximally into the radial neck. The tip of the pin is used to reduce the head and neck fragment. The wire is left in until fracture healing and then removed.

Rarely, the fracture is too unstable or displaced for closed and percutaneous reduction maneuvers. Open reduction is performed cautiously in such instances. There is clearly a higher rate of osteonecrosis and nonunion with open reduction. Loss of motion and poorer outcomes have also been associated with open reduction. A selection bias may affect these results, however, in that only patients with the most severe fractures undergo open reduction. Nonetheless, care must be taken to avoid additional devascularization of the fragment. Fixation is performed with an interosseous technique or pin fixation from the posterolateral corner of the articular surface. The fixation should not violate the ulna to lessen the risk of radioulnar synostosis. After open reduction, the pins should not be removed until healing occurs to avoid nonunion (Figure 10).

Most displaced radial head and neck fractures occur secondary to a valgus stress. Rarely, the displacement

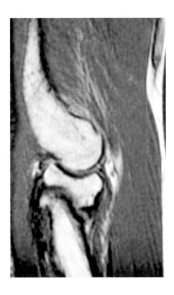

Figure 10 Lateral MRI scan of a radial neck nonunion of a fracture that was treated with open reduction 4 years previously.

can occur secondary to a reduction of an elbow dislocation when the capitellum impacts the radial head and causes the fracture to displace 90° or more. If this is not recognized acutely, near universal poor results occur long term.

Intra-articular fractures in adolescents are rare. However, treatment follows the same criteria used for adults with intra-articular fractures. Fortunately, comminuted fractures rarely occur in pediatric patients. Patients with two- and three-part fractures with greater than 2 mm of step-off should undergo open reduction and internal fixation. Generally, a radial head should never be excised in a skeletally immature trauma patient.

Monteggia Fractures

Although Monteggia fracture-dislocations are rare, they can be challenging to treat. The fracture-dislocation is defined by a radial head dislocation in association with an ulnar fracture. The direction of the radial head dislocation generally follows the apex of the ulnar fracture. Monteggia fracture-dislocations have generally been classified by the direction of the radial head dislocation (Bado classification). Most Monteggia fracture-dislocations are anterior (type I). Type II Monteggia fracture-dislocations are posterior and rare. Type III Monteggia fracture-dislocations are lateral and associated with varus malalignment of the proximal ulna. Type IV Monteggia fracture-dislocations are associated with a fracture of both the radius and ulna. Equivalent Monteggia fracture-dislocations include ulnar shaft fractures with radial head dislocation and traumatic radial head dislocations without associated fracture.

Reducing and stabilizing the ulnar fracture is the key to maintaining radial head reduction. Therefore, in terms of treatment decision making, Monteggia fracture-dislocations may be best classified by the type

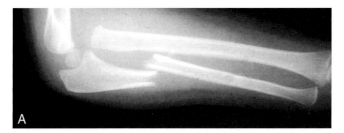
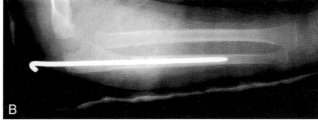

Figure 11 **A,** Preoperative radiograph of a Bado I Monteggia fracture-dislocation. **B,** Postoperative radiograph shows that the fracture was treated by closed reduction and intramedullary nail fixation.

of ulnar fracture. Plastic deformation of the ulna can be treated successfully with closed reduction, as can most incomplete fractures. The problem in patients with plastic deformation of the ulna is more often a missed diagnosis than loss of reduction in a cast. It is imperative that every forearm fracture radiograph is assessed for anatomic alignment of the radiocapitellar and proximal radioulnar joints. Additionally, all Monteggia fracture-dislocations treated with closed reduction must be followed closely during healing for loss of reduction. Complete ulnar fractures can be unstable after closed reduction. Loss of reduction leads to a late-presenting chronic Monteggia fracture-dislocation, which is a challenging and unpredictable injury to treat. Therefore, ulnar stabilization is recommended for complete fractures and some incomplete fractures. Transverse and short oblique fractures can be treated with a smooth intramedullary pin (Figure 11). Long oblique and comminuted fractures can be treated with plate and screw fixation. It is rare for children to have enough comminution to require bone grafting. Treatment of acute Monteggia fracture-dislocations in accordance with these principles almost always leads to a successful outcome (Table 1).

Chronic Monteggia fracture-dislocations are typically the result of either a missed diagnosis or a loss of

reduction. Both problems are potentially avoidable; however, chronic Monteggia fracture-dislocations still occur under the care of well-trained and skilled orthopaedic surgeons and radiologists. Therefore, extra diligence in the assessment of patients with these injuries is highly recommended. Late reconstruction is complex and usually involves an ulnar osteotomy, open reduction of the proximal radioulnar and radiocapitellar joints, and annular ligament reconstruction (Figure 12). Some loss of forearm pronation is expected in patients who undergo late reconstruction. More severe complications

Table 1 | Treatment of Monteggia Fracture-Dislocations in Children According to Ulnar Injury

Type of Injury	Treatment
Plastic deformation	Closed reduction of the ulnar bow and cast immobilization
Incomplete (greenstick or buckle) fracture	Closed reduction and cast immobilization
Complete transverse or short oblique fracture	Closed reduction and Intramedullary Kirschner wire fixation
Long oblique or comminuted fracture	Open reduction and internal fixation with plate and screws

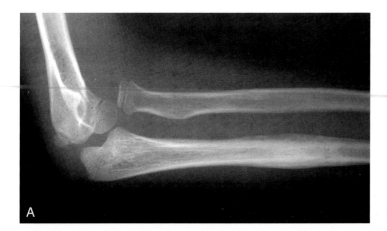
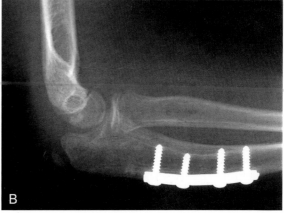

Figure 12 **A,** Preoperative radiograph of a chronic Monteggia lesion with dislocated radial head and ulnar malunion. **B,** Postoperative radiograph shows that the lesion was treated with osteotomy of the ulna, internal fixation, and annular ligament reconstruction.

American Academy of Orthopaedic Surgeons

have been reported to occur in this patient population, including compartment syndrome, loss of radial head reduction, and more marked loss of elbow and forearm motion.

Another complication that occurs in association with chronic Monteggia fracture-dislocations is radial nerve palsy, usually to the posterior interosseous nerve. Generally, this is secondary to contusion and traction ischemia with fracture displacement. Although radial nerve palsy will typically recover spontaneously, the nerve can become entrapped in the joint in association with the radial head buttonholing through the capsule. Due caution must be used with surgical exposure, especially in a patient with chronic Monteggia fracture-dislocation with a persistent radial neuropathy. A congenital dislocation can be misdiagnosed as a chronic Monteggia fracture-dislocation.

Olecranon Fractures

Olecranon fractures are rare injuries in children; when they occur, most are metaphyseal fractures. Olecranon fractures can be associated with other injuries about the elbow, including dislocations, medial epicondyle fractures, or radial neck fractures. Monteggia fracture-dislocations are associated with metaphyseal proximal ulna fractures in varus with lateral dislocation of the proximal radius. Care must to be taken to avoid missing a more complex injury in patients with apparently benign olecranon fractures. Most metaphyseal fractures are well-aligned and can be treated with immobilization in a cast. Most complex injuries may require further evaluation with MRI or arthrography and subsequent surgical intervention. It is important to not miss a complex injury with articular pathology because late reconstruction is challenging.

Intra-articular fractures should be treated with the same principles used to treat adult fractures. Nondisplaced fractures must be monitored closely for displacement during healing. Displaced fractures require open reduction and internal fixation; tension band techniques are used most often. In children and teenagers, use of tension band suture rather than wires is effective and avoids the problem of wire breakage or removal. More comminuted injuries may require plate and screw fixation.

Avulsion fractures of the olecranon are typically associated with osteogenesis imperfecta; therefore, this injury can be the presenting symptom for children with mild osteogenesis imperfecta. The repair techniques for this type of fracture are the same as previously described for other types of olecranon fractures.

Summary

It is important to determine which pediatric shoulder and elbow regions require percutaneous or open reduc-

tion and internal fixation for a successful outcome. Similarly, avoiding complications is imperative. Prompt recognition and treatment are essential in pediatric patients with injuries of the shoulder, elbow, and forearm.

Annotated Bibliography
Shoulder Injuries

Waters PM, Bae D, Kadiyala R: Short-term outcomes after surgical treatment of traumatic posterior sternoclavicular fracture-dislocations in children and adolescents. *J Pediatr Orthop* 2003;23:464-469.

The authors of this retrospective case series reviewed a surgical technique of open reduction and transosseous suture repair of posteriorly displaced sternoclavicular fracture-dislocations. They reported that at an average 22.2-month follow-up, all 13 patients had excellent functional outcomes.

Elbow Injuries

Bae D, Waters PM: Surgical treatment of post-traumatic elbow contracture in adolescents. *J Pediatr Orthop* 2001; 21:580-584.

The authors of this retrospective case series report an average improvement of 53° in flexion/extension arc of motion in patients who underwent extensive surgical release and postoperative rehabilitation including continuous passive motion.

Koudstaal MJ, de Ridder VA, de Lang S, Ulrich C: Pediatric supracondylar humerus fractures: The anterior approach. *J Orthop Trauma* 2002;16:409-412.

The authors of this article outline the surgical technique for open reduction in pediatric patients with supracondylar humerus fractures.

Reitman RD, Waters P, Millis M: Open reduction and internal fixation for supracondylar humerus fractures in children. *J Pediatr Orthop* 2001;21:157-161.

The authors of this study reported that only 65 of 862 patients with displaced supracondylar fractures (8%) required open reduction. The indications were avascular limbs after closed reduction, open fractures, and irreducible fractures. At an average 5.8-month follow-up, the authors reported that 18 elbows were rated as excellent, 8 were rated as good, 3 were rated as fair, and 4 were rated as poor. The authors concluded that highly satisfactory results can be obtained using open reduction to treat severely displaced fractures in children.

Skaggs DL, Hale JM, Bassett J, Kaminsky C, Kay RM, Vernon TT: Operative treatment of supracondylar fractures of the humerus in children: The consequences of pin placement. *J Bone Joint Surg Am* 2001;83:735-740.

The authors of this study reported that lateral entry divergent pins provide stable fixation and avoid medial entry ulnar neuropathy in patients undergoing surgical treatment for displaced supracondylar humerus fractures.

Forearm Injuries

Degreef I, De Smet L: Missed radial head dislocations in children associated with ulnar deformation: Treatment by open reduction and ulnar osteotomy. *J Orthop Trauma* 2004;18:375-378.

In this retrospective review of six children (2 to 6 years of age) with Monteggia fractures that were initially undiagnosed, the authors reported that the missed radial head dislocations ranged from 5 to 59 weeks postinjury. They also reported that open reduction of the radial head combined with a dorsal opening wedge osteotomy of the proximal ulna and fixation with plate and screw resulted in normal range of motion, radial head reduction, and normal axis of the forearm in these patients.

Gicquel PH, De Billy B, Karger CS, Clavert JM: Olecranon fractures in 26 children with mean follow-up of 59 months. *J Pediatr Orthop* 2001;21:141-147.

The authors report the results of a retrospective case series of 26 children with olecranon fractures. Nondisplaced or minimally displaced (< 2mm) fractures were treated successfully with immobilization. Tension band technique open reduction had good clinical results, but some radiographic evidence of displacement was detected at long-term follow-up.

Classic Bibliography

Archibeck MJ, Scott SM, Peters CL: Brachialis muscle entrapment in displaced supracondylar humerus fractures: A technique of closed reduction and report of initial results. *J Pediatr Orthop* 1997;17:298-302.

Bado JL: The Monteggia lesion. *Clin Orthop Relat Res* 1967;50:71-86.

Bernstein SM, McKeever P, Bernstein L: Percutaneous reduction of displaced radial neck fractures in children. *J Pediatr Orthop* 1993;13:85-88.

Campbell CC, Waters PM, Emans JB, et al: Neurovascular injury and displacement in type III supracondylar humerus fractures. *J Pediatr Orthop* 1995;15:47-52.

Fleuriau-Chateau P, McIntyre W, Letts M: An analysis of open reduction of irreducible supracondylar fractures of the humerus in children. *Can J Surg* 1998;41:112-118.

Flynn JC: Nonunion of slightly displaced fractures of the lateral humeral condyle in children: An update. *J Pediatr Orthop* 1989;9:691-696.

Fowles JV, Kassab MT, Moula T: Untreated intra-articular entrapment of the medial humeral epicondyle. *J Bone Joint Surg Br* 1984;66:562-565.

Fowles JV, Sliman N, Kassab MT: The Monteggia lesion in children: Fracture of the ulna and dislocation of the radial head. *J Bone Joint Surg Am* 1983;65:1276-1282.

Gonzalez-Herranz P, Alvarez-Romera A, Burgos J, Rapariz JM, Hevia E: Displaced radial neck fractures in children treated by closed intramedullary pinning (Metaizeau technique). *J Pediatr Orthop* 1997;17:325-331.

Hardacre JA, Nahigian SH, Froimson AI, et al: Fractures of the lateral condyle of the humerus in children. *J Bone Joint Surg Am* 1971;53:1083-1095.

Iyengar SR, Hoffinger SA, Townsend DR: Early versus delayed reduction and pinning of type III displaced supracondylar fractures of the humerus in children: A comparative study. *J Orthop Trauma* 1999;13:51-55.

Jakob R, Fowles JV, Rang M, et al: Observations concerning fractures of the lateral humeral condyle in children. *J Bone Joint Surg Br* 1975;57:430-436.

Josefsson PO, Danielsson LG: Epicondylar elbow fracture in children: 35-year follow-up of 56 unreduced cases. *Acta Orthop Scand* 1986;57:313-315.

Lloyd-Roberts GC, Bucknill TM: Anterior dislocation of the radial head in children: Aetiology, natural history and management. *J Bone Joint Surg Br* 1977;59-B:402-407.

Matev I: A radiological sign of entrapment of the median nerve in the elbow joint after posterior dislocation: A report of two cases. *J Bone Joint Surg Br* 1976;58:353-355.

Metaizeau JP, Lascombes P, Lemelle JL, et al: Reduction and fixation of displaced radial neck fractures by closed intramedullary pinning. *J Pediatr Orthop* 1993;13:355-360.

Millis MB, Singer IJ, Hall JE: Supracondylar fracture of the humerus in children: Further experience with a study in orthopaedic decision-making. *Clin Orthop Relat Res* 1984;188:90-97.

Mintzer CM, Waters PM, Brown DJ, et al: Percutaneous pinning in the treatment of displaced lateral condyle fractures. *J Pediatr Orthop* 1994;14:462-465.

Pirone AM, Graham HK, Krajbich JI: Management of displaced extension-type supracondylar fractures of the humerus in children. *J Bone Joint Surg Am* 1988;70:641-650.

Royce RO, Dutkowsky JP, Kasser JR, et al: Neurologic complications after K-wire fixation of supracondylar humerus fractures in children. *J Pediatr Orthop* 1991;11:191-194.

Shaw BA, Kasser JR, Emans JB, et al: Management of vascular injuries in displaced supracondylar humerus fractures without arteriography. *J Orthop Trauma* 1990;4:25-29.

Shaw BA, Murphy KM, Shaw A, Oppenheim WL, Myracle MR: Humerus shaft fractures in young children: Accident or abuse? *J Pediatr Orthop* 1997;17:293-297.

Voss FR, Kasser JR, Trepman E, Simmons E Jr, Hall JE: Uniplanar supracondylar humeral osteotomy with pre-set Kirschner wires for posttraumatic cubitus varus. *J Pediatr Orthop* 1994;14:471-478.

Zaltz I, Waters PM, Kasser JR: Ulnar nerve instability in children. *J Pediatr Orthop* 1996;16:567-569.

Chapter 25

Fractures of the Forearm, Wrist, and Hand

Donald S. Bae, MD

Introduction

Children use their hands to explore and interact with the world around them. As a result, injuries to the forearm, wrist, and hand are common. Forearm fractures comprise approximately 40% of all childhood long bone fractures, and fractures of the hand make up roughly 25% of all pediatric skeletal injuries. With increased sports participation among younger children, the incidence of forearm, wrist, and hand injuries has risen. Furthermore, recent analyses suggest that increased body weight may be contributing to rising rates of pediatric forearm and wrist fractures. Given the frequency of these fractures, all orthopaedic surgeons should have an understanding of the fundamental concepts of treatment.

Historically, almost all forearm fractures in skeletally immature patients were treated nonsurgically. Recent information regarding functional outcomes, however, has challenged many of the traditional tenets of forearm fracture care. Patients and families often seek more expedient return to activity, with expectations for full return of strength and motion. Furthermore, with the advent of newer instrumentation and techniques of fracture fixation, treatment options have expanded. Rather than provide a comprehensive review of pediatric forearm and hand fractures, the objectives of this chapter are to provide a summary of important core knowledge and to review the recently published information pertaining to the care of these injuries. Particular emphasis is placed on common pediatric fractures.

Diaphyseal Fractures of the Radius and Ulna
General Principles

Diaphyseal fractures of the radius and ulna may be divided into three categories according to the pattern of injury: plastic deformation, incomplete (or greenstick) fractures, and complete fractures. Although each injury type has its own unique features and treatment considerations, several general principles apply.

Normal forearm rotation averages 150° to 180° and occurs around an axis between the proximal radius and distal ulna. Diaphyseal fractures with rotational malalignment will result in a 1° to 2° loss of forearm rotation for every degree of malrotation. Rotational malalignment does not remodel with skeletal growth, and for this reason, should be corrected during treatment to maximize functional outcomes. Angulation may also impede forearm rotation, particularly with involvement of the proximal radial diaphysis. Although prior cadaveric and clinical studies suggest that up to 10° of angulation may be well tolerated without functional limitations, angular deformity greater than 20° may adversely affect forearm pronation and supination.

In the growing child, angular deformity can remodel. Remodeling potential is dependent on several factors, including the amount of growth remaining, distance of the injury from the (distal) physis, severity of angulation, and direction of the deformity. In general, younger patients with fractures close to the physis in the plane of adjacent joint motion have the greatest remodeling potential. Previous studies have established that up to 20° of diaphyseal angulation may remodel in children younger than 8 years. Beyond the age of 10 years, however, angulation of greater than 10° is unlikely to correct spontaneously. Remodeling potential, expected outcome, and the need for fracture manipulation may be better quantified by calculating the axis deviation (the distance between the anatomic and deformed axes of the radius expressed as a percentage of total radius length).

Determining the acceptable limits of deformity is difficult, and there is no consensus on what constitutes an adequate reduction. Furthermore, clinical outcomes of forearm rotation do not always correlate with the degree of malunion. Although each patient merits individual treatment, up to 20° of angulation and bayonet apposition may be accepted in patients younger than 8 years. Up to 10° of angulation is deemed acceptable in patients older than 8 to 10 years. Although some authors suggest that 30° to 45° of malrotation may be acceptable in older and younger patients, respectively, it is important to understand that rotational malalignment does not remodel and should be corrected whenever possible.

Plastic Deformation

Traumatic bowing occurs when forces applied to the skeletally immature radius or ulna exceed the limits of elastic deformation but fall short of the bone's ultimate strength. No obvious cortical disruption may occur, and the clinical and radiographic manifestations of plastic deformation may be subtle (Figure 1). If left uncorrected, plastic deformation may result in limitation of forearm rotation. Some authors have recommended closed reduction and above-the-elbow cast immobilization for fractures with greater than 20° of angulation; others recommend that any acute fracture that limits forearm rotation should be reduced. The technique of reduction involves three-point bending. Constant, gentle pressure is applied over the apex of the deformity, counteracted by opposite forces proximal and distal to the apex. Reductions often require general anesthesia because forces as great as 30 kg maintained for several minutes are often required to achieve adequate correction of deformity.

Greenstick Fractures

Greenstick fractures account for approximately 50% of diaphyseal fractures and typically occur in younger children. Both angular and rotational deformities occur. The typical pattern is one of apex volar angulation combined with supination of the distal fragment. Most greenstick fractures may be successfully treated with closed reduction and above-the-elbow cast immobilization. Closed reduction is performed by reversing the rotational deformity, followed by correction of the angulation. The "rule of thumbs" is often used to guide fracture manipulation because the thumb is directed toward the apex of the deformity during reduction to correct rotation. For example, in an apex volar angulated fracture in which the distal fragment is supinated, directing the thumb volarly will appropriately pronate the distal fragment. A well-molded cast applied with three-point bending, an interosseous mold, and straight ulnar border is critical in maintaining reduction and preventing late displacement.

Bicortical Fractures

Bicortical fractures occur in older children and by definition have a higher predisposition for instability. Closed reduction may be performed by accentuating the deformity, applying traction, and correcting the rotational, angular, and translational deformity. Indications for surgical treatment include irreducible or unstable fractures, segmental fractures, refractures, floating elbow injuries, and neurovascular compromise or soft-tissue swelling that precludes circumferential cast immobilization. Surgical stabilization may be achieved with internal fixation using plate and screw constructs or intramedullary fixation.

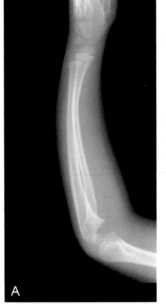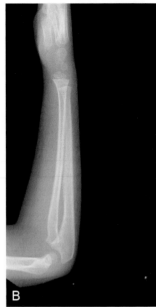

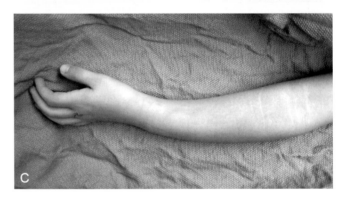

Figure 1 A, Radiograph demonstrating plastic deformation of the radius and ulna. **B,** Radiograph of the unaffected, contralateral forearm is provided for comparison. **C,** Photograph depicting the corresponding clinical deformity, which was associated with limited forearm rotation.

Intramedullary fixation has gained broader acceptance in the treatment of pediatric forearm fractures, and the techniques have been well described. Intramedullary fixation can maintain length and alignment, but does not control rotation and does not provide rigid fixation. For these reasons, postoperative cast immobilization is typically used. The radius fracture can often be stably reduced following intramedullary fixation of the ulna. In such instances, single-bone fixation supplemented with casting will suffice. Internal fixation with plate and screw constructs can also be used, particularly in patients with comminuted fractures or in those nearing skeletal maturity. There continues to be controversy regarding the utility of routine plate removal after bony healing.

Open Fractures

Less than 5% of all pediatric forearm fractures are open injuries. Open fractures are treated by emergent irriga-

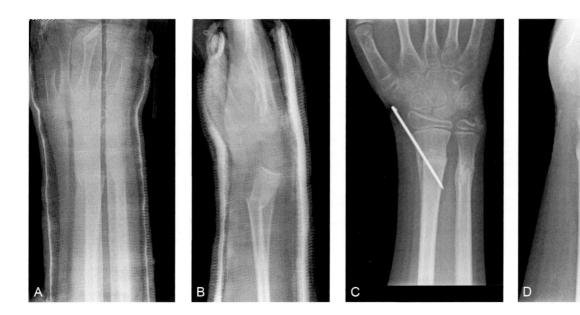

Figure 2 Preoperative AP **(A)** and lateral **(B)** radiographs of an unstable distal radius fracture with progressive apex volar angulation. Because of swelling that occurred after the injury, the cast has been bivalved, which may have contributed to loss of reduction. Postoperative AP **(C)** and lateral **(D)** radiographs after closed reduction and percutaneous pin fixation. Note that this pin enters the distal radius metaphysis proximal to the physis.

tion and débridement with the use of antibiotics in accordance with established principles. In general, open fractures occur as a result of higher-energy mechanisms of injury and may present with more complex fractures and associated soft-tissue and/or neurovascular compromise. Recent reports suggest that with timely débridement and appropriate fracture care following the principles outlined above, most patients will achieve bony healing and acceptable clinical outcomes. Because of the associated soft-tissue injury and periosteal stripping, maintenance of bony alignment can be more difficult. Internal fixation with intramedullary devices or plate and screw constructs results in lower loss of reduction and malunion rates with no significant additional infectious risk in pediatric patients with open fractures.

Distal Radius Fractures
General Principles
Seventy-five percent to 84% of all forearm fractures involve the distal radius. Approximately 15% to 20% of these involve the distal radial physis. Because of the proximity of these fractures to the distal radial physis, remodeling potential is high. In general, closed reduction is recommended in fractures with unacceptable alignment. As with diaphyseal fractures, the parameters defining an acceptable reduction are controversial. In general, 20° to 25° of flexion-extension angulation and 10° of radioulnar deviation may remodel with growth in younger patients. Malrotation will not remodel. Growth potential, the degree of deformity, and the proximity of injury to the physis must all be considered.

Metaphyseal Fractures
Torus (or buckle) fractures commonly occur in the distal radial metaphysis. These injuries are inherently stable because cortical failure occurs in compression. Because of the inherent stability of these fractures, immobilization in a short arm cast or removable wrist splint for 3 weeks provides adequate symptomatic relief and prevents further injury. Recent randomized prospective studies have demonstrated that true torus fractures may be effectively and safely treated with splint immobilization, which can be removed by parents after 3 weeks with no need for subsequent clinical or radiographic evaluation.

Bicortical fractures of the distal radial metaphysis with unacceptable alignment may be treated with closed reduction and above-the-elbow casting. Late displacement, however, may occur in up to 34% of patients; inadequate reduction, poor casting techniques, resolution of soft-tissue swelling, muscle atrophy, and initial periosteal disruption have all been implicated as contributing factors to loss of reduction. Current indications for surgical treatment include irreducible or unstable fractures, open fractures, floating elbow injuries, neurovascular compromise, or soft-tissue swelling that precludes circumferential cast immobilization. Percutaneous smooth pinning may be performed after closed reduction. An oblique pin directed distally to proximally and radial to ulnar and entering the radial metaphysis just proximal to the physis may be used (Figure 2). A second dorsoulnar pin may be used to provide additional stability. Some authors advocate percutaneous pin fixation for all displaced metaphyseal fractures to avoid loss of re-

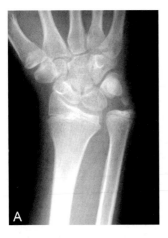
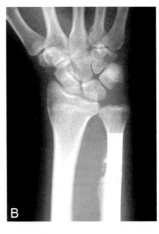

Figure 3 **A,** AP radiograph of the distal radius after previous distal radius physeal fracture demonstrating distal radius growth arrest and ulnar positive variance. **B,** AP radiograph after ulnar epiphysiodesis and shortening osteotomy. Normal ulnar variance has been restored.

duction and the need for remanipulation. However, pin fixation carries with it the concomitant risks of infection and neurovascular injury as well as risks associated with the use of general anesthesia. Randomized, prospective studies comparing the two treatment methods cite similar complication rates and no significant outcomes differences.

Physeal Fractures

Most of these injuries are Salter-Harris type II fractures and are amenable to closed reduction and above-the-elbow cast immobilization. Closed reduction should be performed atraumatically with adequate analgesia and/or anesthesia. Indications for surgical treatment include significant soft-tissue swelling or concomitant neurovascular compromise (for example, compartment syndrome and acute carpal tunnel syndrome) or intra-articular fractures with joint incongruity (for example, Salter-Harris type III fractures). In most patients, percutaneous pin fixation may be performed using a smooth Kirschner wire starting at the radial styloid and engaging the ulnar cortex proximal to the fracture site.

Distal radius growth arrest may occur after physeal fractures. A recent study of 163 physeal fractures with an average 25-year follow-up demonstrated a 4.4% rate of subsequent distal radius growth arrest. Distal ulnar physeal arrest was noted in 50% of patients. Physeal arrest may be caused both by the initial trauma as well as iatrogenic injury. Consequently, late or repeated manipulations of displaced extra-articular physeal fractures should not be performed; instead, observation with the expectation for remodeling is recommended. If there is incomplete correction of deformity with growth, a corrective osteotomy may be performed when the patient reaches skeletal maturity.

Significant radial growth arrest may lead to ulnar overgrowth and altered radial inclination, resulting in abnormal wrist mechanics, ulnocarpal impaction, possible triangular fibrocartilage complex tears, and distal radioulnar joint instability. Depending on patient age, degree of deformity, and arrest pattern, physeal bar resection, radial osteotomy, ulnar epiphysiodesis, and/or ulnar shortening osteotomy may be performed to improve function and prevent progressive deformity (Figure 3).

Wrist Fractures
Scaphoid Fractures

Although the scaphoid is the most commonly fractured carpal bone in children, scaphoid fractures account for fewer than 1% of all upper extremity fractures, most of which involve the scaphoid waist or distal pole and are typically nondisplaced. Thumb spica casting for 2 to 3 months results in successful bony healing in most patients with nondisplaced injuries. Previous studies have suggested that initial above-the-elbow casting for 6 weeks followed by below-the-elbow thumb spica casting may enhance union rates and reduce the risk of late displacement. The treatment options for nondisplaced fractures have expanded with the advent of percutaneous screw fixation techniques. At present, the relative efficacy of screw fixation versus cast immobilization for nondisplaced fractures is unknown; however, early reports suggest no difference in fracture healing and earlier return of motion with screw fixation.

Displaced scaphoid fractures should be treated with anatomic reduction and internal fixation. Nonunion and osteonecrosis of the proximal pole can occur in patients with these injuries. These complications may be treated with open reduction, nonvascularized or vascularized bone graft, and internal fixation.

Hand Fractures
Distal Phalanx Fractures

Extraphyseal fractures of the distal phalanx are extremely common in children and typically result from a crush injury. Bony healing potential is excellent, and the extent of soft-tissue injury guides treatment. In patients with loss of soft tissue, the amputated part may be repaired as a composite graft; conversely, local wound care may allow for healing by secondary intention. Similar clinical outcomes may be expected with these treatment modalities.

Dorsal Salter-Harris type III fractures of the distal phalanx represent the pediatric equivalent of mallet injuries in the adult. Extension splinting for 6 weeks is usually successful. Surgical treatment is considered in patients with large articular fragments associated with volar subluxation of the distal phalanx and distal interphalangeal joint incongruity.

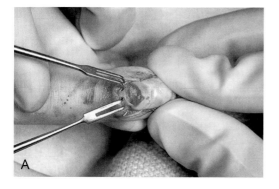

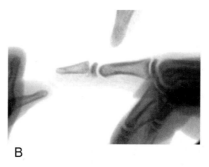

Figure 4 A, Intraoperative photograph of a Seymour's fracture demonstrating the germinal matrix laceration overlying a distal phalangeal physeal fracture. **B,** Lateral fluoroscopic image demonstrating a distal phalangeal physeal fracture with evidence of dorsal soft-tissue interposition at the fracture site.

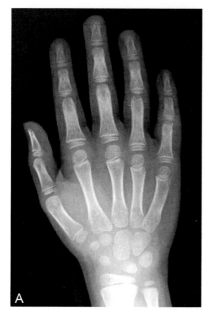

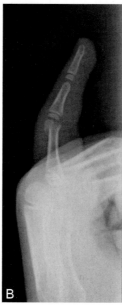

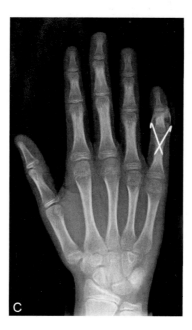

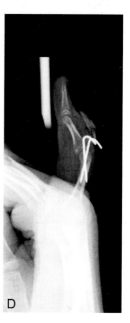

Figure 5 Preoperative AP **(A)** and lateral **(B)** radiographs of a proximal phalangeal neck fracture of the small finger (best demonstrated on the lateral view). Postoperative AP **(C)** and lateral **(D)** radiographs after closed reduction and percutaneous pin fixation. Note the anatomic reconstitution of the subcondylar fossa on the lateral view.

Open physeal fractures of the distal phalanx (the so-called Seymour's fracture) deserve special mention. These physeal fractures are associated with nail bed lacerations and, when displaced, the germinal or sterile matrix may become incarcerated within the fracture site (Figure 4). Closed treatment with reduction maneuvers and extension splinting is unsuccessful as a result of soft-tissue interposition. Treatment involves removing the nail plate, irrigating and débriding the open physeal fracture, removing and repairing the nail bed, and replacing the nail plate beneath the dorsal nail fold. Failure to initiate appropriate and timely treatment may result in infection and long-term growth disturbances of the distal phalanx and nail. Additionally, because these are open fractures, a course of antibiotics is recommended.

Phalangeal Neck Fractures

Phalangeal neck fractures are a characteristic injury of childhood. The mechanism is typically a doorjamb injury in which the phalanx is crushed and the distal fragment is rotated and extended as the hand is withdrawn. In young patients with predominantly cartilaginous phalangeal condyles, the diagnosis is often missed because of innocuous-appearing radiographs depicting only a small fleck or cap of bone. True lateral radiographs of the affected digit are essential to avoid misdiagnosis.

Typically, the distal fragment is displaced dorsally with apex volar angulation. This creates a bony block to interphalangeal joint flexion because the subcondylar fossa is obliterated. Because the phalangeal physis is proximal, these injuries have extremely poor remodeling potential, and the risk of redisplacement after closed reduction is high. For this reason, closed reduction combined with percutaneous pin fixation is recommended for displaced injuries (Figure 5).

Patients with phalangeal neck fractures will often present late with incipient or established malunions. If a lucency is apparent on radiographs, percutaneous osteoclasis followed by closed reduction and pin fixation may be performed. In patients with established malunion, however, corrective osteotomy or subcondylar fossa reconstruction may be necessary to provide adequate interphalangeal joint flexion.

Phalangeal Physeal Fracture

Physeal fractures account for approximately one third of all pediatric hand fractures. Most are Salter-Harris type II injuries and may be treated with closed reduction and immobilization. Care should be taken to correct the rotational as well as the angular and translational deformities. Displaced Salter-Harris type III fractures of the phalanges are typically the result of extensor tendon or collateral ligament avulsions. These fractures, by definition, are intra-articular. Anatomic reduction via closed or open means and smooth wire fixation should be performed in all injuries with articular incongruity or joint instability.

Salter-Harris Type III Fractures of the Thumb Proximal Phalanx

Salter-Harris type III fractures of the thumb proximal phalanx are the pediatric equivalent of adult gamekeeper's injuries. The ulnar collateral ligament is typically attached to the articular fracture fragment, which is avulsed from a radially directed force on the thumb. Open reduction and internal fixation, typically with an oblique Kirschner wire, should be performed to restore articular congruity and joint stability.

Summary

Fractures of the forearm, wrist, and hand are common in children and adolescents. Treatment is predicated by the location and character of the injury, with considerations made for remodeling potential with continued skeletal growth. With adherence to the treatment principles outlined in this chapter and an understanding of injuries that are unique to skeletally immature individuals, treating orthopaedic surgeons may maximize healing potential and functional outcomes.

Annotated Bibliography

General

Khosla S, Melton LJ, Dekutoski MB, Schenbach SJ, Oberg AL, Riggs BL: Incidence of childhood distal forearm fractures over 30 years: A population-based study. *JAMA* 2003;290:1479-1485.

In this population-based study, the authors report that the annual incidence of distal forearm fractures rose from 263.3 to 372.9 per 100,000 between 1969 and 2001. This increase was attributed to changing patterns of physical activity and/or decreased bone density in children.

Skaggs DL, Loro ML, Pitukcheewanont P, Tolo V, Gilsanz V: Increased body weight and decreased radial cross-sectional dimensions in girls with forearm fractures. *J Bone Miner Res* 2001;16:1337-1342.

In this study, 100 girls (4 to 15 years of age) were examined and evaluated with CT. Females with recent forearm fractures tended to be overweight and had smaller cross-sectional areas of the distal radii compared with matched controls.

Diaphyseal Fractures of the Radius and Ulna

Luhmann SJ, Schootman M, Schoenecker PL, Dobbs MB, Gordon JE: Complications and outcomes of open pediatric forearm fractures. *J Pediatr Orthop* 2004;24:1-6.

A retrospective study of 65 patients treated for open forearm fractures revealed 89% good to excellent results and a 17% complication rate. Internal fixation improved bony alignment and avoided repeat manipulations but did not significantly affect outcome.

Vorlat P, De Boeck H: Bowing fractures of the forearm in children: A long term follow-up. *Clin Orthop Relat Res* 2003;413:233-237.

In this study, 11 children were followed for an average of 80 months. One patient had persistent cosmetic deformity and three had limited forearm rotation. Little remodeling occurred after 6 years of age. The authors recommended closed reduction with the patient under general anesthesia for patients older than 6 years with bowing greater than 10°.

Distal Radius Fractures

Cannata G, De Maio F, Mancini F, Ippolito E: Physeal fractures of the distal radius and ulna: Long-term prognosis. *J Orthop Trauma* 2003;17:172-179.

In this study, 163 distal forearm physeal fractures were followed for an average of 25 years. The rate of distal radius and ulnar growth arrest following physeal fracture was 4.4% and 50%, respectively. Symptomatic patients had greater than 1 cm of bony shortening.

McLauchlan GJ, Cowan B, Annan IH, Robb JE: Management of completely displaced metaphyseal fractures of the distal radius in children: A prospective, randomized controlled trial. *J Bone Joint Surg Br* 2002;84:413-417.

In this study, 68 children with completely displaced distal radius fractures were treated either by closed reduction and long arm casting or by additional percutaneous Kirschner wire pinning. The authors reported that 7 of 33 of patients who underwent closed reduction and long arm casting required repeat manipulation. One patient experienced Kirschner wire migration with subsequent malunion. There was no significant difference in the clinical outcome measured 3 months after injury.

Symons S, Rowsell M, Bhowal B, Dias JJ: Hospital versus home management of children with buckle fractures of the distal radius: A prospective, randomized trial. *J Bone Joint Surg Br* 2001;83:556-560.

In this study, 87 patients with distal radius buckle fractures were treated with splint immobilization and either home removal or hospital follow-up. All fractures healed, and there was no difference in clinical outcomes.

Waters PM, Bae DS, Montgomery K: Surgical management of posttraumatic distal radial growth arrest in adolescents. *J Pediatr Orthop* 2002;22:717-724.

The authors presented a case series of posttraumatic distal radius physeal arrests with subsequent ulnar overgrowth, resulting in ulnocarpal impaction, distal radioulnar joint incongruity, and triangular fibrocartilage complex tears. Surgical treatment with corrective osteotomies and soft-tissue repairs is discussed.

Wrist Fractures

Adolfsson L, Lindau T, Arner M: Acutrak screw fixation versus cast immobilization for undisplaced scaphoid waist fractures. *J Hand Surg [Br]* 2001;26:192-195.

In this study, 53 patients with nondisplaced scaphoid fractures were randomized to have either cast immobilization or undergo percutaneous screw fixation. The authors reported that there were no differences between the two groups with regard to union rate or time to union. Patients undergoing surgery had better early range of motion, but no ultimate difference in grip strength when compared with the patients who had cast immobilization.

Toh S, Miura H, Arai K, Yasumura M, Wada M, Tsubo K: Scaphoid fractures in children: Problems and treatment. *J Pediatr Orthop* 2003;23:216-221.

The authors presented a series of 64 scaphoid fractures, including 46 nonunions. Treatment depended on the acuity of injury and fracture displacement. Bony union was achieved in all patients, and all patients had acceptable functional results.

Waters PM, Stewart SL: Surgical treatment of nonunion and avascular necrosis of the proximal part of the scaphoid in adolescents. *J Bone Joint Surg Am* 2002;84:915-920.

Three adolescents with proximal scaphoid nonunions and osteonecrosis were treated with vascularized bone grafting and internal fixation. All healed at a mean of 3.4 months postoperatively. No patient had limiting pain or scapholunate instability on physical or radiographic examination.

Hand Fractures

Al-Qattan MM: Extra-articular transverse fractures of the base of the distal phalanx (Seymour's fracture) in children and adults. *J Hand Surg [Br]* 2001;26:201-206.

In this series of 25 Seymour's fractures, 4 of 18 patients treated with closed reduction developed either infection or flexion deformities. All five patients treated with open reduction and wire fixation healed without complication.

Al-Qattan MM: Phalangeal neck fractures in children: Classification and outcome in 66 cases. *J Hand Surg [Br]* 2001;26:112-121.

In this series of 66 children with 67 phalangeal neck fractures, nondisplaced fractures healed with splint immobilization in almost all patients. The authors reported that displaced injuries had better outcomes when treated with closed reduction and Kirschner wire fixation.

Waters PM, Taylor BA, Kuo AY: Percutaneous reduction of incipient malunion of phalangeal neck fractures in children. *J Hand Surg [Am]* 2004;29:707-711.

The authors described their technique of treating incipient phalangeal neck malunions using percutaneous osteoclasis and Kirschner wire fixation. They reported that 8 patients who underwent this technique achieved fracture healing with normal motion and function.

Classic Bibliography

Flynn JM, Waters PM: Single-bone fixation of bone-bone forearm fractures. *J Pediatr Orthop* 1996;16:655-659.

Friberg KSI: Remodeling after distal forearm fractures in children. *Acta Orthop Scand* 1979;50:537-546.

Gellman H, Caputo RJ, Carter V, Aboulafia A, McKay M: Comparison of short and long thumb-spica casts for non-displaced fractures of the carpal scaphoid. *J Bone Joint Surg Am* 1989;71:354-357.

Price CT, Scott DS, Kurzner ME, Flynn JC: Malunited forearm fractures in children. *J Pediatr Orthop* 1990;10:705-712.

Proctor MT, Moore DJ, Paterson JM: Redisplacement after manipulation of distal radial fractures in children. *J Bone Joint Surg Br* 1993;75:453-454.

Simmons BP, Peters TT: Subcondylar fossa reconstruction for malunion of fractures of the proximal phalanx in children. *J Hand Surg [Am]* 1987;12:1079-1082.

Tarr RR, Garfinkel AI, Sarmiento A: The effects of angular and rotational deformities of both bones of the forearm. *J Bone Joint Surg Am* 1984;66:65-70.

Van der Reis WL, Otsuka NY, Moroz P, Mah J: Intramedullary nailing versus plate fixation for unstable forearm fractures in children. *J Pediatr Orthop* 1998;18:9-13.

Younger ASE, Tredwell SJ, Mackenzie WG: Factors affecting fracture position at cast removal after pediatric forearm fracture. *J Pediatr Orthop* 1997;17:332-336.

Chapter 26

Pediatric Spine Trauma

Daniel Hedequist, MD

Introduction

Pediatric spine injuries, although rare, contribute to significant morbidity and mortality in affected children. Children have unique physiologic characteristics that predispose them to certain injuries; as children approach skeletal maturity, their injury patterns begin to resemble those of the adult population. Spinal fractures represent approximately 5% of all fractures that occur in children. Injuries to the cervical spine account for approximately 60% of all pediatric spinal injuries, followed in frequency by injuries to the thoracic spine and injuries to the lumbar spine. The exact incidence of these injuries is unknown because of underreporting of minor injuries and no reporting of fatal injuries that are not diagnosed. Motor vehicle crashes remain the most common mechanism of spinal injury in children. The mechanism of injury is related to the age of the patient. Spinal injuries to newborns are usually caused by either birth trauma or child abuse, whereas spinal injuries in infants tend to result from motor vehicle crashes. However, in young patients with unexplained injuries, the possibility of child abuse should always be considered. Toddlers and school-age children sustain more spinal injuries because of falls, whereas adolescents tend to have more sports-related spinal injuries than any other group.

Factors Unique to Children

Injuries to the cervical spine are more common in children than in adults secondary to the unique differences in a child's cervical spine. Children have a larger head-to-body ratio compared with adults. Children have increased ligamentous laxity as well as facet joints in the cervical spine which are more horizontal leading, which results in an increase in translation. Children also have immature paraspinal musculature that provides less head control. All of these factors contribute to an increased risk of cervical spine injuries in children compared with adults.

Initial Management

Because of their small body size and relatively large heads, children with suspected spinal injuries require specialized care during immobilization and transport from the site of injury to the emergency department. The initial evaluation of children can be difficult because of their occasional unwillingness or inability to cooperate with an examination; therefore, all children with possible traumatic injuries should be treated as if they have a spinal injury until proved otherwise. The anatomic larger head-to-body ratio of children places them at risk for inadvertent flexion of the cervical spine if they are transported on a standard backboard. Children should be transported on a backboard that either has a cutout for the occiput or that has a mattress to raise the body to prevent inadvertent flexion of the cervical spine (Figure 1). The initial immobilization should occur on a specialized backboard with a cervical collar and sandbags taped to the side of the head. The hospital evaluation begins with a standard history and physical examination followed by appropriate radiographic studies.

Imaging Modalities

The initial imaging test of choice is a series of plain radiographs that include standard AP and lateral radiographs of the affected regions. Children with a documented injury to one area of the spine require radiographic analysis of the entire spine to check for noncontiguous injuries. Most spinal injuries can be diagnosed by high quality plain radiographs. The use of CT has increased over the previous decade and provides more sensitivity to detect injury in the occipital and upper cervical spine. CT may be used as both as a screening examination for patients unable to cooperate with the physical examination and to further delineate fractures seen on plain radiographs. Because of the significant risk to children of radiation exposure, CT should be done using a pediatric protocol to minimize such exposure. The use of MRI has increased the ability of physicians to diagnose injuries that are not readily apparent

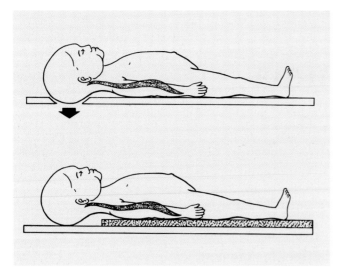

Figure 1 Illustration showing techniques (using an occipital recess or a mattress underneath the body) for avoiding inadvertent flexion in a child's neck during back-board transport. *(Reproduced with permission from Herzenberg JE, Hensinger RN, Dedrick DK, Phillips WA: Emergency transport and positioning of young children who have an injury of the cervical spine: The standard backboard may be hazardous.* J Bone Joint Surg Am 1989;71:15-22.)

on plain radiographs. MRI is a useful screening tool for cervical spine injuries in obtunded patients in the intensive care setting; it is also useful in assessing soft-tissue injuries such as disk herniations or ligamentous injuries that may not be apparent on plain radiographs. MRI is the test of choice for determining and defining injuries to the spinal cord.

The analysis of plain radiographs in children, especially of the cervical spine, may result in several false positive interpretations because of the wide spectrum of radiographic parameters unique to children. Ossification and growth centers (synchondroses) may be mistaken for fracture lines; apparent subluxation of C2 on C3 may be misinterpreted as a ligamentous injury when findings are actually normal; the appearance of an increased atlanto-dens interval may be caused by the presence of cartilage; loss of cervical lordosis may be misread as abnormal; and soft-tissue swelling may be caused by a child crying during radiography rather than by actual soft-tissue trauma. The normal radiographic findings of the cervical spine unique to children are shown in Table 1.

Cervical Spine Injuries
Craniocervical Junction Injuries
Injuries to the craniocervical junction are rare and are frequently underreported because of their high association with fatal outcomes. Atlanto-occipital dislocations in children were believed to be universally fatal injuries; however, because of improvements in emergency care and transport, patients may survive these injuries with variable neurologic deficits. Usually, injuries to the cra-

Table 1 | Normal Radiographic Findings Unique to the Pediatric Cervical Spine	
Increased atlanto-dens interval	> 5 mm abnormal
Pseudosubluxation C2 on C3	> 4 mm abnormal
Loss of cervical lordosis	
Widened retropharyngeal space	> 6 mm at C2; > 22 mm at C6
Wedging of cervical vertebral bodies	
Neurocentral synchondroses	Closure by 7 years of age

niocervical junction are purely ligamentous, highly unstable, and require prompt diagnosis and treatment. The diagnosis of these injuries is often difficult and is made using radiographic studies or MRI (Figure 2). Injury to the craniocervical junction should be considered in patients with unexplained respiratory or neurologic findings resulting from significant trauma. Treatment involves stabilization of the patient with a halo device and an occiput to C2 fusion, preferably with internal fixation.

Atlas Fractures
Injuries to the ring of C1 (also referred to as Jefferson fractures) are uncommon in the pediatric population. The mechanism of injury in a C1 fracture is usually axial loading; most pediatric patients have no neurologic dysfunction given the larger area available for the spinal cord in this region. The diagnosis may be made by findings of excessive overhang of the lateral mass of C1 on C2 on plain radiographs; however, these findings may be subtle and CT is useful in defining the fracture pattern.

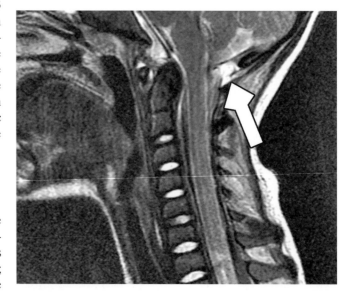

Figure 2 T2-weighted MRI scan of a patient with atlanto-occipital dislocation. The arrow points at an area of increased signal that is consistent with a ligamentous injury.

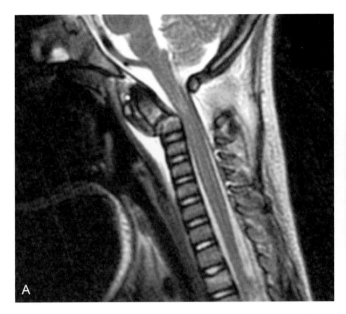
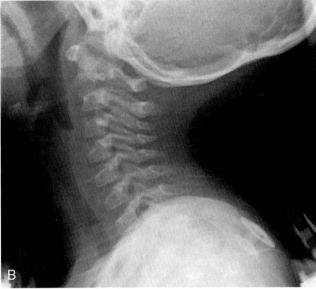

Figure 3 **A,** T2-weighted MRI scan of a patient with an odontoid physeal fracture. **B,** Plain radiograph shows that the fracture has healed in good position after reduction in extension and placement in a halo device for 8 weeks.

Most of these injuries can be treated nonsurgically with an appropriate orthosis such as a cervical collar or a halo device.

Atlantoaxial Injuries

Injuries to the C1-C2 complex are usually ligamentous in nature. Findings of an increased atlanto-dens interval on the lateral radiograph is an indicator of a traumatic injury to this complex. The main stabilizer is the transverse ligament and the secondary stabilizers are the apical and alar ligaments. Patients who have trauma to the neck with pain and spasm and who have an increased atlanto-dens interval on lateral radiographs should be evaluated for this injury. CT scans may show an avulsion of the transverse ligament and MRI scans also show the injury. An atlanto-dens interval of more than 5 mm indicates instability. When the definitive diagnosis of C1-C2 ligamentous instability is made, stabilization of C1 to C2 by posterior arthrodesis is the procedure of choice because of the ligamentous nature of these injuries.

Atlantoaxial Rotatory Subluxation

Rotatory subluxation, manifesting as torticollis, may be posttraumatic or postinfectious. This disorder is caused by attenuation and incompetence of the synovial capsule and/or transverse ligament. Patients present with neck spasm, a "cock robin" position of the head, and an inability to fully rotate the head and neck. The diagnosis may be made clinically. Plain radiographs may be difficult to interpret because a true lateral view of the upper cervical spine cannot be obtained. CT aids in the diagnosis by showing asymmetry of the lateral masses and facets of C1 and C2. Treatment depends on the duration

of symptoms. Patients who have symptoms for less than 1 week should be placed in a soft collar; antispasmodic and anti-inflammatory drugs should be administered. Patients who have symptoms for more than 1 week, or those in whom previous treatment has failed, should be managed with a trial of head-halter traction with physical therapy. Persistent torticollis is managed by halo treatment. If spasm, pain, and rotatory subluxation persist despite these treatment methods, patients must then be treated with a posterior in situ C1-C2 arthrodesis.

Odontoid Fractures

Odontoid fractures in pediatric patients occur as a result of motor vehicle crashes or falls and may be readily diagnosed using a lateral radiograph. These fractures usually occur through the synchondrosis at the base of the dens and represent a physeal injury. Children younger than 5 years of age are most commonly affected because the odontoid physis is closed by the age of 5 years. Most of these injuries are caused by a flexion moment and show anterior displacement (Figure 3). Odontoid fractures may be difficult to diagnose if they are nondisplaced or have spontaneously reduced; in these instances MRI is helpful to document the edema or hematoma around the area of injury. The classic treatment is usually extension or hyperextension to obtain a reduction followed by immobilization in a halo for 8 weeks.

Os Odontoideum

Os odontoideum is believed to be caused by nonunion of an unrecognized odontoid fracture. This disorder is characterized by an apical ossicle separated from the rest of the axis by a transverse gap. Patients with os

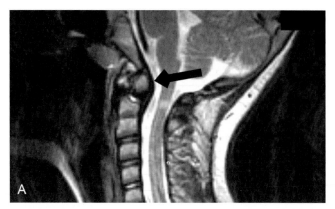
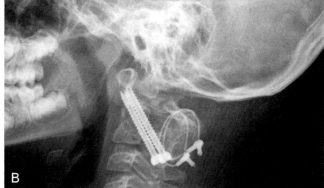

Figure 4 **A,** MRI scan of a gymnast who reported arm numbness after performing a gymnastic routine, which was determined to be caused by C1-2 instability. The arrow shows the os odontoideum; an area of increased signal can be seen in the adjacent spinal cord. **B,** Lateral radiograph of the patient 3 months after posterior C1-C2 fusion with transarticular C1-C2 screws and a Brooks-type fusion were done to treat instability.

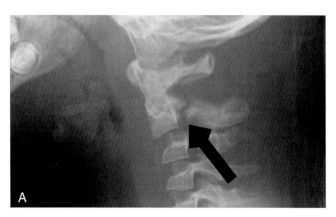
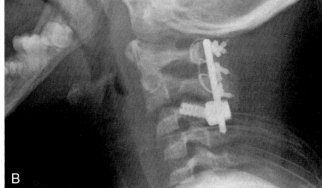

Figure 5 **A,** Lateral radiograph of a patient who presented with neck pain and arm numbness. Note C2 spondylolysis (*arrow*). **B,** Lateral radiograph after fusion of C1-C3 was performed secondary to instability from the defect at C2.

odontoideum may present with neurologic symptoms that may be episodic or transient and are related to cord compression secondary to instability. Instability caused by an os odontoideum may be easily recognized on lateral flexion-extension radiographs because the free dens ossicle moves 8 mm or more with respect to the body of C2. Documented instability puts the upper cervical spinal cord at risk for injury and should be treated by surgical stabilization between C1 and C2 (Figure 4).

Hangman's Fracture

Fractures through the pedicles of C2, referred to as Hangman's fractures, are usually caused by a hyperextension injury in children younger than 8 years. The diagnosis is made using a lateral radiograph on which the fracture lines are visible through the pedicles; excessive angulation and associated forward subluxation of C2 on C3 is usually present. Treatment is closed reduction in extension and placement of a Minerva cast or halo device for approximately 8 weeks. Nonunion may occur with these fractures, either after treatment or if they are unrecognized and treatment is delayed. C2 spondyloly-

sis is believed to be related to fracture that occurred in infancy and did not heal. Instability such as excessive angulation or translation between C2 and C3 should be treated with a posterior arthrodesis or anterior C2-C3 fusion to stabilize the nonunion (Figure 5).

Lower Cervical Spine Injuries

Injuries to the subaxial cervical spine (C3-C7) are more common in adolescent patients because their anatomic features resemble those of an adult. These injuries may be divided into ligamentous injuries, compression fractures, facet injuries, or burst injuries. A pure ligamentous injury may be diagnosed in a child who reports neck pain and has radiographic findings showing a widened distance between adjacent spinous processes; the diagnosis is confirmed by MRI. Alternatively, patients with a documented or suspected ligamentous injury should be treated in a cervical orthosis until they are able to perform voluntary flexion-extension movements during lateral radiographic imaging. If instability is documented with dynamic radiographs, a spinal arthrodesis is used for treatment.

Flexion and axial loading of the spine may result in a compressive injury to the vertebral bodies of the subaxial cervical spine. These injuries are usually stable and in children are rarely associated with injuries to the disks. The diagnosis may be made based on findings of a loss of anterior vertebral height on the lateral radiographs and the presence of a localized kyphosis. After appropriate imaging to clearly define the extent of injury, patients should use a cervical collar for 6 weeks until healing is documented. A series of flexion-extension radiographs should be performed to document stability. Facet injuries, which include unilateral and bilateral facet dislocations, usually occur in adolescent patients. The injuries should be reduced and stabilized. Reduction may be performed either with the patient awake during traction or by open reduction if closed methods are unsuccessful. Once reduction has been obtained, arthrodesis and stabilization should be performed.

Burst fractures of the cervical spine in children usually occur in adolescent patients and are related to an axial load mechanism, such as a diving accident or spear tackling event. Patients may have a neurologic deficit secondary to canal compromise. Patients without neurologic deficit and adequate alignment may be treated with halo immobilization for 6 to 8 weeks followed by flexion-extension radiographs or by arthrodesis with internal stabilization. Patients with neurologic deficits have highly unstable injuries that require surgical stabilization with realignment, stabilization, and arthrodesis. Decompression of the spinal cord may be needed.

Pediatric Halo Placement

The use of a halo vest is important in the treatment of pediatric trauma patients. In general, a halo vest may be used in a child older than 1 year; CT can be used to define skull thickness as well as the presence of open fontanelles or suture lines. MRI-compatible commercial rings and vests are available for pediatric patients and are offered in toddler to adult sizes. Because children have relatively thin skulls, the insertion of halo pins must be done with care. In toddlers and children younger than 8 years, the use of multiple pins is recommended. Pins should be turned only to the point of finger tightness to avoid inner skull penetration. In general, the use of 8 to 12 pins is recommended at a low torque of 2 to 4 inch-pounds; multiple pins are necessary for load sharing at a low torque. The ring should be placed below the maximum head circumference approximately 1 cm above and posterior to the ear helix and eyebrows, with the anterior pins placed above the lateral two thirds of the orbit. The pins should be placed lateral enough to avoid the frontal sinus and supraorbital and supratrochlear nerves and anterior enough to avoid the temporalis muscle. The posterior pins may be turned to finger tightness at locations that are directly diagonal to the ante-

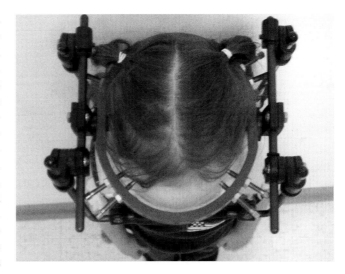

Figure 6 Clinical photograph of a 6-year-old child with a halo device. Notice the use of eight pins with the anterior pins placed directly diagonal to the opposite side posterior pins.

rior pins on the opposite side (Figure 6). The halo is attached to the appropriately sized vest or, if the patient is too small, a plaster vest may be fabricated. Retightening of pins in children younger than 8 years is not recommended to avoid inadvertent skull penetration.

Thoracic and Lumbar Spine Injuries

Injuries in the thoracolumbar region of the spine may be classified based on the mechanism of action. Flexion, distraction, and shear injuries occur in these areas of the spine. Although rare, such injuries may be associated with significant morbidity. Because younger children have much more elasticity in the spinal column than adults, injuries such as periosteal sleeve fractures, endplate fractures, and spinal cord injury without radiologic abnormality (SCIWORA) are seen. The smaller size of children in relationship to automobile lap belts puts them at higher risks for flexion-distraction injuries, the so-called Chance fracture.

Flexion Injuries

Injuries caused by hyperflexion (or compression) may result in single or contiguous anterior vertebral compression fractures. These fractures are commonly caused by falls and can be managed nonsurgically with bracing for comfort for a period of 6 weeks. Multiple fractures may occur because the firmness of the disks transfer all of the force directly to the vertebral bodies resulting in fracture. The loss of vertebral height usually reconstitutes over time with no residual sequela.

Burst fractures may occur in adolescent patients and are usually associated with a high-energy mechanism. Treatment is determined by the presence or absence of neurologic injury as well as the amount of localized kyphosis and canal compromise. Treatment ranges from

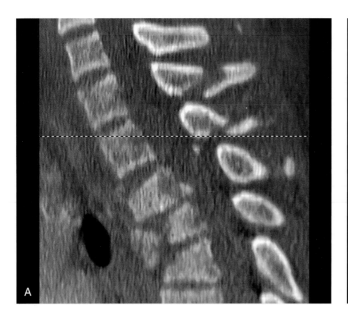

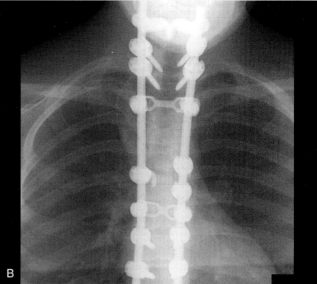

Figure 7 A, CT scan of a patient with an upper thoracic level burst-type injury with associated multiple contiguous fractures and localized kyphosis. **B,** Plain radiograph obtained after instrumented posterior reduction and fusion.

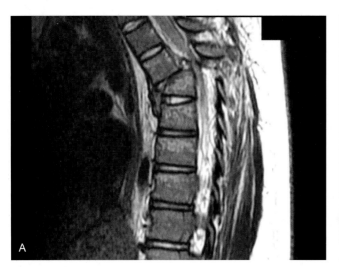

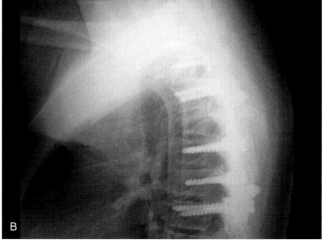

Figure 8 A, MRI scan showing a fracture-dislocation of the upper thoracic spine with injury to the spinal cord resulting in complete paraplegia. **B,** Lateral radiograph of the same patient showing restoration of spinal alignment after posterior instrumented reduction and fusion.

bracing for patients with stable burst fractures to decompression with instrumented reduction and fusion in patients with spinal cord compromise (Figure 7).

Distraction and Shear

High-velocity injuries, such as those resulting from motor vehicle crashes, may cause distraction and shear forces. These injuries are highly unstable and are usually associated with spinal cord injury and traumatic vertebral column displacement. In children younger than 8 years, displacement may occur through the vertebral end plates. In older children, associated bony, ligamentous, and disk injuries frequently occur. Although children who present with incomplete neurologic injuries

have a better prognosis for recovery than adults, the prognosis for patients with an associated complete spinal cord injury remains poor. Treatment consists of realignment and stabilization of the vertebral column by decompression, instrumented reduction, and arthrodesis (Figure 8).

Chance Fractures

Chance fractures are ligamentous or bony injuries resulting from hyperflexion over an automobile lap belt with resultant posterior vertebral element distraction. These flexion-distraction injuries are frequently associated with intra-abdominal injuries which may require laparotomy. A high percentage of flexion-distraction in-

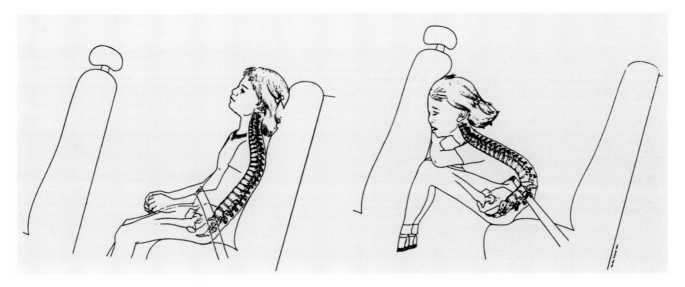

Figure 9 Illustration showing the mechanism of an automotive lap belt injury in a child. *(Reproduced with permission from Chambers H, Akbarnia B: Thoracic, lumbar, and sacral spine fractures and dislocations, in Weinstein S (ed): The Pediatric Spine: Principles and Practice, ed 2. Philadelphia, PA, Lippincott Williams & Wilkins, 2001, p 574.)*

juries are initially missed because the associated intra-abdominal injury masks the spinal fracture. These injuries are often associated with abdominal bruising or a "seat-belt sign" secondary to the lap belt itself. Normally, the lap belt portion of a seat belt contacts the iliac crest when it is in the anatomically correct position; however, in smaller children the lap belt goes above the iliac crest and with sudden deceleration the lap belt causes a hyperflexion moment and resultant flexion-distraction of the spine (Figure 9). Recognition of these injuries is the first step in treatment. The bony and ligamentous injuries may be defined using plain radiographs and CT and MRI scans (Figure 10). Purely ligamentous injuries should be surgically treated and stabilized with instrumentation and arthrodesis, whereas bony injuries may be treated in a hyperextension cast. If the segmental kyphosis prereduction of a bony injury is less than 20° and hyperextension can achieve a closed reduction of the fracture, cast treatment may be applied. An inadequate reduction, the inability to tolerate hyperextension casting, or an unacceptable amount of localized kyphosis, are all factors that indicate the need for surgical reduction with arthrodesis. Surgical treatment of these fractures may be done using posterior compression instrumentation to obtain reduction and to stabilize the spine until arthrodesis is achieved.

Spinal Cord Injury Without Radiographic Abnormality

SCIWORA is more common in the pediatric population than in the adult population. SCIWORA is characterized by a spinal cord injury in a patient with normal radiographic studies. The phenomenon may be related to the increased elasticity of the spinal column or it may be caused by a vascular injury. The cervical cord is most

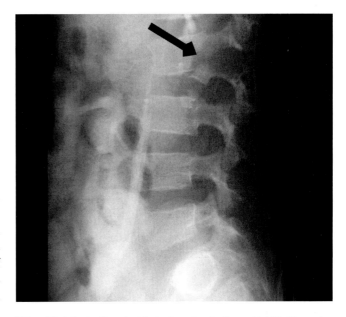

Figure 10 Lateral radiograph of the lumbar spine of a 7-year-old child with an automotive lap belt injury resulting in a Chance fracture. The arrow shows the posterior widening consistent with a flexion-distraction injury.

commonly involved, and the neurologic injury may be complete or incomplete; complete injuries have a poor prognosis. Children with transient neurologic symptoms after trauma and normal radiographic studies should be closely observed because many patients with SCIWORA have a delayed onset of neurologic deficit. MRI can usually delineate cord changes such as swelling, contusion, hemorrhage, infarction, and transection. Somatosensory-evoked potentials also have been useful in diagnosing SCIWORA. Treatment includes preventing further deficit with immobilization of the spine by bracing.

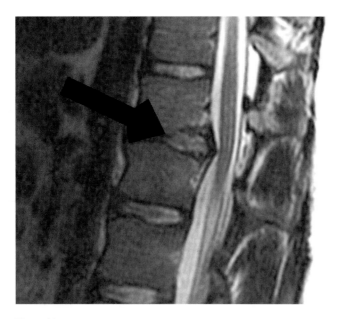

Figure 11 MRI scan of a juvenile patient with a slipped vertebral apophysis at T12-L1. The arrow points to the affected region. Notice the irregularities of the end plates at the posterior corners of T12 and L1.

Slipped Vertebral Apophysis

Slipping of the vertebral apophysis is a traumatic injury seen in adolescent patients, most commonly in boys. This injury involves herniation of a disk with a fragment of cartilaginous ring apophysis; occasionally, bony end plate enters the neural canal. The size of the herniation is variable (Figure 11). The most commonly affected area is usually the lumbar spine, usually the posterior-inferior ring of L4. This condition is analogous to slipped capital femoral epiphysis in regard to the age of patients usually affected and the belief that shear factors play a role in the pathogenesis. The symptoms range from back pain to the presence of clinical radiculopathy. Treatment consists of physical therapy, the use of nonsteroidal anti-inflammatory drugs, and bracing. Patients with neurologic findings or recalcitrant back pain can be treated by removing the protruding disk and bone.

Spondylolysis

Spondylolysis, although usually not caused by a single traumatic event, occurs in 4% to 6% of children and is believed to be related to repetitive microtrauma. Most patients seek treatment during the adolescent growth spurt and commonly have symptoms exacerbated by athletic activity. The pars interarticularis, which is believed to be abnormally loaded with hyperextension of the lumbar spine, is the area affected. The most commonly affected vertebra is L5; less commonly L4 is affected. Symptoms are usually low back pain resulting from hyperextension activities; occasionally nerve tension signs are seen with spondylolisthesis. Treatment fo-

cuses on achieving resolution of back pain. Bracing, physical therapy focusing on hamstring stretching and abdominal strengthening, and the use of nonsteroidal anti-inflammatory drugs are the mainstays of treatment. If these treatment measures are unsuccessful in patients with disabling symptoms, posterolateral arthrodesis between L5 and S1 for L5 spondylolysis is performed. Patients with spondylolysis at L4 or above may be treated by surgical repair of the pars defect. The management of associated spondylolisthesis depends on the amount of vertebral slippage and lumbosacral kyphosis. This treatment ranges from in situ fusion for lower grade spondylolisthesis to partial reduction with instrumentation and anterior grafting through an anterior approach or through posterior lumbar interbody fusion for higher degrees of slippage.

Summary

The treatment of pediatric patients with spine injuries begins with the proper field management and transport to the hospital. The primary evaluation necessitates a thorough history and physical examination followed by standard plain radiographs. Additional imaging of the cervical spine may be done using CT and/or MRI at the discretion of the treating physician. Treatment modalities range from immobilization with the appropriate orthosis to surgical stabilization of the affected area. A systematic evaluation and treatment plan should lead to the appropriate treatment and outcome and limit any potential worsening of the child's condition.

Annotated Bibliography

General

Cirak B, Ziegfeld S, Knight VM, et al: Spinal injuries in children. *J Pediatr Surg* 2004;39:607-612.

A review of 406 pediatric patients with traumatic spinal injuries is presented. Cervical spine injuries were the most common spinal injury. Motor vehicle crashes were the most common mechanism of injury.

Zuckerbraun BS, Morrison K, Gaines B, et al: Effect of age on cervical spine injuries in children after motor vehicle collisions: Effectiveness of restraint devices. *J Pediatr Surg* 2004;39:483-486.

This article presents a retrospective trauma center review of children with cervical spine injuries. The authors address the prevalence of these injuries in younger children and the need for improved restraint devices.

Imaging Modalities

Frank JB, Lim CK, Flynn JM, Dormans JP: The efficacy of magnetic resonance imaging in pediatric cervical spine clearance. *Spine* 2002;27:1176-1179.

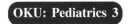

This article shows the cost-effectiveness and clinical accuracy of using MRI of the cervical spine for injury clearance in obtunded, intubated pediatric trauma patients.

Lustrin ES, Karakas SP, Ortiz AO, et al: Pediatric cervical spine: Normal anatomy, variants, and trauma. *Radiographics* 2003;23:539-560.

This article presents a thorough review of normal and abnormal radiographic characteristics found on plain radiographic imaging of the pediatric cervical spine.

Cervical Spine Injuries

Lalonde F, Letts M, Yang JP, Thomas K: An analysis of burst fractures of the spine in adolescents. *Am J Orthop* 2001;30:115-120.

A review of patients who were treated for burst fractures is presented. In patients with neurologic deficits or significant localized kyphosis, surgical treatment was believed to be beneficial.

Lee SL, Sena M, Greenholz SK, Fledderman M: A multidisciplinary approach to the development of a cervical spine clearance protocol: Process, rationale, and initial results. *J Pediatr Surg* 2003;38:358-362.

In this article, the creation of a cervical spine clearance protocol in children was evaluated. The creation of a protocol resulted in a decrease in time for clearance of the cervical spine with no missed injuries.

Wang MY, Hoh DJ, Leary SP, et al: High rates of neurological improvement following severe trauma: Pediatric spinal cord injury. *Spine* 2004;29:1493-1497.

This article is a retrospective review of 121 pediatric patients with traumatic spinal cord injuries. The prognosis for recovery in children is significantly greater than in adults. In this study, some patients with complete deficits showed some neurologic recovery.

Thoracic and Lumbar Spine Injuries

Pang D: Spinal cord injury without radiographic abnormality in children, 2 decades later. *Neurosurgery* 2004; 55:1325-1343.

This article presents a review of SCIWORA as well as an update on the use of MRI for this injury. Injury recognition, verification of injury, and bracing remain the chief modalities of treatment.

Classic Bibliography

Bucholz RW, Burkehead WZ: The pathological anatomy of fatal atlanto-occipital dislocations. *J Bone Joint Surg Am* 1979;61:248-250.

Cattell HS, Filtzer DL: Pseudosubluxation and other normal variants in the cervical spine in children. *J Bone Joint Surg Am* 1965;47:1295-1309.

Fielding JW, Hensinger RN, Hawkins RJ: Os odontoideum. *J Bone Joint Surg Am* 1980;62:376-383.

Herzenberg JE, Hensinger RN, Dedrick DK, Phillips WA: Emergency transport and positioning of young children who have an injury of the cervical spine: The standard backboard may be hazardous. *J Bone Joint Surg Am* 1989;71:15-22.

Mubarak SJ, Camp JF, Vuletich W, et al: Halo application in the infant. *J Pediatr Orthop* 1989;9:612-614.

Pang D, Pollack IF: Spinal cord injury without radiologic abnormalities in children: The SCIWORA syndrome. *J Trauma* 1989;29:654-664.

Phillips WA, Hensinger RN: The management of rotatory atlanto-axial subluxation in children. *J Bone Joint Surg Am* 1989;71:664-668.

Reid AB, Letts RM, Black GB: Pediatric Chance fractures: Association with intra-abdominal injuries and seatbelt use. *J Trauma* 1990;30:384-391.

Steel HH: Anatomical and mechanical consideration of the atlanto-axial articulation. *J Bone Joint Surg Am* 1968;50:1481-1482.

Section 5

Spine

Section Editor:
Mark F. Abel, MD

Chapter 27

Evaluation of Back Pain

John S. Blanco, MD

Mark F. Abel, MD

Introduction

Previously thought to be an unusual complaint indicative of significant pathology, back pain is relatively common in adolescents and children. Although reports on the incidence of pediatric back pain vary depending on the population being studied and the study methodology, recent studies indicate that more than 50% of children will experience back pain by age 15 years, 36% of school age children report episodes of back pain, and 23.6% of adolescent girls in the United States experience back pain more than once a week. In a study of Swedish children ages 6 to 13 years, 18% reported monthly backache, with half of these patients reporting weekly backache. The study found that the prevalence of back symptoms increased with age. No specific factors have been clearly linked to the apparent increased incidence, although factors such as sedentary lifestyles and poor physical conditioning, widespread participation in sports, backpack use in school-age children, a lower threshold for physician referral, and improved access to health care have been considered. One constant is that back pain in the pediatric population can be caused by a variety of conditions, some of which have serious health consequences, and patient evaluation requires a thoughtful, logical diagnostic approach. Although a definitive diagnosis may not be identified in all patients, significant pathology must be ruled out before a diagnosis of idiopathic back pain or back pain of psychosomatic origin can be considered. The reported success rate in identifying the cause of back pain in children ranges from 22% to 84%.

History

The age at presentation is relevant to the differential diagnosis. Children younger than age 10 years rarely have psychosomatic complaints, and their evaluation should be appropriately aggressive. For example, tumors (including those of hematopoietic origin) and infections are causes of back pain in these patients. Older children and adolescents who are involved in sports will often have activity-related pain that may represent soft-tissue

strains, spondylolysis, or spondylolisthesis. Scoliosis and Scheuermann's kyphosis are known causes of back pain in these patients. Even patients with intra-abdominal pathology, such as pyelonephritis, pancreatitis, and appendicitis, can experience back discomfort.

A detailed history should be obtained from the patient and parents. Factors such as the progression of pain; the nature, location, duration, and intensity of symptoms; aggravating circumstances; prior treatment and response; history of recent trauma or inciting activities (such as gymnastics, weight lifting, tackle football); changes in athletic training regimen; systemic illnesses (fever, malaise, weight loss); ability of the child to participate in recreational activities; bowel or bladder symptoms; radiating pain; and changes in gait or posture should be assessed. Pain at night, especially if it awakens the patient from sleep, is an important complaint and traditionally is associated with tumors. Pain of visceral origin typically is not relieved by rest or worsened with activity. Adolescent girls should be asked for any correlation with their menstrual cycle.

The medical history should be assessed to determine if the child is taking any medication such as steroids or has had a susceptibility to illness. Family history is also important to exclude genetic conditions such as neurofibromatosis and to determine if a parent has had back pain. Psychological factors can play a role in pain generation, especially in patients older than age 10 years; therefore, it is important to assess the social history. In a study of the association between psychological stress and musculoskeletal symptoms among Chinese high school students, the prevalence of neck, shoulder, and back complaints was higher in the high stress than in the low stress groups. Thirty-seven percent of patients fitting the high-stress profile reported back pain. According to results of a study of more than 2,000 Icelandic children ages 11 to 16 years, four factors were significantly associated with back pain: older age, morning fatigue, poor eating habits, and inadequate parental support. The importance of these psychosomatic factors, especially in the older age group, is now being realized.

Physical Examination

The physician should have the patient undress sufficiently to adequately assess the body, inspecting for midline spine dimples or hairy patches. Skin lesions such as café-au-lait spots may suggest an underlying disorder (neurofibromatosis). Trunk posture is assessed to determine the presence of physiologic thoracic kyphosis, lumbar lordosis, and lumbosacral alignment. Lateral trunk deviation suggests the presence of scoliosis or a limb-length discrepancy. Long limbs and tall stature may suggest the presence of Marfan syndrome. Gait pattern and movement should be assessed for evidence of weakness or pain. Inspection of gait, including walking on toes and heels and hopping from one foot to the other, provides an assessment of coordination and strength. Flexibility is assessed by examining forward bending, extension, and rotation. Any condition producing inflammation can limit spine motion as a result of muscle spasms. Spondylolysis or spondylolisthesis often is associated with greater pain on extension. Rib or flank rotation during forward bending may indicate the presence of scoliosis. Scoliosometer readings greater than 5° suggest a scoliotic curve greater than 20° and warrant radiographic assessment. Palpation of spinous processes, midline tenderness, and paraspinal muscle discomfort can determine the location of pain. Hip rotation including extremes of external rotation in flexion can reveal sacroiliac pain. An abdominal examination and percussion for flank tenderness may rule out intra-abdominal and retroperitoneal pathology.

A complete neurologic examination, including assessment of strength, reflexes (including abdominal reflexes), and sensation is mandatory. This assessment includes inspection for atrophy or asymmetry in muscle mass, foot deformities such as pes cavus that can be related to spinal cord tethering, or conditions such as Charcot-Marie-Tooth disease (type 1 hereditary sensory-motor neuropathy). Straight-leg raise testing can determine the presence of radiculopathy or may demonstrate hamstring tightness, a common condition associated with overuse back symptoms or spondylolysis and spondylolisthesis.

Diagnostic Studies

Diagnostic studies narrow the differential diagnoses suggested by findings from the history and physical examination. Patients with activity-related back discomfort usually do not require laboratory or radiographic studies and can be treated symptomatically with stretching or physical therapy, nonsteroidal anti-inflammatory drugs (NSAIDs), and activity modification. Follow-up examinations are required to ensure response to these measures. However, because back pain is less frequent in children younger than age 10 years, obtaining radiographs at the initial visit is reasonable. In addition, patients with several weeks of symptoms, night pain, or associated constitutional symptoms warrant radiographs at presentation.

Plain radiographs are often the best initial imaging study. High-quality AP and lateral radiographs with excellent bone detail of the entire spine and pelvis are essential. The radiographic inspection must be methodic and include assessment of the soft-tissue shadows because asymmetry of the psoas shadow can be evidence of an abscess. Calcification in the ureter may be detected. Bony detail is assessed beginning with alignment of the vertebral column and disks. Blastic or lytic bone lesions can be found in the vertebral bodies, pedicles, and posterior elements. A missing or sclerotic pedicle can be evidence of a neoplastic or infectious destructive process. Disk space narrowing and Schmorl's node can indicate the presence of Scheuermann's disease or mechanical deficiencies of the vertebral disk unit. Scoliosis may be present and should be placed in the context of the history or physical examination. Spasm of the paraspinal muscles can cause scoliosis and also can result in flattening of the normal lumbar lordosis. Oblique films of the lumbosacral region can be obtained if a spondylolysis is suspected but should not be obtained routinely. The entire pelvis and sacrum should be visualized because sacroiliitis can be associated with back and/or leg pain. Abnormal bone findings may require more specific imaging with a CT scan for bony detail or MRI to evaluate the bone and adjacent tissues, including the disk and neural elements.

The decision to continue a diagnostic workup when the plain radiographs are normal is based on the history and physical examination. If a bone lesion (such as an infection, tumor, or fracture) is suspected, a technetium bone scan is a sensitive although nonspecific study that will indicate areas of increased bone turnover. If the bone scan is positive, CT can further delineate the area of pathology. Single photon emission CT combines tomographic localization with the sensitivity of a bone scan and has been shown to be sensitive for identifying occult spondylolysis. The presence of upper motor neuron signs or symptoms, such as hyperreflexia, clonus, hypertonia, or loss of abdominal reflexes, warrant an MRI scan of the brain stem and entire spinal cord to rule out intraspinal pathology. Radicular symptoms, weakness, or atrophy may be evaluated with MRI localized to the region of the findings. Electromyography and nerve conduction velocity studies can be helpful to evaluate these neuromuscular abnormalities but often are not tolerated by small children.

Laboratory studies are indicated in patients with back pain and constitutional signs such as fever, weight loss, malaise, and night pain. In these patients, studies such as a complete blood cell count, peripheral smear, erythrocyte sedimentation rate, and C-reactive protein are warranted to complement the imaging studies de-

Table 1 | Differential Diagnosis of Back Pain in Children

Congenital Anomalies	Neoplasms
Tethered cord	Aneurysmal bone cyst
Diastematomyelia	Osteoblastoma
Congenital scoliosis	Osteoid osteoma
Infection	Eosinophilic granuloma
Diskitis	Neurofibroma
Vertebral osteomyelitis	Ewing's sarcoma
Tuberculous spondylitis	Osteogenic sarcoma
Traumatic causes	Chordoma
Fracture	Leukemia
Herniated disk	Lymphoma
Slipped vertebral apophysis	**Spinal cord tumor**
Spondylolysis	Astrocytoma
Overuse injury	Ependymoma
Developmental	**Visceral Causes**
Scheuermann's disease	Pyelonephritis
Scoliosis	Urinary tract infection
Spondylolisthesis	Hydronephrosis
	Pancreatitis
	Ovarian cysts
	Appendicitis
	Inflammatory bowel disease
	Retroperitoneal masses

(Reproduced with permission from Herring JA (ed): Tachdjian's Pediatric Orthopaedics, ed 3. Philadelphia, PA, Saunders, 2002, pp 95-108.)

scribed. Patients in whom intra-abdominal pathology is suspected may require urinalysis, liver function studies, and assessment of amylase levels.

Specific Causes of Back Pain

Age at presentation is a primary determinant of etiology. In patients younger than 6 years, diagnoses such as infection (diskitis, osteomyelitis), neoplasm, and congenital abnormalities such as spinal dysraphism will predominate. In older patients, the more common etiologies will be mechanical causes (such as fractures, disk herniations, overuse injuries, spondylolysis/spondylolisthesis), spinal deformities, and neoplasms. The specific causes of back pain in children and adolescents are listed in Table 1.

Osteovertebral Diskitis

The differentiation between diskitis and contiguous vertebral osteomyelitis may be arbitrary, and some refer to the process as osteovertebral diskitis. The disk is relatively avascular, and the infection probably begins with seeding of the adjacent vertebral end plate. Osteovertebral diskitis or diskitis is rare but can cause back pain in children. Symptoms can include not only back pain but

also abdominal pain, refusal to ambulate, painful limp, and lower extremity discomfort. Approximately one fourth of involved children will have a body temperature greater than 38°C. Erythrocyte sedimentation rate and C-reactive protein will be elevated in almost all patients, and many will appear systemically ill. The typical patient will refuse to bend over, and sitting is painful. Range of motion of the hips, especially in the flexion-extension arc, may elicit pain. Patients are neurologically normal. Radiographs early in the disease process may be unremarkable. Disk space narrowing with vertebral end-plate irregularities and vertebral body erosion eventually can be seen. The diagnosis typically is made with a positive bone scan and/or an MRI scan. Contrast-enhanced MRI will reveal vertebral body changes and any associated abscess formation.

Empiric treatment has consisted of a short course of parenteral antibiotics (for 7 to 10 days) covering *Staphylococcus aureus* followed by oral antibiotics for several weeks, and recovery is reported in most patients. In patients who do not respond to antibiotics within 72 hours, biopsy (CT-guided or direct) for cultures and pathologic tissue evaluation may be required. The differential diagnosis could include diskitis resulting from tuberculosis, fungi, or other bacteria. Neoplasms such as histiocytosis X primarily involve the vertebral body. A paraspinal abscess associated with diskitis may require drainage in the presence of neurologic signs or symptoms. Bracing and bed rest are used for symptomatic relief. Although few long-term studies have been published, some patients will have permanent disk space narrowing with intervertebral fusions and back symptoms.

Spinal Deformities: Scoliosis and Kyphosis

Recent studies show that patients with idiopathic scoliosis frequently report back discomfort. Similarly, patients with rigid kyphosis, such as Scheuermann's kyphosis, often have pain. The source of the pain is largely mechanical overuse. Hamstring tightness is a commonly associated finding. Symptomatic treatment includes stretching of tight hamstrings, core trunk strengthening, aerobic conditioning, and judicious use of NSAIDs. Strengthening of back extensor muscles is often helpful to alleviate the symptoms of kyphosis. For more detailed discussions on Scheuermann's kyphosis and scoliosis see chapter 28.

Neoplasms

Neoplasms of the spine are extremely rare, with a reported incidence of 0.5% of primary bone tumors in the pediatric spine. Most of these lesions are benign and may involve the anterior or posterior columns. Common posterior column benign tumors include osteoid osteoma (Figure 1), osteoblastoma, and aneurysmal bone cyst (Figure 2). Histiocytosis X or eosinophilic granuloma has a predilection for the anterior column with resultant vertebra plana. Primary malignant spinal neoplasms are exceedingly rare and include Ewing's sarcoma and osteosarcoma. Patients with leukemia and lymphoma can present with back pain secondary to spinal column involvement. Leukemia is the most common malignant cause for back pain in children; 6% of patients with acute lymphocytic leukemia have back pain.

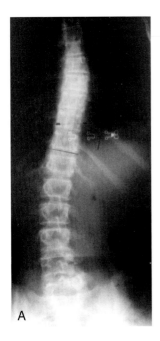
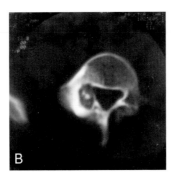

Figure 1 Radiographs of a 13-year-old girl who has painful scoliosis and night pain. **A,** A sclerotic L5 pedicle is seen on an AP spine radiograph. **B,** A CT scan reveals characteristic nidus consistent with osteoid osteoma in the pedicle.

Neuroblastoma is known to metastasize to the thoracic spine in young children.

Patients with neoplastic lesions of the spine will have back pain along with an array of constitutional symptoms including malaise, fever, weight loss, and night pain. Plain radiographs may reveal an osteolytic, osteoblastic, or mixed lesion and, occasionally, diffuse osteopenia. Additional imaging studies, including bone scan, CT, and MRI, usually are warranted. Laboratory work including a peripheral smear may be helpful. In situations involving the commonly occurring benign lesions, such as aneurysmal bone cysts and osteoid osteoma, marginal excision usually is possible after appropriate staging and diagnostic imaging. For example, embolization of an aneurysmal bone cyst or CT localization of an osteoid osteoma can facilitate excision. Resolution of symptoms is expected after treatment with bracing and observation of isolated vertebra plana caused by histiocytosis X. When the diagnosis is in doubt and the only known lesion is in the spine, needle biopsy under CT guidance or formal open biopsy may be required. In patients with metastatic tumors, biopsy of the most accessible lesion should be performed.

Back Pain in the Adolescent

Most sports-related back injuries in the adolescent athlete are self-limited soft-tissue strains. Of these strains, 80% to 90% will resolve over the course of 4 to 6 weeks. In the absence of a specific injury, factors such as a recent change in training regimen, poor off-season

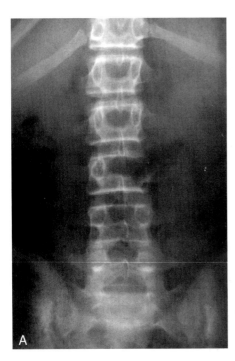
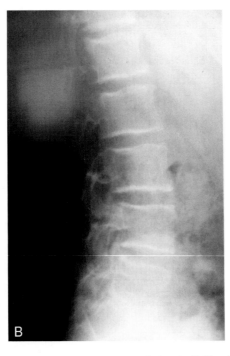
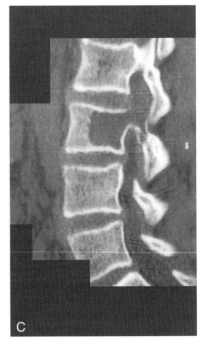

Figure 2 Radiographs of a 14-year-old boy who has back pain of several months' duration and radiculopathy. AP **(A)** and lateral **(B)** radiographs of the lumbar spine reveal a lytic lesion involving the pedicle and vertebral body of L3. **C,** CT scan reveals a lytic process of the posterior elements and vertebral body. The pathology was consistent with aneurysmal bone cyst.

conditioning, hamstring tightness, improper training techniques, and poor equipment all can contribute to backache. Poorly conditioned and sedentary patients also can develop back pain. Other diagnoses to be considered are herniated nucleus pulposus, fractures (end plate), spondylolysis, spondylolisthesis, sacroiliitis, and non–spine-related conditions in the abdomen as described previously. There is also often a history of either repetitive or acute trauma associated with these injuries. The acute inflammation may limit spine mobility. Radicular symptoms may be present with large herniations.

For diffuse back pain suggestive of overuse, a trial of expectant observation with avoidance of stressful activities and use of NSAIDs and physical therapy is a reasonable first-line approach. Therapy should incorporate components of stretching, strengthening, and aerobic conditioning. Radiographs and more sophisticated imaging techniques are not routinely needed for these patients. Imaging studies should be obtained in patients who have experienced an acute traumatic event or those whose symptoms have not improved after several weeks of observation and treatment as described. Any patient with neurologic signs or symptoms requires more urgent evaluation and imaging.

Certain sports have a higher incidence of back injuries than others. Weight lifting can place tremendous stresses on the spine, with disk degeneration a common long-term sequela. Eighty percent of male weight lifters older than 40 years are reported to have disk degeneration. Racquet sports, because of the extensive twisting and rotational moments, lead to a 12% incidence of back injury. Gymnasts and divers, because of hyperextension positioning involved in these sports, have high rates of back injuries and spondylolysis. In general, collision sports such as basketball, rugby, wrestling, tackle football, and ice hockey are associated with higher rates of back injuries. Up to 30% of high school football players miss games as a result of back pain, and 50% of linemen at the professional level report back pain. Back education programs emphasizing proper stretching and lifting techniques can be a helpful adjunct to the standard training regimens of these athletes. A recent study indicated that a back education program involving schoolchildren age 9 to 11 years had lasting efficacy at 1-year follow-up, with a decreased prevalence of neck and back pain and demonstrable retention of learned back care principles.

Spondylolysis and Spondylolisthesis

Spondylolysis, a fracture of the pars interarticularis, is a common occurrence in athletes involved in repetitive flexion-extension and hyperextension activities of the lumbar spine. Spondylolysis can occur in patients involved in all collision sports as well as gymnastics, weight lifting, figure skating, and swimming. The condition typically represents a stress fracture at the L5-S1 level, although it can occur at other levels. Radicular symptoms are uncommon without a concomitant disk herniation or spondylolisthesis. The pain tends to be localized to the L5-S1 facet with paraspinal muscle spasm. Tight hamstrings often are present. Treatment of spondylolysis consists of activity restriction and physical therapy. Bracing can be used in recalcitrant patients. Fusion rarely is necessary and generally is indicated only for progression to higher grade spondylolisthesis. Spondylolisthesis often is associated with greater symptoms and deformity. Both spondylolysis and spondylolisthesis are discussed in more depth in chapter 29.

Herniated Disks and Vertebral Apophysis End-Plate Fracture

Disk herniation is an uncommon cause of leg and/or back pain in the pediatric population, who represent only 1% to 2% of all surgically treated disk herniations. Half of these patients have an acute traumatic inciting event. Many of these patients have underlying congenital anomalies such as transitional vertebrae, spondylolisthesis, and congenital spinal stenosis. There often is a positive family history of disk disease. Predisposing pathology, such as congenital spinal stenosis and lateral recess narrowing, may reduce the effectiveness of nonsurgical treatment.

Slipped vertebral apophyseal injuries (or apophyseal ring fractures) present as sudden onset of pain after an injury or lifting task and often are associated with radiculopathy. Symptoms are similar to those of a herniated disk, but generally are more acute at onset. Male adolescent weight lifters are affected most frequently. The proposed mechanism of injury involves flexion and axial loading of the disk. The resultant disk bulging causes traction on the posteroinferior apophysis, which then avulses and displaces into the spinal canal. The most common site of injury is L4. A CT scan is diagnostic, and surgical treatment may be necessary for large fragments and intractable pain.

Initial treatment of disk herniation or apophyseal end-plate herniation consists of rest, NSAIDs, muscle relaxants, and physical therapy. Epidural steroids may be used for patients in whom initial nonsurgical treatment is unsuccessful. Half of the patients treated nonsurgically will show improvement. Surgery, consisting of microdiskectomy or formal laminectomy with diskectomy, is recommended for those in whom nonsurgical treatment has failed or for patients with significant neurologic deficits. The long-term results of disk excision in this age group have not been well documented.

Backpacks and Back Pain

Backpack use and associated back pain have received significant attention in the lay press as well as in the orthopaedic literature. Attempts to correlate backpack weight, patient gender and age, and method of carrying the backpack with the incidence of reported back pain have produced contradictory results. Although improper use of backpacks can cause alterations in posture and gait, no evidence exists that backpack use is an etiology for scoliosis or kyphosis, nor has it been shown definitively that back pain prevalence is increased with backpack use. Biomechanical studies have determined that 30% of the vertical force generated by a backpack is borne by the low back, whereas the remaining 70% of the vertical load is supported by the upper back and shoulders. A consistent anteriorly-directed force is also exerted on the low back when carrying a backpack. The American Academy of Pediatrics has several recommendations regarding backpack use, including choosing a lightweight backpack with two wide, padded shoulder straps tightened appropriately, a waist strap to distribute the weight more evenly, and back strengthening exercises. An empiric recommendation is that the backpack weight should not exceed 10% to 20% of the student's total body weight. A second set of textbooks and rolling backpacks are other options.

Psychosomatic Causes of Back Pain

In a significant percentage of patients with back pain, no definable etiology is readily apparent, even after a thorough and thoughtful investigation. Several studies have found that a high percentage of school-age and adolescent children will have a variety of somatic complaints including headache, stomachache, morning fatigue, and neck, shoulder, and back pain. These complaints seem to be especially prevalent among preadolescent and adolescent girls. One study found that alcohol use, high caffeine intake, and cigarette smoking were strongly associated with these complaints while support systems including parents and teachers served as protective factors. There may be other family members with back symptomatology or an unstable social environment. Levels of stress as determined by questionnaire have been shown to have a positive correlation with somatic complaints.

When no significant back pathology is discovered or suspected, the treating physician may be left with a psychosomatic etiology or conversion reaction as an explanation for the symptoms. This diagnosis should be one of exclusion after a thorough evaluation has proved negative. Although the factors leading to multiple somatic complaints may not be in the traditional province of orthopaedics, addressing issues such as activity levels, posture, back conditioning, and emotional stress may help to alleviate complaints. A multidisciplinary approach consisting of physicians, psychologists, physical therapists, and parental support often is required to successfully treat this subgroup of patients. Use of pharma-

cologic agents such as muscle relaxants and opiate pain medications is to be avoided. For more on chronic pain syndromes see chapter 4.

Summary

The prevalence of back complaints among the school-age and adolescent population is alarmingly high. Recent studies would seem to indicate that contrary to prior reports, many of these patients will not have a significant or even discernable cause for their complaints. However, a high index of suspicion for a variety of etiologies must be maintained by the evaluating physician to correctly diagnose these patients. Only after a complete history, physical examination, and appropriately ordered tests are obtained can dangerous conditions be excluded and other specific diagnoses be made. Follow-up evaluations should be planned when treating back pain or when the diagnosis is in question. With evidence suggesting that early-onset back pain can lead to adult back pain, it is important to properly educate young patients and their parents on the importance of health, exercise, and proper posture as a means of avoiding back pain.

Annotated Bibliography
General
Herring JA: Back pain, in Herring JA (ed): *Tachdjian's Pediatric Orthopaedics*, ed 3. Philadelphia, PA, WB Saunders, 2002, vol 1, pp 95-108.
This in-depth review of back pain in the pediatric population includes a discussion on treatment of various etiologies of back pain.

Petersen S, Bergstrom E, Brulin C: High prevalence of tiredness and pain in young schoolchildren. *Scand J Public Health* 2003;31:367-374.
A randomized sample of 1,155 Swedish children ages 6 to 13 years indicated that 18% reported monthly back pain, with half of these patients having weekly complaints.

History
Cho CY, Hwang IS, Chen CC: The association between psychological distress and musculoskeletal symptoms experienced by Chinese high school students. *J Orthop Sports Phys Ther* 2003;33:344-353.
The Musculoskeletal Symptom Questionnaire and the Chinese Health Questionnaire were randomly distributed to 550 students in Taiwan. Neck (56%), shoulder (45%), and back (37%) complaints were common and occurred at a higher rate in students characterized as having higher psychological stress.

Kristjansdottir G, Rhee H: Risk factors of back pain frequency in schoolchildren: A search for explanations to a public health problem. *Acta Paediatr* 2002;91:849-854.
Based on a self-administered questionnaire of more than 2,000 Icelandic children, four major factors (age, morning fa-

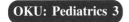

tigue, eating habits, and parental support) emerged as factors associated with back pain.

Diagnostic Studies

Trainor TJ, Wiesel SW: Epidemiology of back pain in the athlete. *Clin Sports Med* 2002;21:93-103.

The authors review the epidemiology of back pain in the athlete as it relates to various types of activities and discuss predisposing factors and general diagnostic and treatment options.

Specific Causes of Back Pain

Cardon GM, DeClercq DL, DeBourdeaudhuij IM: Back education efficacy in elementary schoolchildren: A 1 year follow-up study. *Spine* 2002;27:299-305.

This 1-year follow-up study of 9- to 11-year-old schoolchildren involved in a back education program compared them with a similar group of controls. Not only did the subject students retain the back education principles they had been taught, but these children also had a decreased prevalence of back and neck pain at follow-up.

Garg S, Mehta S, Dormans JP: Langerhans cell histiocytosis of the spine in children. *J Bone Joint Surg Am* 2004;86:1740-1750.

Twenty-three patients with biopsy-proven Langerhans cell histiocytosis of the spine were followed for at least 2 years (average was 9.4 years). There was a high incidence of cervical spine lesions and of multiple site involvement. All patients had resolution of disease at last follow-up. Patient results had no relationship to type of treatment. The authors concluded that the natural history of these lesions is for resolution on their own.

Garron E, Viehweger E, Launay F, Guillaume JM, Jouve JL, Bollini G: Nontuberculous spondylodiscitis in children. *J Pediatr Orthop* 2002;22:321-328.

The authors conducted a retrospective study of 42 children who were treated for nontuberculous spondylodiskitis between 1966 and 1997. The average delay in diagnosis was 42 days. Sixty-one percent of needle biopsies were positive. *S aureus* was found in 55% and *Kingella kingae* in 72%. Thirty-seven patients had no long-term sequelae. Disk fibrosis with subsequent fusion was a frequent finding.

Ghandour RM, Overpeck MD, Huang ZJ, Kogan MD, Scheidt PC: Headache, stomachache, backache, and morning fatigue among adolescent girls in the United States: Associations with behavioral, sociodemographic, and environmental factors. *Arch Pediatr Adolesc Med* 2004;158:797-803.

In a school-based, cross-sectional, national survey of 6th through 10th grade girls, 29% experienced headaches, 20.7% reported stomachaches, 23.6% experience back pain, and 30% report morning fatigue more than once a week.

Mackenzie WG, Sampath JS, Kruse RW, Sheir-Neiss GJ: Backpacks in children. *Clin Orthop* 2003;409:78-84.

A review of the literature regarding backpack usage and back problems indicated that daily use of a heavy backpack, backpack weighing more than 15% to 20% of the child's weight, and improper use of the backpack can alter gait and posture. No evidence exists linking backpack use and the development of spinal deformity.

Negrini S, Carabalona R: Backpacks on! Schoolchildren's perceptions of load, associations with back pain and factors determining the load. *Spine* 2002;27:187-195.

The associations between features of backpack carrying, subjective perceptions of the load, and back pain were assessed in 237 school-age children. Subjectively, backpacks were believed to be too heavy by 79% of children, to cause fatigue by 65% of children, and to cause back pain by 46%.

Sassmannshausen G, Smith BG: Back pain in the young athlete. *Clin Sports Med* 2002;21:121-132.

This article reviews the issue of back pain in the adolescent athlete. Etiologies, diagnostic workup, and initial treatment are discussed. Spondylolysis is particularly discussed.

Sheir-Neiss GI, Kruse RW, Rahman T, Jacobson LP, Pelli JA: The association of backpack use and back pain in adolescents. *Spine* 2003;28:922-930.

A total of 1,126 patients ages 12 to 18 years participated by questionnaire regarding their health, activities, and backpack use. Of 1,122 backpack users, 74% had back pain. Heavy backpack use, female gender, and larger body mass index were associated with back pain.

Siambanes D, Martinez JW, Butler EW, Haider T: Influence of school backpacks on adolescent back pain. *J Pediatr Orthop* 2004;24:211-217.

In a study of 3,498 California students, the authors concluded that backpack weight was predictive for back pain. Girls and students walking to school were also more likely to report back pain.

Van Gent C, Dols JJ, de Rover CM, Hira Sing RA, de Vet HC: The weight of schoolbags and the occurrence of neck, shoulder and back pain in young adolescents. *Spine* 2003;28:916-921.

In a questionnaire-based cross-sectional study of 745 adolescents in the Netherlands, neck, shoulder, and back complaints were reported by 45% of the children. Psychosomatic factors had a higher association with complaints than backpack weight.

Wall EJ, Foad SL, Spears J: Backpacks and backpain: Where's the epidemic. *J Pediatr Orthop* 2003;23:437-439.

In this subjective, retrospective study of 346 children evaluated for back pain only one patient believed the back pain was secondary to backpack usage.

Classic Bibliography

Anderson K, Sarwark JF, Conway JJ, Logue ES, Schafer MF: Quantitative assessment with SPECT imaging of stress injuries of the pars interarticularis and response to bracing. *J Pediatr Orthop* 2000;20:28-33.

Feldman DS, Hedden DM, Wright JG: The use of bone scan to investigate back pain in children and adolescents. *J Pediatr Orthop* 2000;20:790-795.

Papagelopoulos PJ, Shaughnessy WJ, Ebersold MJ, Bianco AJ, Quast LM: Long-term outcome of lumbar discectomy in children and adolescents sixteen years of age or younger. *J Bone Joint Surg Am* 1998;80:689-698.

Ramirez N, Johnston CE, Browne RH: The prevalence of back pain in children who have idiopathic scoliosis. *J Bone Joint Surg Am* 1997;79:364-368.

Richards BS, McCarthy RE, Akbarnia BA: Back pain in childhood and adolescence, in Zuckerman JD (ed): *Instr Course Lect* 1999;48:525-542.

Chapter 28

Scoliosis: Classification and Treatment

Mark F. Abel, MD

John S. Blanco, MD

Introduction

This chapter focuses on the classification of scoliosis, a condition associated with several disorders. Clinicians must recognize that scoliosis is a clinical sign. Thorough patient assessment is necessary to establish a possible cause and to exclude underlying conditions such as tumors, infection, and primary disturbances of the muscular and/or nervous systems. Some of these relationships are discussed in chapter 27. This chapter will emphasize management of idiopathic scoliosis; management of other specific causes of scoliosis are discussed in other chapters.

Spinal Alignment

Scoliosis refers to a frontal plane (coronal) deviation of the spine of greater than 10° measured using the Cobb method. The central sacral vertical line (CSVL) formed by a perpendicular to the iliac wings and bisecting the L5 vertebra normally should remain centered on the vertebrae up to the skull. The CSVL is used to assess frontal balance and should meet, in parallel, the C7 plumb line (Figure 1). Sagittal spinal measurements are variable with normal values for thoracic kyphosis ranging from 20° to 45° and for lumbar lordosis from 30° to 60° (Figure 2). In the sagittal plane, the vertical plumb line should pass from C2 through C7 and pass through or near the posterior-superior end plate of S1. However, scoliosis is a three-dimensional deformity that includes, in addition to frontal deformity, sagittal plane deviations such as thoracic hypokyphosis and apical vertebral rotation with rib cage deformities. The transverse plane deformity or rib hump is reflected by the scoliosometer measurement or radiographically by the pedicle asymmetry. A scoliosometer measurement of greater than 5° is often used as a threshold value for the need to obtain radiographs, assuming that active treatment with bracing should be started for curves greater than 20°. This screening method has approximately a 2% to 5% false negative rate in missing curves greater than 20° with scoliosometer readings of less than 5°, but the false positive rate is as high as 50% (curves less than 20° with a

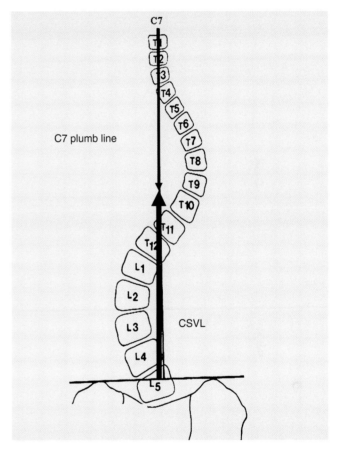

Figure 1 Coronal compensation exists when the C7 plumb line and the center sacral vertical line meet. The stable vertebrae are bisected by the CSVL. *(Reproduced with permission from Mason DE, Carango P: Spinal decompensation in Cotrel-Dubousset instrumentation. Spine 1991;16(suppl 8):S394-S403.)*

scoliosometer reading over 5°). The value of the scoliosometer as a screening tool has been questioned because of this high false positive rate. Surgical treatment of scoliosis is intended to restore coronal balance and preserve or correct sagittal profiles of the spine.

Scoliosis Classification Systems

Several classification systems are used to differentiate types of scoliosis. The Scoliosis Research Society has

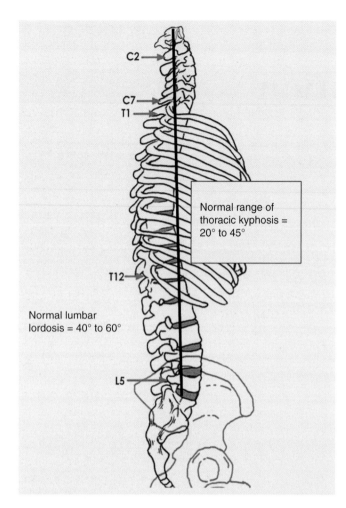

Figure 2 Sagittal alignment: the vertical plumb line passes through C1 to S1. *(Reproduced with permission from O'Brien MF, Kuklo T, Blanke KM, Lenke LG (eds): Spinal Deformity Study Group: Radiographic Measurement Manual. Memphis, TN, Medtronic Sofamor Danek USA, 2004.)*

Labels in figure:
C2
C7
T1
Normal range of thoracic kyphosis = 20° to 45°
T12
Normal lumbar lordosis = 40° to 60°
L5

Table 1 | Scoliosis Research Society Classification: Location of Curve Apex

Curve Type	Apex
Cervical	C2 to C6
Thoracic	T2 to T11/12 disk
Thoracolumbar	T12 to L1
Lumbar	L1-2 disk to L4

Table 2 | Etiologic Classification

Idiopathic Scoliosis
  Infantile 0 to 3 years
  Juvenile 3 to 10 years
  Adolescent older than 10 years
Neuromuscular
  Myelomeningocele
  Muscular dystrophy/myopathies
  Friedrich's ataxia
  Hereditary-sensory neuropathies
Congenital Scoliosis
  Formation defects
  Segmentation defects
Other Causes
  Neurofibromatosis
  Marfan syndrome
  Posttraumatic (paralytic)
  Postlaminectomy
  Radiation-induced
  Limb-length discrepancy
  Inflammatory (reactive)

adopted two classification systems, one based on the location of the apical vertebra and another based on etiology (Tables 1 and 2). Generally, scoliosis is considered to be rigid or structural in nature. Exceptions are scoliosis resulting from limb-length discrepancies or other causes of pelvic obliquity (such as muscle contractures) and reactive scoliosis resulting from an inflammatory condition such as a tumor, infection, or muscle strain. In addition, classification can be based on etiology. Idiopathic scoliosis is the largest grouping, and other causes can be associated with neuromuscular conditions such as cerebral palsy, muscular dystrophies and myopathies, and myelomeningocele. Congenital malformation, often occurring as part of a syndrome, can lead to growth abnormalities of the spine and scoliosis. These topics are covered in more depth in chapter 31; the behavior of the spinal deformity is unique to the underlying condition.

Two conditions commonly associated with scoliosis are Marfan syndrome and neurofibromatosis. Dystrophic and nondystrophic types of scoliosis and ky-phoscoliosis occur in patients with neurofibromatosis. The dystrophic types are associated with rigid short curves, often with scalloped vertebra and penciling of the ribs. These curves are prone to progress rapidly; therefore, fusion and instrumentation should be done early, frequently before adolescence. Furthermore, anterior and posterior fusions are often required because of curve rigidity and poor fusion rates. Nondystrophic curves are treated in the same way as idiopathic scoliosis. Because of the high frequency of intraspinal anomalies (neurofibromas and dural ectasia), preoperative MRI is necessary.

Marfan syndrome is caused by an autosomal dominant defect in the fibrillin gene. In addition to generalized ligamentous laxity, patients with Marfan syndrome often have cardiac abnormalities such as thinning of the aorta and aortic valve regurgitation. Thus, a thorough cardiac assessment is mandatory. Other complicating features of Marfan syndrome include multiple curves along the vertebral column and a high propensity for curve progression. Progression is common even when a brace is worn. Complications from surgery include bleeding, pseudarthrosis, dural leak, and, commonly, late progression below the area of instrumentation.

Imaging

Typically radiographs are obtained in the PA projection on 36-inch cassettes to assess the Cobb angles, the CSVL, the neutrally rotated vertebrae, the stable vertebrae, and the apical deviation (Figure 1); all of these factors may be used for surgical planning. The PA radiograph is chosen over the AP view to limit radiation exposure of the breast tissue. The PA view is repeated at regular intervals, typically every 4 to 6 months in growing children, to determine progression rates. An increase of at least 5° in the Cobb measure is generally accepted as evidence of curve progression. Lateral radiographs usually are obtained on the initial visit to ensure that there is not an asymptomatic spondylolysis and to evaluate sagittal alignment. Only when planning surgery are radiographs obtained to assess flexibility. The typical radiographs to assess flexibility are supine AP projections with side bending to the right and left or traction radiographs. Techniques for these projections have not been standardized. Supine spine radiographs are used for young children and for patients with neuromuscular or other conditions that preclude standing. In many of these patients, traction radiographs may be obtained instead of bending radiographs to assess the flexibility of the spasm.

CT, including reformatted multiplanar images, is useful to show bone anatomy, especially in patients with congenital scoliosis or when severe deformity makes assessment of bone landmarks difficult. In addition, CT has been used to assess chest wall dimensions in patients with infantile and congenital scoliosis.

MRI is indicated for the following situations: (1) neurologic abnormalities such as weakness, atrophy, or upper motor neuron findings; (2) severe pain; (3) young patients (infantile or juvenile scoliosis) with curves greater than 20°; (4) atypical patterns, such as left thoracic curves, short angular curves, congenital scoliosis, or severe deformity (>70°); and (5) when rapid progression (>1°/month) is noted. MRI is performed to rule out intraspinal pathology such as tethered cord, syringomyelia, or spinal tumors as a cause of scoliosis.

Idiopathic Scoliosis

Idiopathic scoliosis is the most common spinal deformity that develops in otherwise healthy children. Subtypes of idiopathic scoliosis are based on the age at diagnosis, with infantile scoliosis occurring between birth and age 3 years, juvenile scoliosis occurring between ages 3 and 10 years, and adolescent idiopathic scoliosis occurring after age 10 years (Table 2).

Adolescent idiopathic scoliosis, if defined as the presence of a curve greater than 10°, has a prevalence of 2% to 3% in the population at risk (between ages 10 and 16 years). The prevalence drops below 0.1% for curves greater than 40°. A polygenetic interaction is suspected but the etiology remains unclear. The diagnosis of idiopathic scoliosis is made after excluding all other causes. Characteristically, female to male ratios are equal for small curves but rise to 10:1 for curves over 30°. The typical curve pattern is right thoracic, left lumbar. However, other patterns exist and are presented as radiographic classifications. Left thoracic curve patterns are distinctly unusual and occasionally associated with underlying syndromes or syringomyelia. A left thoracic curve is adequate indication for MRI.

The characteristics and demographic patterns of juvenile idiopathic scoliosis tend to be similar to those of adolescent idiopathic scoliosis; infantile scoliosis affects more males than females and is characterized by more left thoracic curve patterns. Calculation of the rib-vertebral angle difference (RVAD) at the apex has been reported to predict infantile idiopathic scoliosis prone to progression (RVAD > 20°).

Patients with idiopathic scoliosis frequently are asymptomatic, although mild back pain occurs in adolescents (see chapter 27). Trunk asymmetry often is noted incidentally by parents or health care providers. Other complaints include discontent over body image because of the trunk shift or the rib hump. Patients with idiopathic scoliosis do not have neurologic complaints; if present, other diagnoses should be considered. Scoliosis must never be assumed to be idiopathic until a complete history and physical examination has excluded other diagnoses.

In patients with adolescent idiopathic scoliosis, curve progression is related to growth rate. During the adolescent growth spurt, curve progression is believed to average 1° per month. Therefore, assessment of physical maturity becomes crucial for planning bracing or surgical treatment. Growth remaining and maturity are assessed by considering the age of menarche, Tanner stage, Risser sign, and the presence of triradiate cartilage. Girls at high risk for curve progression are premenarchal, Tanner stage 2 to 3 or less, Risser grade 0, and have open triradiate cartilage. Each of these criteria exists before or near the peak adolescent growth velocity. In general, curves are more likely to progress in girls than in boys, but boys often will have considerable growth in Tanner stages 3 and 4 and even after Risser grade 2, necessitating longer follow-up. Ideally, patients should be followed with serial height measurements and radiographs every 4 to 6 months until the pubertal growth spurt is over.

Classification

Attempts to classify adolescent idiopathic scoliosis for the purpose of planning and evaluating surgical treatments were initiated with the King-Moe classification (Figure 3). This radiographic classification was based primarily on the frontal plane deformity and the relative size and flexibility of the thoracic and lumbar components. The Lenke radiographic classification was proposed in 2001 (Table 3 and Figure 4) with parameters including location of the dominant curve, the relative magnitude of the lesser curves, deviation of the apical lumbar vertebra, and the associated sagittal profile. Six types were identified: primary thoracic, double thoracic, double major (thoracic/lumbar), triple major, thoracolumbar/lumbar, and thoracolumbar/lumbar curves with a structural thoracic component. Modifiers are used to grade the deviation of the apical lumbar vertebra from the CSVL and the sagittal deformity of the thoracic spine. This new radiographic classification system is being used by several outcome study groups and is frequently referenced in the literature.

Natural History

Natural history studies show that untreated adolescent idiopathic scoliosis results in a higher incidence of back pain and discontent with body image than is found in control patients. Curves greater than 50° at skeletal maturity can progress in adult life (average 1°/yr), and curves greater than 60° can be associated with asymptomatic but measurable declines in pulmonary function tests. Hypokyphosis worsens the impact of scoliosis on pulmonary function tests. Despite the adverse effects of severe scoliosis on pulmonary function tests, scoliosis surgery has not been shown conclusively to have a positive effect on the outcome of these tests. Treatments of idiopathic scoliosis, whether nonsurgical bracing or surgical, are chosen based on the severity of the deformity, the patient's age or state of maturity (pubertal growth phase), and the location of the apex.

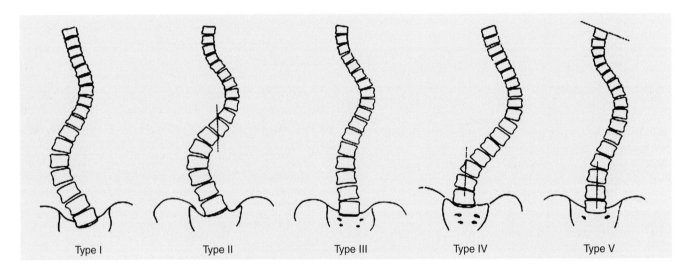

Type I   Type II   Type III   Type IV   Type V

Figure 3   King-Moe classification. Type I: lumbar dominant; type II: thoracic dominant/lumbar flexible; type III: primary thoracic; type IV: thoracic, T4 tilted into curve; and type V: double thoracic. *(Reproduced from Grayhack J: Idiopathic scoliosis: Surgical management, in Sponseller P (ed): Orthopaedic Knowledge Update: Pediatrics 2. Rosemont, IL, American Academy of Orthopaedic Surgeons, 2002, p 308.)*

Table 3 | Lenke Classification of Idiopathic Scoliosis*

Type	Proximal Curve	Main Thoracic	Thoracolumbar/Lumbar	Curve Type
1	Nonstructural	Structural[†]	Nonstructural	Main Thoracic
2	Structural	Structural[†]	Nonstructural	Double Thoracic
3	Nonstructural	Structural[†]	Structural	Double Major
4	Structural	Structural[†]	Structural	Triple Major
5	Nonstructural	Nonstructural	Structural[†]	Thoracolumbar/Lumbar
6	Nonstructural	Structural[†]	Structural[†]	Thoracolumbar/Lumbar-Main Thoracic

*The Lenke classification system also included modifiers to describe the associated thoracic sagittal profile and deviation of the apical lumbar vertebra (see Figure 4)

[†]Major; largest Cobb measurement, always structural

(Reproduced with permission from Lenke LG, Betz RR, Haher TR, et al: Multisurgeon assessment of surgical decision-making in adolescent idiopathic scoliosis: Curve classification, operative approach, and fusion levels. Spine 2001;26(21):2347-2353.)

Nonsurgical Treatment

Bracing has been the traditional nonsurgical treatment for idiopathic scoliosis. However, the use of braces is controversial because compliance is unpredictable and effectiveness has been assessed primarily through uncontrolled observational studies. Nevertheless, bracing is believed to be the most effective nonsurgical treatment for adolescent scoliosis. Bracing is indicated for growing children showing curve progression (greater than 5° increase) up to or beyond a curve of 20°. Furthermore, bracing commonly is prescribed for growing adolescents even in the absence of proven curve progression if the curve is between 25° and 40° at presentation. Bracing is discontinued if the curve reaches surgical dimensions (45° to 50°) or when growth has stopped and skeletal maturity is reached. However, bracing of curves greater than 40° in the infant or the juvenile patient is certainly acceptable to allow for further trunk growth, recognizing that surgical treatment probably will be recommended in the future. Studies suggest that maintenance of the Cobb angle is the best that can be expected as an end result of brace treatment, and improvement in curve magnitude with treatment should not be an expected outcome. For adolescent idiopathic scoliosis, a relative contraindication to brace treatment is thoracic hypokyphosis. Patients with juvenile onset scoliosis and curves over 35° in patients who are Risser grades 0 to 1 are most at risk for failure of brace treatment.

Wide variation exists not only in the method of brace fabrication but also in the duration of brace use, with ranges from 12 to 23 hours per day. From the existing studies, bracing is most effective when applied before the adolescent growth phase, before the curves reach 30°, when in-brace correction of at least 25% is achieved, and when worn for more than 16 hours per day. Spinal braces come in various forms; however, the thoracolumbosacral orthosis is used most commonly to control curves when the apex is at or below T7. Night bending braces are also prescribed, except for the treatment of double major curves. The cervical thoracolum-

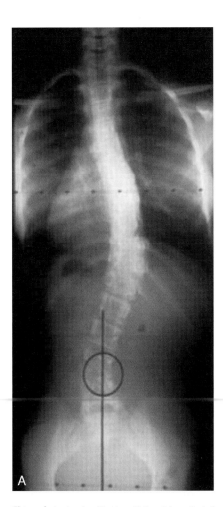
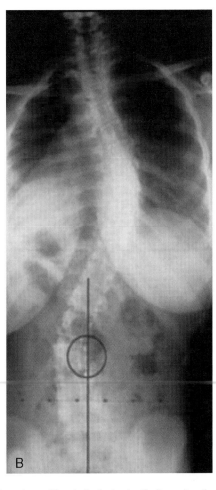
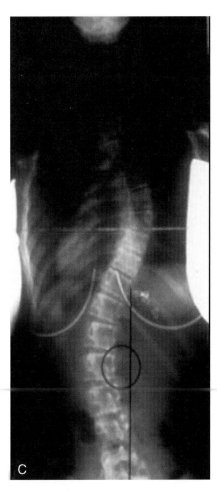

Figure 4 Lenke classification of idiopathic scoliosis lumbar spine modifiers. In the Lenke classification system, the six frontal curve patterns are further described using lumbar modifiers (A, B, and C) to denote the severity of the lumbar curve. **A,** The modifier A is used when the CSVL passes between the pedicles of the apical lumbar vertebra. **B,** The modifier B is used when the CSVL passes between the wall of the pedicle and the side of the apical vertebra. **C,** The modifier C is used when the apical lumbar vertebra is off of the CSVL. *(Reproduced from Lenke L, Kim YJ: Classification of adolescent idiopathic scoliosis, in Newton PO (ed): Adolescent Idiopathic Scoliosis. Rosemont, IL, American Academy of Orthopaedic Surgeons, 2004, p 31.)*

American Academy of Orthopaedic Surgeons

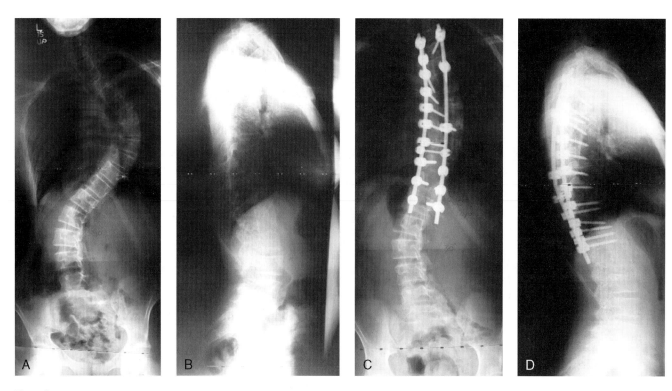

Figure 5 Preoperative AP **(A)** and lateral **(B)** radiographs of a 12-year-old girl with idiopathic scoliosis and double major curve (Lenke 3 or King-Moe 2); 90° right thoracic and 55° left lumbar pattern are noted. Postoperative AP **(C)** and lateral **(D)** radiographs show the patient after anterior release and posterior selective thoracic instrumentation with multiple pedicle screws. Residual scoliosis is acceptable with balanced 30° curves and preservation of lumbar motion.

bosacral orthosis or Milwaukee brace exerts forces on the upper thorax when the curve apex is above T7. Few data exist to confirm the effectiveness of brace use for these high thoracic curves.

Another form of nonsurgical treatment is casting for infantile forms of scoliosis, but again, evidence comes from uncontrolled studies. Alternative methods offered as treatment of scoliosis include physical therapy, chiropractic manipulations, dietary adjustments, and electrical stimulation. Physical therapy often is prescribed if back pain and stiffness are associated with scoliosis. However, physical therapy and other methods of therapy have never been proven to alter the natural progression of scoliosis.

Surgical Treatment

The indications for surgical treatment of idiopathic scoliosis are largely predicated on the adverse natural history of curves in adult life, but are tempered by the fact that there currently is no cure for the condition, and treatment means fusion of the spine. Therefore, curves greater than 45° to 50° in growing adolescents are usually treated with surgery (instrumentation and fusion) (Figure 5). However, marked trunk imbalance may lead to surgical management of a 40° curve at the thoracolumbar junction in a patient of similar age (Figure 6), whereas double major curves of approximately 45° may be acceptable in a skeletally mature patient.

The natural history of early-onset scoliosis, particularly before age 5 years, is especially malignant because alveolar multiplication is ongoing from birth to age 4 to 5 years. Scoliosis at this early age can hinder pulmonary alveolar growth, ultimately leading to significant cardiopulmonary impairment with restrictive lung disease and, possibly, cor pulmonale. Beyond age 5 years, lung capacity is mostly a function of thoracic cage growth and expansion of existing alveoli. Therefore, the adverse effects of thoracic scoliosis are particularly pronounced in young children, especially with infantile onset.

Attempts to maximize trunk height and thus pulmonary function have been made through the use of expandable growth rods without fusion in young children (younger than age 8 years) with scoliosis. Reports of this technique show average spine lengthening of 2.0 to 3.5 cm over the instrumented segments and maximum lengthening rarely exceeding 5 cm. Therefore, growth rods will allow a limited amount of growth but will require many surgical treatments occurring at intervals of 6 to 9 months. Because of these limitations, other fusionless techniques are being investigated.

Expansion thoracoplasty using opening wedge thoracostomy with insertion of a titanium rib expansion device has been developed over the past 15 years. Results for children with fused ribs and congenital bars have been encouraging, with growth produced in the spine as well as the thorax. Expanding the indications for this

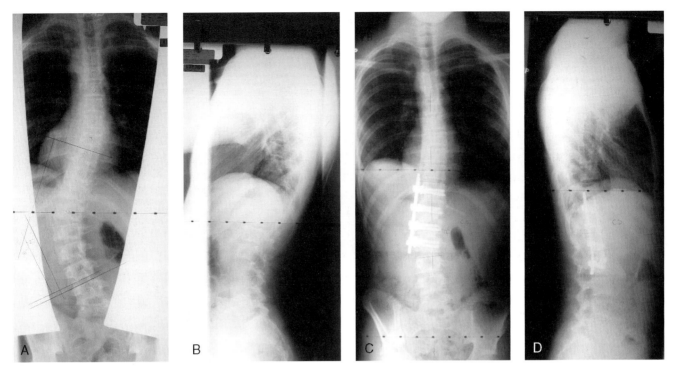

Figure 6 Radiographs of a 14-year-old boy with adolescent idiopathic scoliosis. **A,** 45° left thoracolumbar curve (Lenke 5). **B,** The trunk was coronally off balance to the left. AP **(C)** and lateral **(D)** radiographs after surgery were performed using an anterior approach with anterior instrumentation.

procedure to children with infantile idiopathic scoliosis and associated thoracic insufficiency is being adopted.

Surgical Complications in Idiopathic Scoliosis

Complications following treatment of adolescent idiopathic scoliosis are rare. Medical complications most commonly include the syndrome of inappropriate antidiuretic hormone release and ileus. This syndrome can be exacerbated by the use of hypotonic intravenous solutions postoperatively. Ileus is common after surgery and is related to the length of the operation, the use of narcotics, and hypotension. In most instances, ileus resolves within 48 hours. Early and late infections occur with a frequency of up to 5%. Infections are minimized by the use of perioperative antibiotics and by attention to sterile surgical techniques. Successful management of infections may include implant removal, débridement, primary wound closure, and administration of antibiotics.

Other complications include implant failure and pseudarthrosis, with rates of up to 3%. Local autograft and allograft typically are used to treat adolescent idiopathic scoliosis. One report promotes the use of local autograft alone with no pseudarthrosis over 6-year average postoperative follow-up. Another recent report corroborated previous studies showing that stable correction at a minimum 2-year postoperative follow-up can be achieved with cancellous allograft and with demineralized bone matrix plus autologous marrow aspirate. However, the most sustained Cobb correction occurred

in the group using autologous iliac crest graft and demineralized bone matrix plus marrow. Pseudarthrosis is diagnosed by pain in the area of instrumentation, more than 10° loss of correction, or implant failure or fracture (Figure 7 and Table 4).

Neurologic injury following surgical treatment of idiopathic scoliosis fortunately is rare, with a reported incidence of 0.4%. Spinal cord injury can be related to mechanical compression from an implant or bone, excessive tension, and vascular compromise or cord hypoperfusion alone. Avoidance of spinal cord injury is enhanced by spinal cord monitoring with somatosensory- evoked potentials and motor-evoked potentials and use of the wake-up test if neural monitoring is not available. Furthermore, mean arterial pressure should be maintained at greater than 70 mm Hg in high-risk patients.

Blood loss is an expected result of surgery for spinal deformity; however, strategies implemented preoperatively, intraoperatively, and postoperatively have been developed to reduce the need for allogeneic transfusion. The following techniques are commonly used despite the ongoing cost assessments. Autologous donation of red blood cells has been shown to effectively reduce the need for allogeneic transfusions. Autologous donation combined with recombinant erythropoietin can result in rapid recovery of red cell mass. Intraoperative blood salvage using cell-saver machines to recycle suctioned blood is done routinely. To complement the cell saver, some degree of hypotension and intraoperative position-

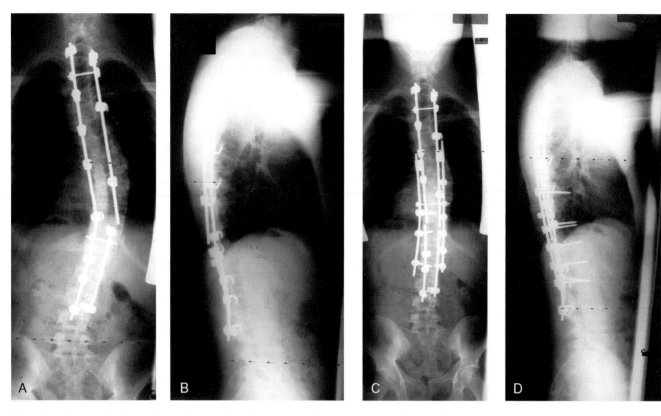

Figure 7 Radiographs of a 20-year-old patient treated with adolescent onset scoliosis who was treated with surgery. The patient had back pain and a pseudarthrosis presenting as a rod fracture with curve progression 3 years after the initial instrumentation. AP **(A)** and lateral **(B)** radiographs show the broken rods; AP **(C)** and lateral **(D)** radiographs after revision surgery included removal of apical hooks, a posterior element osteotomy at the deformity apex, distal pedicle fixation to L2, and linkage to the proximal rods.

Table 4 | Surgical Complications in Adolescent Idiopathic Scoliosis

Complication	Approximate Frequency
Infection (early)	1% to 2%
Infection (late)	Up to 5%
SIADH*	5% to 33%
Coagulopathy	1%
Ileus	3% to 6%
Neurologic defects (complete and incomplete)	0.4% to 0.7%
Pseudarthrosis	3%

Syndrome of inappropriate antidiuretic hormone release

ing is used to reduce abdominal pressure. Postoperative blood salvage and recycling is also available. More recently, pharmacologic methods have been used to reduce blood loss. Antifibrinolytic agents including episolon aminocaproic acid and apoprotein, a proteinase inhibitor, have been shown to reduce perioperative blood loss.

Instrumentation

A steady evolution of instrumentation systems has occurred since the inception of the Harrington and Dwyer systems in the early 1960s. The goal of surgery is to stop curve progression and to obtain an anatomically aligned and balanced spine in all anatomic planes with fusion of as few segments as possible. Fusion for severe deformity is a compromise, with correction of deformity being chosen over spinal mobility. Biomechanical factors that increase construct stiffness include rod diameter, number of anchors, and anchor configuration (Table 5). Anchors placed in compression will increase stiffness as will anterior column grafting and support if diskectomy is performed. Correction forces used in deformity surgery include cantilevering, segmental rotation, transverse traction, and distraction and compression to produce kyphosis or lordosis, respectively, and to tilt the vertebra in the frontal plane. Two-rod systems are typically used posteriorly with hooks, wires, and/or screws to anchor to the spine. However, the instrumentation also may be applied to the anterior column. Precise indications for choosing posterior or anterior instrumentation have not been developed.

Pedicle screw anchors recently have been used more often than hooks and wires, with reports showing greater correction with perhaps fewer levels included in the fusion, but the cost is two to three times greater. Neurologic injuries have not increased with pedicle screw use. In vivo studies show that up to 3 mm of medial intrusion

Table 5 | Mechanical Factors Increasing Construct Stiffness in Scoliosis-Long Segment Fusions

Rod diameter
Number of anchors
Compression toward the apex
Interbody grafts
Cross-linking

into the canal is comparable to what typically occurs with dorsal intrusion using a sublaminar hook. Nevertheless, insertion of pedicle screws requires an understanding of the pedicle anatomy as it varies along the length of the spine. The spinal cord shifts to the concavity, making screw insertion riskier at the concave apex. For thoracic curves, the highest risk area lies between T6 and T9 on the concave side where there are relatively narrow pedicles and the spinal cord is closest to the medial wall. The pedicle screw technique appears to reduce the rib prominence more effectively so that thoracoplasty has not been performed as often in recent years.

Criteria for choosing fusion levels are still evolving for different patterns of adolescent idiopathic scoliosis. In general, when the lumbar curve is more flexible than the thoracic curve, such as in Lenke 1 or King-Moe II curves, selective fusion of thoracic curves leads to acceptable balance and outcomes over the intermediate term (2 to 15 years). If the lumbar curve is large, then attempts are made to stop the fusion at L3 rather than extending to L4. However, guidelines for discontinuing the instrumentation are not definitive because well-controlled outcome studies are not available.

Anterior approaches to the spinal column have become common for the release of rigid segments (often defined as > 70° on standing films or > 50° on bending films) as well as for instrumentation (Figure 5). Anterior approaches are also used to obliterate the physeal end plates in prepubertal children when crankshaft progression is a concern. In patients with idiopathic scoliosis, thoracolumbar curves (Lenke 5 and 6 curves) are often addressed with thoracoabdominal approaches and anterior instrumentation using either single- or double-rod fixation (Figure 6). Anterior instrumentation can exaggerate kyphosis; therefore, it often is used with interbody grafts of bone or mesh cages. In addition, anterior thoracic instrumentation had been introduced with the idea that greater correction can be achieved with fewer segments fused. However, complications related to thoracic instrumentation include a higher pseudarthrosis rate, which is associated with screw pull-out that occurs in weak and small vertebral bone. It has been reported that anterior thoracic instrumentation led to worsening of pulmonary function tests in the short term. Additionally, surgeons must recognize that the position of the aorta is more posterior and lateral in the scoliotic thoracic spine. Reports of vascular injury are rare; nevertheless, a pedicle screw that is too lateral or a vertebral body screw that is too long could produce catastrophic vascular injury. For advanced and rigid deformities, pedicle subtraction or Smith-Petersen osteotomies may be required. In all instances fusion depends on thorough facet excision and bone grafting. Surgical techniques for specific diagnoses will be covered separately in other chapters.

Surgical outcome commonly has focused on the technical aspects of correcting the radiographic deformity. More recently, however, health assessments have been done with the Scoliosis Research Society questionnaire and Medical Outcomes Study Short Form-36, showing that pain and self-image are adversely perceived in scoliosis patients independent of curve severity, suggesting that factors other than Cobb measurement are also at the root of patient concerns. Studies suggest that pain seems to improve following surgery with short follow-up. What remains unclear is the rate of early or late trunk decompensation resulting from inappropriate choice of fusion levels, connective tissue laxity, or later degeneration. Surgeons operate under the assumption that without treatment severe curves (generally accepted as those greater than 45°) will progress. However, no long-term surgical outcome studies are available to compare with the existing 30-year natural history studies. Furthermore, the conclusions drawn from the longest surgical studies may not be generalized because surgical techniques have continually evolved. Longer-term, multicenter studies with control patients and more comprehensive outcome measurements are needed to understand the true impact of surgical treatment on scoliosis.

Summary

Because scoliosis is a clinical sign, the underlying diagnosis must be ascertained. Idiopathic scoliosis occurs in otherwise healthy patients. If curve progression begins before age 5 years, pulmonary development and cardiopulmonary function can be severely compromised. Adolescent onset rarely is associated with clinically significant cardiopulmonary compromise.

The outcomes from brace treatment and surgical treatment have not been studied in controlled trials. Therefore, ideal indications and precise outcomes are not known. The evidence suggests that bracing is less effective for curves greater than 35° and that curves greater than 50° tend to progress in adult life. How surgical treatment compares with untreated scoliosis in terms of symptoms has not been ascertained by long-term studies. Instrumentation techniques have continuously evolved to include more rigid, multisegmental fixation.

Annotated Bibliography
General
Dobbs MB, Weinstein SL: Infantile and juvenile scoliosis. *Orthop Clin North Am* 1999;30:331-341.

The diagnosis and treatment of scoliosis in the infantile and juvenile age groups is reviewed. These authors found that once a deformity has proved to be progressive, surgical intervention is likely to be necessary because brace treatment is less effective in these patients.

Little DG, Song KM, Katz D, Herring JA: Relationship of peak height velocity to other maturity indicators in idiopathic scoliosis in girls. *J Bone Joint Surg Am* 2000; 82:685-693.

Height velocity data obtained from clinical height measurements for girls who had idiopathic scoliosis were compared with the data for adolescents who did not have scoliosis. The height velocity plot grouped by peak height velocity showed a high peak and a sharp decline with values similar to those in normal populations. Height velocities generated from clinical height measurements for patients with idiopathic scoliosis document the growth peak and reliably predict cessation of growth. Knowing the timing of the growth peak provides valuable information on the likelihood of progression to a magnitude requiring spinal arthrodesis.

Scoliosis Classification Systems
Jones KB, Erkula G, Sponseller PD, Dormans JP: Spine deformity correction in Marfan syndrome. *Spine* 2002; 27:2003-2012.

This retrospective review of patients with Marfan syndrome who underwent surgery for primary scoliosis (n = 26), kyphosis (n = 7), or deformity secondary to previous surgery (n = 6) showed high complication rates. The complications included increased blood loss and rates of infection (10%), dural tear (8%), instrumentation fixation failure (21%), pseudarthrosis (10%), and coronal (8%) and sagittal (21%) curve decompensation. One patient died of valvular insufficiency 11 weeks after surgery. The authors concluded that the cardiopulmonary condition of patients with Marfan syndrome should be evaluated presurgically. Imaging should include CT to assess bony adequacy for fixation and MRI to evaluate dural ectasia.

Lenke LG, Betz RR, Clements D, et al: Curve prevalence of a new classification of operative adolescent idiopathic scoliosis: Does classification correlate with treatment. *Spine* 2002;27:604-611.

A retrospective multicenter consecutive case review of surgical adolescent idiopathic scoliosis showed that all 606 patients were classifiable by this system.

Lenke LG, Betz RR, Harms J, et al: Adolescent idiopathic scoliosis: A new classification to determine extent of spinal arthrodesis. *J Bone Joint Surg Am* 2001;83-A: 1169-1181.

A new classification system was developed with three components: curve type (1 through 6), a lumbar spine modifier (A, B, or C), and a sagittal thoracic modifier (-, N, or +).

Imaging
Dobbs MB, Lenke LG, Szymanski DA, et al: Prevalence of neural axis abnormalities in patients with infantile idiopathic scoliosis. *J Bone Joint Surg Am* 2002;84:2230-2234.

The records of 46 consecutive patients seen between 1992 and 2000 at three spinal deformity clinics were retrospectively reviewed to determine the incidence of neural axis abnormalities in patients with infantile scoliosis. All patients were evaluated with a total spine MRI protocol and 10 patients (21.7%) were found to have a neural axis abnormality. Eight of the 10 patients needed neurosurgical intervention for treatment of the abnormality. The high prevalence of neural axis abnormalities led to a recommendation that all patients with infantile idiopathic scoliosis who have a curve measuring 20° or more have a total spine MRI evaluation at the time of presentation.

Idiopathic Scoliosis
Asher M, Min LS, Burton D, Manna B: Scoliosis research society-22 patient questionnaire: Responsiveness to change associated with surgical treatment. *Spine* 2003;28:70-73.

Fifty-eight patients, average age 16 years and average Cobb size 63°, completed the Scoliosis Research Society-22 outcomes questionnaire preoperatively and at 3- (within 4 months), 6- (5 to 8 months), 12- (9 to 16 months), and 24-month (22 to 36 months) intervals postoperatively. Self-image was significantly improved at 3 months and maintained improvement through 24 months. Function was significantly decreased at 3 months but returned to baseline by 6 months. Pain was significantly worse at 3 months but improved at 6, 12, and 24 months. The Scoliosis Research Society-22 questionnaire was believed to be responsive to changes in the postsurgical period.

Bridwell KH, Shufflebarger HL, Lenke LG, Lowe TG, Betz RR, Bassett GS: Parents' and patients' preferences and concerns in idiopathic adolescent scoliosis: A cross-sectional preoperative analysis. *Spine* 2000;25:2392-2399.

A multicenter cross-sectional study was conducted to assess parents' and patients' concerns and preferences regarding surgery for idiopathic scoliosis. Ninety-one sets of parents and patients were separately asked to complete questionnaires regarding the patients' upcoming surgery. The greatest concern was neurologic deficit, and the least concern was location and appearance of the scar. The highest expectation and main reason for having the surgery was to reduce future pain and disability as an adult.

Freidel K, Petermann F, Reichel D, Steiner A, Warschburger P, Weiss HR: Quality of life in women with idiopathic scoliosis. *Spine* 2002;27:E87-E91.

The health-related quality of life of 226 female patients with idiopathic scoliosis was compared with that in age-matched general population norms using either the Medical Outcomes Study Short-Form-36 or the Berner Questionnaire for Well-Being. Patients with idiopathic scoliosis were less happy with their lives than the age-matched general population norm. Adult patients reported more psychologic and physical impairment than in the population norm. These results were largely independent of age and Cobb angle.

Kuklo TR, Owens BD, Polly DW Jr: Perioperative blood and blood product management for spinal deformity surgery. *Spine J* 2003;3:388-393.

This article reviews current blood management strategies. Techniques were organized into preoperative, intraoperative, and postoperative categories, and results were reviewed and well referenced.

Mineiro J, Weinstein SL: Subcutaneous rodding for progressive spinal curvatures: Early results. *J Pediatr Orthop* 2002;22:290-295.

This study retrospectively reviewed records of 11 patients with progressive early-onset scoliosis who underwent consecutive distraction of subcutaneous rods. At surgery, the average patient age was 5.6 years, with a mean Cobb angle of 74°. Subcutaneous rodding halted curve progression in all patients. At an average of 5.1 years after surgery, one patient showed no deterioration of the curve and nine patients showed an improvement of 40% or more. Spinal growth in all 11 patients ranged from 0.5 to 4.5 cm (mean 2.0). Early results indicate that subcutaneous rodding with consecutive distraction allows correction of progressive early-onset scoliosis.

Richards BR, Emara KM: Delayed infections after posterior TSRH spinal instrumentation for idiopathic scoliosis: Revisited. *Spine* 2001;26:1990-1996.

A retrospective analysis of medical records from 489 patients with scoliosis 2 or more years after surgery showed 23 (4.7%) had delayed infections. Spontaneous drainage occurred in 15 patients, fluctuance in 6, and pain and fever in 2. Sedimentation rate averaged 48 mm/h. All patients had instrumentation removed. Cultures at the time of removal grew *Propionibacterium acnes* in 12 patients, *Staphylococcus epidermidis* (or coagulase-negative *Staphylococcus*) in 4, *Micrococcus varians* in 1, and *S aureus* in 1. Five patients had negative cultures. After removal, all patients received parenteral antibiotics, followed by oral antibiotics in 21 patients.

Weinstein SL, Dolan LA, Spratt KF, Peterson KK, Spoonamore MJ, Ponseti IV: Health and function of patients with untreated idiopathic scoliosis: A 50-year natural history study. *JAMA* 2003;289:559-567.

At 50-year follow-up, 117 untreated patients with late onset idiopathic scoliosis were compared with 62 age- and sex-matched volunteers. The estimated probability of survival was not significantly different. Twenty-two of 98 patients (22%) reported shortness of breath during everyday activities compared with 8 of 53 volunteers (15%). An increased risk of shortness of breath was also associated with the combination

of a Cobb angle greater than 80° and a thoracic apex. Sixty-six of 109 patients (61%) reported chronic back pain compared with 22 of 62 volunteers (35%) ($P = 0.003$). The authors concluded that untreated late-onset idiopathic scoliosis causes little physical impairment other than back pain and cosmetic concerns.

Instrumentation

Belmont PJ Jr, Klemme WR, Robinson M, Polly DW Jr: Accuracy of thoracic pedicle screws in patients with and without coronal plane spinal deformities. *Spine* 2002;27: 1558-1566.

This retrospective observational study evaluated 399 transpedicular thoracic screws using postoperative CT to examine the in vivo accuracy of placement in patients with and without coronal plane spinal deformities. In patients with coronal plane spinal deformities, penetration of the pedicle wall and the anterior vertebral cortex was increased at T9 to T12 and overall. There were no neurologic or vascular complications. Fully contained screw accuracy in patients with coronal plane spinal deformities was less than in patients without these deformities at T9 to T12 and overall. Penetration of the anterior vertebral cortex was more frequent in patients with coronal plane spinal deformities than in those without.

Edwards CC, Lenke LG, Peelle M, Sides B, Rinella A, Bridwell KH: Selective thoracic fusion for adolescent idiopathic scoliosis with C modifier lumbar curves: 2- to 16-year radiographic and clinical results. *Spine* 2004;29: 536-546.

A retrospective clinical and radiographic review was conducted to evaluate outcome of selective thoracic fusion for adolescent idiopathic scoliosis with compensatory lumbar curves. For all 44 patients the compensatory minor lumbar C-modifier curves meant that the apical lumbar vertebra was deviated off the center sacral line. A mean 36% thoracic correction was closely matched by a 34% lumbar correction at latest follow-up. Most spontaneous lumbar correction occurred in the segments above the apical vertebra. The authors conclude that satisfactory results can be achieved with selective thoracic fusion in the presence of C-modifier lumbar curves.

Suk SI, Lee SM, Chung ER, Kim JH, Kim WJ, Sohn HM: Determination of distal fusion level with segmental pedicle screw fixation in single thoracic idiopathic scoliosis. *Spine* 2003;28:484-491.

A retrospective study was conducted to determine the exact distal fusion level in the treatment of single thoracic idiopathic scoliosis (King-Moe types 3 and 4) with segmental pedicle screw fixation. The authors believed that fusion should be to the neutral vertebra unless the neutral vertebra was too distal to the true end vertebra of the curve. In this case excellent balance could be achieved by fusing one short of the neutral vertebra. The evidence from this study is weak to support conclusions but it is one of the few studies to assess fusion relative to the neutral vertebra as a frame of reference.

Chapter 29

Spondylolysis, Spondylolisthesis, and Pediatric Disk Disease

Travis Hunt, MD

Christopher I. Shaffrey, MD

Spondylolysis and Spondylolisthesis

Spondylolysis is an acquired condition that is thought to be a stress fracture of the pars interarticularis caused by repetitive hyperextension. It occurs in 6% of individuals in the general population and in up to 53% of those in Eskimo populations. Spondylolysis occurs more commonly in males than females, with a ratio of almost 6 to 1. Soccer players, football players, wrestlers, and gymnasts have a greater predisposition to developing this lysis of the pars interarticularis. When spondylolysis is radiographically visible, an associated spondylolisthesis may occur in up to 25% of patients.

Spondylolisthesis refers to the forward slippage of one vertebra on another. It most often occurs in the lumbar spine and is classified by severity, etiology, and potential for progression. The incidence of spondylolisthesis differs in regard to gender and race based on the underlying cause. Heredity and environmental factors play a role in the development of spondylolisthesis.

Progression of spondylolisthesis has been associated with the adolescent growth spurt, lumbosacral kyphosis, and greater amount of initial slippage on presentation. Younger age (decreased skeletal maturity), vertebra slippage of greater than 50%, vertebra slippage angle greater than 40° to 50° (0° to 10° is normal), female gender, dome-shaped sacrum, and a dysplastic lumbosacral junction all are associated with an increased risk of progressive spondylolisthesis. Significant progression is uncommon in adulthood.

Classification

Spondylolisthesis was classified into five groups based on etiology described by Newman in 1963 and later by Wiltse, Newman, and Macnab, which distinguishes congenital, isthmic, traumatic, pathologic, and iatrogenic (Table 1).

Dysplastic or congenital spondylolisthesis is the result of a congenital defect at the L5-S1 articulation. The pars interarticularis may be poorly formed but is intact. Typically, abnormal facet orientation and/or a dome-shaped sacral promontory is present, and the normal buttress effect is not present. Progression is common in patients with congenital spondylolisthesis because the dysplastic facets permit the superior vertebral body to slip forward over the inferior vertebral body. Anterior translation results in stenosis of the exiting nerve root in the neuroforamen and can present as a radiculopathy. Severe neurologic conditions such as cauda equina can occur in patients with dysplastic spondyloptosis because the nerve roots become entrapped by the lamina, the intact pars interarticularis, and the sacral dome.

The Wiltse, Newman, and Macnab classification system describes lytic or isthmic spondylolisthesis as a defect of the pars interarticularis, which is thought to be the result of a stress fracture. These defects typically present in adolescents and are the most common subtype in this age group. It has been reported that 85% to 95% of spondylitic defects occur at the L5 level, whereas the next most commonly affected level is L4 (5% to 15%). In patients with isthmic spondylolisthesis, males are more commonly affected than females, and the most common level of involvement is L5-S1. However, among patients with high-grade isthmic spondylolisthesis, females are affected four times more commonly than males, the highest rates of which occur

Table 1 | Wiltse Newman, and Macnab Classification System for Spondylolisthesis

Dysplastic (congenital)
    Articular processes with transverse orientation
    Facet articulations with a sagittal orientation
    Anomalies of the lumbosacral junction
Isthmic
    Lytic lesion of the pars interarticularis
    Elongated pars
    Acute fracture of the pars
Degenerative
Traumatic
Pathologic
Iatrogenic

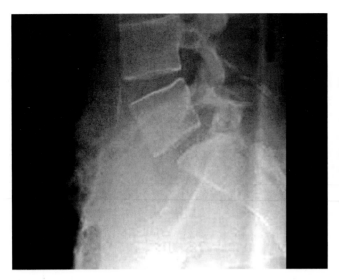

Figure 1 Radiograph showing traumatic spondylolisthesis in a teenage patient.

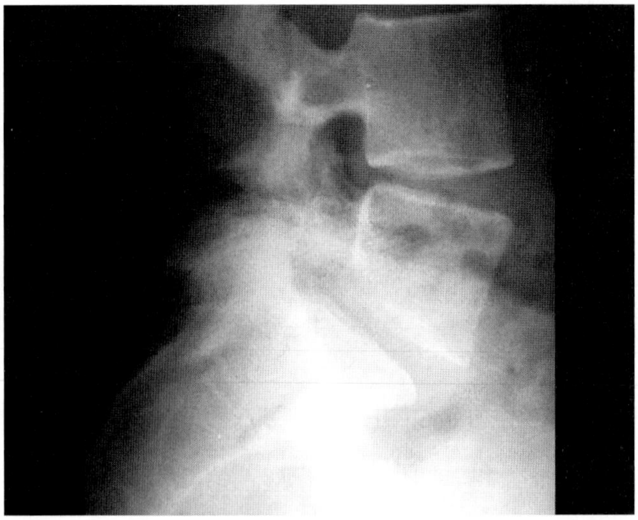

Figure 2 Spot lateral radiograph of the lumbosacral junction showing grade 1 spondylolisthesis and an L5 pars interarticularis defect.

among Alaskan female Eskimos. Hereditary factors appear to play a role in isthmic conditions because an increased incidence among first-degree relatives ranging from 19% to 69% has been cited in different series.

The other types in the Wiltse, Newman, and Macnab classification system are degenerative, traumatic, pathologic, and iatrogenic or postoperative. Traumatic spondylolisthesis is the result of a single high-energy injury and is a variant of spinal fracture-dislocation. These forms of injury are not common in either children or adults. Forces producing the lesion have been postulated to be hyperflexion in patients with pure dislocations and hyperflexion in combination with compression or axial translation in patients with significant fractures. A traumatic spondylolisthesis is extremely unstable and is often associated with a progression of displacement and risk of neurologic deficit. Listhesis of the involved segment is more likely to occur at L4-5 or L5-S1 than the upper lumbar segments. Treatment of traumatic spondylolisthesis generally consists of open reduction internal segmental fixation and fusion (Figure 1).

Pathologic spondylolisthesis can be divided into local and systemic processes that compromise the integrity of the intervertebral articulation. Local pathologic spondylolisthesis is secondary to a focal process at the involved level such as a spinal tumor. Systemic pathologic spondylolisthesis is the result of a generalized bone or connective tissue disorder such as osteogenesis imperfecta, Ehlers-Danlos syndrome, or Marfan syndrome.

Degenerative spondylolisthesis does not occur in children or adolescents. It typically presents in adults in the sixth and seventh decades of life and is more common in females and at the L4-5 level. It can be associated with other degenerative conditions such as spinal stenosis and scoliosis.

Marchetti and Bartolozzi developed a system that essentially distinguishes spondylolisthesis as dysplastic (congenital) or acquired (isthmic). This system acknowledges that patients with isthmic spondylolisthesis typically have normal vertebral structure; therefore, the spondylolisthesis is less likely to progress. Conversely, patients with dysplastic listhesis typically have abnormal vertebral architecture; therefore, the spondylolisthesis is more likely to progress. The 2004 Spine/Scoliosis Research Society spondylolisthesis summary statement recommended the use of this classification system.

The Meyerding classification is the most commonly used radiographic system for measuring spondylolisthesis. It is based on the percentage of translation of the cranial vertebra in relation to the caudal vertebra. The superior end plate of the inferior vertebrae is divided into quarters, and the amount of translation is recorded, based on which quadrant displacement occurs. Spondyloptosis describes 100% translation and is most often associated with deformity and neurologic deficits (Figure 2).

As the L5 vertebral body slides forward over the sacrum, the L5 body tilts into kyphosis. The kyphosis is quantified using the slippage angle that is measured by drawing a line perpendicular to a line drawn along the posterior aspect of the sacral vertebral body and measuring the angle between that and a line parallel to the inferior end plate of L5. Spondylolisthesis with slippage angles greater than 50% is likely to progress.

Evaluation

Patients with spondylolysis and spondylolisthesis most often present with back pain that is largely mechanical in nature; therefore, it is worse with activity and improves with rest. The pain typically localizes to the lum-

Meyerding Classification

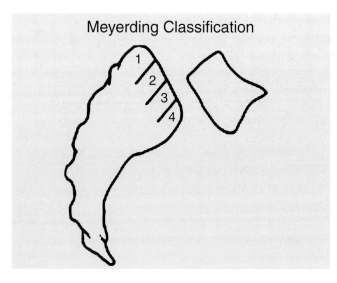

Figure 3 Schematic representation of the Meyerding classification for measuring spondylolisthesis. *(Reproduced with permission from Ganju A: Isthmic spondylolysthesis. Neurosurg Focus 2002;13:1-6.)*

bosacral area of the slip and is often worse on the side of the spondylosis.

Physical examination findings in patients with isthmic spondylolisthesis can include paraspinal muscle spasms, reduced lumbar mobility, and tight hamstrings. Hyperextension and rotation may aggravate symptoms as may single-leg stance while leaning backward. Patients with high-grade spondylolisthesis can have stooped posture with flexion at the hips and knees and can walk with a waddling gait. The flexed posture and hyperlordosis are compensation for the impending or real lumbosacral kyphosis at the level of the spondylolisthesis. Forward flexion in a patient with concomitant radiculopathy can reduce tension on the involved nerve root.

Diagnostic Studies

Radiographic evaluation begins with plain radiographs including AP, lateral, and bilateral oblique radiographs. On plain oblique radiographs, the defect in the pars interarticularis has been described as resembling the collar on a Scottish terrier (Scotty dog sign). A spot lateral view of the lumbosacral junction is the most sensitive view, disclosing the defect in 84% of patients. Bone scanning is often positive in patients with new lesions, but it is often negative in patients with long-term lesions. Bone scanning may be helpful in confirming the presence of symptomatic pars interarticularis lesions by showing evidence of increased activity at the defect. CT is more sensitive than plain radiography or nuclear medicine studies for identifying pars interarticularis lesions, but it is not considered 100% sensitive or specific. Single photon emission CT has advantages over bone scanning and plain radiography in this patient population. Single photon emission CT has greater sensitivity

than specificity for demonstrating a pars interarticularis defect. MRI has a less defined role for imaging pars interarticularis lesions, but it can help evaluate other associated pathology such as disk herniation, disk degeneration, annular disruption, or the presence of infection or tumor. This associated pathology can be the main source of symptoms in some patients (Figure 3).

Conservative Treatment

Most incidences of spondylolysis are found incidentally, are asymptomatic, and require no treatment. Occasionally, these lesions can be associated with significant low back pain, as is often the case with adolescents and young adults who ultimately present to spine surgeons with reports of severe, focal, low back pain that prevents participation in sports activities. All treatment options aim to relieve pain, optimize physical function, and possibly promote bony healing of the underlying defect of the pars interarticularis.

Reviews of the literature regarding standard treatment of spondylolysis can be confusing because the natural history of symptoms has not been clearly defined. Considerable debate exists over the indications for nonsurgical treatment, including the indications for bracing, the type of brace that is best tolerated and best relieves symptoms, the value of physical therapy, and the period required to define a failure of nonsurgical therapy.

Generally, spondylolysis will respond to nonsurgical treatment, including bracing, physical therapy with hamstring stretching, and activity restriction. The only absolute surgical indication is clear progression to a spondylolisthesis. Intolerable pain that does not respond to nonsurgical modalities is a relative indication for fusion.

In children who have significant or complete resolution of symptoms after conservative measures, a gradual reconditioning program is initiated before allowing them to return to routine sports activities. A physical therapy program focusing on stretching the lumbodorsal fascia and strengthening the paraspinous and abdominal musculature without hyperextension of the spine is performed. After reconditioning, the asymptomatic patient is allowed a gradual return to full activity.

Surgical Treatment

Indications for surgery include uncontrolled pain or major symptoms despite activity modification and bracing, slippage greater than 50% on initial presentation or progressive slippage from 25% to 50%, a slippage angle greater than 30% with significant growth remaining, and the presence of significant nerve root irritation causing sciatica, scoliosis, or progressive neurologic deficit.

Selected young patients with spondylolysis who do not respond to nonsurgical management may be considered for a primary repair of the pars interarticularis defects. Decompression alone has been associated with a

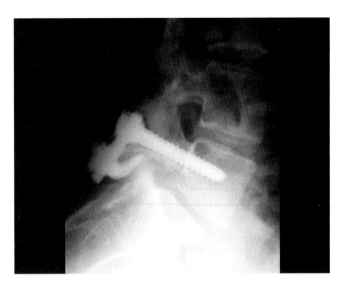

Figure 4 Radiograph showing spondylolisthesis treated with a compression hook and screw construct.

high rate of progression in the pediatric population. Primary repair can be performed by wiring, screw fixation, or both. Compression pedicle screw and hook constructs have also been described with favorable results (Figure 4). The advantage of such procedures is that they are intended to preserve the facet joint and motion of the affected segment. Early disk degeneration commonly occurs in patients with spondylolysis and spondylolisthesis and should be identified before surgery. If any question exists about the disk versus the pars interarticularis as a pain source, direct pars interarticularis injection with local anesthetic may help differentiate the source of pain. In patients with disk degeneration, a fusion should be performed. In patients with substantial disk degeneration or segmental instability, posterolateral fusion with or without instrumentation is the procedure of choice.

Noninstrumented (in situ) posterolateral fusion is an option in some patients with spondylolysis and spondylolisthesis. This procedure has been shown to reduce symptoms in 70% to 100% of patients, although overall fusion rates are slightly lower and can range from 40% to 100%. Fusion rates are lower in patients with higher-grade spondylolisthesis, especially in those with an increased slippage angle. Traditionally, noninstrumented procedures were managed with spica casting until the fusion consolidated. The use of a thoracic lumbosacral orthotic brace with a thigh extension in the postoperative period is not uncommon.

The advent and success of transpedicular instrumentation and fusion for other spinal disorders has led to their use in most patients with spondylolisthesis. Posterior segmental instrumentation and fusion can be performed with or without reduction and has the advantage over noninstrumented fusion in that it permits correction of the slippage angle and thereby improves body

posture and mechanics. Instrumentation increases fusion rate in patients with higher-grade spondylolisthesis while allowing full neural decompression. The treatment of high-grade spondylolisthesis may require the use of interbody fusion via a transforaminal or anterior approach combined with posterior instrumentation to relieve symptoms by decompression. The goals of an interbody fusion in patients with high-grade spondylolisthesis are to decompress neural elements, improve alignment, and obtain a solid fusion.

Most patients with spondylolysis or isthmic spondylolisthesis are asymptomatic and do not present to physicians. For symptomatic patients, nonsurgical measures that include activity restriction, physical therapy, and bracing usually control symptoms. Surgical intervention is reserved for patients who clearly fail nonsurgical management, those with progressive slippage, and those with significant or progressive neurologic deficit. The range of such procedures depends on the age of the patient, the presence of neurologic deficit, and the specific type of lesion present.

Pediatric Disk Disease

Disk problems are rare in patients younger than 19 years, with an incidence of 0.2% to 3.2% of patients admitted to the hospital for the treatment of sciatic type pain. In many patients, a herniated nucleus pulposus or slipped apophysis is most typically related to some antecedent factor such as trauma, tumor, genetics, or congenital anomaly. Overall, there appears to be no difference in gender distribution for pediatric disk disease, except that the incidence appears to be higher in preadolescent girls than preadolescent boys.

Classification and Evaluation

Sharpey's fibers connect the disk to the ring apophysis, and this attachment is stronger than the junction between the ring and the vertebral body. Therefore, the osteocartilaginous junction is a weak point until it becomes ossified. As a result, herniation of disk material with the bony apophysis (referred to as a slipped vertebral apophysis) can occur in children, as opposed to adults in whom the pathology is almost exclusively the result of migration of disk contents.

Diagnostic Studies

Children with a herniated disk or slipped vertebral apophysis most often present with low back pain, stiffness, and radicular symptoms. Radicular symptoms alone are infrequent. These patients require a thorough examination and imaging studies, including radiography, CT, and MRI to evaluate for the presence of a potential underlying pathology.

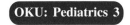

Conservative Treatment

Conservative treatment of pediatric disk disease is warranted in the acute phase. A short duration of rest in addition to nonsteroidal anti-inflammatory drugs or a steroid taper is usually effective in alleviating acute symptoms. Physical therapy, including massage and other modalities such as gentle stretching, is also helpful. Bracing has not been demonstrated to help with the natural history of pediatric disk disease and is therefore not recommended.

Surgical Treatment

Surgical intervention may be considered after failure of conservative treatment or in patients with cauda equina syndrome and consists of decompression of the affected nerve roots. Appropriate studies such as MRI are required to identify the presence of ring fractures, disk degeneration, and sequestered disk material. In patients with healthy disks and ring fractures, decompression of the hernia or ring fracture is sufficient, and complete diskectomy is not warranted. Spinal fusions are only indicated in patients with concomitant spondylolisthesis. Overall, outcomes have been reported to be good, with 95% good to excellent results and a 21% reoperation rate reported at 34-year follow-up.

Summary

A slipped vertebral apophysis in pediatric patients may present in the same manner that a herniated disk presents in adults. All pediatric patients with a slipped vertebral apophysis should be evaluated for potential underlying pathologies. After a thorough evaluation, most patients should initially be managed conservatively. If a patient fails to respond to conservative treatment, then surgical decompression may be warranted.

Annotated Bibliography

Beutler WJ, Fredrickson BE, Murtland A, Sweeney CA, Grant WD, Baker D: The natural history of spondylolysis and spondylolisthesis: 45-year follow-up evaluation. *Spine* 2003;28(10):1027-1035.

This prospective study of spondylolysis and spondylolisthesis was initiated in 1955 with a radiographic and clinical study of 500 first-grade children. The authors reported that there appeared to be a marked slowing of slippage progression with each decade. They also found that patients with pars interarticularis defects follow a clinical course that is similar to that of the general population and that no patients had reached 40% slippage.

Labelle H, Roussouly P, Berthonnaud E, et al: Spondylolisthesis, pelvic incidence, and spinopelvic balance: A correlation study. *Spine* 2004;29(18):2049-2054.

This retrospective study demonstrated that pelvic anatomy may play a role in the progression of spondylolisthesis. The authors found that an increased pelvic incidence may predispose some patients to not only development of spondylolisthesis but progression as well.

Lundin DA, Wiseman D, Ellenbogen RG, Shaffrey CI: Direct repair of the pars interarticularis for spondylolysis and spondylolisthesis. *Pediatr Neurosurg* 2003;39(4): 195-200.

The authors described their experience with five patients who were treated with direct pars interarticularis repair. They reported that the advantage of direct pars interarticularis repair over intertransverse fusion with or without segmental instrumentation involves the preservation of the anatomic integrity and motion of the affected segment. The authors concluded that direct pars interarticularis repair is a safe and effective modality to treat select groups of patients with spondylolysis and low-grade spondylolisthesis.

Mardjetko S, Albert T, Andersson G, et al: Spine/SRS spondylolisthesis summary statement. *Spine* 2005;30(6 suppl):S3.

The Scoliosis Research Society recommends the classification scheme proposed by Marchetti and Bartolozzi. This system is based on etiology and most clearly distinguishes between developmental and acquired forms of spondylolisthesis. It highlights the pathogenesis of the different types of spondylolisthesis and therefore potentially has the most relevance to natural history, risk of progression, and implications for treatment.

Ward CV, Latimer B: Human evolution and the development of spondylolysis. *Spine* 2005;30(16):1808-1814.

The authors compared normal spinal architecture with that of patients with spondylolysis and found that normal individuals had a significantly greater increase in interfacet dimensions progressing down the spine from L4 to S1 than patients with spondylolysis.

Classic Bibliography

Buck JE: Direct repair of the defect in spondylolisthesis: Preliminary report. *J Bone Joint Surg Br* 1970;52(3):432-437.

Ebersold MJ, Quast LM, Bianco AJ Jr: Results of lumbar discectomy in the pediatric patient. *J Neurosurg* 1987;67(5):643-647.

Freeman BL III, Donati NL: Spinal arthrodesis for severe spondylolisthesis in children and adolescents: A long-term follow-up study. *J Bone Joint Surg Am* 1989; 71(4):594-598.

Gaines RW, Nichols WK: Treatment of spondyloptosis by two stage L5 vertebrectomy and reduction of L4 onto S1. *Spine* 1985;10(7):680-686.

Gill GG, Manning JG, White HL: Surgical treatment of spondylolisthesis without spine fusion. *J Bone Joint Surg Am* 1955;37:493-520.

Kurihara A, Kataoka O: Lumbar disc herniation in children and adolescents: A review of 70 operated cases and their minimum 5-year follow-up studies. *Spine* 1980;5(5):443-451.

Lonstein JE: Spondylolisthesis in children: Cause, natural history, and management. *Spine* 1999;24(24):2640-2648.

Marchetti PG, Bartolozzi P: Classification of spondylolisthesis as a guideline for treatment, in Bridwell KH, DeWald RL (eds): *The Textbook for Spinal Surgery*, ed 2. Philadelphia, PA, Lippincott-Raven, 1997, pp 1211-1254.

Meyerding HW: Spondylolisthesis. *Surg Gynecol Obstet* 1932;54:371-377.

Molinari RW: Complications in the surgical treatment of pediatric high-grade, isthmic dysplastic spondylolisthesis: A comparison of three surgical approaches. *Spine* 1999;24(16):1701-1711.

Newman PH: The etiology of spondylolisthesis. *J Bone Joint Surg Br* 1963;45:39-59.

Poussa M, Schlenzka D, Seitsalo S, et al: Surgical treatment of severe isthmic spondylolisthesis in adolescents: Reduction or fusion in situ. *Spine* 1993;18:894-901.

Saraste H: Long-term clinical and radiological follow-up of spondylolysis and spondylolisthesis. *J Pediatr Orthop* 1987;7(6):631-638.

Schollner D: One stage reduction and fusion for spondylolisthesis. *Int Orthop* 1990;14(2):145-150.

Turner RH, Bianco AJ Jr: Spondylolysis and spondylolisthesis in children and teen-agers. *J Bone Joint Surg Am* 1971;53(7):1298-1306.

Wiltse LL, Newman PH, Macnab I: Classification of spondylolysis and spondylolisthesis. *Clin Orthop* 1976;117:23-29.

Wynne-Davies R, Scott JH: Inheritance and spondylolisthesis: A radiographic family survey. *J Bone Joint Surg Br* 1979;61-B(3):301-305.

Zamani MH, MacEwen GD: Herniation of the lumbar disc in children and adolescents. *J Pediatr Orthop* 1982;2(5):528-533.

Chapter 30

Pediatric Kyphosis

Vincent Arlet, MD

Dietrich Schlenzka, MD, PhD

Introduction

Pediatric kyphosis is known to have different etiologies; postural kyphosis and Scheuermann's kyphosis are the most common. Other etiologies such as postlaminectomy kyphosis, congenital kyphosis, postinfectious conditions, chondrodysplasia, or posttraumatic kyphosis are less common and are listed in Table 1. For the orthopaedic surgeon, Scheuermann's kyphosis represents the most classic form of kyphosis for which a therapeutic decision must be made. However, indications for treatment of Scheuermann's kyphosis are not well codified and remain rare because the natural history of the disease is in most cases benign.

Normal Sagittal Alignment

The normal sagittal alignment of the spine varies from birth to old age. In the teenager or adolescent, the normal gravity line should be dropped from the odontoid process, cross the thoracolumbar junction, and fall between the femoral heads and S2. Such sagittal balance is essential for the patient to stand with minimal effort. Abnormal sagittal balance is observed when the spinal column cannot compensate to keep the gravity line between the femoral heads and the sacrum. Positive sagittal balance occurs when the gravity line falls in front of the femoral heads, and negative sagittal balance occurs when the gravity line falls posterior to the sacrum. These two considerations are important because a negative sagittal balance may be observed in patients with neuromuscular conditions and who have weak hip extensors, and a positive sagittal balance may be observed in patients with developmental delay or a rigid kyphotic lumbar spine. Most patients with Scheuermann's kyphosis are in the negative sagittal balance group.

The thoracic spine should be in slight kyphosis with a Cobb angle ranging from 20° to 45° between T2 and T10. The thoracolumbar spine should be straight between T10 and L2, and the lumbar spine between L2 and the sacrum should show more lordosis than thoracic kyphosis.

Table 1	Etiology of Kyphosis
Postural kyphosis
Idiopathic kyphosis
Scheuermann's kyphosis
Thoracic
Thoracolumbar
Neuromuscular conditions
Paralytic
Spastic
Spinal cord tumor
Postlaminectomy kyphosis
Posttraumatic kyphotic deformity
Connective tissue disorders
Congenital kyphosis
Postinfectious (tuberculosis)

Abnormal Kyphosis

The location of the deformity must be determined before assessment of the absolute amount of kyphotic deformity. For instance, a thoracolumbar kyphotic deformity of 20° between T10 and L3 is highly abnormal, whereas a thoracic kyphosis of 55° between T2 and T12 would be considered normal by some surgeons.

However, absolute numbers can be given to indicate excessive kyphosis: a thoracic kyphosis in excess of 45° to 55° is abnormal, and a thoracolumbar kyphosis in excess of 15° is also abnormal. At the lumbosacral spine there should be more lordosis than thoracic kyphosis.

Scheuermann's Kyphosis
Historical Background

Scheuermann's kyphosis is a thoracic hyperkyphosis resulting from wedged vertebrae that develop during adolescence. It was first described in 1921 as being different from postural kyphosis on the basis of spine rigidity (Figure 1). Its etiology is believed to be a developmental error in collagen aggregation leading to a disturbance of the enchondral ossification of the vertebral end plates.

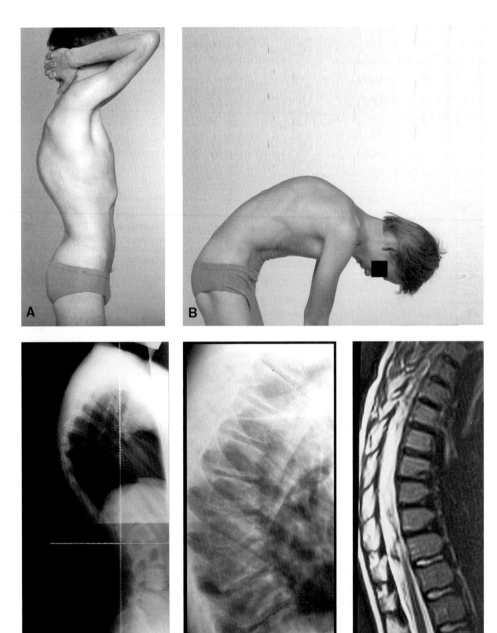

Figure 1 **A** and **B,** Photographs showing the typical aspect of a patient with Scheuermann's kyphosis in whom the deformity is clinically rigid. **C,** Weight-bearing radiograph showing increased kyphosis. **D,** Spot radiograph showing irregularities of the end plates. **E,** MRI scan showing consecutive vertebral wedging and dehydrated disks. *(A through D, Reproduced with permission from Arlet V, Schlenzka D: Scheuermann kyphosis: Surgical management. Eur Spine J 2005;14(9):817-827.)*

This disturbance causes wedge-shaped deformation of the vertebrae and increased kyphosis. Genetic, hormonal, and mechanical etiologies have been discussed, and an autosomal dominant pattern of inheritance now is accepted. The incidence of Scheuermann's kyphosis is estimated to be between 1% and 8%, with a ratio of boys to girls between 2:1 and 7:1.

Clinical Presentation and Patient Assessment

Patients are brought to a physician because the parents are concerned that the child's back is hunched over or because of back pain. Patients have a rigid hyperkyphosis in the midthoracic or lower thoracic spine (Figure 1)

and a compensatory hyperlordosis of the cervical and/or lumbar spine. Mild secondary scoliosis with minimal or no rotation at all may be present.

Knowledge of a family history of kyphotic deformity is important because patients with Scheuermann's kyphosis often have a genetic predisposition. The physical examination must look for any rigidity of the spine, which is a hallmark that distinguishes postural kyphosis from other pathologic kyphotic deformities. Assessment of any hamstring tightness, a thorough neurologic examination, and assessment of range of motion of different joints including the neck are key points of the examination.

Weight bearing and lateral radiographs of the whole spine, spot films, and lateral shoot-through radiographs with the patient positioned on a sand bag will be required. Additional imaging studies such as CT or MRI usually are required before surgical intervention is begun.

The hallmark of the diagnosis is rigidity of the spine. This rigidity is best assessed by asking a patient in the prone position to hyperextend the back and lift the head. Hamstring tightness is common. Neurologic findings are very rare. Pain may occur in the region of the kyphosis or in hyperlordotic areas above or below the main deformity.

Radiographically, Scheuermann's kyphosis is characterized by an increased kyphosis with compensatory lumbar hyperlordosis (Figure 1, *C*). A classic finding is wedging of three consecutive vertebrae (> 5°), with endplate irregularities, loss of disk space height, and Schmorl's nodes (Figure 1, *D*). Aside from these typical features, some authors have considered any vertebral wedging as a sign of Scheuermann's kyphosis. MRI (Figure 1, *E*), which should be requested before surgery, shows a premature dehydration in the intervertebral disks and an irregularity of ossification in the vertebral bodies.

The differential diagnosis of Scheuermann's kyphosis is made radiographically. Postural kyphosis has no wedging of the vertebral bodies and is supple; however, congenital kyphosis with a defect of segmentation can mimic Scheuermann's kyphosis and is difficult to distinguish because the bony bar of the defect of segmentation may be seen only in late adolescence. The extreme rigidity along with the lack of visible disk space on radiographs and MRI will confirm the diagnosis. Clinicians must be aware that spinal cord tumor may present in teenagers in the form of pure kyphosis.

Natural History

Patients usually have pain or deformity (Figure 2). Symptoms are common during the early teenage years and, in most instances, decrease in late adolescence or early adulthood. Half of the patients in one study had thoracic pain while teenagers, and only 25% had pain after achieving skeletal maturity. An increase in the incidence of disabling back pain in adults was reported in another study, and pain was, therefore, considered a classic indication for surgery in this age group. In a report on the natural history of Scheuermann's disease over a 32-year period, the condition appeared to be benign in most patients. Affected patients seemed to have more back pain than healthy control patients; however, the pain rarely interfered with daily activities or professional career. However, the reported series usually involved the mild form of the disease (average kyphotic deformity of 71°), and authors of other series report severe thoracic pain in patients with more severe kyphotic deformities (> 75°). Cardiorespiratory conditions may occur in patients with very severe deformities (kyphosis > 100°). However, most patients experienced an increase in functional lung capacity.

Treatment

Nonsurgical Treatment

Nonsurgical treatment (exercise, bracing, casting) classically is indicated during the growth period if thoracic kyphosis exceeds 45° and radiologic signs of the disease are present. Exercise has not been shown to improve kyphosis; however, it does have the advantage of increasing the patient's awareness of the condition. Bracing and casting are of value only in patients with a mobile kyphotic deformity and with a sufficient amount of growth remaining. One year of remaining growth usually is acceptable to begin orthopaedic treatment. Curves greater than 75° have a higher failure rate. Bracing and/or casting is known to become ineffective in patients whose curves are Risser grade 4 or 5. However, in the largest nonsurgical treatment series, compliant patients treated with the Milwaukee brace achieved stabilization or a small improvement in their deformity. Thirty percent of patients with initial curves greater than 75° required surgery. Because of the high rate of noncompliance with Milwaukee brace treatment, other braces, such as the modified Boston or the modified Milwaukee, have been tried and shown to be effective. Brace treatment usually must be continued a minimum of 18 months to have an effect on vertebral wedging.

Surgical Treatment

A neurologic complication associated with Scheuermann's kyphosis is a formal indication for surgery. Such complications are rare and require neurologic decompression through an anterior thoracotomy or a posterolateral decompression.

Apart from these exceptional neurologic complications, there are no evidence-based criteria for surgical treatment. According to the literature, surgical treatment should be considered in patients with a kyphotic deformity greater than 75°, significant pain that has not responded to nonsurgical measures, and/or respiratory problems resulting from severe kyphosis, usually greater than 100°.

Because the natural history of Scheuermann's kyphosis tends to be benign, indications for surgery must be evaluated on a case-by-case basis, keeping in mind the potential complications of the surgery. The preoperative workup should focus on the patient's pain and/or cosmetic concerns and attempt to identify the patient's motivation. Stiff hamstrings, a popliteal angle of less than 30°, and any subtle neurologic findings should be assessed during the clinical examination. The impor-

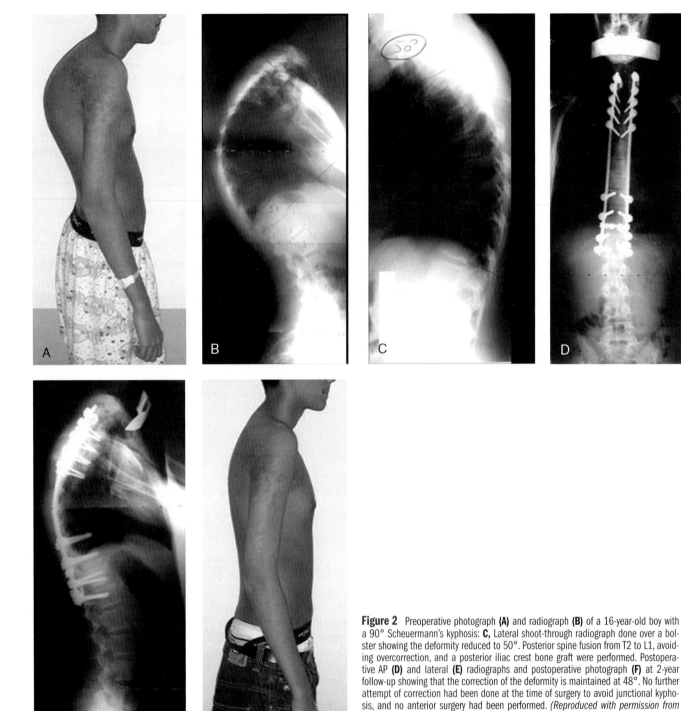

Figure 2 Preoperative photograph **(A)** and radiograph **(B)** of a 16-year-old boy with a 90° Scheuermann's kyphosis: **C,** Lateral shoot-through radiograph done over a bolster showing the deformity reduced to 50°. Posterior spine fusion from T2 to L1, avoiding overcorrection, and a posterior iliac crest bone graft were performed. Postoperative AP **(D)** and lateral **(E)** radiographs and postoperative photograph **(F)** at 2-year follow-up showing that the correction of the deformity is maintained at 48°. No further attempt of correction had been done at the time of surgery to avoid junctional kyphosis, and no anterior surgery had been performed. *(Reproduced with permission from Arlet V, Schlenzka D: Scheuermann kyphosis: Surgical management. Eur Spine J 2005;14(9):817-827.)*

tance of tight hamstrings as a possible cause of sagittal decompensation recently has been emphasized. Radiographs include long-cassette weight-bearing scoliosis films and a hyperreduction film best obtained as a lateral shoot-through as described previously (Figure 2). Pulmonary function tests are not necessary because function usually is normal or even increased. MRI before surgery is recommended to rule out any excep-

tional thoracic disk herniation, epidural cyst, and possible spinal stenosis. These exceptional circumstances have been described in various reports of neurologic complications. MRI will also assess the lumbar spine disks because, in some patients, disk degeneration in the lumbar spine may explain the pain rather than the deformity itself. The surgeon also should look for a possible spondylolysis, which frequently is observed in these

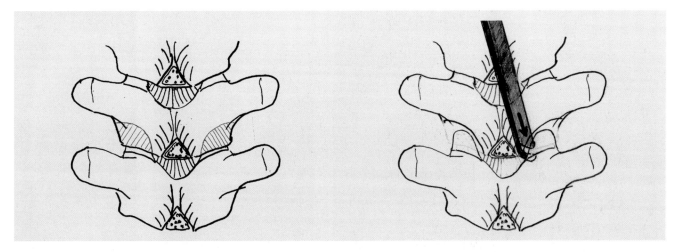

Figure 3 Schematic representation of the Ponte procedure in which the superior and inferior facets and the ligamentum flavum are removed at the apex of the deformity. *(Reproduced with permission from Arlet V, Schlenzka D: Scheuermann kyphosis: Surgical management. Eur Spine J 2005;14(9):817-827.)*

patients. Because surgery is also done to improve posture, clinical photographs may be useful for documentation (Figure 2, *A*).

Several questions must be answered before surgical decisions are made. Does the curve need an anterior release, what levels are to be included in the spine fusion, which technique of correction should be used, and how much correction should be performed?

Classic indications for anterior release are curves that do not correct over a sandbag to less than 50°. However, with the advent of modern and stiff posterior instrumentation, along with spine shortening techniques, this theory may not hold true (Figure 2).

The posterior shortening procedure will remove the superior and inferior facets at the apex of the deformity to help reduce the curve (Figure 3). Posterior fusion alone, however, may result in progression over time, as was first pointed out after simple Harrington posterior instrumentation. The long-term result of surgery with pedicle screw instrumentation is not known. Because the incidence of late surgical site pain is in the range of 5% to 10% in patients with segmental posterior instrumentation and removal of that instrumentation may lead to recurrence of the deformity even with a solid posterior fusion, anterior fusion of large and stiff Scheuermann's kyphosis may be safer for a long-lasting correction. In adult patients with Scheuermann's kyphosis and anterior bony bridging, anterior release will, of course, be necessary.

With modern segmental instrumentation, performance of an anterior release in the surgical candidate with Scheuermann's kyphosis currently is questionable. It is not known whether posterior surgery alone will hold with an extended follow-up of several decades.

How many levels should be fused posteriorly? The current recommendation is to include the entire kyphotic Cobb angle and stop distally above the first lordotic disk. The minimum number of vertebrae that must be fused for a thoracic Scheuermann's kyphosis with an apex at T8 is usually from T2 down to L1 or even L2. In patients with a thoracolumbar Scheuermann's kyphosis, the fusion may have to extend distally as low as L3.

Which techniques of posterior correction should be used? The spine shortening technique of Ponte should be well known in patients with stiff curves where correction is not feasible (Figure 3). The surgeon will remove the posterior spinous processes at the apex, remove the ligamentum flavum, and perform complete superior and inferior facet resection. These posterior resections have to be done at the apex of the curve after the different implants have been inserted.

The spinal instrumentation should consist of a strong foundation of pedicle screws, supplemented with laminar hooks if necessary in the lumbar spine and in the upper thoracic spine (Figures 2 and 4). There may be no need for instrumentation of the apex of the deformity. Hooks alone at the apex of the kyphosis or at the distal end of the construct can be potentially dangerous because they can compress the spinal cord at the apex of the deformity or pull out distally.

In situ bending may be used to fine tune the final correction or to undo what appeared to be too much correction. The literature does not seem to favor one technique over the other. Normalization of the thoracic kyphosis below 50° in the 40° to 50° range currently seems to be the goal to avoid postoperative imbalance. Posterior bone grafting from the iliac crest is recommended after thorough spinal decortication of the posterior elements to achieve a thick fusion mass.

With the advent of strong segmental posterior instrumentation, indications for postoperative bracing have relaxed. During the era when Harrington rods were used primarily, postoperative bracing was advised for a period of several months. Currently, bracing often

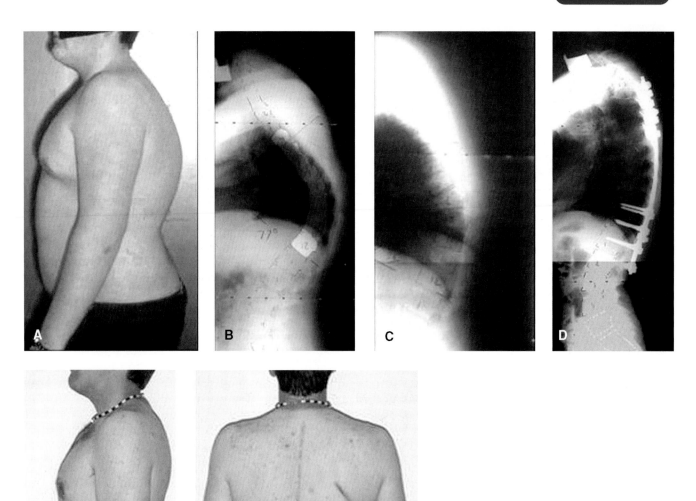

Figure 4 A, Preoperative photograph of a 15-year-old boy with rigid low Scheuermann's disease. **B,** The deformity was 77° using the Cobb angle method. **C,** Lateral shoot-through radiograph done over a bolster showing the deformity reduced to 58°. Because of the rigidity of the deformity and the patient's weight, an anterior release and posterior instrumentation were performed on the same day. Postoperative radiograph **(D)** and photographs **(E** and **F)** at 2-year follow-up show correction of the deformity; note also that the patient has lost a considerable amount of weight. *(Reproduced with permission from Arlet V, Schlenzka D: Scheuermann kyphosis: Surgical management. Eur Spine J 2005;14(9):817-827.)*

is not prescribed, as in patients after surgery for scoliosis. Forces are, however, totally different in patients with Scheuermann's kyphosis, and in active teenagers willing to resume physical activities as soon as possible regardless of the doctor's advice, bracing for the first 3 months after surgery is a reasonable choice.

Complications of Surgery

Neurologic complications can arise during the correction maneuvers because of a rare but unknown intracanal complication or from a complication resulting from surgical technique. The exact rate of neurologic complications in surgery for Scheuermann's kyphosis is not known but probably is higher than for idiopathic

scoliosis. Other complications, such as death, infection, and gastrointestinal obstruction, are common to any corrective procedure for spinal deformities.

Junctional kyphosis occurs in 20% to 30% of patients (Figure 5), and some series report an incidence higher than 50%. In the pathogenesis of junctional kyphosis, it was initially believed that the passage of sublaminar wires as in the Luque technique would result in disruption of the superior and infraspinatous ligaments with partial removal of the ligamentum flavum. Persistence of this complication even with the use of modern instrumentation that takes such structures into account prompted other plausible explanations: (1) fusion that is too short, stopping short of the first lordotic disk at the

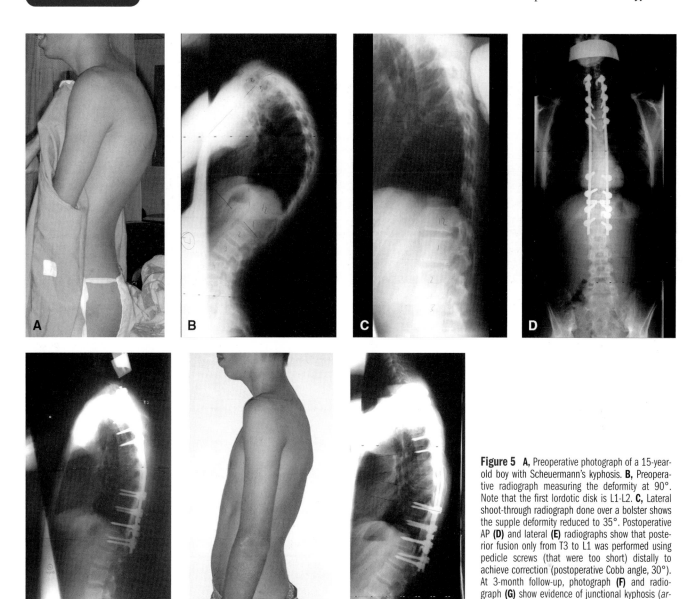

Figure 5 **A,** Preoperative photograph of a 15-year-old boy with Scheuermann's kyphosis. **B,** Preoperative radiograph measuring the deformity at 90°. Note that the first lordotic disk is L1-L2. **C,** Lateral shoot-through radiograph done over a bolster shows the supple deformity reduced to 35°. Postoperative AP **(D)** and lateral **(E)** radiographs show that posterior fusion only from T3 to L1 was performed using pedicle screws (that were too short) distally to achieve correction (postoperative Cobb angle, 30°). At 3-month follow-up, photograph **(F)** and radiograph **(G)** show evidence of junctional kyphosis (*arrow*), with rotation of the distal vertebra around the distal pedicle screws that were too short. *(Reproduced with permission from Arlet V, Schlenzka D: Scheuermann kyphosis: Surgical management. Eur Spine J 2005;14(9):817-827.)*

bottom with a resultant distal junctional kyphosis; (2) fusion that is too short proximally and does not include the entire kyphosis on the top with a resultant proximal junctional kyphosis and a goose neck appearance; and (3) hypercorrection. The kyphosis should not be corrected to more than 50% of its initial value (Figure 5). Postoperative brace use in a patient with Scheuermann's kyphosis may help prevent distal junctional kyphosis.

Results of surgery for Scheuermann's kyphosis can be analyzed according to the two major indications for which the surgery was performed: pain and cosmetic deformity. All series report between 60% and 90% improvement in the amount of back pain. One author reported a marked improvement in the Oswestry Disability score from an average of 23 preoperatively to 6.6 at follow-up. However, neck pain did not seem to have improved after surgery. Interestingly, no relationship seemed to exist between the amount of correction and the amount of residual back pain. Most series report a very high satisfaction rate, up to 96%. Most surgical series report a correction from an average initial Cobb angle of 70° to 75° to 40° to 45° at the last follow-up, or between 40% and 50% of correction.

Summary

In most patients, Scheuermann's kyphosis is a self-limited condition that remains benign and requires observation or exercise. In patients with a skeletal maturity level of Risser grade 3 or less, treatment with a cast or brace can be attempted, with the knowledge that in most instances the spine deformity will remain identical to what it was at the onset of treatment.

Indications for surgery in patients with Scheuermann's kyphosis should be considered for each patient individually. Spinal cord compression is rare and an absolute indication for surgery in adults. Other indications are based on the amount of deformity and its acceptance by the patient. Most authors agree that curves above 70° to 75° are an indication for surgery. Pain, especially in an adult, may represent another reason for surgery. New techniques such as video-assisted thoracoscopic anterior release and fusion, mini-open approaches, stiff third-generation segmental instrumentation, and posterior osteotomies have resulted in fewer formal open anterior releases. Proper selection of levels and avoidance of overcorrection will avoid complications such as junctional kyphosis. Most patients will have satisfactory results after surgery.

Annotated Bibliography
Abnormal Kyphosis
Arlet V, Liang J, Ouellet J: Is there a need for anterior release for 70-90 degrees thoracic curves in adolescent scoliosis. *Eur Spine J* 2004;13:740-745.

In this study, 19 patients whose thoracic curves were measured between 70° and 90° had posterior surgical correction with a third-generation stiff spinal segmental instrumentation. Postoperatively, the thoracic Cobb angle was measured at 34.8° (range, 25° to 45°), which represents a correction rate of 54% (range 40.0% to 67.1%), and it remained unchanged at the most recent follow-up (35°). Therefore, with adequate posterior release and the use of third-generation segmental instrumentation, there is no need for anterior release even for patients with curves in the 70° to 90° range.

Scheuermann's Kyphosis
Arlet V, Schlenzka D: Scheuermann kyphosis: Surgical management. *Eur Spine J* 2005;14(9):817-827.

This is a literature review on the surgical treatment of Scheuermann's kyphosis. Indications should be assessed patient by patient for curves greater than 75°. The fusion should include the entire Cobb angle and stop above the first lordotic disk. Frequent complications such as junctional kyphosis can be avoided with proper surgical technique, level selection, and avoidance of hypercorrection. The role of anterior release is no longer clear with the advent of strong posterior instrumentation.

Hosman AJ, de Kleuver M, Anderson PG, et al: Scheuermann kyphosis: The importance of tight hamstrings in the surgical correction. *Spine* 2003;28:2252-2259.

In this review of 33 patients with Scheuermann's kyphosis who underwent surgical correction, 16 patients had tight ham-

strings (popliteal angle > 30°) and 17 did not. Patients with tight hamstrings had a significantly greater risk of postoperative imbalance ($P < 0.05$). These patients can be classified as "lumbar compensators" and as such are prone to overcorrection and imbalance.

Hosman AJ, Langeloo DD, de Kleuver M, Anderson PG, Veth RP, Slot GH: Analysis of the sagittal plane after surgical management for Scheuermann's disease: A view on over correction and the use of an anterior release. *Spine* 2002;27:167-175.

A cohort of 33 patients who had undergone surgery for Scheuermann's kyphosis were reviewed, Group A, posterior technique (n = 16); Group B, anteroposterior technique (n = 17). At follow-up evaluation (4.5 ± 2 years) there was no difference in curve morphometry, correction, sagittal balance, average age, and follow-up period between groups A and B. The authors believe that surgeons should aim at a correction within the high normal kyphosis range of 40° to 50°, providing good results and, particularly in flexible adolescents and young adults, minimizing the necessity for an anterior release.

Papagelopoulos PJ, Klassen RA, Peterson HA, Dekutoski MB: Surgical treatment of Scheuermann's disease with segmental compression instrumentation. *Clin Orthop Relat Res* 2001;386:139-149.

In this study, 21 patients with Scheuermann's kyphosis underwent surgery to treat a progressive kyphotic deformity of 50° or greater. All patients had posterior spine arthrodesis with segmental compression instrumentation. Seven patients with rigid kyphosis had combined anterior and posterior spine arthrodesis. The mean preoperative thoracic kyphotic curve of 68.5° improved to 40° at the most recent follow-up, with an average loss of correction of 5.75°. The authors concluded that posterior arthrodesis and segmental compression instrumentation seems to be effective for correcting and stabilizing kyphotic deformity in patients with Scheuermann's disease.

Poolman RW, Been HD, Ubags LH: Clinical outcome and radiographic results after operative treatment of Scheuermann's disease. *Eur Spine J* 2002;11:561-569.

This prospective study evaluated radiographic findings, patient satisfaction, and clinical outcome, and reported complications and instrumentation failure after surgical treatment of Scheuermann's kyphosis using combined anterior and posterior spondylodesis. Significant correction was maintained at 1- and 2-year follow-up but recurrence of the deformity was observed at the final follow-up. The late deterioration of correction in the sagittal plane was caused mainly by removal of the posterior instrumentation, and occurred despite radiographs, bone scans, and thorough intraoperative explorations demonstrating solid fusions. The indication for surgery in patients with Scheuermann's kyphosis is questionable, and surgery should be limited to patients with kyphosis greater than 75° who have failed nonsurgical treatment.

Soo CL, Noble PC, Esses SI: Scheuermann kyphosis: Long-term follow-up. *Spine J* 2002;2:49-56.

Sixty-three patients were evaluated at a mean of 14 years after treatment (10 to 28 years) using a specially designed questionnaire. During the cohort study, the patients had been treated using three different modalities: exercise and observation, Milwaukee bracing, and surgical fusion using the Harrington Compression System. At time of follow-up there were no differences in marital status, general health, education level, work status, degree of pain, and functional capacity between the various curve types, treatment modalities, and degrees of curve. Patients treated by bracing or surgery had improved self-images, and patients with kyphotic curves exceeding 70° at follow-up had an inferior functional result.

Tribus CB: Transient paraparesis: A complication of the surgical management of Scheuermann's kyphosis secondary to thoracic stenosis. *Spine* 2001;26:1086-1089.

The author of this article reported on a 16-year-old boy with progressive Scheuermann's kyphosis measuring 80° from T7 to T12 who underwent an anterior-posterior spinal fusion. During the instrumentation posteriorly, somatosensory-evoked potential monitoring became markedly abnormal. This was followed by a wake-up test that demonstrated the patient's inability to move either of his lower extremities. All instrumentation was removed and neurologic recovery was observed. Postoperatively, CT myelography was performed, which demonstrated severe thoracic stenosis from T8 to T10. Repeat surgery (laminectomy and posterior spinal instrumentation) was performed 1 week later without any complications. The author currently obtains a thoracic MRI scan before the surgical correction of any patient with Scheuermann's kyphosis.

Classic Bibliography

Ascani E, LaRosa G: Scheuermann's kyphosis, in Weinstein SL (ed): *The Pediatric Spine: Principles and Practice.* New York, NY, Raven Press, 1994, pp 557-585.

Bernhardt M, Bridwell KH: Segmental analysis of the sagittal plane alignment of the normal thoracic and lumbar spines and thoracolumbar junction. *Spine* 1989;14: 717-721.

Bradford DS, Moe JH, Montalvo FJ, Winter RB: Scheuermann's kyphosis and roundback deformity: Results of Milwaukee brace treatment. *J Bone Joint Surg Am* 1974;56:740-758.

Bradford DS, Moe JH, Montalvo FJ, Winter RB: Scheuermann's kyphosis: Results of surgical treatment by posterior spine arthrodesis in twenty-two patients. *J Bone Joint Surg Am* 1975;57:439-448.

Lowe TG, Kasten MD: An analysis of sagittal curves and balance after Cotrel-Dubousset instrumentation for kyphosis secondary to Scheuermann's disease: A review of 32 patients. *Spine* 1994;19:1680-1685.

Murray PM, Weinstein SL, Spratt KF: The natural history and long-term follow-up of Scheuermann kyphosis. *J Bone Joint Surg Am* 1993;75:236-248.

Newton PO, Shea KG, Granlund KF: Defining the pediatric spinal thoracoscopy learning curve: Sixty-five consecutive cases. *Spine* 2000;25:1028-1035.

Otsuka NY, Hall JE, Mah JY: Posterior fusion for Scheuermann's kyphosis. *Clin Orthop Relat Res* 1990; 251:134-139.

Montgomery SP, Erwin WE: Scheuermann's kyphosis: Long-term results of Milwaukee braces treatment. *Spine* 1981;6:5-8.

Reinhardt P, Basset GS: Short segmental kyphosis following fusion for Scheuermann's disease. *J Spinal Disord* 1990;3:162-168.

Sorenson KH: *Scheuermann's Kyphosis: Clinical Appearance, Radiography, Etiology and Prognosis.* Copenhagen, Denmark, Munsksgaard, 1964.

Speck GR, Chopin DC: The surgical treatment of Scheuermann's kyphosis. *J Bone Joint Surg Br* 1986;68: 189-193.

Sturm PF, Dobson JC, Armstrong GW: The surgical management of Scheuermann's disease. *Spine* 1993;18: 685-691.

Wenger DR, Frick SL: Scheuermann kyphosis. *Spine* 1999;24:2630-2639.

Chapter 31

Congenital Anomalies of the Spine

John P. Dormans, MD

Leslie Moroz, BA

Introduction

Anomalies in the formation and segmentation of vertebrae and ribs can lead to asymmetric growth of the spine and progressive deformity. Although some deformities have little effect on patients' lives and do not require treatment, the natural history of other more serious anomalies should be known and carefully monitored for signs of progression with the goal of maintaining spinal balance and stability throughout growth. Surgical intervention is sometimes indicated to prevent curve progression, to reestablish alignment and balance in those with established deformity, and to prevent neurologic compromise.

Failures of formation and segmentation may produce right/left asymmetry in the frontal plane of the vertebral body leading to scoliosis, or the asymmetry may be anterior/posterior in the sagittal plane leading to kyphosis. Many spine deformities are three-dimensional, with both coronal and sagittal components that should be considered in evaluation and management. In a series of 584 patients with congenital spinal deformities, 81% of patients had scoliosis, 13% had kyphosing scoliosis, and 6% had kyphosis. Estimates of the incidence of congenital scoliosis in the general population range from 1% to 4%. Congenital kyphosis is less common.

The segmentation defects of cervical vertebrae seen in Klippel-Feil syndrome are reported to occur in about 0.7% of the population. However, the incidence of vertebral anomalies in the cervical spine is much higher among patients with anomalies in other regions of the spine. In a study of 1,215 children with congenital scoliosis or kyphosis, it was reported that 298 patients (25%) were noted to have a segmentation defect of at least one level in the cervical spine.

Although the genetic and developmental etiology of congenital spine deformities remains mostly unknown, progress is being made. Vertebral defects can arise from the disruption of genes involved in development, environmental insults during gestation, or a combination of both factors. Clinical studies have provided evidence that congenital vertebral anomalies arise from disruptions in somatogenesis, the process by which the axial skeleton is formed during embryogenesis. In a radiographic analysis of 81 patients with vertebral anomalies, it was reported that 57 patients (70%) had multiple adjacent vertebral defects. Furthermore, 8 of the 19 children with Klippel-Feil syndrome (42%) also had a thoracic or lumbar vertebral malformation. This pattern is consistent with the continuous process of somite formation such that multiple, contiguous vertebral defects would be distributed along the craniocaudal axis of the spine. The neurologic anomalies associated with vertebral anomalies may share a common etiology or could be secondary to disruptions in somatogenesis.

The higher incidence of idiopathic scoliosis reported among families of children with congenital scoliosis has led investigators to explore the role of genetic defects as a predisposing factor for the development of spine deformities. One condition involving congenital vertebral defects for which the genetic etiology is known is spondylocostal dysplasia. Spondylocostal dysplasia is the association of vertebral anomalies with rib or sternal abnormalities, sometimes also associated with diastematomyelia, meningocoele, or underlying cardiovascular abnormalities, which has been mapped to chromosome 19q13.1-q13.3. Sequencing and analysis of the gene encoding the notch ligand delta-like 3 (DLL3) in families with spondylocostal dysplasia has provided evidence of the importance of the notch signaling pathway and its components in patterning the mammalian axial skeleton. A recent study that used an induced mutation of the notch ligand *DLL3* gene in a mouse model has shown that the mutation has different effects on the expression of cycling and stage-specific genes involved in somite formation. These findings suggest that the deformities seen in human spondylocostal dysplasia may arise from unique and specific disruptions of genes expressed during somatogenesis.

Clinical Evaluation

Most children with congenital spine deformities present at an early age. In some patients, the deformity can be

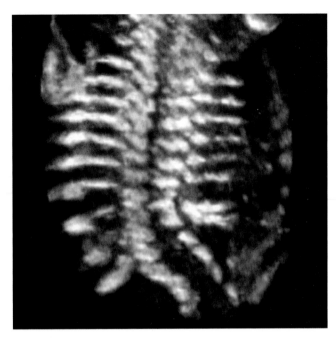

Figure 1 Prenatal ultrasound showing congenital spine deformity.

detected on prenatal ultrasonography (Figure 1). Young children may present with a mild deformity or instability, or anomalies may be found incidentally on radiographs. Although vertebral anomalies are infrequently the cause of torticollis in infants and young children, it was reported that in a series of 288 children, osseous anomalies accounted for approximately 6% of children who present with signs of head tilt and limited range of motion. Occasionally, patients present with advanced deformity. In patients with severe congenital kyphosis or anomalies of the cervical spine, signs of neurologic compromise sometimes occur.

A careful history should be obtained with particular attention given to a family history of spine deformities, spina bifida, dysraphic problems, and maternal exposure to teratogens. Assessment should include evaluation of spine and shoulder symmetry; rib or lumbar prominences; head tilt; cervical, thoracic, and lumbar range of motion and flexibility; pelvic tilt; limb-length differences; calf and thigh circumference differences; and cavus foot deformity. Signs of associated intraspinal anomalies are sometimes apparent on physical examination. The presence of hair patches, dimples, nevi, tumors, or asymmetrical or absent abdominal reflexes may be indicative of spinal dysraphism. MRI is indicated to define defects of the neural axis, particularly prior to spinal surgery for congenital deformity. Physical findings characteristic of patients with Klippel-Feil syndrome or atlanto-occipital fusion include a short, broad neck; torticollis; scoliosis; low hairline posteriorly; high scapula; and jaw anomalies. Sprengel deformity is seen in about one third of patients with Klippel-Feil syndrome.

The prevalence of cervical spine instability in patients with Down syndrome has been widely reported. In a study of 70 children with Down syndrome, 43 (61.4%) had hypermobility of the atlanto-occipital junction, 15 (21.4%) had atlantoaxial instability, whereas none had subaxial cervical spine instability. Children with Down syndrome and an osseous anomaly are at increased risk for future neurologic compromise. Although the incidence of neurologic compromise among patients with Down syndrome is low, a careful history and physical examination can help assess a child's risk. One study reported on a series of 34 patients with Down syndrome and craniovertebral junction abnormalities and found that 20 patients had osseous anomalies of the cervical spine, the most common of which was os odontoideum (12 patients) followed by atlantal arch hypoplasia and bifid anterior or posterior arches (8 patients). The patients in this series most often presented with torticollis or pain. Patients who participate in sports should also be closely monitored.

Congenital anomalies are frequently associated with other organ system problems. In a series of 126 children with congenital spine deformity, it was reported that 64 children (55%) had associated organ defects. In this series, 7 of 14 children (50%) with congenital kyphosis and 55 of 103 children (53.4%) with congenital scoliosis had associated organ defects, either isolated or associated with a syndrome. The incidence of congenital heart disease (particularly ventricle and atrial septal defects and patent ductus arteriosus) in patients with congenital spine deformity was 26%, and the incidence of genitourinary anomalies (most often renal hypoplasia, horseshoe kidney, and single kidney) was 21%. Although symptoms of other system involvement are not always present in patients with spine deformity, the high incidence of associated problems warrants a thorough examination to detect other anomalies. Patients with Klippel-Feil and/or congenital scoliosis should have a screening renal ultrasound and cardiac evaluation and/or echocardiogram.

Careful evaluation of pulmonary function is important in this patient population. Thoracic insufficiency syndrome has been described extensively and is defined as the inability of the thorax to support normal respiration or lung growth. Patients with thoracic insufficiency syndrome comprise a small subset of patients with congenital scoliosis, but the exact incidence is unknown. Thoracic volume in these patients is restricted by the physical limitations of the thorax because of congenital rib fusions or, less commonly, the absence of ribs. Patients usually present with a history of respiratory symptoms (fatigability, frequent respiratory infection, increased respiratory rate, or need for supplemental oxygen). Thoracic cage mobility may be diminished and pulmonary function impaired. Thoracic hypoplasia can be evaluated by measuring the circumference of the

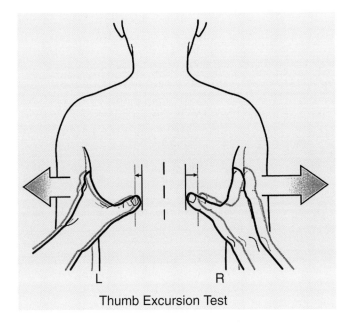

Thumb Excursion Test

Figure 2 Schematic representation of the thumb excursion test, which can be used to determine the degree of unilateral loss of secondary breathing. The examiner encircles the base of the chest with fingers anterior to the anterior axillary line and thumbs equidistant from the spine. Motion of the thumbs away from the spine on inhalation is an indication of the secondary breathing mechanism. *(Reproduced with permission from Campbell R, Smith M, Mayes T: The characteristics of thoracic insufficiency syndrome associated with fused ribs and congenital scoliosis. J Bone Joint Surg Am 2003; 85A(3):399-408.)*

chest. Loss of chest wall mobility is determined by the thumb excursion test, a measure of the expansion of the chest during a deep breath (Figure 2). Pulmonary function testing can quantify lung volume. Thoracic insufficiency syndrome can be progressive, and children noted to have decreased thoracic volume because of rib and vertebral anomalies should be routinely examined for signs of worsening deformity and decreased lung function.

Careful neurologic examination is indicated in infants and children with congenital spine deformity. It is estimated that between 20% and 40% of patients with congenital spine deformities also have a congenital anomaly of the neural axis. Neurologic deficits may be associated with vertebral anomalies secondary to the spine deformity or congenital abnormalities of the neural axis.

Differential Diagnosis

Recent studies indicate that between 38% and 55% of patients with vertebral anomalies present with a constellation of defects that constitute a syndrome (Table 1). The VATER and Goldenhar syndromes are most frequent among infants and children with congenital scoliosis. Vertebral anomalies, anorectal anomalies, tracheoesophageal fistula, and renal and vascular anomalies together comprise the VATER syndrome, or, if cardiac and limb defects are also included, VACTERL syndrome. The spectrum of oculo-auriculo-vertebral defects

that comprise Goldenhar's syndrome include partially formed or completely absent ears, eye growths or an absent eye, and an asymmetric mouth or chin, usually affecting one side of the face only (hemifacial microsomia). Children with Goldenhar's syndrome may have hearing loss, weakness in the smaller side of the face, a shift in the soft palate to the unaffected side of the face, or a tongue that is smaller on the affected side of the face. Klippel-Feil syndrome is also associated with syndactyly or hypoplastic thumb, congenital cervical stenosis, and hearing loss, which may occur in as many as 30% of these children. There are two subtypes of Jarcho-Levin syndrome associated with congenital spine deformity: spondylothoracic dysplasia, which is characterized by flared ribs and spondylocostal dysplasia, which is characterized by fused or missing ribs.

Scoliosis is a common orthopaedic manifestation of type 1 neurofibromatosis, although far less common among children with type 2 neurofibromatosis. Although the presentation and natural history of many curves associated with neurofibromatosis is similar to that of adolescent idiopathic scoliosis, a smaller subset of children with neurofibromatosis present with a dystrophic curve, usually early in childhood, the natural history of which is relentless progression. Radiographic findings in patients with dystrophic curves may mimic those of congenital scoliosis, but on closer examination are different. Plain radiographs may show distorted ribs and vertebral anomalies such as scalloping, defective pedicles, vertebral body dislocation, and enlargement of the neural foramina. Tan-colored (café-au-lait) spots larger than 5 mm are the trademark cutaneous markings of neurofibromatosis; the presence of neurofibromas, optical glioma, freckling in the groin and axillae, hamartoma of the iris (known as Lisch nodules), osseous lesions such as nonossifying fibromas, congenital pseudarthrosis of the tibia or ulna, or a family history of neurofibromatosis are other characteristics that can confirm the diagnosis. In a study of 459 patients with neu-

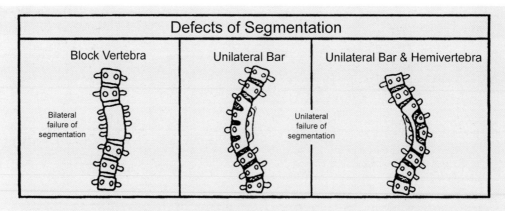

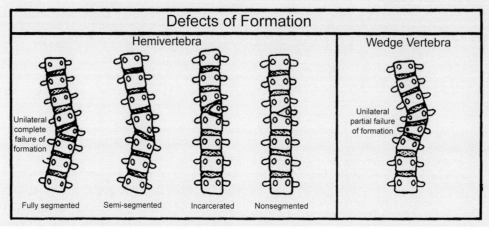

Figure 3 Classification of congenital vertebral anomalies resulting in scoliosis. Defects of segmentation include block vertebra, unilateral bar, and unilateral bar with contralateral hemivertebra. Defects of formation include unilateral complete or partial failures of formation. *(Reproduced with permission from McMaster MJ: Congenital scoliosis, in Weinstein SL (ed): The Pediatric Spine: Principles and Practices. New York, NY, Raven Press, 1994, pp 227-244.)*

rofibromatosis, 327 (71.2%) had a positive family history, whereas 132 (28.8%) had no positive family history for type 1 neurofibromatosis.

The differential diagnosis for young children with kyphotic deformity includes kyphosis caused by tuberculosis or other infection, achondroplasia, Scheuermann's kyphosis, and trauma.

Diagnostic Imaging

When evaluating a patient with confirmed or suspected congenital scoliosis, the first step is to characterize bony abnormalities with high-quality radiographs. Picture archiving and communications systems have improved our ability to obtain high-definition images of the spine. Careful evaluation of the vertebrae and disk spaces is essential for defining the area of the spine involved, the pattern of deformity, and the specific type of anomalous malformation. Congenital vertebral anomalies have been classified as defects of formation and defects of segmentation (Figure 3). Most children have a mixture of both types of deformity, with one type predominating. Incomplete failure of formation results in a wedge vertebra when height asymmetry is noted but both pedi-

cles are present. Failure of formation leading to hemivertebra results in one of three types of abnormality: a fully segmented vertebra with growth cartilage and disk spaces above and below, a partially segmented vertebra with the hemivertebra partially fused to one adjacent vertebra and separated by growth cartilage and a disk space between the other adjacent vertebra, or an unsegmented hemivertebra that is partially fused to both adjacent vertebra. A butterfly vertebra is characterized by a central defect in the vertebral body that results in two contralateral hemivertebrae at the same level. Hemimetameric segmental displacement or shift is a multilevel pattern of vertebral anomalies characterized by two contralateral hemivertebrae separated by at least one normal vertebra. Contralateral hemivertebrae, either at different levels or the same level, can result in a relatively balanced spine and favorable natural history depending on the location of the deformity.

Examples of failures of segmentation are bilateral or unilateral unsegmented fibrous, cartilaginous, or bony bars between adjacent vertebrae. Bilateral failure of segmentation results in a block vertebra. Unilateral defects in segmentation result in a unilateral fusion bar on

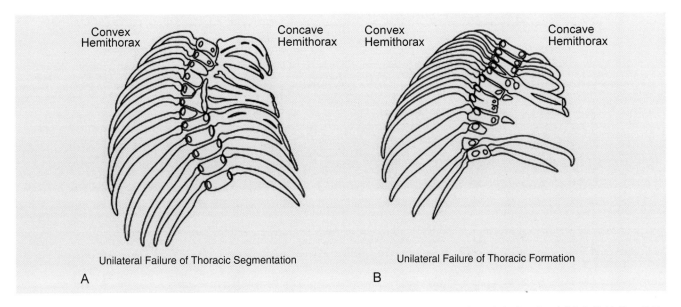

Figure 4 Schematic representation of unilateral failure of thoracic segmentation **(A)** and formation **(B)**. *(Reproduced with permission from Campbell R, Smith M, Mayes T: The characteristics of thoracic insufficiency syndrome associated with fused ribs and congenital scoliosis. J Bone Joint Surg Am 2003;85A(3):399-408.)*

the concave side of the curve. Unilateral fusion bars occasionally occur opposite a hemivertebra and result in particularly severe progression.

Primary thoracic deformity may result from vertebral anomalies with associated fused or absent ribs and is categorized accordingly as unilateral failure of thoracic formation or segmentation (Figure 4). The tethering effect exerted on the spine from rib anomalies can produce a secondary deformity of the rib cage. In patients with the most severe deformities, a windswept thorax results from the combination of severe lordosis and rotation.

Vertebral anomalies associated with kyphosis are divided into failures of formation (type I), failures of segmentation (type II), mixed anomalies (type III), and rotatory/congenital dislocation of the spine (type IV) (Figure 5). Type I defects range from asymmetric or symmetric involvement in the anterior third to half of the vertebral body to aplasia of the pars or facet joint. The thoracic or thoracolumbar regions are most often affected, the angle of the curve is usually acute, and the defects may be associated with instability, rapid progression, and neurologic loss. Type II defects vary according to the depth of ossification. The anomaly is not always a true bar, but rather a defect of the perivertebral structures, most often in the lumbar or thoracolumbar region. Type II anomalies usually involve more vertebrae and thus produce a more gradual curve than type I anomalies.

Anomalies in the cervical spine include the same patterns of failures of segmentation, formation, and mixed anomalies. Klippel-Feil syndrome is most often characterized by failures of segmentation in the cervical spine. The spectrum of involvement ranges from two fused vertebrae to the entire cervical spine, which is apparent as areas of fusion on plain AP, lateral, open-mouth, and flexion-extension radiographs.

Os odontoideum, a free ossicle, is most likely the result of nonunion, which can lie in the line of the formerly intact process, be displaced, or be fused to surrounding structures such as the clivus. The conventional wisdom is that os odontoideum is actually a result of unrecognized trauma to the odontoid process rather than a congenital anomaly. Over time, os odontoideum can result in atlantoaxial instability, potentially leading to myelopathy.

Evaluation of cervical spine radiographs includes several measurements that can be drawn to define the relative positions of bony landmarks (Figure 6). Basilar invagination is defined by the extent of protrusion of the odontoid process into the foramen magnum observed on lateral radiographs. Protrusion of the odontoid above McRae's line, drawn from the posterior rim of the foramen magnum to the tip of the clivus, is another indication of basilar impression. In patients with basilar impression, the odontoid protrudes more than 5 mm beyond McGregor's line, drawn from the upper surface of the posterior edge of the hard palate to the most caudal point of the occiput. Varying degrees of fusion between atlas and occiput, usually anteriorly, can be detected on flexion-extension radiographs and CT scans.

Atlantoaxial instability is assessed using atlanto-dens interval (ADI) and the Power's ratio. The ADI is the space between the anterior border of the dens and the posterior edge of the anterior ring of the atlas. For children age 7 years and younger, the accepted ADI is no greater than 4 mm; for children age 8 years and older, the accepted ADI is no greater than 3 mm. The Power's

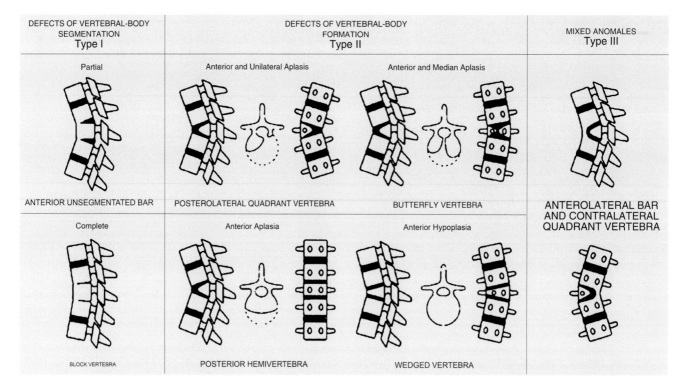

Figure 5 Classification of congenital vertebral anomalies resulting in kyphosis (type IV not shown). Defects of segmentation include an anterior unsegmented bar and a block vertebra. Defects of formation include unilateral complete or partial failures of formation. A mixed defect is characterized by an anterolateral unsegmented bar with a contralateral hemivertebra. *(Reproduced with permission from McMaster MJ, Singh H: Natural history of congenital kyphosis and kyphoscoliosis. J Bone Joint Surg Am 1999;81A(10): 1367-1383.)*

ratio is the length of the line from the basion to the posterior margin of the atlas divided by the length of the opisthion to the anterior arch of the atlas; a ratio greater than one suggests atlantoaxial instability. Because of the atypical relative position of cervical spine anatomy in patients with Down syndrome, radiographic changes are not always accompanied by clinical evidence of instability.

The space available for the spinal cord (SAC) can be directly measured on sagittal and axial MRI to detect spinal cord compression and neurologic impingement. A line drawn from the posterior margin of the odontoid to the anterior margin of the posterior ring of C1 is measured to assess SAC. The SAC is inversely related to ADI. In normal patients, the SAC is usually not less than 13 mm.

MRI or fine-cut CT helps determine the full extent of vertebral anomalies, particularly in young children whose vertebrae are still largely cartilaginous, and is an essential part of preoperative planning. In a series of 31 patients, plain radiographs and three-dimensional CT scans revealed that additional abnormalities were present in more than 50% of the patients when advanced CT scans were examined.

For patients with thoracic deformity, changes in the width and depth of the rib cage can be appreciated using CT scans. The milliampere-second settings for CT

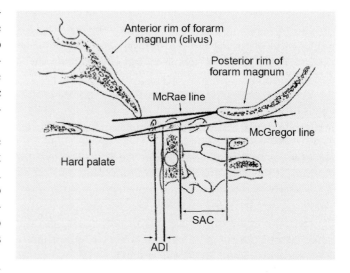

Figure 6 Schematic representation of McRae's line, which is drawn between the posterior rim of the foramen magnum and the tip of the clivus, and McGregor's line, which is drawn from the superior surface of the posterior edge of the hard palate to the caudal-most point of the occiput. The ADI is defined as the region between the anterior border of the dens and the posterior edge of the anterior ring of the atlas. The SAC is defined as the region between the posterior margin of the odontoid and the anterior margin of the posterior ring of C1. *(Adapted with permission from Horn BD, Dormans JP: Evaluation of the cervical spine in children, in Clark C (ed): The Cervical Spine. Philadelphia, PA, Lippincott Williams & Wilkins, 2005, pp 403-414.)*

should be decreased to the appropriate level for children to decrease radiation exposure. One study re-

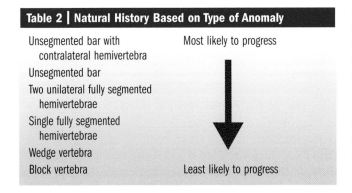

Table 2 | Natural History Based on Type of Anomaly

Unsegmented bar with contralateral hemivertebra	Most likely to progress
Unsegmented bar	
Two unilateral fully segmented hemivertebrae	
Single fully segmented hemivertebrae	
Wedge vertebra	
Block vertebra	Least likely to progress

ported that the lifetime radiation risk of children may be increased, even with a single axial CT study, because of the young age of the patients at the time of exposure and also organ radiosensitivity. The benefits of obtaining advanced imaging usually far outweigh the risks, but care should be taken to minimize the radiation exposure whenever possible.

MRI should be performed to detect intraspinal anomalies. In a series of 126 patients with congenital spine deformity, intraspinal anomalies were identified in 56% of the patients with congenital kyphosis; among the patients with congenital scoliosis, intraspinal anomalies were present in 29% of those with failure of formation, 40% of those with failure of segmentation, and 40% of those with mixed defects. Anomalies most often seen include Chiari type 1 malformation, diastematomyelia, tethered spinal cord, syringomyelia, low conus, and intradural lipoma. Diastematomyelia in particular has been noted to occur more often in patients with scoliotic curves with an unsegmented bar with a contralateral hemivertebra. A recent advance in diagnostic imaging technology with applications in the evaluation of congenital spine deformities is the use of periodically rotated overlapping parallel lines with enhanced reconstruction (PROPELLER) MRI, which uses multiple shots to disperse motion artifacts and has the potential to eliminate the need for sedation under general anesthesia.

Natural History

The risk associated with vertebral malformations is asymmetric spine growth. Coronal plane deformity may progress with further loss of spine balance and possibly eventual cardiothoracic compromise; in addition to these concerns, sagittal plane deformities pose neurologic risks. The natural history of congenital scoliosis depends on the type (Table 2) and location of the vertebral anomalies. The presence of a unilateral unsegmented bony bar on one side of the spine can create a tethering effect. Asymmetric growth and deformity may be provoked by the inhibition of longitudinal growth by the absence of growth cartilage and the presence of ex-

tra growth potential associated with a unilateral hemivertebra. In a series of 251 patients with congenital scoliosis, it was reported that the curves of patients with a unilateral unsegmented bar (with or without a contralateral hemivertebra) progressed most rapidly, followed by patients with a hemivertebra, wedged vertebra, and block vertebra. In patients with bilateral failure of segmentation (block vertebra), butterfly vertebra, and hemimetameric shifts (two contralateral hemivertebrae separated by at least one normal vertebra), spine balance is more likely to be maintained.

The natural history of congenital kyphosis depends on the type of deformity and number of vertebrae involved. Progression occurs throughout growth, usually with the peak growth velocity occurring with adolescence. Type III anomalies (mixed deformity) usually result in the most rapid progression, followed by type I anomalies (failure of formation). Estimates of the rate of deterioration for type I deformity range from 7° to 9° per year until skeletal maturity. Type II vertebral anomalies (unilateral anterior fusion bars) have a better prognosis: progression is approximately 5° per year until skeletal maturity. Type II anterolateral bars result in more severe kyphosis with more rapid deterioration than midline anterior bars. Although the Cobb angle measures the extent of sagittal deformity from the end vertebrae of the curve, it does not reflect the behavior of the spine around the apex of the curve where there is the greatest risk of spinal cord compression. For curves with similar Cobb angles, a patient with a type I deformity is at greater risk for developing a short, sharp apex and neurologic complications than a patient with a type II deformity that results in a gradual curve. In a series of 112 children with congenital kyphosis, it was reported that anterior spinal cord compression led to neurologic compromise in 11 children (10%); 7 of the 11 patients had a type I anomaly, and 4 could not be classified. Neurologic deficit is not usually found in patients with type II deformity. Although the location of the vertebral anomaly does not correspond to the severity of kyphosis, spinal cord compression infrequently occurs in spinal curves with an apex below T11.

The natural history of the global deformity of the thorax associated with thoracic insufficiency syndrome is uncertain. In a study of more than 500 children with severe spine and rib deformities, it was proposed that the concave hemithorax acts as a lateral tether, promoting the unbalanced growth of the spine already underway because of vertebral deformities. In a series of 16 patients, it was reported that patients with fused ribs tended to have greater spinal curve progression for each of the five types of congenital spine deformities, except unilateral bar with contralateral hemivertebra. Progression of thoracic deformity can correspond to progressive thoracic insufficiency, resulting in apparent or occult severe restrictive lung disease and ventilator dependency either early in life or once compensatory mechanisms are no longer sustainable.

For individuals with anomalies of the cervical spine, instability and neurologic compromise are most often associated with anomalies in the upper segments (occiput to C3). Instability resulting from vertebral anomalies in the cervical spine may be progressive, and risks include compression of the spinal cord and compromise of the vertebral artery. Anomalies in the lower segment of the cervical spine can lead to degenerative changes such as decreased range of motion and occasionally myelopathy.

Functional Assessment

According to the results of the Pediatric Outcomes Data Collection Instrument (PODCI) scores and functional assessments with congenital scoliosis, patients with congenital scoliosis and patients with congenital kyphosis differ from children without orthopaedic conditions with respect to their activity performance, comfort, and possibly self-image. Responses from 56 patients with congenital scoliosis or kyphosis to questions about upper extremity function, mobility, sports and physical function, comfort or pain, and global function (an average of the previous scores) yielded significantly lower scores than in the "normal" patient group. However, the PODCI scores of children with congenital deformity did not differ significantly from those children with idiopathic scoliosis.

Nonsurgical Treatment

The most appropriate treatment is determined by the natural history of the type of anomalies present, an assessment of the potential for asymmetric growth and the projected loss of spine balance, and the risk for eventual neurologic compromise. Children with mild congenital scoliosis or kyphosis with a favorable natural history may not require treatment; but children with vertebral anomalies that are prone to progress should be closely monitored with radiographs until skeletally mature, and those with unacceptable progression should be treated. Likewise, surgical correction may not be indicated for patients with mild thoracic insufficiency syndrome, but pulmonary function should be monitored along with diagnostic imaging studies to quantify existing thoracic insufficiency and also to detect progression. The frequency of radiographic assessment should correspond with suspicion of progression (natural history) based on the type and location of the deformity and patient age.

The potential for growth in a particular region can be estimated by assessing the growth cartilage on either side of an abnormal vertebra. Spinal curves progress more quickly during times of rapid growth, particularly between the ages of 2 to 3 years and during adolescence. An increased rate of deterioration after age 10

years has been reported. Radiographic measurement of the deformity every 4 to 6 months during these critical periods enables the surgeon to detect the rate of progression and plan appropriate surgical intervention if necessary.

Because spinal curves produced by congenital anomalies are generally less flexible than idiopathic curves, bracing is rarely effective in managing the primary curve. Orthotic management may be used in some patients with long flexible curves to achieve spinal balance through the normal vertebrae adjacent to the pathologic vertebrae at the apex of the curve. Compensatory or secondary spinal curves are also occasionally managed with bracing. However, long-term bracing during active growth can have a deleterious effect on the immature rib cage, and the growth of the thoracic cavity and can result in chest wall deformities. Bracing to improve alignment in the cervical spine is ineffective, and the symptoms of degenerative changes are usually managed without surgical intervention.

For children with cervical spine instability associated with Down syndrome, a set of radiographic guidelines has been proposed to assess the risk for future neurologic compromise and determine appropriate management (Table 3).

Surgical Treatment

The goals of surgical treatment of congenital scoliosis and kyphosis are either to halt asymmetric growth and thereby prevent progressive spinal imbalance or to correct the existing deformity. For children with congenital kyphosis, particularly that associated with failures of formation (types I) or mixed deformity (type III), there is a high risk of neurologic compromise associated with progression. Thus, the goal of surgical treatment is to directly address the threat of spinal cord compression. For children with anomalies of the cervical spine and instability, the goal of surgical intervention is to achieve stability and thereby decrease the risk of neurologic compromise.

For patients with congenital scoliosis or kyphosis, prophylactic surgery can prevent spinal curve progression. In situ anterior and/or posterior hemiepiphyseodesis, usually with associated hemiarthrodesis, is a surgical option for addressing asymmetric growth, thus preventing unacceptable deformity (Figure 7). More aggressive surgical approaches to congenital scoliosis are being more widely described, particularly for patients who have not reached skeletal maturity. Hemivertebra excision and anterior and/or posterior osteotomy/ vertebrectomy with or without instrumentation are indicated in some patients with severe deformity. For children with type II kyphosis (anterior failure of segmentation), correction is rarely the goal; however, anterior osteotomy is occasionally indicated in patients with

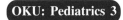

Table 3 | Recommended Guidelines for Evaluating the Cervical Spine in Children With Down Syndrome

Atlanto-dens Interval

< 4.5 mm	Full, unrestricted activity
> 4.5 mm and < 10 mm and neurologically normal	Limit high-risk activities*
> 4.5 mm and neurologic deficit	Limit activities
	Neurologic consultation
	MRI
	Normal study: observation
	Signal changes within spinal cord: surgical stabilization
> 9.9 mm	Surgical fusion

Occipitoatlantal Mobility

Normal	Full, unrestricted activity
> 2 mm motion and neurologically normal	Limit high-risk activities*
> 2 mm motion and neurologic deficit	Limit activity
	Neurologic consultation
	MRI
	Normal study: observation
	Signals changes in spinal cord: surgical fusion

Subaxial Cervical Spine Degenerative Changes

Neurologically normal	Observation
Pain without neurologic deficit	Symptomatic treatment
Neurologic deficit	Neurologic consultation
	Electromyography and nerve conduction velocity studies
	MRI
	Disk excision and fusion

*Boxing, diving, football, gymnastics, ice hockey, rugby, soccer, and wrestling
(Reproduced with permission from Pizzutillo PD, Herman MJ. Cervical spine issues in Down syndrome. J Pediatr Orthop 2005;25(2):253-259.)

severe deformity. Although most of these approaches appear to be safe in experienced hands, the risks and benefits should be carefully assessed, especially when excellent results are achieved with more conservative surgical procedures.

All surgical procedures carry the risk of affecting overall spine length. Although trunk height may be further reduced by progression of a deformity and the development of a secondary spinal curve, surgical intervention may also limit growth potential. Depending on the type and location of the vertebral anomaly and pattern and flexibility of the spinal curve, it may be possible to surgically reduce the degree of deformity. However, major corrections may increase the risk of neurologic injury. MRI to detect intraspinal anomalies prior to surgery is essential. Intraspinal anomalies should be addressed prior to correction and fusion. High-quality neuromonitoring, including somatosensory-evoked potentials, transcranial motor-evoked potentials, and electromyography, should be used during surgery.

Congenital Scoliosis

Early in situ focal arthrodesis is usually indicated for infants or children with unilateral unsegmented bars. For younger children, arthrodesis of the involved segment of the spine should often be anterior and posterior. One of the risks associated with posterior fusion alone in skeletally immature patients is the crankshaft phenomenon. This is defined as continued progression of greater than 10° of the Cobb angle caused by continuing anterior growth of the spine in the presence of a posterior fusion. One study reported that the crankshaft phenomenon was observed in 8 of 54 skeletally immature patients (15%) during 12 years of follow-up (until skeletal maturity). The crankshaft phenomenon was more likely to be observed in patients who were younger at the time of surgery and in those with spinal curves with an initial measurement of greater than 50°.

Postoperative immobilization with orthosis, cast, or more rarely in a halo vest, may be used for noninstrumented patients. Instrumentation is used to achieve correction, stabilize the arthrodesis, and balance the spine in older patients with flexible or less severe curves. However, neurologic risks (overdistraction or direct injury to the spinal cord or roots) are greater for instrumentation in children with congenital scoliosis than in those with idiopathic scoliosis. The risk of spinal cord ischemia can be reduced in anterior procedures by preserving the segmental vessels and by avoiding excessive lengthening of the spine with distraction maneuvers.

For children with progressive deformity associated with a fully segmented hemivertebra who are younger (≤ 5 years of age), convex anterior and posterior hemiepiphyseodesis and arthrodesis may allow for continued growth on the concave side of the curve and thus prevention of the progression of deformity; in some patients, it may allow a gradual improvement of the deformity. Preoperative imaging of the three dimensions of the anomalous vertebra is an integral part of surgical planning.

Anterior or posterior osteotomy and/or vertebrectomy with or without instrumentation and fusion may be indicated for patients with severe rigidity, fixed pelvic obliquity, or decompensated deformities. However, the neurologic risks are greater for these procedures. Transpedicular eggshell osteotomy has also been described as a potential approach to treating older patients with multiple anomalies and multiplanar deformities. Screws or hooks are placed above and below the osteotomy site, transpedicular decancellation of the body is carried out as close to the end plates as possible, and the correction maintained by means of internal fixation. One study reported obtaining an average correction of 38° in the sagittal plane and 28.7° in the coronal plane in three patients treated with this technique. If this technique is used, excess growth cartilage associated with the

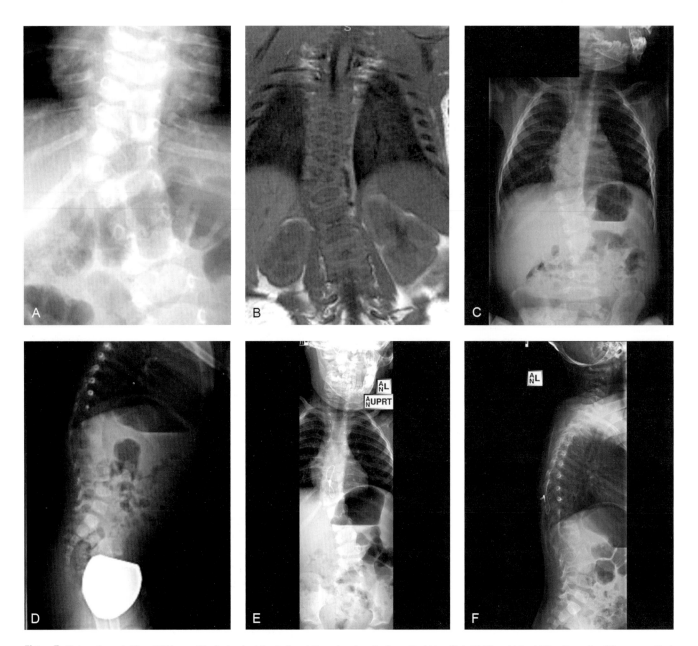

Figure 7 Plain radiograph **(A)** and MRI scan **(B)** of a hemivertebra in the midthoracic spine of a 6-month-old boy. Plain AP **(C)** and lateral **(D)** radiographs of the same patient at age 18 months show 49° thoracolumbar scoliosis. Plain AP **(E)** and lateral **(F)** radiographs 1 year after anterior-posterior hemiarthrodesis of the right side of the involved thoracic spine and posterior instrumentation with sublaminar titanium cable and bone graft show correction to 28°.

hemivertebra must be removed. Additionally, care must be taken to avoid displacing residual fragments of the vertebra into the spinal cord during correction.

Reports of hemivertebra excision are appearing more frequently in the literature. The goal of hemivertebra excision is to directly address and improve spinal imbalance. Ideally, correction can be achieved, and future asymmetric growth can be prevented. This technique should be reserved for patients who are at high risk for progression of the curve and spinal imbalance if the more traditional in situ fusion or hemiepiphysiodesis and fusion techniques have already been attempted. The best indication for excision is a fully segmented

hemivertebra at the lumbosacral junction. Resection may be posterior, anterior, or combined, and approaches to instrumentation vary.

Reports of combined anterior and posterior hemivertebra excision have shown good postoperative correction with little deterioration. Estimates of the mean postoperative curve correction obtained in hemivertebra resections in all parts of the spine range from 59% to 67% of the initial curve, with little loss of correction at least 24 months postoperatively. Hemivertebra resection via a posterior approach minimizes surgical exposure with similar potential for correction, but may be a more difficult and risky procedure. In a case series of three children who were followed for an average of 12.8 years after single-stage posterior thoracolumbar hemivertebra excision and instrumentation, it was reported that spinal curve correction ranged from 23° to 36°, with an average total 3.7° loss of correction at last follow-up. The neurologic risks of hemivertebra excision are greater than those of hemiepiphysiodesis, and repeated surgery is sometimes necessary to correct implant failures or to address progressing asymmetric growth.

The goal of lumbosacral hemivertebra resection is to make the lumbar vertebra parallel to S1 and eliminate pelvic obliquity. One technique for addressing pelvic obliquity in patients with lumbosacral spine hemivertebrae consists of instrumentation with pelvic fixation following anterior and posterior excision of a hemivertebra at the lumbosacral junction. A cable construct connects the adjacent normal vertebra to the ilium with screws and provides an alternative construct for achieving fixation in the smaller and more porous bones of young children. One study reported that correction was achieved and maintained throughout a follow-up period of at least 3 years in each of three patients treated with hemivertebra excision, pelvic fixation, and bilateral posterior fusion.

For children with thoracic insufficiency syndrome associated with fused ribs and congenital scoliosis, thoracoplasty and opening wedge thoracostomy with instrumentation for longitudinal lengthening can enable growth and provide increased thoracic spinal height, depth, and width. One study reported an average thoracic spine growth rate of 8 mm/yr (average follow-up, 4.2 years) in 21 patients with congenital scoliosis and fused ribs who underwent expansion thoracoplasty with vertical, expandable prosthetic titanium rib (Figure 8). The growth rate on the concave side averaged 7.9 mm/yr and 8.3 mm/yr on the convex side. In a subsequent series, the results of management with vertical, expandable prosthetic titanium rib implants on scoliosis and thoracic insufficiency were reported in 27 patients (average age, 3.2 years; age range, 0.6 to 12.5 years) with fused ribs and congenital scoliosis that was progressing at an average rate of 15°/yr. In this series, scoliosis decreased from an average 74° to 49° at the time of last follow-up (mean follow-up, 5.7 years), and statistically significant increases in the volume of vital capacity were reported in all patients. Although the long-term pulmonary function of children treated with vertical, expandable prosthetic titanium rib technique remains unknown, the early results are encouraging.

Congenital Kyphosis

Although progression can be monitored without surgery for some patients who experience failure of segmentation, surgical treatment is indicated for most children

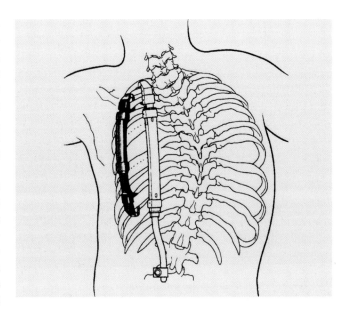

Figure 8 Schematic representation of a vertical, expandable prosthetic titanium rib device implanted after opening wedge thoracostomy in a patient with congenital vertebral anomalies and fused ribs. Gradual correction promotes thoracic growth to increase height, depth, and width. (*Reproduced with permission from Campbell RM, Smith MD, Mayes TC, et al: The effect of opening wedge thoracostomy on thoracic insufficiency syndrome associated with fused ribs and congenital scoliosis. J Bone Joint Surg Am 2004;86A(8):1659-1674.*)

with kyphosis. For children younger than 5 years with curves less than 55°, posterior fusion allows for some spontaneous correction of the deformity with growth. However, the extent of growth within the segment is unpredictable, and the overall magnitude of correction is often small. Instrumentation is used in some patients to provide stabilization rather than correction because of the increased neurologic risk associated with correction, especially when using distraction maneuvers. There is debate about whether routinely extending the fusion mass is necessary, particularly in patients with instrumentation. Posterior fusion may also be indicated for older children with a failure of segmentation resulting in less severe curves (< 50°), although further correction of the deformity is not anticipated. Anterior decompression is performed in patients in whom neural structures are compromised.

Anterior and posterior fusion is usually necessary to provide stability in older patients with kyphosis greater than 55°. Instrumentation may be used to provide fixation, although for patients with large angular curves, it can be difficult to apply. Correction of kyphosis carries a high risk of paraplegia, particularly in patients with type I deformity (hemivertebrae). However, for some patients with severe deformities, correction can be achieved with anterior strut graft and posterior fusion. Vascularized rib grafts in particular have been shown to heal quickly and provide stability, whereas free fibular or rib strut grafts are sometimes slow to heal and occasionally fracture.

Osteotomy is rarely indicated for patients with congenital kyphosis. However, in some patients with failure of segmentation that results in high-angle, long, rigid curves, anterior osteotomy and anterior-posterior fusion with instrumentation can be used to achieve correction. Osteotomy may be a better option in a younger patient with a cartilaginous bar. Likewise, vertebral resection is also rare, but for some patients with severe deformities that are present at the time of birth and with hemivertebra situated posterior and close to the spinal cord, excision with a short arthrodesis may be indicated to avoid paraparesis or paraplegia. Loss of correction throughout growth is likely following vertebral excision, and the additional procedures may be necessary to extend the fusion mass with future growth.

Congenital Cervical Spine Anomalies

Clinical evidence of instability or neurologic symptoms and radiographic evidence of spinal cord compression, narrowing of the spinal canal (< 13 mm), or basilar invagination are indications for surgical management of infants and children with vertebral anomalies in the cervical spine. Surgical stabilization is achieved with posterior fusion in most patients. Some patients with irreducible subluxation and basilar invagination, those in whom abnormal soft tissue acts as a mass, or those with congenital stenosis of the cervical canal, anterior and/or posterior decompression may be necessary. Fixation with instrumentation can provide additional stability.

Summary

A variety of congenital vertebral anomalies pose risks to spine balance and progressive deformity because of asymmetric spine growth. Classifying and understanding the pathoanatomy of the anomaly are key to determining the likely natural history of the deformity. Treatment for children with congenital vertebral anomalies is best defined in the context of the natural history of the deformity, but the safety of the treatment is the most important consideration. Only techniques that have been proved to be safe should be used, and high-quality spinal cord monitoring is essential.

Annotated Bibliography

General

Erol B, Tracy MR, Dormans JP, et al: Congenital scoliosis and vertebral malformations: Characterization of segmental defects for genetic analysis. *J Pediatr Orthop* 2004;24:674-682.

Eighty-four instances of vertebral segmentation disorders were evaluated radiologically, and genetic analysis was done for 39 patients. Groups of congenital vertebral defects for clinical genetic studies were proposed based on the extent of contiguous defects and craniocaudal location.

Hedequist D, Emans J: Congenital scoliosis. *J Am Acad Orthop Surg* 2004;12:266-275.

The authors review the classification, diagnosis, and management of congenital scoliosis.

Kusumi K, Mimoto MS, Covello KL, Beddington RS, Krumlauf R, Dunwoodie SL: Dll3 pudgy mutation differentially disrupts dynamic expression of somite genes. *Genesis* 2004;39(2):115-121.

The authors describe the different effects of the DLL39(pu) mutation on cycling and stage-specific genes, findings that provide an explanation for the complex deformities observed in patients with spondylocostal dysplasia.

Maisenbacher MK, Han JS, O'Brien ML, et al: Molecular analysis of congenital scoliosis: A candidate gene approach. *Hum Genet* 2005;116:416-419.

The authors present the first molecular study of congenital scoliosis by analysis of the candidate gene *DLL3*, a homozygous delta-like 3 mutation of which is associated with spondylocostal dysostosis type 1. One novel missense variant is described, but no novel or previously described mutations were present in the cohort, indicating that *DLL3* mutations may not be a major cause of congenital scoliosis.

Clinical Evaluation

Basu PS, Elsebaie H, Noordeen MH: Congenital spinal deformity: A comprehensive assessment at presentation. *Spine* 2002;27:2255-2259.

In a series of 126 patients with congenital spine deformity, 64 patients (55%) had organ defects. Organ defects were more common among patients with mixed vertebral defects. The most common anomalies were cardiac (26%) and urogenital (21%).

Campbell RM Jr, Smith MD, Mayes TC, et al: The characteristics of thoracic insufficiency syndrome associated with fused ribs and congenital scoliosis. *J Bone Joint Surg Am* 2003;85:399-408.

The authors define the clinical and radiographic characteristics of thoracic insufficiency and discuss diagnostic criteria and treatment goals.

Diagnostic Imaging

Belmont PJ Jr, Kuklo TR, Taylor KF, Freedman BA, Prahinski JR, Kruse RW: Intraspinal anomalies associated with isolated congenital hemivertebra: The role of routine magnetic resonance imaging. *J Bone Joint Surg Am* 2004;86:1704-1710.

Of 76 patients with at least one hemivertebra who underwent MRI, 29 had an isolated hemivertebra, and 47 had a complex hemivertebral pattern. Eight of the 29 patients with an isolated hemivertebra (28%) and 10 of the 47 patients with a complex hemivertebral pattern (21%) had an intraspinal anomaly that was detected with MRI. Overall, an abnormal finding on the history or physical examination demonstrated an accuracy of 71%, a sensitivity of 56%, a specificity of 76%,

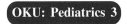

a positive predictive value of 42%, and a negative predictive value of 85% for the diagnosis of an intraspinal anomaly.

Brenner DJ, Elliston CD: Estimated radiation risks potentially associated with full-body CT screening. *Radiology* 2004;232(3):735-738.

The authors used estimates of cancer mortality incidence associated with atomic bomb associated radiation exposure and calculated doses of radiation to exposed organs from CT to estimate the lifetime risks of CT studies.

Facanha-Filho FA, Winter RB, Lonstein JE, et al: Measurement accuracy in congenital scoliosis. *J Bone Joint Surg Am* 2001;83:42-45.

This assessment of the accuracy of measurements of spinal curves in patients with congenital scoliosis reported that an accuracy of ± 3° can be expected in 95% of patients.

Forbes KP, Pipe JG, Bird CR, Heiserman JE: PROPELLER MRI: Clinical testing of a novel technique for quantification and compensation of head motion. *J Magn Reson Imaging* 2001;14:215-222.

This comparison of PROPELLER (Periodically Rotated Overlapping ParallEL Lines with Enhanced Reconstruction) MRI and conventional MRI reported that motion artifact was less commonly seen on PROPELLER MRI than conventional MRI ($P < 0.001$) and was preferred over conventional MRI by all radiologists who participated in the study for all subjects ($P < 0.05$).

Newton PO, Hahn GW, Fricka KB, Wenger DR: Utility of three-dimensional and multiplanar reformatted computed tomography for evaluation of pediatric congenital spine abnormalities. *Spine* 2002;27(8):844-850.

In a retrospective comparison of 31 sets of plain radiographs and advanced imaging studies of congenital pediatric spine deformities, multiplanar reformatted and three-dimensional CT images allowed identification of unrecognized malformations in 17 of 31 patients (54.8%).

Functional Assessment

Lerman JA, Sullivan E, Haynes RJ: The Pediatric Outcomes Data Collection Instrument (PODCI) and functional assessment in patients with adolescent or juvenile idiopathic scoliosis and congenital scoliosis or kyphosis. *Spine* 2002;27:2052-2058.

In this study, 102 patients with adolescent idiopathic scoliosis, 47 with congenital scoliosis without kyphosis, 9 with congenital kyphosis, and a control group without spine deformity completed the Pediatric Outcomes Data Collection Instrument. Scores from patients with congenital scoliosis were lower than those of the control group in all categories except happiness. All category scores were significantly lower than those of the control group for patients with congenital kyphosis.

Nonsurgical Treatment

Pizzutillo PD, Herman MJ: Cervical spine issues in Down syndrome. *J Pediatr Orthop* 2005;25(2):253-259.

The authors provide a review of cervical spine instability in children with Down syndrome, guidelines for clinical and radiographic evaluation, and recommendations for management.

Surgical Treatment

Campbell RM Jr, Hell-Vocke AK: Growth of the thoracic spine in congenital scoliosis after expansion thoracoplasty. *J Bone Joint Surg Am* 2003;85:409-420.

At an average duration of follow-up of 4.2 years, 21 children with congenital scoliosis and fused ribs after expansion thoracoplasty with use of a vertical, expandable titanium prosthetic rib showed significant growth of the concave side of the thoracic spine (an increase in length of 7.9 mm/yr or 7.1%/yr) and the convex side (8.3 mm/yr or 6.4%/yr) compared with the baseline lengths.

Campbell RM Jr, Smith MD, Mayes TC, et al: The effect of opening wedge thoracostomy on thoracic insufficiency syndrome associated with fused ribs and congenital scoliosis. *J Bone Joint Surg Am* 2004;86:1659-1674.

In this study, 27 patients with congenital scoliosis and a mean increase in curve magnitude of 15°/yr associated with fused ribs of a concave hemithorax had an opening wedge thoracostomy with primary longitudinal lengthening with use of a chest-wall distractor known as a vertical, expandable prosthetic titanium rib and repeat lengthenings of the prosthesis performed at intervals of 4 to 6 months. At a mean follow-up of 5.7 years postoperatively, there was a decrease in the mean curve of scoliosis, an improvement in the space available for the lung, and a mean increase in thoracic spine height of 0.71 cm/yr. In a group of patients who had sequential testing, all increases in the volume of vital capacity were significant. The most common complication was asymptomatic proximal migration of the device through the ribs in seven patients.

Cil A, Yazici M, Alanay A, Acaroglu RE, Uzumcugil A, Surat A: The course of sagittal plane abnormality in the patients with congenital scoliosis managed with convex growth arrest. *Spine* 2004;29:547-553.

Of 11 children with congenital scoliosis treated with convex growth arrest, the coronal plane deformities were an average 58° (range, 36° to 105°) before surgery and 52° (13° to 107°) at the final follow-up. Six curves improved, and five stabilized. At the end of the follow-up, sagittal Cobb angle of the abnormal segments remained stable in seven patients and deteriorated in four; none of the four patients required any reconstructive spine procedure for kyphosis during follow-up.

Deviren V, Berven S, Smith JA, Emami A, Hu SS, Bradford DS: Excision of hemivertebrae in the management of congenital scoliosis involving the thoracic and thoracolumbar spine. *J Bone Joint Surg Br* 2001;83:496-500.

The authors report the results of 10 consecutive patients who underwent excision of thoracic or thoracolumbar hemivertebrae for either angular deformity in the coronal plane or both coronal and sagittal deformity. The mean preoperative coronal curve was 78.2° (range, 30° to 115°) and was corrected to 33.9° (range, 7° to 58°) postoperatively, a mean correction of 59%. Preoperative coronal decompensation of 35 mm was improved to 11 mm postoperatively.

Hosalkar HS, Luedtke LM, Drummond DS: New technique in congenital scoliosis involving fixation to the pelvis after hemivertebra excision. *Spine* 2004;29:2581-2587.

The authors report the use of a technique for hemivertebra excision followed by fixation of the adjacent normal vertebra to the ilium with screws and cables in three young children with hemivertebrae at the lumbosacral junction. All patients had solid fusion and well-balanced spine at latest follow-up.

Kesling KL, Lonstein JE, Denis F, et al: The crankshaft phenomenon after posterior spinal arthrodesis for congenital scoliosis: A review of 54 patients. *Spine* 2003;28:267-271.

A Cobb angle increase of more than 10°, the crankshaft phenomenon, was seen in 8 of the 54 patients (15%) included in this study. The authors noted a positive correlation with earlier surgery and larger (> 50°) curves.

Kim YJ, Otsuka NY, Flynn JM, Hall JE, Emans JB, Hresko MT: Surgical treatment of congenital kyphosis. *Spine* 2001;26:2251-2257.

The authors conducted a retrospective review of 26 patients with congenital kyphosis and kyphoscoliosis treated surgically. They observed a low pseudarthrosis rate with or without routine augmentation of fusion mass if instrumentation was used. They also noted that gradual correction of kyphosis may occur with growth in patients younger than 3 years with failure of segmentation and mixed type deformities after posterior fusion, but it appears to be unpredictable. Additionally, they reported that the risk of neurologic injury with anterior and posterior fusion for kyphotic deformity was associated with greater age, more severe deformity, and preexisting spinal cord compromise.

Klemme WR, Polly DW Jr, Orchowski JR: Hemivertebral excision for congenital scoliosis in very young children. *J Pediatr Orthop* 2001;21:761-764.

The authors report on a series of six children younger than 34 months who underwent single-anesthetic sequential anterior and posterior hemivertebral excision. The mean postoperative curve correction was 67% (range, 52% to 84%), and the average correction at final follow-up was 70% (range, 50% to 85%). No neurologic or other significant complications were reported.

McMaster MJ, Singh H: The surgical management of congenital kyphosis and kyphoscoliosis. *Spine* 2001;26:2146-2155.

In this study, 9 of 11 patients age 5 years and younger with kyphosis less than 55° who were managed surgically with posterior arthrodesis were observed to have a mean correction of 15° at 11-year follow-up.

Mikles MR, Graziano GP, Hensinger AR: Transpedicular eggshell osteotomies for congenital scoliosis using frameless stereotactic guidance. *Spine* 2001;26(20):2289-2296.

Three children with congenital multiplanar curves underwent one-stage posterior transpedicular eggshell osteotomy. The average coronal correction of the major curve was 28.7° (range, 22° to 33°). The average correction of lateral displacement from the center of the trunk was 4.8 cm (range, 3.0 to 7.5 cm).

Nakamura H, Matsuda H, Konishi S, Yamano Y: Single-stage excision of hemivertebrae via the posterior approach alone for congenital spine deformity: Follow-up period longer than ten years. *Spine* 2002;27:110-115.

Three children with thoracolumbar hemivertebra region and two children with lumbosacral hemivertebra underwent single-stage excision of the hemivertebra via a posterior approach. For patients with a thoracolumbar hemivertebra, scoliosis improved from 49° ± 6° to 22.3° ± 3.5° (54.3% correction). The correction ratio for kyphosis was 67.4%. Loss of scoliotic curvature correction was 3.7° at an average follow-up of 12.8 years. The correction ratio for patients with a lumbosacral hemivertebra was 32.5%.

Ruf M, Harms J: Posterior hemivertebra resection with transpedicular instrumentation: Early correction in children aged 1 to 6 years. *Spine* 2003;28:2132-2138.

In this study, 28 children between 1 and 6 years of age with congenital scoliosis were treated with hemivertebra resection by a posterior-only approach with transpedicular instrumentation. The mean initial Cobb angle was 45°, 14° after surgery, and 13° at a mean follow-up of 3.5 years. Compensatory cranial curve was 17° before surgery and 5° after surgery, compensatory caudal curve was 22° preoperatively and 8° postoperatively. The angle of kyphosis was 22° before surgery and 10° after surgery. Two patients required additional surgery during the course of follow-up to treat new developing deformities.

Classic Bibliography

Ballock RT, Song KM: The prevalence of nonmuscular causes of torticollis in children. *J Pediatr Orthop* 1996;16(4):500-504.

Bulman MP, Kusumi K, Frayling TM, et al: Mutations in the human delta homologue, DLL3, cause axial skeletal defects in spondylocostal dysostosis. *Nat Genet* 2000;24(4):438-441.

Danisa OA, Turner D, Richardson WJ: Surgical correction of lumbar kyphotic deformity: Posterior reduction "eggshell" osteotomy. *J Neurosurg* 2000;92:50-56.

Hensinger RN, Lang JE, MacEwen GD: Klippel-Feil syndrome: A constellation of associated anomalies. *J Bone Joint Surg Am* 1974;56:1246-1253.

Lawhon SM, MacEwen GD, Bunnell WP: Orthopaedic aspects of the VATER association. *J Bone Joint Surg Am* 1986;68:424-429.

McGaughran JM, Harris DI, Donnai D, et al: A clinical study of type 1 neurofibromatosis in north west England. *J Med Genet* 1999;36(3):197-203.

McMaster MJ, Ohtsuka K: The natural history of congenital scoliosis: A study of two hundred and fifty-one patients. *J Bone Joint Surg Am* 1982;64:1128-1147.

McMaster MJ, Singh H: Natural history of congenital kyphosis and kyphoscoliosis: A study of one hundred and twelve patients. *J Bone Joint Surg Am* 1999;81:1367-1383.

Shahcheraghi GH, Hobbi MH: Patterns and progression in congenital scoliosis. *J Pediatr Orthop* 1999;19(6):766-775.

Taggard DA, Menezes AH, Ryken TC: Treatment of Down syndrome-associated craniovertebral junction abnormalities. *J Neurosurg* 2000;93(2 suppl):205-213.

Thompson AG, Marks DS, Sayampanathan SR, Piggott H: Long-term results of combined anterior and posterior convex epiphysiodesis for congenital scoliosis due to hemivertebrae. *Spine* 1995;20:1380-1385.

Tredwell SJ, Newman DE, Lockitch G: Instability of the upper cervical spine in Down syndrome. *J Pediatr Orthop* 1990;10(5):602-606.

Index

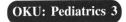

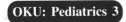

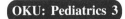